SERIES EDITORS

R. C. G. Russell MS FRCS
Consultant Surgeon, The Middlesex Hospital, London, UK

Henry A. Pitt MD
Professor of Surgery, Medical College of Wisconsin, Milwaukee, USA

ART EDITOR

Gillian Lee FMAA, HonFIMI, AMI, RMIP
Gillian Lee Illustrations, 15 Little Plucketts Way, Buckhurst Hill, Essex

Operative Cardiac Surgery

FIFTH EDITION

Edited by

Timothy J Gardner MD
William Maul Measey Professor of Surgery
University of Pennsylvania School of Medicine
Division of Cardiothoracic Surgery
Hospital of the University of Pennsylvania
Philadelphia, Pennsylvania, USA

Thomas L Spray MD
Alice Langdon Warner Professor of Surgery
Department of Cardiothoracic Surgery
University of Pennsylvania School of Medicine
and Division Chief of Cardiothoracic Surgery
The Children's Hospital of Philadelphia
Philadelphia, Pennsylvania, USA

A member of the Hodder Headline Group
LONDON

This fifth edition published in 2004 by
Arnold, a member of the Hodder Headline Group,
338 Euston Road, London NW1 3BH

http://www.arnoldpublishers.com

Distributed in the United States of America by
Oxford University Press Inc.,
198 Madison Avenue, New York, NY10016

Whilst the advice and information in this book are believed to be true and
accurate at the date of going to press, neither the author[s] nor the publisher
can accept any legal responsibility or liability for any errors or omissions
that may be made. In particular (but without limiting the generality of the
preceding disclaimer) every effort has been made to check drug dosages;
however it is still possible that errors have been missed. Furthermore,
dosage schedules are constantly being revised and new side-effects
recognized. For these reasons the reader is strongly urged to consult the
drug companies' printed instructions before administering any of the drugs
recommended in this book.

British Library Cataloguing in Publication Data
A catalogue record for this book is available from the British Library

Library of Congress Cataloging-on-Publication Data
A catalog record for this book is available from the Library of Congress

ISBN 0340 75974 7

1 2 3 4 5 6 7 8 9 10

Commissioning Editor: Joanna Koster
Production Controller: Lindsay Smith
Cover Designer: Sarah Rees
Project Management: Nora Naughton, Sam Gear

Typeset by Phoenix Photosetting, Chatham, Kent
Printed and bound in Italy

What do you think about this book? Or any other Arnold title?
Please send your comments to feedback.arnold@hodder.co.uk

Contents

Section III: Surgery for Valvular Heart disease

Section IV: Surgery for Heart Failure

Section V: Thoracic Aortic Disease

Contributors

Michael A Acker MD
Section of Cardiac Surgery, Division of Cardiothoracic Surgery,
Department of Surgery, University of Pennsylvania, School of
Medicine, Philadelphia, Pennsylvania, USA

Gabriel S Aldea MD
Professor and Chief of Adult Cardiac Surgery, Department of
Cardiothoracic Surgery, University of Washington School of
Medicine, Seattle, Washington, USA

Robert H Anderson BSc MD FRCPATH
Joseph Levy Professor of Paediatric Cardiac Morphology, Institute of
Child Health, University College, London, UK

John H Arnold MD FACS
Staff Physician, Department of Thoracic and Cardiovascular Surgery,
The Cleveland Clinic Foundation, Cleveland, Ohio, USA

J E Arrowsmith MD MRCP FRCA
Consultant in Cardiothoracic Anaesthesia and Intensive Care,
Department of Anaesthesia, Papworth Hospital National Health
Service Trust, Cambridge, UK

Erle H Austin III MD
Professor of Surgery, University of Louisville School of Medicine,
Chief of Cardiothoracic Surgery, Kosair Children's Hospital, Louisville
Kentucky, USA

Carl Lewis Backer MD
AC Buehler Professor of Surgery, Division of Cardiovascular Thoracic-
Surgery, Children's Memorial Hospital, Professor of Surgery,
Northwestern University Feinberg Schoool of Medicine, Chicago,
Illinois, USA

Vinay Badhwar MD
Chairman, Tampa Bay Heart Institute, St Petersburg, Florida, USA

Joseph E Bavaria MD
Associate Professor of Cardiothoracic Surgery, University of
Pennsylvania School of Medicine, Director, Thoracic Aortic Surgery
Program, University of Pennsylvania Medical Center, Philadelphia,
Pennsylvania, USA

Friedhelm Beyersdorf MD FETCS
Professor of Surgery, Department of Cardiovascular Surgery, Albert-
Ludwigs University Freiburg, Freiburg, Germany

Jay K Bhama MD
Surgical Resident, Division of General Surgery, Michael E DeBakey
Department of Surgery, Baylor College of Medicine, The Methodist
DeBakey Heart Center, Houston, Texas, USA

David P Bichell MD
Director of Cardiovascular Surgery, Children's Hospital San Diego,
Calforina, USA

Steven F Bolling MD
Professor of Surgery and Attending Surgeon, Section of Cardiac
Surgery, University of Michigan Medical School, Ann Arbor,
Michigan, USA

Robert Sutart Bonser FRCP FRCS
Honorary Senior Lecturer of Surgery, University of Birmingham
School of Medicine, Consultant Surgeon, Cardiothoracic Surgical
Unit, Queen Elizabeth Hospital, Birmingham, UK

Edward L Bove MD
Professor of Surgery and Head, Section of Cardiac Surgery,
University of Michigan Medical School, Director of Pediatric Cardiac
Surgery, University of Michigan Medical Center, Ann Arbor,
Michigan, USA

Edward M Boyle Jr MD
Cardiothoracic Surgeon, Heart Institute of the Cascades, Bend,
Oregon, USA

Charles R Bridges MD SCD
Assistant Professor of Surgery, University of Pennsylvania School of
Medicine, Chief, Division of Cardiothoracic Surgery, Pennsylvania
Hospital, Philadelphia, Pennsylvania, USA

Christian PR Brizard MD
Cardiac Surgical Unit, Royal Children's Hospital, Melbourne, Australia

Gerald D Buckberg MD
Professor of Surgery, School of Medicine at UCLA, Los Angeles,
California, USA

Brian F Buxton MB MS FRACS FRCS
Professor of Cardiac Surgery, University of Melbourne, School of
Medicine, Melbourne, Victoria, Australia, Director of Cardiac Surgery
Austin Hospital, Heidelberg, Victoria, Australia

Robert Cesnjevar MD
Cardiothoracic Surgeon, Zentrum Fuer Herzchirurgie,
Universitaetsklinik Erlangen–Neuremberg, Erlangen, Germany

Duke Cameron MD
Chief of Pediatric Cardiac Surgery, Professor of Surgery,
The Johns Hopkins Medical Institutions, Baltimore, Maryland, USA

Walter Randolph Chitwood Jr MD
Chairman of Surgery, East Carolina University Brody School of Medicine, Cardiothoracic Surgeon, Department of Surgery, University Health Systems of Eastern North Carolina, Greenville, North Carolina, USA

Gideon Cohen MD MSc PhD
Assistant Professor, Division of Cardiac Surgery, Univesity of Toronto Faculty of Medicine, Staff Surgeon, Division of Cardiovascular Surgery, The Schulick Heart Centre, Toronto, Ontario, Canada

Gordon A Cohen MD PHD
Senior Lecturer, Department of Cardiothoracic Surgery, University College London, Consultant Cardiothoracic Surgeon, Cardiothoracic Unit, Great Ormond Street Hospital for Children National Health Service Trust, London, UK

Lawrence H Cohn MD
Virginia and James Hubbard Professor of Cardiac Surgery, Harvard Medical School, Chief of Cardiac Surgery, Brigham and Women's Hospital, Boston, Massachusetts, USA

Joseph S Coselli MD
Professor and Chief, Division of Cardiothoracic Surgery, Michael E DeBakey Department of Surgery, Baylor College of Medicine, The Methodist DeBakey Heart Center, Houston, Texas, USA

Delos M Cosgrove MD
Chairman, Department of Thoracic and Cardiovascular Surgery, The Cleveland Clinic Foundation, Cleveland, Ohio, USA

Tirone E David MD
Professor of Surgery, University of Toronto, Faculty of Medicine, Chief, Division of Cardiovascular Surgery, Toronto General Hospital, Toronto, Ontario, Canada

William M DeCampli MD PHD
Associate Professor of Surgery, University of Pennsylvania School of Medicine, Cardiothoracic Surgeon, The Children's Hospital of Philadelphia, Philadelphia, Pennsylvania, USA

G Michael Deeb MD
Professor of Surgery, Section of Cardiac Surgery, University of Michigan, Ann Arbor, Michigan, USA

Marc R De Leval MD FRCS
Professor of Cardiothoracic Surgery and Consultant Cardiothoracic Surgeon, Cardiothoracic Unit, Great Ormond Street Hospital for Children National Health Service Trust, London, UK

Pedro J Del Nido MD
Professor of Surgery, Harvard Medical School, Senior Associate in Cardiac Surgery, Children's Hospital, Boston, Massachusetts, USA

Martin J Elliott MD FRCS
Senior Lecturer of Surgery, Institute of Child Health, University College, Consultant Cardiothoracic Surgeon, Cardiac Unit, Great Ormond Street Hospital for Children National Health Service Trust, London, UK

James I Fann MD
Assistant Professor of Cardiothoracic Surgery, Stanford University School of Medicine, Surgeon of Cardiothoracic Surgery, Stanford University Medical Center, Stanford, California, USA

Bruce G French FRACS
Head and Cardiothoracic Surgeon, Department of Cardiothoracic Surgery, Liverpool Hospital, Liverpool, New South Wales, Australia, Cardiothoracic Surgeon, Royal Prince Alfred Hospital , Camperdown, New South Wales, Australia

Timothy J Gardner MD
William Maul Measey Professor of Surgery, University of Pennsylvania School of Medicine, Division of Cardiothoracic Surgery, Hospital of the University of Pennsylvania, Philadelphia, Pennsylvania, USA

J William Gaynor MD
Assistant Professor of Surgery, University of Pennsylvania School of Medicine, Assistant Surgeon, Department of Cardiothoracic Surgery, The Children's Hospital of Philadelphia, Philadelphia, Pennsylvania, USA

Frank L Hanley MD
Professor of Cardiothoracic Surgery, Stanford University School of Medicine, Director, Pediatric Heart Center, Lucille Packard Children's Hospital, Stanford, California, USA

Michael S Hanna MD FACC
Assistant Clinical Professor of Medicine, Director, Electrophysiology Laboratory, Pennsylvania Hospital, Philadelphia, Pennsylvania, USA

Susan Harrocks RN BN
Clinical Nurse Manager, Cardiac Surgical Research Unit , The Prince Charles Hospital, Brisbane, Queensland, Australia

Roland Hetzer MD PHD
Professor of Surgery, Humboldt University of Berlin, Chairman, Deutsches Herzzentrum, Berlin, Head, Department of Cardiothroacic and Vascular Surgery, Berlin, Germany

Keith A Horvath MD
Associate Professor of Cardiothoracic Surgery, Department of Surgery, Northwestern University Medical School, Attending Surgeon, Department of Surgery, Northwestern Memorial Hospital, Chicago, Illinois, USA

Clifford Frederick Hughes AO MBBS FRACS FACC FACS
Clinical Associate Professor, Division of Surgery, University of Sydney Faculty of Medicine, Head, Cardiothoracic Surgical Unit, Royal Prince Alfred Hospital , Baird Insititue for Applied Heart and Lung Surgical Research, Sydney, New South Wales, Australia

Jennifer C Hirsch MD
Section of Cardiac Surgery, Department of Surgery, The University of Michigan School of Medicine, Ann Arbor, Michigan, USA

Erik W L Jansen MD PhD
Department of Cardiothoracic Surgery, Utrecht University, University Medical Center, Heart–Lung Institute, Utrecht, The Netherlands

Tom R Karl MD MS
Director of Cardiothoracic Surgery and Professor of Surgery,
University of California, San Francisco, School of Medicine, Professor
of Pediatric Cardiothoracic Surgery, UCSF Medical Center, San
Francisco, California, USA

John D Kneeshaw MB CHB FRCA
Consultant in Cardiothoracic Anaesthesia and Intensive Care,
Department of Anaesthesia, Papworth Hospital National Health
Service Trust, Cambridge, UK

Stephen J Korkola MD
Chief Resident, Cardiovascular Surgery, The Montreal Children's
Hospital, McGill University Health Center, Montreal, Canada

Irving L Kron MD
Chair, Department of Surgery, and Chief, Division of Cardiothoracic
Surgery, University of Virginia Medical Center, Charlottesville,
Virginia, USA

François Lacour-Gayet MD
Professor of Surgery, University of Colorado, Chairman
Cardiothoracic Infant Department, The Children's Hospital, Denver,
Colorado, USA

David T M Lai FRACS
Carl and Leah McConnell Cardiovascular Surgical Research Fellow,
Department of Cardiothoracic and Vascular Surgery, Stanford
University School of Medicine, Stanford, California, USA

Hillel Laks MD
Professor and Chief of Cardiothoracic Surgery and Director of Heart
and Heart-Lung Institute, UCLA School of Medicine, Los Angeles,
California, USA

Yves LeCompte MD
Head Surgeon, Department of Pediatric Cardiology, Institut Jacques
Cartier, Massy, France

Scott A Lemaire MD
Assistant Professor of Surgery, Division of Cardiothoracic Surgery,
Michael E DeBakey Department of Surgery, Baylor College of
Medicine, The Methodist DeBakey Heart Center, Houston, Texas, USA

Bruce W Lytle MD
Surgeon, Department of Thoracic and Cardiovascular Surgery, The
Cleveland Clinic Foundation, Cleveland, Ohio, USA

Peter B Manning MD
Associate Professor of Pediatric Cardiothoracic Surgery, University of
Cincinnati College of Medicine, Director of Cardiothoracic Surgery,
Children's Hospital Medical Center, Cincinnati, Ohio, USA

Patrick G Magee MB CHB FRCS
Consultant Surgeon, Department of Cardiothoracic Surgery, London
Chest Hospital, London, UK

Patrick M McCarthy MD
Surgical Director, Kaufman Center for Heart Failure, Department of
Thoracic and Cardiovascular Surgery, The Cleveland Clinic
Foundation, Cleveland, Ohio, USA

Bonnie L Milas MD
Assistant Professor of Anesthesia, Department of Anesthesia,
University of Pennsylvania School of Medicine, Philadelphia,
Pennsylvania, USA

D Craig Miller MD
Thelma and Henry Doelger Professor of Cardiovascular Surgery,
Department of Cardiothoracic Surgery, Stanford University School of
Medicine, Stanford, California, USA

Rohinton J Morris MD
Associate Professor of Surgery, Division of Cardiothoracic Surgery,
University of Pennsylvania Health System, Presbyterian Medical
Center, Philadelphia, Pennsylvania, USA

L Wiley Nifong MD
Assistant Professor and Director of Surgical Research and Robotics,
Department of Surgery, Division of Cardiothoracic Surgery, The Brody
School of Medicine at East Carolina University, Greenville, North
Carolina, USA

Mark F O'Brien FRACS FRCS
Cardiac Surgeon and Director of Cardiac Surgical Research, The
Prince Charles Hospital, Brisbane, Queensland, Australia

Miralem Pasic MD PHD
Professor of Cardiac Surgery, Humboldt University Berlin, Deutsches
Herzzentrum, Berlin, Germany

J R Pepper MA MChir FRCS
Professor of Cardiothoracic Surgery, Department of Surgery, Imperial
College of Science, Technology and Medicine, Consultant
Cardiothoracic Surgeon, Department of Surgery, Royal Brompton
Hospital, London, UK

Mark D Plunkett MD
Assistant Professor of Surgery, Division of Cardiothoracic Surgery,
University of California, Los Angeles, UCLA School of Medicine,
Pediatric Cardiac Surgeon, Division of Cardiothoracic Surgery, UCLA
Medical Center, Los Angeles, California, USA

John D Puskas MD MS
Associate Professor of Surgery, Division of Cardiothoracic Surgery,
Emory University School of Medicine, Attending Cardiothoracic
Surgeon, Department of Surgery, Crawford Long Hospital of Emory
University, Atlanta, Georgia, USA

V Mohan Reddy MD
Assistant Professor, Children's Hospital, Indiana University,
Indianapolis, Indiana, USA

J Mark Redmond MD FRCS
Consultant Pediatric Cardiac Surgeon, Our Lady's Hospital for Sick
Children, Crumlin, Dublin, Ireland

Bruce A Reitz MD
Norman E Shumway Professor and Chairman, Department of
Cardiothoracic Surgery, Stanford University School of Medicine,
Stanford, California, USA

Mark D Rodefeld MD
Assistant Professor of Surgery, Section of Cardiothoracic Surgery, Indiana University School of Medicine, James Whitcomb Riley Hospital for Children, Indianapolis, Indiana, USA

Alfredo J Rodrigues MD PhD
Assistant Professor of Cardiothoracic Surgery, School of Medicine of Ribeirão Preto, University of São Paulo, São Paulo, Brazil

Joseph S Savino MD
Associate Professor of Anesthesia, University of Pennsylvania School of Medicine, Section Chief of Cardiovascular Thoracic Anesthesia and Intensive Care, Department of Anesthesia, Hospital of the University of Pennsylvania, Philadelphia, Pennsylvania, USA

Hartzell V Schaff MD
Stuart W Harrington Professor of Surgery, Division of Cardiovascular Surgery, Mayo Clinic, Professor of Surgery, Division of Cardiovascular Surgery, Saint Mary's Hospital , Rochester, Minnesota, USA

Erez Sharoni MD
Cardiothoracic Surgery, Rabin Medical Center, Bielinson Campus, Petach Tikva, Sackler School of Medicine, Tel Aviv, Israel

Irving Shen MD
Assistant Professor of Surgery, Section of Pediatric Cardiac Surgery, Doernbecher Children's Hospital, Oregon Health Sciences University, Portland, Oregon, USA

Thomas L Spray MD
Alice Langdon Warner Professor of Surgery, Department of Cardiothoracic Surgery, University of Pennsylvania School of Medicine, Division Chief of Cardiothoracic Surgery, The Children's Hospital of Philadelphia, Philadelphia, Pennsylvania, USA

Christopher D Smith MBBS FRACS
Lecturer, Department of Surgery, University of Queensland, Consultant Cardiothoracic Surgeon, Princess Alexandra Hospital, Brisbane, Queensland, Australia

Iva A Smolens MD
Section of Cardiac Surgery, University of Michigan, Ann Arbor, Michigan, USA

Christo I Tchervenkov MD
Professor of Surgery, McGill University Faculty of Medicine, Director of Cardiovascular Surgery, The Montreal Children's Hospital, Montreal, Quebec, Canada

Steven S L Tsui BA MB BCH MA MD FRCS (Eng) FRCS (C-Th)
Consultant Cardiothoracic Surgeon, Papworth Hospital National Health Service Trust, Cambridge, UK

Ross M Ungerleider MD
Professor of Surgery, Chief, Pediatric Cardiac Surgery, Section of Pediatric Cardiac Surgery, Doernbecher Children's Hospital, Oregon Health Sciences University, Portland, Oregon, USA

Edward D Verrier MD
Vice Chairman of Surgery and Chief of Cardiothoracic Surgery, Department of Surgery, University of Washington Medical Center, Seattle, Washington, USA

Pascal R Vouhé MD
Professor of Cardiac Surgery, Paris V University, Consultant Cardiac Surgeon, Department of Pediatric Cardiac Surgery, Necker Hospital Group for Sick Children, Paris, France

John Wallwork FRCS(ED) MB CHB FRCS FRCP MA
Consultant Cardiothoracic Surgeon and Director of Transplantation, Department of Cardiac Administration, Papworth Hospital National Health Service Trust, Cambridge, UK

Richard D Weisel MD
Professor and Chair, Division of Cardiac Surgery, University of Toronto, Faculty of Medicine, Staff Surgeon, Division of Cardiovascular Surgery, University Health Network, Toronto General Hospital, Toronto, Ontario, Canada

Francis C Wells FRCS
Associate Lecturer of Surgery, University of Cambridge School of Clinical Medicine, Consultant Surgeon, Cardiothoracic Surgical Unit, Papworth Hospital National Health Service Trust, Cambridge, UK

David M Williams MD
Professor of Radiology, University of Michigan School of Medicine, Director, Vascular and Interventional Radiology, University of Michigan Medical Center, Ann Arbor, Michigan, USA

David Zeltsman MD
Assistant Professor of Surgery, Division of Thoracic Surgery, Thomas Jefferson University, Jefferson Medical College, Philadelphia, Pennsylvania, USA

Contributing medical artists

Angela Christie MMAA RMIP
14 West End Avenue, Pinner, Middlesex, HA5 1BJ

Peter Cox NDD MMAA RMIP
PCA Designs Ltd., 1 Church Lane, Ledbury, Herefordshire, HR8 1DL

Patrick Elliott BA(Hons) ATC MMAA MIMI RMIP
46 Stone Delf, Fulwood, Sheffield, S10 3QX

Gillian Lee FMAA HonFIMI AMI RMIP
Gillian Lee Illustrations, 15 Little Plucketts Way, Buckhurst Hill, Essex, IG9 5QU

Gillian Oliver FMAA RMIP
7 Princess Street, Stotfold, Hitchin, Herts, SG5 4EP

Denise Smith BA(Hons) MMAA RMIP
Dawson Weir House, Rochdale Road, Todmorton, Lancashire, OL14 7LU

Phoenix Photosetting
Badger Road, Lordswood, Chatham, Kent ME5 8TD

We are also indebted to the following for allowing us to use or adapt artwork drawn originally by them for inclusion in the book:

Chapter 8
Beth Croce CMI, Austin and Repatriation Medical Centre, Cardiac Surgery Publishing Office, Austin Campus HSB/5, Heidelberg, Victoria, 3084 Australia

Chapter 31
Joseph A. Pangrace, Senior Medical Illustrator, Cleveland Clinic Foundation, Department of Medical Illustration, Cleveland, Ohio, USA

Chapter 33
Tanya Leonello, Medical Illustration and Graphics, 1301 Granger Avenue, Ann Arbor, MI 48104, United States of America

Chapter 34
Scott Weldon, MA, Supervisor, Medical Illustrator, Division of Cardiothoracic Surgery, Baylor College of Medicine and Carol Pienta Larson, BSF

Preface

Twenty-one years have passed since the publication of the 4th Edition of Operative Cardiac Surgery. That volume in Rob & Smith's respected and durable multi-volume textbook series of Operative Surgery was the first edition to separate cardiac surgery procedures from those operations encompassed in the broader field of Thoracic Surgery. The 4th Edition, Cardiac Surgery, contained 60 separate chapters dealing with the full spectrum of adult and pediatric cardiac surgery techniques and procedures that encompassed this specialty in the early 1980s. While the 60 chapters of this 5th Edition of Cardiac Surgery also comprise an entire volume, the range of topics in this current Edition accurately reflect the impressive progress of cardiac surgery in all directions over the past two decades.

The Section on Operative Management now includes a chapter on the use of echocardiography in heart surgery, a diagnostic tool that has become so important in our management before, during and after surgery. The Section on Surgery for Ischemic Heart Disease includes 2 chapters on revascularization techniques and procedures performed on the beating heart and without the patient being placed on the heart-lung machine. The exciting array of options for heart valve surgery, including routine techniques for valve repairs and valve-sparing procedures, as well as the use of limited access approaches, are described in the Section on Surgery for Valvular Heart Disease. The numerous advances and exciting developments in Surgery for Heart Failure, including not only heart transplantation, but expanded options for mechanical assistance and reconstructive surgery in the failing heart are presented in the chapters describing operative procedures for heart failure. A five-chapter Section is devoted to the important recent developments in Thoracic Aortic Surgery, where so much progress and innovation have occurred over the last decade.

In the twenty-three chapters covering Surgery for Congenital Heart Disease, impressive enhancement of surgical capabilities in this challenging subspecialty of cardiac surgery are well demonstrated. In general, surgery for congenital heart disease has had the most impressive advances in innovative operative procedures for very young infants. While the full range of operations for patients with congenital heart abnormalities are presented in these chapters, what is perhaps most impressive are those chapters describing surgical procedures that are now routinely performed in newborn and infant children during the first few days or weeks of life.

As much as these chapters reflect the advances in cardiac surgery over the past two decades, we believe that what especially distinguishes this 5th Edition are the outstanding illustrations that accompany every chapter and all of the descriptions of operative procedures. The authors and contributors include many experienced and credible cardiac surgeons from around the world. The descriptions of the operative techniques and other aspects of current approaches to heart surgery for the full spectrum of cardiac conditions are well prepared. What is most unique in this volume, however, is the brilliant art work that illustrates with such clarity and simplicity the anatomical and technical features of the operative procedures.

We are honored to have had the opportunity to edit this 5th Edition in such a respected series of operative texts. We thank all of the editors and contributors, and we especially acknowledge the daunting contributions of Gillian Lee who provided superb leadership in the creation of the illustrations.

Timothy J Gardner, MD
Thomas L Spray, MD

SECTION I

Operative Management

Anesthetic techniques

JOHN D. KNEESHAW MB, CHB, FRCA
Consultant in Cardiothoracic Anaesthesia and Intensive Care, Department of Anaesthesia, Papworth Hospital, National Health Service Trust, Cambridge, UK

J. E. ARROWSMITH MD, MRCP, FRCA
Consultant in Cardiothoracic Anaesthesia and Intensive Care, Department of Anaesthesia, Papworth Hospital, National Health Service Trust, Cambridge, UK

The aim of anesthesia for cardiac surgery is to maintain cardiovascular stability while ensuring an adequate depth of anesthesia. Patients presenting for cardiac surgery may be suffering from coronary artery disease, acquired valvular disease, congenital lesions, or lesions of the great vessels. In the developed world, approximately 70 per cent of cardiac surgical procedures involve patients with coronary artery disease and are designed to revascularize ischemic myocardium. Many of these patients will have impaired ventricular function, seen in its most extreme form in those patients with end-stage disease presenting for cardiac transplantation or the implantation of ventricular assist devices. Patients with cardiac disease are more vulnerable to the adverse hemodynamic effects of anesthetic agents. They are less able to compensate for the effects of these agents because of their disease process and because of concomitant drug therapy, such as beta-blockade. Anesthesia in these patients should always be directed to maintaining hemodynamic stability and should promote a positive myocardial oxygen balance.

Coexisting systemic disease is also common in patients presenting for cardiac surgery. Hypertension, diabetes mellitus, peripheral vascular disease, cerebrovascular disease, renal disease, and pulmonary disease are frequently encountered, as increasing numbers of high risk and/or elderly patients are being considered for surgical treatment. Intercurrent systemic disease may be encountered in any population of surgical patients, but the effect of systemic disease in cardiac surgery and anesthesia is often magnified by the profound physiological changes associated with the surgery and, in particular, with cardiopulmonary bypass (CPB). Therefore, the anesthetist involved in cardiac surgery must have a thorough understanding not only of the pathophysiology of cardiac disease, CPB, and the surgical procedures involved, but also of the management of patients with a wide range of systemic disease processes.

In addition to the above factors, cardiac surgery, anesthesia, and CPB involve complex equipment. This situation carries an increased risk of hazard to the patient. The anesthetist undertaking the care of patients undergoing cardiac surgery should be trained in cardiovascular anesthesia and should be familiar with the complex hemodynamic and other monitoring modalities which must be used to maintain patient safety. Increasingly, the ability to acquire and interpret transesophageal echocardiographic (TEE) images is becoming the role of the cardiac anesthetist. In the future, the ability to use TEE will become an essential part of the training of cardiovascular anesthetists.

PATIENT ASSESSMENT

A thorough preoperative evaluation of the cardiac surgical patient by the anesthetist is essential. Information gathered during this assessment allows the anesthetist to tailor perioperative management to the specific needs of the individual patient. In many centers, this evaluation is conducted on the day before surgery. In recent years, however, the trend has been towards assessment of elective patients in 'preadmission' clinics held a week or more before surgery. Such an approach permits additional clinical investigations to be performed without delaying surgery, alerts support services (e.g. transfusion) to likely demand, and provides the option to admit the patient to the hospital on the day of surgery rather than the day before.

In all elective patients, and in the majority of emergency cases, the patient will have already undergone extensive investigation, and the diagnosis will have been established. For this reason, preoperative assessment invariably begins with a review of the patient's medical notes. This information and correspondence should, ideally, provide the patient's presenting complaint, investigations, and therapeutic interventions, as well as details of past medical, surgical, and anesthetic encounters; current and past drug therapy; adverse drug reactions or interactions; and consumption of alcohol and tobacco. Direct questioning and physical examination of the patient gives the anesthetist the opportunity to confirm the presence, progression, and severity of documented symptoms and signs of the primary cardiac disease, and other significant coexisting morbidity. Furthermore, significant and previously undocumented disease or new intercurrent illness may be excluded. The presence of factors known to be associated with increased perioperative mortality and morbidity should be documented. Such factors include patient age, congestive cardiac failure, obesity (defined as body mass index (BMI) > 35 kg/m^2), peripheral vascular disease, aortic atheromatous disease, renal insufficiency, arterial hypertension, diabetes mellitus, unstable angina, chronic pulmonary disease, neurological disease, and previous cardiac surgery. The presence of these and other risk factors in combination with the type of surgical procedure planned forms the basis of risk indices such as the Parsonnet score and, more recently, the Stroke Risk Index and EuroSCORE. Although still widely used, scoring systems such as the American Society of Anesthesiologists severity of disease score is of limited value in predicting risk or outcome in cardiac surgery.

Symptoms of cardiorespiratory disease, such as angina pectoris, dyspnea, orthopnea, declining exercise tolerance, or (pre)syncope, should be actively sought. A recent or rapid progression in symptom severity, particularly the onset of angina at rest (New York Heart Association class IV), should alert the anesthetist to the potential for perioperative ventricular dysfunction. In addition, documentation of any history or symptoms suggestive of gastroesophageal reflux is important, because of the increased risk of regurgitation and pulmonary aspiration during induction of anesthesia. Furthermore, a history of other upper gastrointestinal pathology, such as hiatus hernia, may contraindicate the intraoperative use of TEE. A brief review of other symptoms should then be conducted to elicit any history of neurological, metabolic, endocrine, renal, hepatic, or hematological disease. If subscription to a particular religious or cultural belief system (e.g. Jehovah's Witnesses) has the potential to influence any aspect of perioperative management, this situation should be comprehensively documented and, if necessary, be taken into account during discussions about risk and informed consent.

The anesthetist should briefly review any history of previous surgical procedures, focusing on the indication for surgery, the outcome, and any anesthetic-related morbidity. Patients who have previously undergone cardiac surgery should be specifically questioned about perioperative events and postoperative progress. A patient's own recollection of the duration of postoperative ventilation, the need for cardiac or renal support, and the duration of critical care dependency and hospitalization provides useful information. When available, the records of previous anesthetics and critical care unit admissions should be examined for documentary evidence of adverse events or airway management difficulties.

An accurate record of current and recent prescribed drug administration, including dosage and route of administration, should be made. Cardiovascular drugs commonly prescribed in this population include aspirin, nitrates, anticoagulants beta-adrenoceptor antagonists, angiotensin converting enzyme inhibitors, digoxin, diuretics, potassium and calcium channel blockers. The use of other drugs such as insulin, oral hypoglycemics, histamine antagonists, proton-pump inhibitors, bronchodilators, corticosteroids, or psychotropic agents is not uncommon. The medication history should include drugs taken on an 'as required,' or PRN, basis; proprietary, or 'over-the-counter,' medicines; and nonprescribed, or 'recreational,' drugs. A history of allergic or other idiosyncratic reaction to a particular drug (e.g. suxamethonium) or class of drug (e.g. penicillins) should be sought and documented.

Routine physical examination should focus on the cardiovascular and respiratory systems. As previously discussed, the principle purpose is to confirm previous findings, to assess the extent of disease progression, and to exclude new pathology. At a minimum, this exam should include measurement of heart rate and rhythm, arterial blood pressure, and respiratory rate; examination of the peripheral pulses and neck vessels; and auscultation over the carotid arteries, precordium, and lung fields. Examination of the state of dentition (including documentation of the location of any permanent dental prostheses), extent of jaw opening, and cervical spine mobility should allow prediction of difficulties with airway management and tracheal intubation. The Allen's test should be performed in both arms to assess the adequacy of the ulnar collateral circulation. Allen's test is mandatory if a radial artery is to be harvested for use as a revascularization conduit.

In the presence of neurological disease, documentation of the extent and severity of any existing impairment is important. If necessary, formal examination of both the peripheral (muscle tone and power, reflexes, coordination, and sensation) and central (cranial nerves and cognitive function) nervous system should be undertaken.

Preoperative investigations can be conveniently considered in two groups – those that are performed routinely in most cardiac surgical patients and those that are performed in specific circumstances dictated by the patient's cardiac pathology and medical history. As many investigations are not without risk, investigations should not be needlessly repeated. An automated blood count; coagulation studies; determination of blood group; measurement of serum electrolytes, urea, and creatinine; a plain chest radiograph; a 12-lead electrocardiogram (ECG); and cardiac catheterization should be regarded as routine preoperative investigations in virtually all cardiac surgical patients. The blood count should exclude significant anemia and quantitative leucocyte and platelet abnormalities. Coagulation studies are essential in patients treated with heparin or warfarin. Seemingly trivial prolongation of the activated partial thromboplastin time may indicate the presence of an otherwise asymptomatic coagulopathy that may place the patient at risk of excessive perioperative hemorrhage. Such a finding, in the absence of anticoagulant administration, should prompt further hematological evaluation.

Chronic diuretic therapy may produce total body depletion of sodium, potassium, and other ions, as well as elevation of serum urea. The serum potassium concentration does provide some indication of total body stores but is a poor index of intracellular potassium stores. Hypokalemia (serum potassium concentration less than 3.5 mmol/L) is a common finding in cardiac surgical patients and is frequently associated with hypomagnesemia. Although normal plasma concentrations of urea and creatinine virtually exclude significant renal pathology, they give no indication of renal reserve. A plain posteroanterior chest radiograph provides information about the boney anatomy of the chest, heart size, and pulmonary vasculature.

The ECG provides documentary evidence of cardiac rate and rhythm and acts as a preoperative baseline. The ECG remains the investigation of choice for detecting myocardial ischemia and, in addition, may provide information about conduction anomalies, previous transmural myocardial infarction, and chamber hypertrophy or enlargement.

Left heart catheterization typically includes coronary angiography and left ventriculography. This test provides information about coronary vascular anatomy, the sites and severity of coronary stenoses, aortic and mitral valve function, ventricular morphology and function, and regional ventricular wall motion. Direct measurement of intracavity pressures, such as left ventricular end-diastolic pressure, provides indirect evidence of ventricular function, whereas measurement of transcardiac pressure gradients allows the severity of stenotic lesions to be quantified. In cases in which a communication exists between the pulmonary and systemic circulations, serial blood sampling allows computation of shunt fraction. The cardiac anesthetist must not only be familiar with the techniques and complications of cardiac catheterization, but also have the ability to place the findings in their clinical context.

Exercise stress (treadmill) testing is frequently used as a means of screening patients with symptoms suggestive of myocardial ischemia. In addition to providing information about the severity and anatomical basis of ischemia, this test gives some indication of physiological reserve. In most centers, stress testing is performed as a prelude to coronary angiography.

Transthoracic (precordial) echocardiography is frequently used to define cardiac anatomy and assess both ventricular and valvular function. Color Doppler echocardiography is used to estimate blood flow velocity from which transvalvular gradients, valve orifice area, pulmonary artery pressure, and cardiac output can be derived. The noninvasive nature of transthoracic echocardiography makes it a useful tool for monitoring the progress of cardiac disease and assisting in determining both the timing and type of surgical intervention. The development of biplane and, more recently, multiplane probes has prompted the use of TEE as both a preoperative diagnostic tool and an intraoperative monitor of cardiac function. In most centers, TEE has expanded the role of the anesthetist to include that of echocardiographer. Echocardiography is discussed in more detail in Chapter 2. Additional investigations such as respiratory function tests, arterial blood gas analysis, carotid angiography and ultrasonography, creatinine clearance, and permanent pacemaker evaluation should be conducted as appropriate.

In the emergency situation, conduct of the full range of preoperative investigations may not be possible before surgery. Moreover, the results of tests already conducted may not be at hand, and documentation may be limited to the current illness. In this situation, the anesthetist should elicit information directly from the patient, family members, and referring physicians and assess the condition of the patient by physical examination and interpretation of clinical investigations. The desire for complete preoperative assessment, hemodynamic monitoring, and optimization using supportive measures has to be balanced against the need to expedite surgery.

PERIOPERATIVE MONITORING

Perioperative physiological monitoring should be regarded as an adjunct to, rather than a replacement for, continuous clinical assessment of the patient. Modern monitoring systems are claimed to improve patient safety and facilitate accurate documentation of intraoperative events. Monitoring of the cardiac surgical patient should, at a minimum, comply with established published guidelines, be commenced before the induction of anesthesia, and be continued into the period of recovery.

All anesthetic equipment, including emergency equipment, should be thoroughly checked before use. Anesthetic gas delivery systems must be fitted with an oxygen analyzer, an oxygen supply failure alarm, and a capnometer. The use of airway pressure monitoring and some measure of exhaled tidal volume are recommended. Continuous measurement of heart rate, ECG, pulse volume or arterial pressure, peripheral hemoglobin-oxygen saturation, and end-tidal carbon dioxide tension is mandatory.

1 The ECG is used as a monitor of electrical activity, rate, rhythm, conduction abnormalities, electrolyte disturbances, and ischemia. The standard five-lead configuration, comprising four standard limb leads and one precordial lead, is the preferred system. Continuous display of leads II and V_5 (fifth left intercostal space in the anterior axillary line) is recommended. The former provides the best information about atrial activity, whereas the latter is the best single precordial lead for the detection of left ventricular ischemia. The widest bandpass filter (typically 0.05–100 Hz; 'diagnostic mode') should be selected to reduce artefactual amplification of ST-segment changes. This figure demonstrates the effect of filter selection on the ST segment, showing the apparent change in ST segment between diagnostic and monitor modes. Application of the monitor mode produces artefactual 1-mm ST-segment depression. This figure has been reproduced with permission from Mark, J.B. 1998. *Atlas of Cardiovascular Monitoring*. New York, NY: Churchill Livingstone.

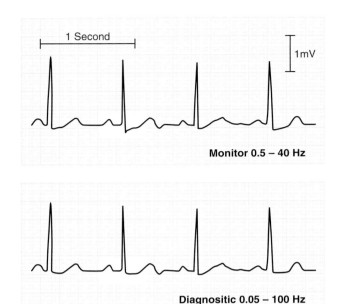

Monitor 0.5 – 40 Hz

Diagnositic 0.05 – 100 Hz

1

Although automated, intermittent noninvasive blood pressure (NIBP) monitoring is adequate for the majority of general surgical procedures, it is not suitable for use during cardiac surgery. Measurement cycles may last up to 90 seconds and fail to capture rapid changes in blood pressure or more subtle variations, such as pulsus alternans or cyclical variations caused by dysrhythmia and mechanical ventilation. Most NIBP devices accurately measure mean arterial pressure (MAP). At low arterial pressure (MAP less than 45 mm Hg), NIBP tends to overestimate pressure, whereas at high pressure (MAP greater than 150 mm Hg), NIBP tends to underestimate pressure. Furthermore, oscillometric NIBP monitoring relies on the presence of a pulsatile pressure, rendering it useless during CPB.

In adult patients, systemic arterial and, frequently, central venous pressure (CVP) monitoring is commenced before induction of anesthesia. All invasive pressure monitoring equipment and tubing should be primed with saline, rigorously deaired, and checked for leaks in advance. The length of pressure monitoring lines should be minimized to ensure that the pressure waveform is not adversely affected by resonance and over-damping. In many centers, the use of heparinized saline has been abandoned because of the incidence of heparin allergy. Transducers should be firmly secured to the operating table and calibrated such that the zero reference point lies at the midcardiac level. Simultaneous numerical and pressure waveform displays are essential — the former presents systolic, diastolic, and mean pressure in a readable format, whereas the latter allows waveform analysis (i.e. subtle beat-to-beat pressure variations, *cv* waves, cannon waves, artefacts during blood sampling and line flushing).

Although virtually any peripheral artery may be used for arterial pressure monitoring, the distal radial artery of the nondominant arm is the most frequently used. Typically, a 20G or 22G cannula is sited under aseptic conditions and

local anesthesia by either direct insertion over a hollow stylet or use of the modified Seldinger technique. If the nondominant radial artery is to be used as a coronary revascularization conduit, arterial pressure monitoring must be established in either the dominant arm or a common femoral artery. An 18G or 20G cannula, 8–12 cm in length, should be used to cannulate the femoral artery. Many anesthetists prefer to retain the ability to use NIBP monitoring during surgery both as a backup system and to verify the results of invasive monitors during periods when arterial pressure is pulsatile.

Continuous CVP monitoring is an essential component of perioperative monitoring in the cardiac surgical patient. In addition to providing indirect evidence about intravascular volume, the CVP waveform, in conjunction with the ECG, can be used to diagnose cardiac rhythm disturbances or epicardial pacemaker problems. A number of central veins, including the internal jugular, basilic, subclavian, and common femoral veins, may be used as a site for cannulation for CVP monitoring and central administration of drugs. The subclavian route has the disadvantage of being within the surgical field and having a higher rate of complications associated with cannulation. The right internal jugular vein, which has a superficial course in the neck, is easily identified and is the first choice of most cardiac anesthetists. In most institutions, the modified Seldinger technique is used to place multi-lumen central catheters; some anesthetists, however, prefer to use one or more single-lumen cannulae introduced over a stylet.

Although many techniques have been described for internal jugular vein cannulation, the following general principles apply to all techniques. Continuous ECG monitoring is essential, as Seldinger wires and catheters may induce dysrhythmias as they enter the heart. Excessive 'head down' tilt and neck rotation should be avoided, particularly in the compromised patient. Topical disinfectant should be widely applied and the site covered with sterile drapes. In the conscious patient, adequate local anesthesia should be obtained before proceeding. Regardless of the method used to locate the vein, care should be taken to avoid carotid, pleural, or vertebral vessel puncture. Because of the risk of kinking, sheering, and unwinding, Seldinger wires should not be withdrawn once the tip has been inserted beyond the end of the introducer needle. If more than one catheter is required (e.g. a central venous and a pulmonary artery catheter), additional wires should be sited by separate vein puncture before any catheter is inserted. In cases in which vein identification is in doubt (e.g. in the presence of markedly elevated CVP, severe tricuspid regurgitation, or cannon atrial waves), direct manometric pressure measurement at the needle hub should be considered before proceeding.

Considerable debate exists as to whether central venous cannulation should be performed before or after the induction of anesthesia. Ultimately, the condition of the patient, institutional or departmental guidelines, and the anesthetist's preference will determine when central venous cannulation is performed.

The pulmonary artery flotation catheter provides the anesthetist with the opportunity to directly measure pulmonary artery pressure and pulmonary artery occlusion or 'wedge' pressure, an estimate of left atrial pressure. Modifications of the basic catheter design allow intermittent or continuous measurement of cardiac output by the thermodilution technique using the Stewart-Hamilton equation

$$Q = \frac{V.(T_B - T_I).K}{\int_0^\infty \Delta T_B(t)dt}$$

in which Q is the cardiac output (L/minute), V is the volume of injectate (mL), T_B is blood temperature, T_I is initial injectate temperature, K is the catheter-specific computation constant, and the divisor is the integral of temperature change with respect to time.

In combination with other measurements, a number of hemodynamic variables such as left ventricular stroke volume and systemic and pulmonary vascular resistance may be calculated. Simultaneous measurement of hemoglobin concentration and both arterial and mixed venous oxygen saturation allows calculation of oxygen delivery, oxygen consumption, and, therefore, the oxygen extraction ratio.

2 Pressure waveforms recorded from a pulmonary artery (PA) catheter passing from the right atrium to the PA are shown here. The venous *a*, *c*, and *v* waves are recorded from both the right atrium and PA wedge positions. The PA catheter is usually placed through a hemostatic introducer sited in a central vein using the technique described above. The high probability of catheter-induced dysrhythmia during placement mandates continuous ECG monitoring. Before insertion, each vascular lumen should be flushed with saline, the balloon checked to confirm proper inflation and deflation, and pressure monitoring tubing connected to the distal lumen. The catheter is passed through the introducer sheath into the right atrium, where characteristic *a*, *c*, and *v* pressure waves are observed. The balloon is inflated with air and the catheter advanced until it passes into the right ventricle. Passage of the catheter across the tricuspid valve may be aided by positioning the patient head-down. The right ventricular pressure waveform is pulsatile and characterized by a marked increase in systolic pressure and a diastolic pressure similar to the right atrial pressure. The catheter is then advanced into the main PA, a procedure frequently associated with premature ventricular beats. Passage of the catheter across the pulmonary valve may be aided by positioning the patient head-up and on the right side. As PA systolic pressure is similar to right ventricular systolic pressure, the measurement of a diastolic pressure higher than right ventricular diastolic pressure is usually used to confirm successful PA catheterization. In case of uncertainty, examination of the diastolic pressure waveform allows PA pressure to be distinguished from right ventricular pressure. Ventricular filling causes right ventricular pressure to rise during diastole, whereas PA pressure falls after pulmonary valve closure. Further insertion of the catheter causes the balloon to wedge in a proximal PA. The pulmonary artery pressure waveform is replaced by *a*, *c*, and *v* pressure waves that resemble left atrial pressure. After insertion, the balloon should be deflated to prevent pulmonary infarction. For the same reason, the catheter should be withdrawn 5–8 cm at the onset of CPB. This figure has been modified with permission from Mark, J.B. 1998. *Atlas of Cardiovascular Monitoring*. New York, NY: Churchill Livingstone.

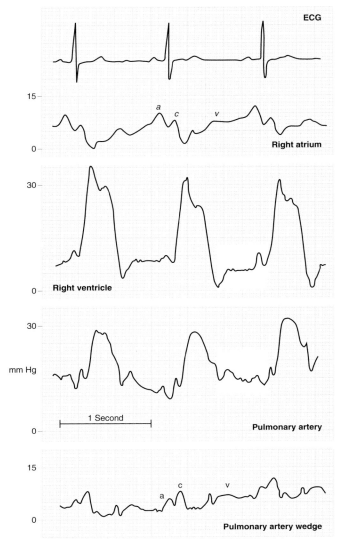

For many years, the intraoperative use of the pulmonary artery catheter has been regarded as routine in many institutions, particularly in North America. A recently published and widely publicized investigation of outcomes following pulmonary artery catheterization in intensive care patients at five US institutions has prompted a more rational evaluation of the use of these devices. An extensive review of available published evidence supporting the use of pulmonary artery catheters in a wide variety of clinical settings has resulted in the publication of a consensus statement. The consensus group was made up of representatives from the Society for Critical Care Medicine, the American Association of Critical Care Nurses, the American College of Chest Physicians, the American College of Critical Care Medicine, the American Thoracic Society, and the European Society of Intensive Care Medicine. Currently, available evidence suggests that the routine use of a pulmonary artery catheter in low-risk cardiac surgical patients does not improve patient outcome. The use of pulmonary artery catheters in high-risk cardiac surgical patients remains controversial, as unequivocal evidence of improved patient outcomes is lacking. Use of the pulmonary artery catheter assumes that the operator is competent in its deployment and the correct interpretation of hemodynamic data obtained. Of concern, evidence exists suggesting that knowledge of the basic principles of pulmonary artery catheterization is, at best, suboptimal.

2

Following induction of anesthesia, monitoring of inhaled oxygen and nitrous oxide, and end-tidal carbon dioxide, and volatile anesthetic concentration agent is established. In addition, the use of continuous airway pressure monitoring should alert the anesthetist to airway obstruction, changes in pulmonary compliance, and inadvertent breathing system disconnection. Catheterization of the urinary bladder and the use of a graduated urine collection system allows both urine output and quality to be monitored.

Accurate temperature measurement is essential during the perioperative period. Typically, devices using bead thermistors are used to monitor both central (nasopharyngeal, bladder, tympanic) and peripheral (cutaneous) temperature. Although most devices are capable of measuring steady-state temperature with a high degree of accuracy,

their physical properties and anatomical placement may lead to inaccuracies during periods when temperature is changing.

Continuous physiological monitoring is supplemented by intermittent arterial blood analysis to establish pulmonary or oxygenator gas exchange, acid–base status, serum electrolyte and glucose concentrations, hematocrit, and activated whole blood clotting time. The use of advanced monitors of coagulation, such as thromboelastography, has yet to gain widespread acceptance in routine practice. The provision of additional pressure transducers and monitoring lines (so-called diagnostic lines) facilitates direct or intracavity pressure monitoring within the cardiac chambers and great vessels.

3 This figure illustrates the typical arrangement of perioperative monitors for cardiac surgery. Specialized monitoring techniques, particularly those developed for central nervous system monitoring (e.g. transcranial Doppler sonography, processed electroencephalography, cerebral near infrared spectroscopy, somatosensory evoked potentials, jugular bulb oximetry), remain largely experimental. TEE = transesophageal echocardiography; HME = heat and moisture exchanger/airway filter; PAC = pulmonary artery catheter; IPPV = intermittent positive-pressure ventilation.

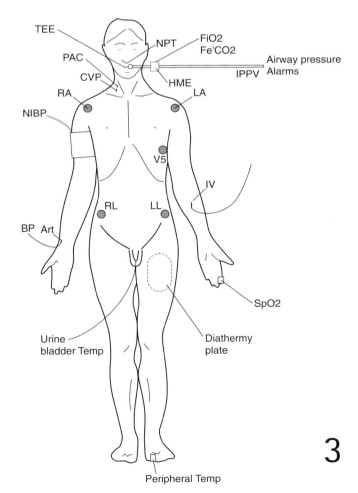

3

CONDUCT OF ANESTHESIA

General principles

The stated aim of anesthesia in all patients with cardiovascular disease is the maintenance of cardiovascular stability while ensuring an adequate depth of anesthesia. These aims are particularly challenging in patients presenting for cardiac surgery. This dilema exists because the great range of ages and disease processes result in widely differing responses to anesthetic agents from one patient to another. As a consequence, anesthetic drug dosages must be tailored to the requirements of the individual patient and, in many cases, titration of the drug to the desired effect is required.

Preoperative preparation

Historically, patients undergoing general anesthesia for all surgery underwent a period of 8–12 hours of starvation from solids and liquids because of fears of aspiration of gastric contents during induction of anesthesia. This practice led, in some patients, to relative dehydration in the immediate preoperative period. Currently, in many institutions, the period of preoperative starvation has been reduced, such that elective anesthesia is not induced within 4–6 hours after the last intake of food, and clear oral fluids are allowed up to 3 hours before the induction of anesthesia. Routine cardiovascular drug therapy should be administered up to and including the morning of surgery with the exception of loop diuretics and digoxin. Diabetic patients should not be given oral hypoglycemics or full doses of insulin on the day of surgery. The anesthetist may wish to prescribe additional drugs on the morning of surgery, and these medications might include histamine blockers such as ranitidine or proton pump inhibitors such as omeprazole to reduce gastric acid production. Patients taking long-term oral corticosteroids may require extra intravenous doses of replacement steroids. Traditionally, premedication for cardiac surgery consisted of substantial doses of opiates, often administered with an anticholinergic agent such as hyoscine. The aim of this premedication was to induce anxiolysis and to reduce the doses of induction agents required for anesthesia. Worldwide, huge variation exists in premedicant drugs administered with an increased use of benzodiazepine tranquilizers. Phenothiazine drugs remain popular for premedication, especially in pediatric practice. No evidence exists to suggest that any particular combination of premedicant drugs is ideal for cardiac surgery; but clearly, anxiolysis is beneficial, and antisialagogues are useful in pediatric practice.

Following premedication, most cardiac surgical patients should be given oxygen by facemask, and this treatment should be continued during transfer to the induction room. During this transfer, the patient should be in a comfortable position. Those patients who, because of their disease process, prefer the sitting position, such as patients with any degree of left ventricular failure or cardiac tamponade, should not be forced to assume a supine position.

Induction of anesthesia

Institutional practice varies widely on the location of the patient for the institution of invasive monitoring and for the induction of anesthesia. Some centers favor moving the patient to the operating room for the establishment of monitoring and for the induction of anesthesia. In other institutions, monitoring lines are placed when the patient is in a reception room, and the patient is moved to the operating room for the induction of anesthesia. In other centers, monitoring is established, and anesthesia is induced in a separate anesthetic room before transfer to the operating room. Each of these strategies has advantages and disadvantages. The use of the operating room for the whole of the anesthetic procedure has the advantage that monitoring is not discontinued at any stage during the course of the procedure, but the disadvantage is that the turnover time in that operating room may be prolonged. Also, the operating room in which preparations for surgery are being made may be a noisy and frightening environment for the awake patient. The use of anesthetic or induction rooms allows the anesthetist to work in a quieter environment and may reduce the turnover time for the operating room. However, this strategy has the disadvantage that monitoring must be discontinued when the anesthetized patient is transferred to the operating room.

The patient's identity and the presence of adequate documentary consent and other documentation, including relevant investigations, should be checked before the anesthetic procedure is begun, as should the availability of an adequate supply of crossmatched bank blood. Before the induction of anesthesia, the anesthetist will establish intravenous access with a large i.v. cannula, and invasive monitoring is established as previously described.

A wide variety of anesthetic drugs and drug cocktails have been described to produce anesthesia for cardiac surgery. Although many of these drug regimes have strong proponents, no evidence exists that any one technique can be claimed to be the method of choice for patients with cardiovascular disease. From the 1960s, high-dose morphine anesthesia was advocated for cardiovascular stability; this technique, introduced by Lowenstein, remained popular until the 1970s, when Stanley suggested a high-dose fentanyl technique for both the induction and maintenance of anesthesia. This high-dose fentanyl technique has been widely used and meets the criterion of producing hemodynamic stability. Unfortunately, opiate-alone anesthesia is associated with a significant risk of awareness, especially at the time of the onset of CPB. The use of high-dose opiate anesthesia also leads to persistent postoperative respiratory depression, which necessitates prolonged positive pressure ventilation in an intensive care unit (ICU). Much cardiac anesthesia throughout the world is still opiate based, but in almost all centers, opiates are now combined with other agents to produce a more balanced form of anesthesia.

Induction of anesthesia may be accomplished with intravenous induction agents, such as propofol, thiopentone, or one of the available benzodiazepines. Each of these agents has advantages and disadvantages, but great care should be exercised with the administration of bolus doses of induction agents such as propofol or thiopentone, which may produce a fall in blood pressure secondary to reduced left ventricular contractility and a reduction in systemic vascular resistance. Etomidate and ketamine have also been used. Etomidate has gained some popularity, because it may offer improved cardiovascular stability. Ketamine, however cannot be recommended for routine use because of a tendency to unwanted sympathetic stimulation and a tendency to produce unwanted postoperative psychological sequelae. In some centers, inhalational induction of anesthesia is gaining popularity. The volatile agent sevoflurane is achieving some favor because of its apparent cardiovascular stability.

In most centers, induction of anesthesia is achieved by combining small doses of the chosen induction agent with a moderate dose (fentanyl 10–30 µg/kg) of opiate. Neuromuscular blockade is achieved with a nondepolarizing agent such as pancuronium bromide (0.15 mg/kg) or vecuronium bromide (0.15 mg/kg). Ventilation is assisted until the neuromuscular blockade achieved is adequate for endotracheal intubation. An endotracheal tube is placed and its correct location confirmed by inspection, auscultation, and capnometry. The lungs should be ventilated to normocapnia to minimize cardiovascular instability and to maintain autoregulation of cerebral blood flow.

The depth of anesthesia must be adequate to obtund the hemodynamic responses to intubation. Hypertension and tachycardia are to be avoided, especially in patients with ischemic heart disease. These intubation responses can usually be avoided simply by adequate anesthesia, but some institutional protocols allow for small bolus doses of an induction agent, opiate, or lignocaine just before intubation. Some institutions still favor the use of local anesthetic spray to the vocal cords before intubation. This practice requires laryngoscopy, which is itself associated with unwanted hemodynamic effects.

If the procedure so far has been conducted in an anesthetic or induction room, the patient is transferred to the operating room, invasive monitoring is re-established, and ventilation of the lungs is resumed. At this stage, the anesthesiologist should make a complete check of the patient and all of the anesthesia monitoring equipment, including drug infusions, before allowing the patient to be prepared and draped for surgery.

Maintenance of anesthesia before cardiopulmonary bypass

Anesthesia may be maintained with either a volatile anesthetic agent or by the continuous infusion of hypnotic agents.

Table 1.1 *A sample anesthetic regimen for adult cardiac surgery*

Premedication	
Morphine sulphate	0.3 mg/kg (i.m.) 1 h preinduction
Hyoscine HBr	5 µg/kg (i.m.) 1 h pre-induction
Preinduction	
If required to produce sedation during placement of venous and arterial cannulae	
Midazolam	1–5 mg (i.v.)
Or	
Diazepam	2.5–10 mg (i.v.)
Induction	
Propofol infusion	10 mg/kg per h for 5 min, reducing to 4 mg/kg per h over 15 min
Fentanyl	2–15 µg/kg
Pancuronium bromide	0.15 mg/kg
Maintenance	
Propofol infusion	3–4 mg/kg per h
Morphine sulphate	0.2 mg/kg (i.v.) after separation from cardiopulmonary bypass
Antagonism of residual neuromuscular blockade	
Neostigmine	2.5 mg (i.v.)
Glycopyrrolium	0.5 mg (i.v.)
Postoperative sedation	
Propofol infusion	2 mg/kg per h
Morphine infusion	1–3 mg/h

There is an increasing trend in the developed world towards the use of total intravenous anesthesia, either combined with one of the established opiates or combined with an infusion of the more recently introduced, rapidly metabolized, ultra–short-acting opiate, remifentanil. This i.v. infusion approach has the advantage that it can be used throughout the CPB period and continued into the postoperative period for sedation in the ICU. A sample anesthetic regimen, as used by the authors, is shown in Table 1.1.

Nitrous oxide is now recognized as a drug with significant myocardial depressant properties and is used infrequently in cardiac anesthesia. If nitrous oxide is to be used, its administration should be stopped well before the onset of CPB to prevent the expansion of any bubbles that may be introduced into the circulation at the time of cannulation. For cases in which nitrous oxide is not used, the patient's lungs are ventilated with oxygen-enriched air, with or without a volatile agent. Some authorities recommend that the air should also be discontinued before the onset of CPB so that any air bubbles that are introduced into the circulation will be rapidly absorbed. Baseline measurements should be made of arterial blood gases and electrolytes, especially potassium, as well as of whole blood activated clotting time, well before heparinization and establishment of bypass.

A hemodynamic response may occur to the onset of surgery and especially to sternotomy. Although adequate depth of anesthesia will frequently obtund these responses, blood pressure control with additional doses of anesthetic agents or by the infusion of a vasodilator drug such as glyceryl trinitrate or sodium nitroprusside may be required. These hemodynamic responses to surgery may be particularly marked in non-beta-blocked patients. Most anesthetists attempt to control the systemic blood pressure during the period of dissection before CPB, and many anesthetists aim for a mean arterial pressure between 65 and 85 mm Hg. Anticoagulation for CPB is most frequently achieved with a dose of 300 IU/kg of unfractionated heparin. This dose should be increased to 400 or even 500 IU/kg in the presence of aprotinin or in patients with recent heparin exposure. Following heparinization, the whole blood activated clotting time is monitored. This time should, in general, be greater than 400 seconds (or three times the baseline measurement), and this figure should be achieved before cannulation for bypass. Control of the blood pressure during cannulation of the aorta is required to minimize aortic trauma, and in many institutions the mean arterial pressure is reduced to approximately 60–65 mm Hg at this stage.

Anesthesia during cardiopulmonary bypass

CPB is the use of a pump and an oxygenator to take over the function of the heart and lungs during surgery. The onset of CPB is associated with profound changes in patient physiology beyond the bounds of normal homeostatic compensation. Marked alterations in the distribution, metabolism, and elimination of anesthetic drugs also occur.

Before the institution of CPB, the anesthetist should discuss the choice of priming solutions with the perfusionist and ensure that the function of the heart-lung machine and its associated monitoring has been checked. At the onset of CPB, the patient's blood volume is mixed with the priming solution of the bypass circuit. In adult practice this is usually a crystalloid solution. The onset of bypass is invariably associated with a profound decrease in mean arterial pressure due to hemodilution, which produces a sudden decrease in the viscosity of the circulating blood. A secondary vasodilatation, which may be associated with the introduction of nonpulsatile flow, may occur. The overall effect is a decrease in peripheral blood flow with relative preservation of the central circulation. Hepatic, renal, cerebral, and skeletal perfusion have all been shown to be reduced during CPB. These effects are more marked if systemic hypothermia is used for the duration of CPB.

Ventilation of the patient's lungs should not be discontinued until bypass is fully established with a pump flow rate of at least 2.4 L/minute per m^2 if the patient is normothermic. CPB produces dilution of all the components of blood, redistribution and changes in protein binding of many anesthetic agents. Reduced drug elimination occurs due to impaired hepatic flow and also impaired renal clearance. Some drugs, such as fentanyl, are sequestered in poorly perfused tissues, such as adipose and lung tissue. For most drugs, at the onset of CPB a reduction in plasma concentration of the drug occurs, followed by a gradual rise in plasma concentration. This effect is most marked with lipophilic drugs with large volumes of distribution and less marked for hydrophilic, polarized drugs (e.g. neuromuscular blocking agents) with smaller volumes of distribution.

Until the recent past, the period following the onset of CPB was associated with an increased risk of awareness. This situation was almost always associated with anesthetic techniques that used opiate drugs as sole agents. If anesthesia is to be maintained by the continuous infusion of an hypnotic agent, such as propofol, this drug should be continued throughout CPB. If maintenance anesthesia is being produced by a volatile agent, this technique can be achieved by directly adding vapor to the pump oxygenator gas supply. The minimum alveolar concentration for the volatile anesthetic agent is likely to be reduced because of reduced metabolism and elimination. Concerns about the risk of awareness at the onset of CPB have led to some institutional protocols advocating the administration of drugs such as benzodiazepines and neuromuscular blocking agents at the onset of CPB. In most centers, however, an adequate depth of anesthesia is ensured by the continuous administration of adequate doses of anesthetic agents (either intravenous or volatile).

The following checklist is suggested for the anesthetist at the time of the institution of CPB.

- Check with the perfusionist to ensure that full bypass flow has been achieved
- Discontinue ventilation of the lungs
- Turn off all i.v. fluid infusions
- Turn off all vasoactive drug infusions
- Check the patient's pupils for size and equality
- Check to ensure that anesthetic drugs are being administered (i.v. infusion or volatile via pump)
- Note volume of urine passed pre-bypass, and zero the collection for the bypass period
- Secure the transesophageal echo probe

During CPB, the anesthetist should remain in the operating room to monitor the patient and to deal with any unforeseen events. The mean arterial pressure should be monitored as an indication of cerebral perfusion pressure. The cerebral perfusion pressure during bypass may be the difference between the mean arterial pressure and the right atrial or superior vena cava pressure. If the venous cannulation is inadequate for drainage of the superior vena cava system, then the CVP may be elevated in such a way as to reduce cerebral perfusion pressure. Throughout the period of CPB, urinary output, temperature, arterial blood gases, coagulation, glucose, and hematocrit should also be monitored.

Separation from cardiopulmonary bypass

If a hypothermic bypass technique has been used, the patient should be adequately rewarmed before attempting to discontinue bypass. The heart rate should be adequate, and the rhythm should be regular (preferably sinus). If an epicardial pacing is required, this system should be attached and its function verified before bypass is discontinued. Arterial blood gases and serum electrolytes should be within the normal physiological ranges.

Intermittent positive pressure ventilation of the lungs is recommended and a visual check should be made to ensure adequate re-expansion of both lungs. The lower lobe of the left lung is often slow to re-expand after bypass, and persistent lobar collapse is a significant cause of morbidity in the postoperative period.

The anesthetist should have blood or other colloid solutions immediately available for transfusion, if required, once bypass has been discontinued. Any antidysrhythmic or vasoactive drugs that may be required should be prepared as infusions and, if necessary, started just before separation from bypass. The use of standardized concentrations of vasoactive and other drugs in an institution simplifies their preparation and reduces the risk of error (Table 1.2). During separation from CPB, the anesthetist should monitor the heart by direct inspection and by monitoring the systemic arterial pressure and cardiac filling pressures.

After discontinuation of bypass and venous decannulation, protamine sulphate is given in a dose of 3 mg/kg to reverse the residual heparinization. In some institutional protocols, protamine is not administered until the arterial inflow cannula has also been removed. In some patients, the administration of protamine may be associated with severe hypotension, and most anesthetists administer an initial test dose (10 mg).

In the post-bypass period, while the surgeon is securing hemostasis, the whole blood activated clotting time should be measured to check that it has returned to normal, and arterial blood gases should be within normal physiological limits. Some anesthetists will add positive end-expiratory pressure to ventilation in the operating room; certainly, this strategy should be considered if the partial pressure of arterial oxygen-to-fraction of inspired oxygen ratio is less than 250 mm Hg (35 KPa) after discontinuation of bypass.

Table 1.2 *Example dilutions and dosage regimens for some commonly used vasoactive drugs as used in the authors' hospital*

Drug	Dilution	Concentration	Loading dose	Maintenance
Dopamine	400 mg/250 mL D5%	1.6 mg/mL	NA	3–15 µg/kg per min
Adrenaline	5 mg/250 mL D5%	20 µg/mL	NA	0.5–5 µg / kg per min
Isoprenaline	1 mg/250 mL D5%	4 µg/mL	NA	0.1–1.5 mg/kg per min
Noradrenaline	8 mg/50 mL D5%	160 µg/mL	NA	1–10 mg/kg per min
Phenylephrine	10 mg/50 mL NS	200 µg/mL	NA	3–20 mg/kg per min
Enoximone	100 mg/40 mL NS	2.5 mg/mL	0.2–0.4 mg/kg	50–300 mg/kg per min
Milrinone	10 mg/50 mL D5%	200 µg/mL	50 µg/kg	0.35–0.75 mg/kg per min
Esmolol	2.5 G/250 mL D5%	10 mg/mL	1 mg/kg	150–500 mg/kg per min
Amiodarone	1.2 G/500 mL D5%	2.4 mg/mL	4 mg/kg	12 mg/kg per 24 h
Lignocaine	1G/250 mL D5%	4 mg/mL	1–1.5 mg/kg	1–2 mg/kg per h
Procainamide	1G/250 mL D5%	4 mg/mL	10–15 mg/kg	1–5 mg/kg per h
Antidiuretic hormone	10 IU/50 mL D5%	0.2 IU/mL	NA	0.2–2.5 IU/h
Sodium nitroprusside	50 mg/250 mL D5%	200 µg/mL	NA	0.3–6 mg/kg per min
Glyceryl trinitrate	25 mg/50 mL NS	500 µg/mL	NA	10–75 µg/kg per min

D5% = 5% dextrose solution, NA = not applicable, NS = normal saline solution.

IMMEDIATE POSTOPERATIVE CARE

On completion of surgery, the patient is transferred to the ICU, where cardiorespiratory support and invasive monitoring are continued into the recovery period. Hemodynamic stability should be achieved before the patient leaves the operating room and be maintained throughout transfer. For this reason, mechanical assistance, epicardial pacing, and infusions of anesthetic, vasoactive, inotropic, and anti-arrhythmic drugs should be continued. The surgeon, scrub nurse, and operating department technician do not usually assist the anesthetist during transfer.

In most centers, a portable, battery-operated device is used to monitor the ECG, arterial blood pressure, and peripheral oxygen saturation during transfer. Unless the patient's trachea has been extubated in the operating room, mechanical ventilation must be continued until the patient is connected to a ventilator in the ICU. Although portable gas-driven ventilators are available, most anesthetists prefer to continue ventilation manually.

On arrival in the ICU, physiological monitoring and mechanical ventilation should be recommenced as soon as possible. The anesthetist must ensure that hemodynamic stability has been maintained, that appropriate ventilator settings have been selected, and that ventilation is adequate. Before leaving the ICU, the anesthetist should convey a brief resumé of the patient's medical history and intraoperative course to the ICU staff. This summary should include details of the surgical procedure performed and any complications or difficulties encountered, the type of anesthesia used, any known drug allergies, intraoperative fluid administration, blood product use, urine output, the rate of ongoing drug infusions, the requirement for cardiac pacing, and the results of recent blood gas and electrolyte analyses.

In most centers it is usual to continue mechanical ventilation and infusions of sedative drugs until the following criteria are met:

- The patient is hemodynamically stable on minimal pharmacological and mechanical support.
- Pulmonary gas exchange is adequate and acid–base status satisfactory.
- Core body temperature is above 35.5°C.
- No significant hemorrhage continues.
- Urine output is adequate.
- Residual neuromuscular blockade is absent or has been antagonized.

Thereafter, sedative drugs are gradually withdrawn, and the patient is weaned from mechanical ventilation. Before tracheal extubation, protective airway reflexes must be present, and measures of respiratory performance (respiratory rate, tidal volume, vital capacity, maximum negative inspiratory pressure, and arterial blood gases) are compatible with spontaneous respiration.

FURTHER READING

Association of Anaesthetists of Great Britain and Ireland. 1997. *Checklist for anaesthetic apparatus 2*. Hampshire: Alresford Press.

Association of Anaesthetists of Great Britain and Ireland. 1999. *Management of anaesthesia for Jehovah's witnesses*. Hampshire: Alresford Press.

Connors, A.F. Jr., Speroff, T., Dawson, N.V., et al. 1996. The effectiveness of right heart catheterization in the initial care of critically ill patients. *Journal of the American Medical Association* **276**, 889–97.

Estafanous, F.G., Barash, P.G., Reves, J.G. (ed.) 1994. *Cardiac anesthesia. Principles and clinical practice*. Philadelphia, PA: JB Lippincott.

Nashef, S.A., Roques, F., Michel, P., et al. 1999. European system for cardiac operative risk evaluation (EuroSCORE). *European Journal of Cardiothoracic Surgery* **16(1)**, 9–13.

Newman, M.F,, Wolman, R., Kanchuger, M., et al. 1996. Multicenter preoperative stroke risk index for patients undergoing coronary artery bypass graft surgery. Multicenter Study of Perioperative Ischemia (McSPI) Research Group. *Circulation* **94(9 Suppl II)**, 74–80.

Echocardiography for cardiac surgery

JOSEPH S. SAVINO MD
Associate Professor of Anesthesia, University of Pennsylvania School of Medicine; Section Chief of Cardiovascular Thoracic Anesthesia and Intensive Care, Department of Anesthesia, Hospital of the University of Pennsylvania, Philadelphia, Pennsylvania, USA

BONNIE L. MILAS MD
Assistant Professor of Anesthesia, Department of Anesthesia, University of Pennsylvania School of Medicine, Philadelphia, Pennsylvania, USA

HISTORY

Transesophageal echocardiography (TEE) is the most significant advance in intraoperative monitoring for cardiac surgery since the advent of the pulmonary arterial catheter. TEE provides functional and anatomical information that is not redundant with other diagnostic modalities. TEE anatomical assessment uses high-resolution images to depict cardiac and intravascular structures. The images are displayed as a cine and recorded on VHS tape, although other electronic mediums are being explored. Anatomical and functional information pertaining to the myocardium, intracardiac masses, and blood vessels permit a detailed depiction of the spatial relationships of structures within the mediastinum before a surgeon's commitment to sternotomy and cardiopulmonary bypass. TEE functional data permits real-time, on-line measures of regional and global ventricular systolic function, ventricular diastolic function, valvular diastolic and systolic function, intracavitary and intravascular blood flow velocity, and ventricular chamber size and filling. Color flow Doppler interrogates blood flow velocities in all chambers of the heart and communicating vessels, enabling the creation of a blood flow velocity map superimposed onto the two-dimensional (2-D) image of the beating heart. The real-time display of color flow maps is extensively used in the intraoperative assessment of valvular function, intracardiac shunts, and diseases of the aorta. The spectral display of pulsed wave and continuous-wave Doppler remains useful for the quantitative measure of valvular gradients, continuity equation, velocity flow profiles, and peak velocity measures of regurgitant and stenotic lesions.

PRINCIPLES AND JUSTIFICATION

A few general principles regarding image generation, interpretation of data, and limitations of the system are useful in understanding TEE in the clinical setting. 2-D imaging is most effectively achieved when the ultrasound beam is orthogonal to the tissue planes. Doppler measure of blood flow velocity is dependent on the incident angle ϕ produced by the Doppler signal and vector of blood flow. Blood flow velocity is a function of the difference between reflected ultrasound frequency and the transmitted frequency and the cosine ϕ. The instrumentation assumes that blood flow is parallel to the Doppler signal and that the cosine $\phi = 1$ (i.e. $\phi = 0°$ or $180°$). Transmitral blood flow velocity normally moves away from the transducer in the esophagus, rendering quantitative measures reliable and reproducible. Mitral regurgitation produces blood flow toward the transducer. Color Doppler depicts the direction and amplitude of blood flow velocity using a color scheme selected by the user. Conventionally, blue depicts blood flow moving away from the transducer (negative Doppler Shift), whereas red depicts blood flow moving toward the transducer (positive Doppler Shift). Color flow Doppler uses a pulsed wave technology in which the ability to unambiguously measure high velocity is limited (Nyquist limit). When the velocity limit is exceeded, the Doppler signal will alias and produce a mosaic of colors. Continuous-wave Doppler is not limited by pulse frequency and can measure high velocities displayed on a spectral grid. However, continuous-wave technology does not allow range-gating of the signal and cannot be converted to a color map. Continuous-wave Doppler interrogation is used to measure high velocities produced by stenotic or regurgitant jets between two chambers.

The transesophageal window produces high-resolution images because the ultrasound signal travels through soft tissue (low acoustic impedance) enabling deep penetration.

INSTRUMENTATION

The TEE probe is a modified gastroscope in which the optics have been removed and a high-frequency transducer and associated electronics and cables have been placed. The TEE scope may be turned with torque, flexed, or moved laterally. In addition, the ultrasound transducer may be rotated (0° to 180°) within its encasement without external movement of the probe (Multiplane probe).

Probe insertion and manipulation may lead to significant injury, and precautions are necessary to minimize the risk. Most perioperative TEEs are performed in anesthetized and intubated patients who cannot respond to pain or discomfort caused by excessive probe impingement of soft tissue. Before insertion, the TEE probe is inspected for damage or breakage of the encasement. Then the probe is lubricated, inserted into the mouth, and passed posteriorly into the esophagus. The stomach is entered for the commonly used transgastric views. Manufacturers' recommendations for probe cleaning and maintenance should be heeded with a systematic approach to instrument processing.

Contraindications for TEE are disorders of the mouth, esophagus, and stomach that could preclude safe passage of the probe. Esophageal strictures, diverticula, webs, and cancer may result in significant injury, as TEE passage is not optically guided. Abnormal displacement of the esophagus, such as occurs with a large aortic aneurysm, is associated with increased risk. Ultrasound is not known to cause significant cellular injury. However, high-frequency ultrasound transducers produce heat, and most machines contain a fail-safe 'turn-off' switch, should the transducer temperature exceed a preset limit. Esophageal burns from TEE are unusual. However, in the arena of cardiac surgery, even mild degrees of warming may be counterproductive. The warm transducer may warm adjacent structures in the mediastinum (e.g. posterior wall of the left ventricle), which is particularly problematic if circulatory management requires hypothermia and cooling of the myocardium. Although physical injury from TEE is uncommon, when it occurs, the consequences may be devastating and life threatening.

COMPREHENSIVE EXAMINATION

1 In an attempt to standardize the intraoperative TEE examination, a consensus document defining the guidelines for perioperative TEE was developed through the combined efforts of the American Society of Echocardiography and the Society of Cardiovascular Anesthesiologists. The guidelines describe a series of 20 anatomically directed images. The TEE examination is conducted by inserting the probe to the appropriate depth in the esophagus (~30 cm) and generating an image. The images and spatial relationships between the transducer and the anatomical structures govern further movement of the probe. Approximate multiplane angle is indicated by the icon adjacent to each view. No order to the sequence of the examination has been established. This figure has been reproduced with permission from Shanewise, J.S., Cheung, A.T., Aronson, S., et al. ASE/SCA guidelines for performing a comprehensive intraoperative multiplane transesophageal echocardiography examination: recommendations of the American Society of Echocardiography Council for Intraoperative Echocardiography and the Society of Cardiovascular Anesthesiologists Task Force for Certification in Perioperative Transesophageal Echocardiography. *Anesthesia and Analgesia* 89, 870–84, 1999 and *Journal of the American Society of Echocardiography* 12, 884–900, 1999.

Guidelines for performing a comprehensive intraoperative multiplane examination enhance communication among practitioners, institutions, educators, and researchers across disciplines. A common platform for data measurement is available to all users in the industry. Quality improvement programs with assessment of technical quality and completeness are being developed at individual sites or among participating centers within a consortium. The consistency of image acquisition and description will facilitate education across specialties, communication within and between centers, and provide a basis for investigation, potentially leading to outcomes-based research. Most users of TEE in the operative setting believe that this expensive and invasive technology makes a difference in outcome. Although TEE has clearly changed the practice of cardiac surgery, a paucity of evidence demonstrates that patient outcome is actually improved. Finally, TEE images are stored in the analogue or digital domain using VHS tape or digital medium. Although cumbersome and inefficient, VHS tape has proven to be practical and has been accepted throughout the industry. With the advent of the electronic revolution, TEE images are increasingly being stored in the digital domain, allowing electronic transmission of data and storage and compression of data with minimal loss of information. This situation can only occur if the industry has identified a set of 'standard' images to guide data acquisition.

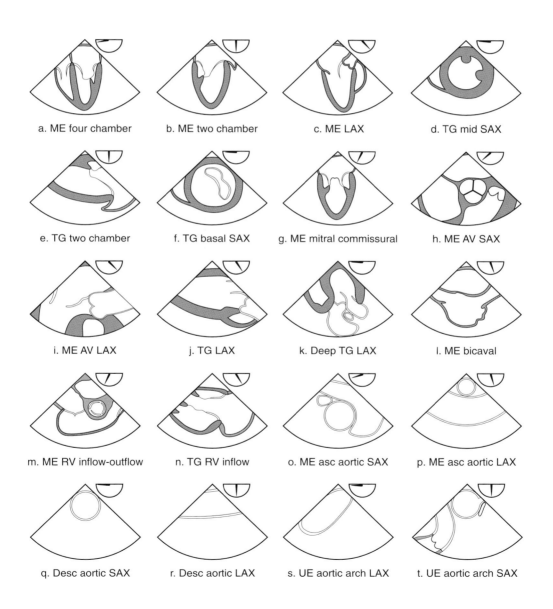

a. ME four chamber b. ME two chamber c. ME LAX d. TG mid SAX

e. TG two chamber f. TG basal SAX g. ME mitral commissural h. ME AV SAX

i. ME AV LAX j. TG LAX k. Deep TG LAX l. ME bicaval

m. ME RV inflow-outflow n. TG RV inflow o. ME asc aortic SAX p. ME asc aortic LAX

q. Desc aortic SAX r. Desc aortic LAX s. UE aortic arch LAX t. UE aortic arch SAX

1

Left ventricle

2a–e The regional assessment of left ventricular function attempts to correlate myocardial anatomy and wall motion with coronary blood flow. The left ventricle is segmented into 16 regions. The longitudinal axis of the left ventricle is described as basal, mid-, or apical. The four-chamber view show the three septal and three lateral segments (Figure 2a). Two-chamber views show the three anterior and three inferior segments (Figure 2b). Long-axis (LAX) views show the two anteroseptal and two posterior segments (Figure 2c). Short-axis (SAX) views show all six segments at the mid level (Figure 2d). Basal SAX views show all six segments at the basal level (Figure 2e). These figures have been reproduced with permission from Shanewise, J.S., Cheung, A.T., Aronson, S., *et al.* ASE/SCA guidelines for performing a comprehensive intraoperative multiplane transesophageal echocardiography examination: recommendations of the American Society of Echocardiography Council for Intraoperative Echocardiography and the Society of Cardiovascular Anesthesiologists Task Force for Certification in Perioperative Transesophageal Echocardiography. *Anesthesia and Analgesia* **89**, 870–84, 1999 and *Journal of the American Society of Echocardiography* **12**, 884–900, 1999.

The basal and mid-levels of the left ventricle are circumferentially divided into six segments, and the apical level is divided into four segments.

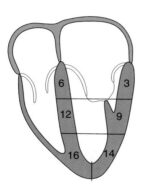

a. ME four-chamber view

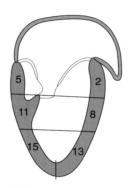

b. ME two-chamber view

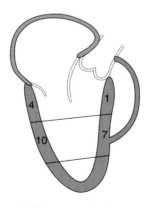

c. ME long-axis view

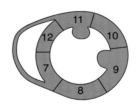

d. TG mid – short-axis view

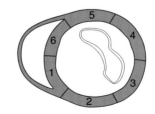

e. TG basal short-axis view

Key

Basal Segments	Mid Segments	Apical Segments
1 = Basal Anteroseptal	7 = Mid Anteroseptal	13 = Apical Anterior
2 = Basal Anterior	8 = Mid Anterior	14 = Apical Lateral
3 = Basal Lateral	9 = Mid Lateral	15 = Apical Inferior
4 = Basal Posterior	10 = Mid Posterior	16 = Apical Septal
5 = Basal Inferior	11 = Mid Inferior	
6 = Basal Septal	12 = Mid Septal	

2

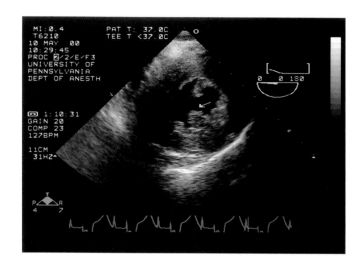

3 Transgastric (TG) SAX view with arrow depicting anterolateral papillary muscle.

3

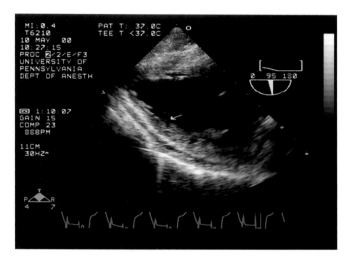

4 TG two-chamber view with arrow depicting anterior wall of left ventricle.

4

5 TG apical SAX view depicting diastole.

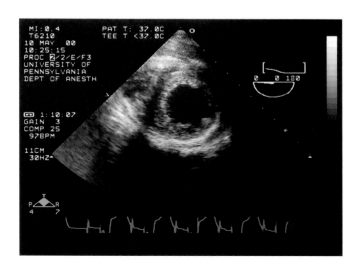

5

6 TG apical SAX view depicting systole. Wall motion is scored based on wall thickening and percent endocardial excursion using the following scale: normal (wall thickening greater than 30 percent), mild hypokinesis (10–30 percent thickening), severe hypokinesis (less than 10 percent thickening), akinesis (no thickening), and dyskinesis (paradoxical motion). Endocardial excursion is the measure of radial shortening between the endocardium and the centroid of the left ventricle. Endocardial excursion is affected by translational motion of the heart during contraction and respiration. Decreased systolic wall thickening and endocardial motion characterize segmental myocardial dysfunction. Regional hypokinesis is most often caused by myocardial ischemia or infarction. Less common causes include stunning, tethering from adjacent infarction, or prosthetic material. With acute infarction, the wall thickness during diastole may be normal, but displays abnormal thickening and endocardial motion or excursion. Over time, the affected segments become thinned and echogenic due to fibrosis and scarring. Transmural myocardial infarctions (Q waves) demonstrate akinesis and thinning, whereas nontransmural infarctions (non–Q wave) may demonstrate hypokinesis with little or no myocardial thinning. The affected myocardial segments detract from overall left ventricular function and result in decreased ejection fraction. The velocity of circumferential fiber shortening is an alternative method to assess regional function, but this information is not often used clinically and requires off-line analysis.

Prolonged ischemia or acute myocardial infarction with successful reperfusion may result in myocardial stunning, whereby a segmental wall motion abnormality can persist for 24–72 hours without irreversible injury. Hibernating myocardium is a persistent wall motion abnormality due to chronic hypoperfusion that is reversed by re-establishing blood flow. Nonetheless, persistent new hypokinesis or akinesis after cardiopulmonary bypass is myocardial ischemia until proven otherwise.

Myocardial ischemia produces abnormal diastolic relaxation, with spectral Doppler of the left ventricular inflow often demonstrating decreased E velocity (i.e. passive left ventricular filling). Mitral regurgitation due to papillary muscle dysfunction or rupture, ventricular septal defect, ventricular free wall rupture, ventricular aneurysm or pseudoaneurysm, pericardial effusion or tamponade, or right ventricular (RV) infarction are conditions associated with infarction that are readily diagnosed with TEE.

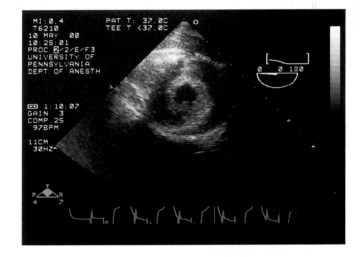

6

7 TG apical SAX view using automated border detection to provide on-line measure of fractional area change (FAC), a measure of area ejection fraction often used as a surrogate for left ventricular ejection fraction in patients with near-normal left ventricular geometry.

EDA = End-diastolic area
ESA = End-systolic area.

$$FAC = EDA\text{–}ESA\ /\ EDA.$$

Left ventricular aneurysms, masses, or scarring may render this technique less accurate in estimating global function. Assessment of global function should be performed at basal, mid-, and apical levels. Automated techniques enable the continuous measure and recording of FAC while the transducer is in a stable position. Longitudinal shortening of the left ventricle can be appreciated by TEE through assessment of the apical displacement of the mitral annulus.

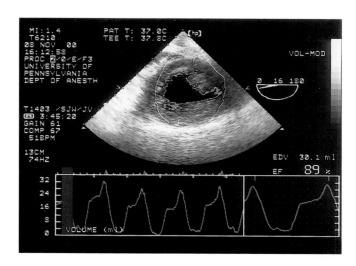

7

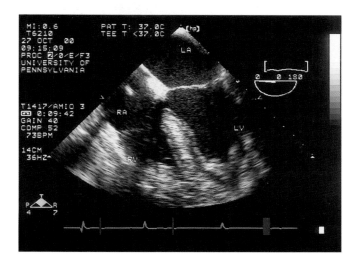

8

Right ventricle

8 Midesophageal (ME) four-chamber view. The asymmetrical crescent-shaped cavity of the RV does not lend itself to 2-D quantification measurements using techniques applied to the left ventricle. A formal segmented model of the RV based on distribution of coronary blood flow has not been established. The four walls of the RV are the anterior, lateral, inferior, and RV outflow tract. Wall motion abnormalities of the RV are more difficult to detect and quantify compared to those of the left ventricle. Flattening of the normally convex septum frequently accompanies RV pressure overload.

Aortic valve, aortic root, and left ventricular outflow tract

9 ME aortic valve (AV) LAX view demonstrating diameters of AV annulus sinuses of Valsalva and sinotubular junction. Short- and long-axis images of each of the following structures of left ventricular outflow are necessary in all patients undergoing cardiac surgery: left ventricular outflow tract (LVOT), AV annulus, cusps, sinuses of Valsalva, coronary ostia, sinotubular junction, and proximal aorta.

The aortic root and ascending aorta are imaged from the ME and TG windows.

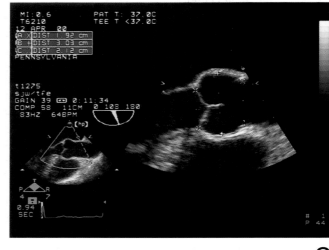

9

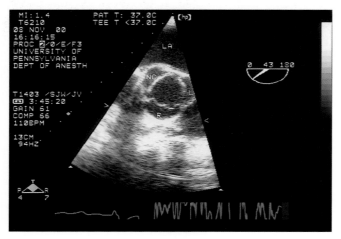

10a

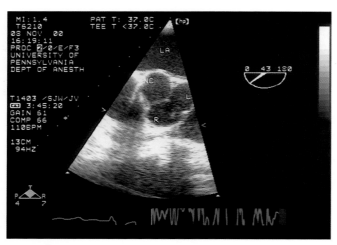

10b

10a, b The ME AV SAX view, at the level of the aortic cusps, permits measurement of the area of the AV orifice by planimetry. Systole (Figure 10a); diastole (Figure 10b).

11 Color flow Doppler is applied to this ME AV SAX view to detect aortic regurgitation and to assess the size and location of the regurgitant orifice. The TEE probe can be advanced or withdrawn to image the LVOT, coronary ostia, sinuses of Valsalva, sinotubular junction, or ascending aorta. The ME AV LAX view (110°–130°) provides the ideal window for measurement of the aortic annulus, sinuses of Valsalva, sinotubular junction, and proximal ascending aorta (Figure 9). The most anterior aortic cusp is the right coronary cusp. The posterior cusp in this view may be either the left or the noncoronary cusp, depending on the image plane. If a coronary ostium is clearly identified, then the posterior cusp is the left coronary cusp. These measurements help plan surgical management, including the size of the prosthesis or homograft to be used. Color flow Doppler is used for the detection and quantification of aortic regurgitation within the LVOT. The ME ascending aortic SAX also permits direct measurement of aortic root and ascending aortic diameters. Two TG views used to evaluate AV dysfunction align the Doppler beam near parallel to the flow through the AV. Doppler quantification of flow velocities through the AV and the LVOT permits measurement of AV area and gradients (mean and peak). Normal LVOT and AV velocities are less than 1.5 m/s. Subvalvular obstruction produced by hypertrophic cardiomyopathy or systolic anterior motion produces early closure of the AV and the typical 'dagger' shape of the flow velocity profile.

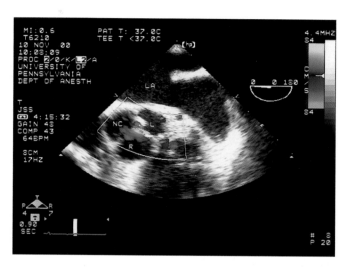

11

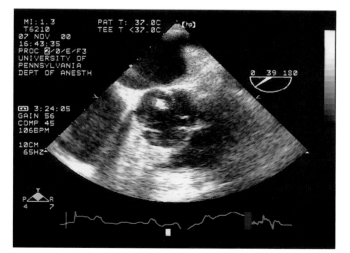

12

AORTIC STENOSIS

12 ME AV SAX. 2-D Echocardiographic imaging of the stenotic AV typically reveals areas of increased echogenicity consistent with calcification, immobile leaflets, and a small systolic orifice. Planimetry may prove difficult due to severe calcification and acoustic shadowing.

13 ME AV SAX view with arrow depicting vegetation on bicuspid AV. Congenital bicuspid AVs are common. The 'acquired' bicuspid AV due to calcific disease and fusion of one of the three commissures make it appear similar to a raphe. The truly congenital bicuspid valve orifice in systole typically appears elliptical rather than triangular. Rheumatic AV changes result in commisural fusion, increased echogenicity, and systolic cusp doming. These changes are similar to those associated with calcific aortic stenosis and are not pathognomonic for rheumatic disease. Regardless of the etiology, direct measurement of the valve area from SAX views by planimetry is feasible. Left ventricular hypertrophy (left ventricular wall thickness greater than 11 mm) is common with preserved systolic function until late in the course of the disease. The echocardiographic examination must verify the exact locus of LVOT obstruction. An increased left-ventricle-to-aortic-pressure gradient may occur from aortic stenosis, a subvalvular membrane, systolic anterior motion, or another congenital anomaly.

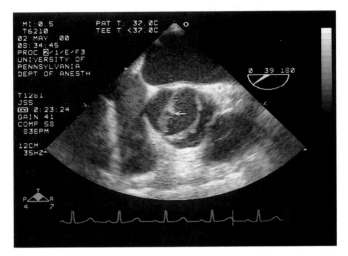

13

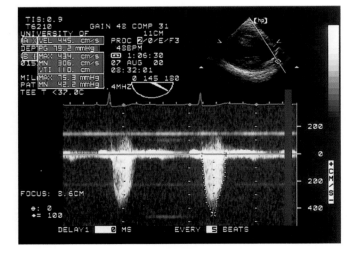

14

14 TG LAX view with continuous-wave Doppler through stenotic AV. The severity of valvular stenosis is determined by using pulsed or continuous-wave Doppler to estimate transvalvular gradient. The maximum transaortic pressure gradient is calculated from the maximum aortic jet velocity using the following modified Bernoulli equation:

$$\Delta Pmax = 4V^2max$$

The mean pressure gradient can be calculated by digitizing the spectral velocity curve and averaging the instantaneous gradients over the systolic ejection period. This process permits the calculation of the mean velocity, and hence, the mean pressure gradient.

The maximum Doppler gradient is the maximum 'instantaneous' gradient and is always greater than the peak-to-peak gradient measured by cardiac catheterization. Pressure gradients are dependent on flow rate. Thus, pressure gradients increase when transaortic stroke volume increases (e.g. pregnancy, exercise, anxiety, aortic regurgitation) and decrease when transaortic stroke volume decreases (e.g. hypovolemia, left ventricular dysfunction, mitral regurgitation).

The AV area can be calculated based on the principle of continuity of flow using the following simplified continuity equation:

$$AVA = CSA_{LVOT} \times (V_{LVOT}/V_{AV})$$

AVA represents the stenotic AV area, *CSA* is the cross-sectional area (cm^2) of the LVOT, and *V* is blood flow velocity in the LVOT and AV, respectively.

Attention to technical details is necessary to obtain accurate data for calculation of transaortic pressure gradients and AV areas. The measurement of peak aortic pressure gradient requires the measurement of the peak velocity. The most common error in underestimating the AV pressure gradient is malalignment (i.e. nonparallel alignment) of the Doppler signal with the blood flow vector. The locus of measurement of the LVOT diameter (CSA $_{LVOT} = \pi \, (D/2)^2$) and V$_{LVOT}$ should be the same. Small errors in outflow tract diameter can lead to large errors in cross-sectional area.

AORTIC REGURGITATION

The echocardiographic assessment of aortic regurgitation includes determination of the severity and etiology of the regurgitation, the effect of the regurgitant lesion on ventricular size and function, and the presence of associated findings. Aortic regurgitation may be due to abnormalities of the root or cusps. The same disease processes affecting the aortic cusps and causing valvular stenosis are associated with aortic regurgitation (e.g. bicuspid AV, rheumatic disease, senile calcification).

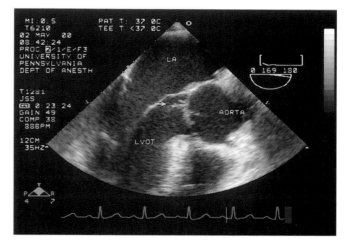

15

15 Myxomatous valvular disease produces redundant, and often prolapsing, cusps. This ME AV LAX view demonstrates a prolapsing AV with vegetations (*arrow*).

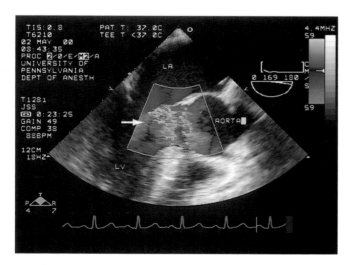

16

16 ME AV LAX view demonstrating severe aortic regurgitation (arrow). Endocarditis of the AV produces aortic regurgitation either due to cusp or annular destruction. Vegetations and abscesses are common.

17 ME AV LAX view. Dilatation of the aortic root with normal cusp morphology can lead to aortic regurgitation owing to the lack of normal supporting structures. Causes of aortic root dilatation include hypertension, collagen-vascular disorders (e.g. Marfan's syndrome, Ehlers-Danlos syndrome), rheumatoid arthritis, syphilitic aortitis, mycotic aneurysm, and poststenotic dilatation associated with aortic stenosis.

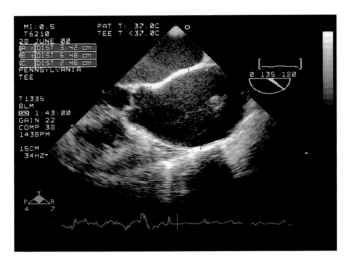

17

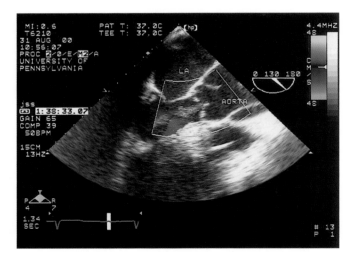

18

18 ME AV LAX view. Aortic dissection produces an intimal flap in the lumen of the aorta (dissection flap detected in aortic root). Para-aortic hematoma is common. Blood flow may exist in the true and false lumen. Aortic dissection may produce aortic regurgitation as a result of annular dilation or undermining of the aortic annulus by the intimal flap.

Ascending aortic aneurysm frequently produces valvular insufficiency with dilatation of the sinotubular junction (Figure 17). Changes in the left ventricle depend upon the duration of the disease. When exposed to volume overload, the left ventricle responds by slow, progressive dilation. In the presence of increasing aortic regurgitation and chronic volume overload, left ventricular systolic dysfunction ensues with decreasing ejection fraction and left ventricular dilatation. In acute aortic regurgitation (aortic dissection or AV endocarditis), the ventricular chamber size may be normal; however, the left ventricular end-diastolic pressure is increased due to the accommodation of increased left ventricular volume.

19 Color Doppler flow mapping of the aortic regurgitation velocity permits semiquantitative assessment of severity. The width of the aortic regurgitation velocity jet is compared to the width of the LVOT at the origin of the jet, immediately adjacent to the AV. Aortic regurgitation jet width of less than 30 per cent of the LVOT width is considered mild (Figure 18), 30–60 per cent is moderate, and the ME AV LAX view in this figure demonstrates severe aortic regurgitation (greater than 60 per cent). Length of the regurgitant jet correlates poorly with angiographic grade.

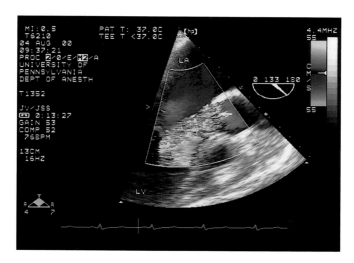

19

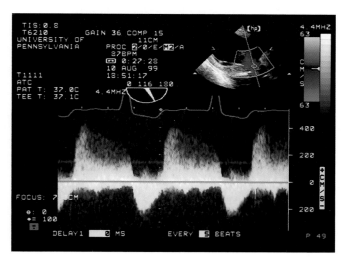

20

20 TG LAX view with continuous-wave Doppler producing high-velocity diastolic flow signal. The continuous-wave Doppler spectral recording of aortic regurgitation typically reveals an increased velocity flow of 3–5 m/s. Optimal alignment of the continuous-wave signal to obtain a parallel intercept angle is usually obtained from the deep TG window (inverted image) or the TG LAX view of the left ventricle (image angle rotated 110°–130°). The shape of the continuous-wave Doppler time–velocity integral depends on the time-varying, instantaneous pressure gradient across the valve in diastole. Spectral Doppler display of acute aortic regurgitation appears similar to severe chronic insufficiency (steep deceleration slope with a short pressure half-time), even when moderate in severity. This situation is due to the inability of the left ventricle to compensate for the acute increase in volume. These spectral signals should only be used as a complementary tool to color flow Doppler in the estimation of grade, because they are affected by other confounding variables.

MITRAL VALVE AND LEFT ATRIUM

Advances in the surgical correction of the disorders of the mitral valve have been possible, in part, because of the introduction of TEE. Mitral annular calcifications, restrictive or excessive motion of mitral valve leaflets, size of the mitral valve anulus, and the integrity of the subvalvular apparatus can be determined with accuracy and precision in the operating room before commitment to cardiopulmonary bypass. TEE has a vital role in the design of the surgical repair.

MITRAL REGURGITATION

The most common causes of mitral valve systolic dysfunction (i.e. mitral regurgitation) are ischemic heart disease, myxomatous degeneration, endocarditis, and rheumatic heart disease. The etiology of mitral regurgitation is often not discernible without a TEE. Surgical correction of mitral regurgitation is guided by whether leaflet motion is normal, excessive, or restrictive. Most mitral valve repairs include an annuloplasty ring in an effort to buttress the atrioventricular membrane along the free wall of the left ventricle.

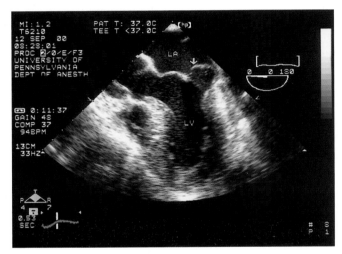

21a

21a, b ME four-chamber view demonstrating prolapse of posterior mitral leaflet. Severe mitral regurgitation (Figure 21b).

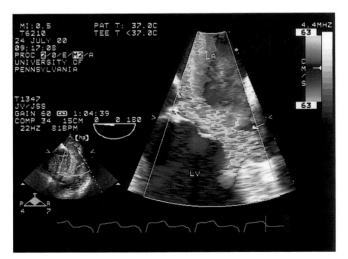

21b

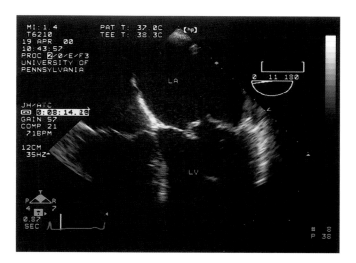

22a

22a, b
ME four-chamber view. Prolapse of anterior and posterior mitral valve leaflets (Figure 22a). Severe mitral regurgitation (Figure 22b).

The choice to repair a regurgitant mitral valve is dependent on the complexity of the lesion and the associated risk of a 'failed repair.' A focal defect of the posterior leaflet with a normal anterior leaflet is associated with a much greater rate of successful repair compared to that associated with endocarditis affecting both leaflets. TEE interrogation of the mitral valve includes the SAX and LAX views. The LAX view of the mitral valve permits quantitation of the grade of mitral regurgitation and a detailed anatomy of the left atrium, mitral valve annulus, mitral valve leaflets, LVOT, and subvalvular apparatus. Occasionally, calcium and prosthetic material within the mitral valve will shadow more distant structures and prevent effective imaging of chordae and papillary muscles. Preoperative mitral regurgitation may be significantly reduced in severity after induction of general anesthesia when the heart is subjected to the unloading effects of inhalational and intravenous anesthetics. Severity of mitral regurgitation is graded on a scale of 1+ to 4+ based on the size of the regurgitant jet using color Doppler. A large (greater than 8 cm^2) jet area with increased velocity suggests severe mitral regurgitation.

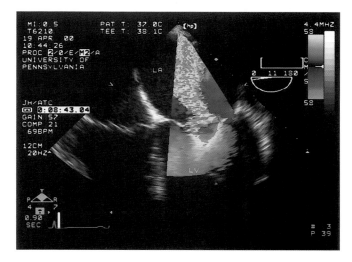

22b

23 ME two-chamber view demonstrating eccentric mitral regurgitation. Severe regurgitation may manifest as eccentric jets that impinge the wall of the left atrium producing a small jet area that 'hugs' the atrial wall. Systolic reversal of pulmonary vein blood flow velocity suggests severe mitral regurgitation.

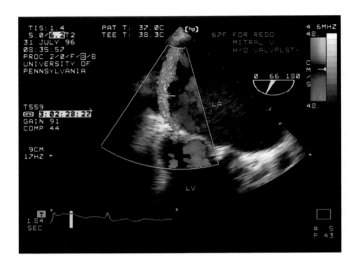

23

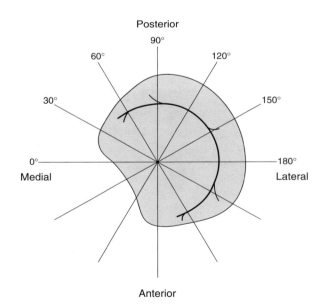

24 The SAX view of the mitral valve more closely resembles a surgeon's perspective from a left atriotomy. This figure has been reproduced with permission from Shanewise, J.S., Cheung, A.T., Aronson, S., *et al.* ASE/SCA guidelines for performing a comprehensive intraoperative multiplane transesophageal echocardiography examination: recommendations of the American Society of Echocardiography Council for Intraoperative Echocardiography and the Society of Cardiovascular Anesthesiologists Task Force for Certification in Perioperative Transesophageal Echocardiography. *Anesthesia and Analgesia* **89**, 870–84, 1999 and *Journal of the American Society of Echocardiography* **12**, 884–900, 1999.

24

25 TG basal SAX view. ME SAX view with color Doppler demonstrating regurgitant orifice. With colorflow Doppler, the locus of the regurgitant orifice can be identified within the mitral valve, thereby directing surgical repair to the functional lesion, which may not be easily discernible in the flaccid, arrested heart. Both the SAX and LAX views are important immediately after mitral valve repair to detect residual mitral regurgitation and structural abnormalities. Diastolic function in a newly repaired mitral valve is assessed by measuring a transmitral valve mean and peak pressure gradient and calculating the mitral valve area using the pressure half-time. The peak gradient is measured using the transmitral flow velocity generated by passive filling of the left ventricle (E Wave) and applying the following modified Bernoulli equation: $\Delta P = 4 V^2$.

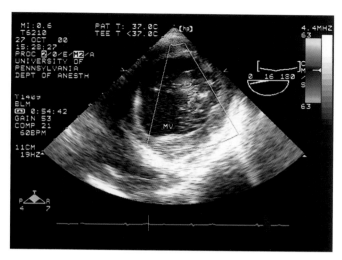

25

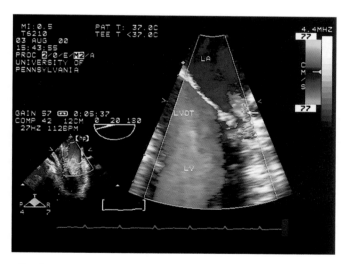

26

26 ME four-chamber view demonstrating eccentric mitral regurgitation (*arrow*). Residual mitral regurgitation after mitral repair is not uncommon. Mild to moderate mitral regurgitation detected under the influence of general anesthetics might revert to severe mitral regurgitation and symptomatic pulmonary edema in the exercising patient. The mechanisms of failed repair include persistent excessive leaflet motion, prolapse, perforation, and a spectrum of disorders producing malcoaptation of the anterior and posterior leaflets. Systolic anterior motion of the mitral valve tends to occur in patients with an excessively long (i.e. edge-to-annulus) posterior leaflet. Systolic anterior motion produces mitral regurgitation and obstruction of the LVOT. Hypovolemia and vasodilatation exacerbate systolic anterior motion. Treatment includes volume administration and (if persistent) reinitiation of cardiopulmonary bypass and a sliding posterior valvuloplasty or mitral valve replacement may be necessary.

The maximum allowable mitral regurgitation after repair is controversial. Many clinicians will accept 1+ mitral regurgitation, especially if reinitiation of cardiopulmonary bypass and recross-clamping poses a significantly increased risk (e.g. elderly, concomitant ischemic disease, decreased ejection fraction).

MITRAL STENOSIS

The most common cause of mitral stenosis is rheumatic heart disease. The obstructed diastolic filling of the left ventricle results in an increased transmitral gradient and transmitral flow velocities. The transmitral gradient can be calculated using the modified Bernoulli equation $\Delta P = 4 V^2$. The mitral valve area can be estimated using the following method of pressure half-time:

$$MVA\ (cm_2) = \frac{220}{P\frac{1}{2}t}$$

The pressure half-time is estimated using spectral Doppler through the mitral valve during diastole. The decay in velocity after the peak E wave is dependent on the left atrial-left ventricular pressure difference. The pressure half-time is the time elapsed for the peak transmitral pressure (peak E wave) gradient to decrease by 50 per cent. In the presence of aortic regurgitation, pressure half-time underestimates the severity of mitral stenosis (overestimates mitral valve area by underestimating pressure half-time). Patients who undergo mitral valve surgery for mitral stenosis typically have an established diagnosis before surgery. However, the intraoperative TEE does provide anatomical information regarding structural abnormalities of the mitral valve and adjacent structures. Although most stenotic rheumatic mitral valves are treated with valve replacement, there are several sites in the United States that have attempted to repair rheumatic mitral stenosis through a process of decalcification and débridement. The long-term efficacy of such a procedure remains controversial.

27 Prosthetic valve replacements are associated with technical complications that are readily detected and quantified by the postcardiopulmonary bypass TEE. Normal function of a mechanical valve would include signature closing jets that must be differentiated from perivalvular or intravalvular leaks. In this figure, a deep TG LAX view demonstrates a perivalvular leak from the prosthetic valve in the aortic position. Perivalvular leaks typically produce high velocity, high variance jets emanating external to the sewing ring. Intravalvular leaks are associated with abnormal leaflet function. Doppler across a prosthetic valve measures the instantaneous transvalvular pressure gradient (peak and mean).

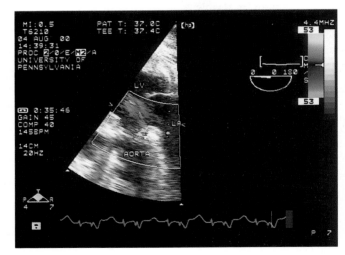

27

TRICUSPID VALVE, RIGHT ATRIUM AND INTERATRIAL SEPTUM, AND PULMONARY ARTERY

28 ME bicaval with blood flow through patent foramen ovale (arrow). TEE of the right atrium and tricuspid valve is a reliable method of detecting atrial septal defects, sinus venosus defects, anomalous insertion of pulmonary veins, dilated coronary sinus (e.g. persistent left-sided vena cava), and abnormalities of the tricuspid valve. Insertion of a coronary sinus cardioplegia cannula can be facilitated by direct imaging. Patent foramen ovale is common and diagnosis is established using 2-D color Doppler and/or contrast echocardiography.

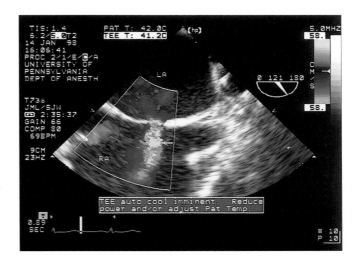

28

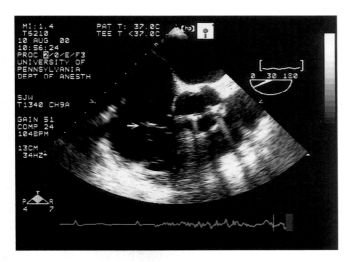

29

29 ME AV SAX view. Dilated right atrium with flail portion of tricuspid valve (arrow).

30 ME four-chamber view demonstrating moderate tricuspid regurgitation (arrow). The grade of tricuspid regurgitation is qualitatively based on the size of the regurgitant jet in the right atrium (Figures 29 and 30). Vegetations appear as mobile densities on leaflets or chordae, and abscess formation is not uncommon. TEE assessment of the pulmonary artery is used to determine the presence of pulmonic regurgitation, should a Ross procedure be indicated. TEE may detect large saddle thrombi in the pulmonary artery, but it lacks the sensitivity for the diagnosis of pulmonary embolism.

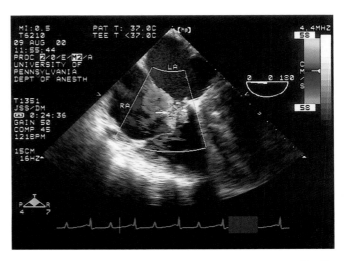

30

Thoracic aorta

AORTIC ANEURYSM

31 ME ascending aorta SAX view demonstrating aneurysm. Patients presenting with aortic aneurysm for elective repair have generally had their diagnosis confirmed by a variety of diagnostic modalities (e.g. transthoracic echocardiogram, computed tomography, magnetic resonance imaging, angiography) before presenting for surgery. Emergency surgery is typically performed for rupture, rapid expansion, or symptoms of pain or malperfusion. Aortic aneurysms with diameters greater than 5.5 cm or in the setting of rapidly increasing dimensions is an indication for surgery. The purpose of a precardiopulmonary bypass TEE would be to confirm the precise location and extent of the aneurysm, assess the integrity of the AV (for root or ascending aortic aneurysm), exclude chronic aortic dissection, measure aortic dimensions for sizing of grafts or valved conduits, and assess ventricular function. Postcardiopulmonary bypass TEE is aimed at assessing repair and detecting occult complications, such as malperfusion, dissection, residual intracavity air or debris, and aortic regurgitation. New regional wall motion abnormalities may suggest ischemia from air emboli or a technical deficiency in the anastomosis of the coronary ostia onto the graft conduit. Aneurysmal dilation of the aortic root/ascending aorta increases lateral tension on the aortic commissures, which can result in distortion of the aortic cusps and aortic regurgitation.

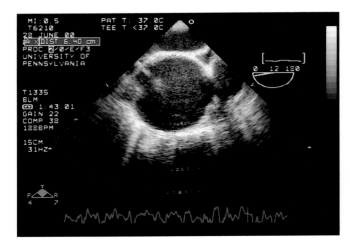

31

AORTIC DISSECTION

TEE offers significant advantages in the diagnosis of acute aortic dissection (Table 2.1). The decision between emergency surgery and medical therapy hinges on several factors, including type A versus type B dissection, malperfusion syndrome, bleeding, hemodynamic instability, and refractory pain. Detection of involvement of the ascending aorta requires repair via sternotomy, whereas a type B dissection may be treated medically or via left thoracotomy in the unstable patient. The management of patients with suspected acute ascending aortic dissection has changed significantly with the advent of TEE. Immediate admission from the emergency room or referring hospital to the cardiac surgery suite permits expedient diagnosis and treatment of this often-lethal disease. Clinical suspicion is based on chest and/or back pain, widened mediastinum on chest radiograph, murmur of aortic regurgitation, and/or evidence of malperfusion (e.g. stroke, loss of pulses) or pericardial effusion. The patient is monitored appropriately in anticipation of cardiac surgery. Once in the operating room, induction of general anesthesia and tracheal intubation is often necessary, after which a TEE probe is inserted and the diagnosis confirmed. Bypassing the delay and risk associated with obtaining CAT scans, MRI, or angiograms in often poorly monitored settings can be life-saving.

Table 2.1 *Diagnostic tests for acute aortic dissection*

	Transesophageal echocardiography[a]	Computed tomography[a]	Magnetic resonance imaging[a]	Angiography[b]
Sensitivity	98%	94%	98%	88%
Specificity	98%	83%	87%	85%
Ionizing radiation	–	+	–	+
Expediency	+	–	–	–
Operating room location	+	–	–	–
Left ventricular function	+	–	–	–
Arch imaging	–	+	+	+
Pericardial fluid	+	+	+	–
Aortic regurgitation	+	–	–	+

[a]Nienaber, C.A., von Kodolitsch, Y., Nicholas, V., *et al.* 1993. The diagnosis of thoracic aortic dissection by non-invasive imaging procedures. *New England Journal of Medicine* **328**, 1–9.

[b]Chirillo, F., Cavallini, C., Longhini, C., *et al.* 1994. Comparative diagnostic value of transesophageal echocardiography retrograde aortography in the evaluation of thoracic aortic dissection. *American Journal of Cardiology* **74**(6), 590–5.

32 Descending aorta SAX view. Aortic dissection with pleural effusion, probably hemothorax. The hallmark of aortic dissection is a linear, mobile echogenic density (i.e. intimal flap (arrow)) within the lumen of the aorta. Undulating motion of the flap can be associated with systole.

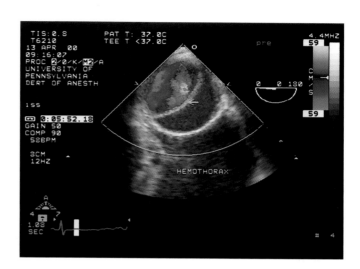

32

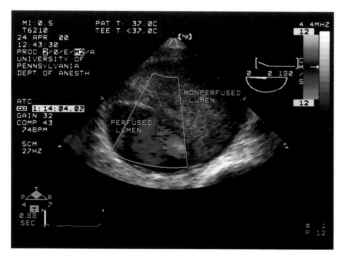

33

33 Descending aorta SAX view. Aortic dissection with thrombosed false lumen.

Color flow Doppler may detect blood flow within a true (endothelial/atherosclerotic lined) and/or false lumen. An entry site (fenestration) between the true and false lumen is often identified. The absence of a discrete flap does not exclude the diagnosis of dissection. Intramural hematoma is never a normal finding and implies significant injury to the integrity of the aortic wall (e.g. dissection, transection, or disruption). Hematoma may appear as an echogenic mass within the media or adjacent to the aorta, contained by echogenic adventitia. Caution should be used to avoid misinterpretation due to ultrasound artifacts such as reverberation artifact and beam-width artifact in oblique image planes. Transthoracic imaging of the suprasternal notch may reveal a limited dissection in the portion of the aortic arch that is not readily accessible by TEE. Ultrasound examination of the carotid arteries may detect dissection or compression. Magnetic resonance imaging, computed tomography, or angiographic evaluation is warranted if the diagnosis is equivocal.

Aortic dissection may expand with compression of the true lumen, propagation into major branch vessels, rupture, or thrombosis. Dilation of the aortic root leads to aortic regurgitation (Figure 18). Extension of the dissection flap into the aortic root can result in a flail aortic cusp due to inadequacy of supporting structures. Coronary ostial occlusion produces severe ventricular dysfunction. Aortic rupture into the pericardium or pleural space is often fatal. However, if the rupture is contained by adjacent structures, a pericardial effusion/tamponade or pleural effusion can be detected and tolerated by the patient until emergency surgery corrects the defect.

Initial echocardiographic assessment should focus on detection of an intimal flap to confirm the diagnosis of aortic dissection. A TG SAX view of the left ventricle determines if the pericardium contains blood and permits assessment of regional and global ventricular function. The ME AV SAX view provides images of AV integrity and the detection of aortic regurgitation. Compression of the coronary ostia or inclusion of the ostia in the false lumen affects surgical management. Color flow Doppler imaging can be used to verify flow within the proximal right and left coronary arteries. ME SAX views of the ascending aorta will often display an intimal flap. ME AV LAX views assess aortic regurgitation, the detection of an intimal flap, and the ability to measure size of the aortic root and ascending aorta, should replacement/repair be necessary. The descending aorta and the distal aortic arch are evaluated by rotating the probe to the patient's left from the ME transducer position. The left pleural space is easily imaged and evaluated for a pleural effusion. On initiation of cardiopulmonary bypass, the adequacy of arterial inflow into the true lumen and carotid arteries can be assessed using hand-held transducers.

FURTHER READING

Salgo, I.S., Savino, J.S. 1998. Transesophageal echocardiography. In Longnecker, D.E., Tinker, J.H., Morgan, G.E., (eds), *Principles and practice of anesthesiology*, 2nd edition. Philadelphia, PA: Mosby–Year Book, 829–58.

Savino, J.S. 1996. Transesophageal echocardiographic evaluation of native valvular disease and repair. *Critical Care Clinics* 12, 321–81.

Savino, J.S, Cheung, A.T. 1996. Rheumatic mitral stenosis. In Oka, Y., Konstadt, S. (eds), *Clinical transesophageal echocardiography: a problem-oriented approach*. Philadelphia, PA: Lippincott–Raven, 3–30.

Savino, J.S., Salgo, I.S. 1997. Monitoring the anesthetized patient. In Longnecker, D.E., Murphy, F.L. (eds), *Dripps, Eckenhoff and Vandam's introduction to anesthesia*, 9th edition. Philadelphia, PA: WB Saunders, 48–62.

Shanewise, J.S., Cheung, A.T., Aronson, S., *et al.* 1999. ASE/SCA guidelines for performing a comprehensive intraoperative multiplane transesophageal echocardiography examination: recommendations of the American Society of Echocardiography Council for Intraoperative Echocardiography and the Society of Cardiovascular Anesthesiologists Task Force for Certification in Perioperative Transesophageal Echocardiography. *Anesthesia and Analgesia* 89, 870–84, and *Journal of the American Society of Echocardiography* 12, 884–900.

Weyman, A.E. 1994. *Principles and practice of echocardiography*, 2nd edition. Philadelphia, PA: Lea & Febiger.

Cardiopulmonary bypass: access and technical options

IRVING L. KRON MD
Chair, Department of Surgery, and Chief, Division of Cardiothoracic Surgery, University of Virginia Medical Center, Charlottesville, Virginia, USA

CHRISTOPHER D. SMITH MBBS, FRACS
Lecturer, Department of Surgery, University of Queensland, and Consultant Cardiothoracic Surgeon, Princess Alexandra Hospital, Brisbane, Queensland, Australia

HISTORY

The development of cardiopulmonary bypass can be largely attributed to the pioneering of John Gibbon, who demonstrated its first successful use in animals in the 1930s and performed the first successful human open heart operation in 1953, when he repaired an atrial septal defect using cardiopulmonary bypass. However, after several subsequent deaths, he became discouraged by the results and postponed its subsequent human use. At approximately the same time, C. Walton Lillehei began using controlled cross-circulation from parent to child to allow intracardiac repairs. In 1965, John Kirklin used a modified Gibbon heart-lung machine for intracardiac repair in a series of patients, heralding the era of cardiopulmonary bypass. Since this early work, progressive developments have occurred in materials used and in surgical techniques to improve the safety, reliability, and efficacy of cardiopulmonary bypass.

PRINCIPLES AND JUSTIFICATION

1 During cardiopulmonary bypass, systemic de-oxygenated venous blood drains into the extracorporeal circuit and passes via a venous reservoir to a pump, which propels blood through a membrane oxygenator, allowing gas transfer, before returning to the systemic arterial circulation. The pump therefore diverts the flow of blood through the heart and lungs while providing oxygenated systemic blood to maintain organ perfusion. A heat exchanger allows for control of body temperature and permits core cooling and rewarming as required. Multiple access ports are in the circuit to add perfusate and drugs, provide cardioplegia, salvage blood from the surgical field, and obtain blood samples.

Cardiopulmonary bypass is indicated when an empty heart is required for intracardiac repair, when cardiac mechanical arrest is needed, when cardiac manipulation requires circulatory support, and when deep hypothermia is needed to allow for a period of systemic circulatory arrest. Anticoagulation is required to prevent blood clotting in the extracorporeal circuit, and 200–400 units/kg heparin is administered systemically before cannulation to maintain an activated clotting time (ACT) of greater than 400 seconds during bypass. Occasionally, patients who receive preoperative heparin develop heparin 'resistance' due to deficiency of antithrombin III and may require administration of fresh frozen plasma to replenish these levels. The ACT is monitored every 20–30 minutes during bypass to ensure that adequate anticoagulation is maintained.

Required flow rates for cardiopulmonary bypass depend on the patient's body surface area and temperature. At 37°C, flow of 2.2 L/m² per minute is required for adequate perfusion. Oxygen consumption is reduced, however, by 50 per cent for every 10°C drop in temperature. At 20°C, a 30-minute period of circulatory arrest can be safely tolerated. A guide to the adequacy of tissue perfusion can be achieved by measurement of the mixed venous oxygen saturation. Some degree of hypothermia is used in most operations, because this provides a margin of safety in the event of unexpected cessation of flow. Although arterial perfusion pressure does not necessarily equate to tissue perfusion, a perfusion pressure of greater than 50 mm Hg is recommended. Higher perfusion pressures are used in the presence of generalized atherosclerosis, especially when renovascular or cerebrovascular disease is present. It is imperative that the surgeon has a sound working knowledge of the bypass circuit, a specific plan for the conduct of cardiopulmonary bypass during the procedure, and clear communication with the other members of the operative team.

PREOPERATIVE ASSESSMENT AND PREPARATION

Cardiopulmonary bypass is a flexible tool, and its implementation needs to be individualized to the patient and the planned procedure. The surgeon must have a clear plan of the operation, including the conduct of cardiopulmonary bypass management and contingencies for unplanned events. To do this, the surgeon must consider the operative access needed, the requirements to facilitate the planned procedure (e.g. cardioplegia, hypothermic circulatory arrest), and patient factors, which affect the establishment and conduct of cardiopulmonary bypass. Assessment of the patient must include a thorough history and physical examination. Comorbidities, such as ventricular dysfunction, renal impairment, cerebrovascular disease, and peripheral arterial disease, must be identified. The chest radiograph and coronary angiograms must be inspected for aortic calcification. Calcification in the aorta that is noted on x-ray or at catheterization should alert the surgeon to the possibility of significant aortic disease.

In the patient who is undergoing redo surgery, the previous operative record must be reviewed, the posteroanterior and lateral chest x-ray inspected, and the angiograms assessed to determine the risk of right ventricular or graft injury on re-entry.

ANESTHESIA

General anesthesia with muscle relaxation and endotracheal intubation is required for procedures that involve cardiopulmonary bypass. Intraoperative monitoring includes multi-lead electrocardiography, continuous arterial pressure monitoring, pulmonary artery catheterization, and transesophageal echocardiography. Patients who undergo these procedures are particularly sensitive to the myocardial and hemodynamic effects of anesthetic agents, and thoughtful induction of anesthesia is required to optimize the myocardial supply-demand ratio, by minimizing myocardial depression and avoiding hypertension and tachycardia. An individualized combination of narcotics, sedatives, and inhalational agents is used to induce and maintain anesthesia. Initiation of cardiopulmonary bypass acutely changes circulating drug concentrations as a result of the dilutional effect of the priming volume. Systemic hypothermia may reduce anesthetic requirements. During the rewarming phase, however, inadequate anesthesia can occur, with the risk of intraoperative awareness. Accordingly, additional intravenous agents are typically administered at these times.

OPERATION

Incision and access

2a In the majority of operations that require cardiopulmonary bypass, access is via the median sternotomy. The actual skin incision may begin inferior to the suprasternal notch to reduce the length of the external scar after surgery.

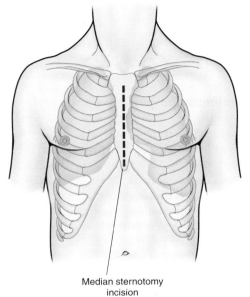

Median sternotomy incision

2a

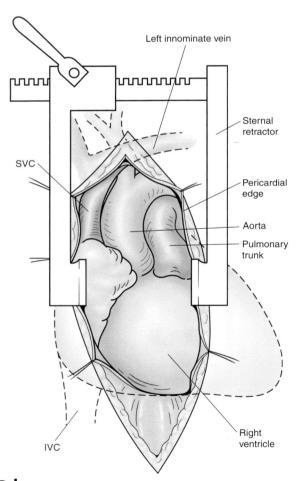

Left innominate vein

Sternal retractor

SVC

Pericardial edge

Aorta

Pulmonary trunk

Right ventricle

IVC

2b

2b After sternal division, a sternal retractor is placed with the ratchet positioned at the upper end of the wound. The pericardium is opened vertically down to its attachment at the diaphragm. The thymic remnant is mobilized by separating its lobes. The inferior aspect of the left innominate vein is visualized. Absence of hypoplasia of this vein indicates the possibility of a persistent left SVC. The short, wide thymic vein and its tributaries may require clipping and division. The pericardium is separated from the diaphragm inferiorly by a transverse incision, avoiding entry into the pleural spaces. Frequently, a pleuropericardial branch of the internal mammary artery is encountered at this point. A pericardial well is created by placement of pericardial retraction sutures. This maneuver allows exposure of the ascending aorta up to the origin of the innominate artery and the right atrium. Gentle digital palpation of the ascending aorta is performed to ascertain the presence of calcification. Inflammation or immobility of the aortic adventitia suggests underlying atherosclerotic disease. If aortic atheromatous disease is suspected, epiaortic echocardiography can be performed to assess the extent, to guide placement of the cannula and aortic clamp, or to confirm the requirement for an alternative cannulation site.

Aortic cannulation pursestrings

3a A satisfactory position for arterial cannulation is usually just proximal and to the left of the innominate artery origin. The region at the immediate base of the innominate artery origin should be avoided, as atheromatous disease frequently occurs at this point. If the ascending aorta is short and/or more room is required below the cannulation site, the pericardium can be mobilized to expose the aortic arch for cannulation. The planned cannulation should be at a site that is accessible for repair should unexpected bleeding occur.

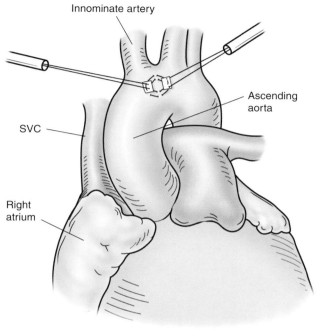

3a

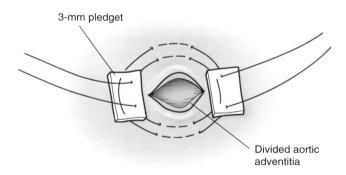

3b

3b Two opposing diamond-shaped pursestrings are placed using two double-armed 3/0 polypropylene sutures, each with a 3-mm Teflon pledget. The depth of the bites should be into the media of the aortic wall, but not full thickness. The size of the pursestring should be one third greater than the diameter of the cannula tip. Division of the adventitia within the pursestring is an important step to allow smooth insertion of the cannula.

Venous cannulation pursestring

4 For operations that do not involve entry into the right heart or exposure of the mitral valve, a single two-stage cavoatrial cannula provides adequate exposure and ease of insertion. A 3/0 polypropylene pursestring suture is placed in the right atrial appendage. The pursestring should be of generous size to accommodate the venous cannula. One should avoid the areas of the appendage that abut the right atrioventricular groove and the sinoatrial junction, as these areas are often thin walled and tear easily, and repair at these sites risks injury to the right coronary artery and sinoatrial node, respectively. Systemic heparinization is achieved by injecting heparin into the right atrium within the atrial pursestring. If retrograde cardioplegia is to be administered, a 4/0 polypropylene pursestring is placed in the anterior aspect of the right atrium for insertion of a coronary sinus cannula. Although desirable, placement of pursestrings is not an essential maneuver before cannulation, and in the emergent situation cannulae can be placed and held in position to initiate bypass, with placement of pursestrings subsequently.

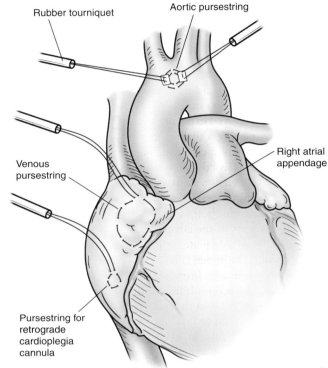

Rubber tourniquet

Aortic pursestring

Venous pursestring

Right atrial appendage

Pursestring for retrograde cardioplegia cannula

4

Arterial cannulation

5a, b The appropriate arterial cannula size depends on the required flow; however, as a general guide, a 24-Fr is suitable for a for a body surface area (BSA) of greater than 2 m^2, a 22-Fr for a BSA of 1.5–2.0 m^2, and a 20-Fr for a BSA of less than 1.5 m^2. Before proceeding with arterial cannulation, one should ensure that the systolic arterial blood pressure is below 100 mm Hg and that an adequate ACT is confirmed. Improved exposure to the cannulation site can be obtained by placing a tonsil forceps on the aortic epicardial fat pad, which is retracted caudally by an assistant. A No. 15 blade scalpel is passed into the aorta to create a transverse incision that is equal to the diameter of the cannula. The cannula is held against the blade of the scalpel, and as the blade is removed, the cannula tip is passed into the aortotomy in a single movement. If the adventitia has been divided and the aortotomy is of adequate length, the cannula should pass smoothly into the lumen (Figure 5a). Under no circumstance should the cannula be inserted with force, as this carries the risk of aortic dissection. If the cannula does not pass easily, it should be removed and the aortotomy gently dilated before reinsertion is attempted. If the cannula cannot be inserted despite this, or if uncontrolled bleeding occurs around the cannula because the aortotomy has extended beyond the pursestring, the cannula can be removed, the pursestrings tied, and a new site selected. Confirmation of the intraluminal position of the cannula is confirmed by the cannula filling with arterial blood and by transducing arterial pressure after connection to the arterial line. Once the cannula is in place, the pursestrings are snugged tight, the cannula is secured to one of the purse- string tourniquets, and the arterial line is connected, ensuring that the line is free of air (Figure 5b).

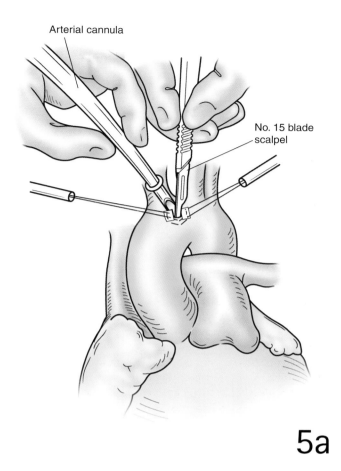

Arterial cannula

No. 15 blade scalpel

5a

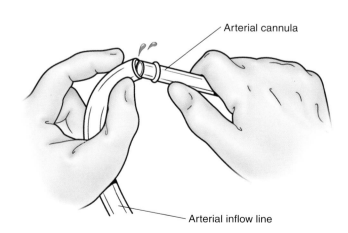

Arterial cannula

Arterial inflow line

5b

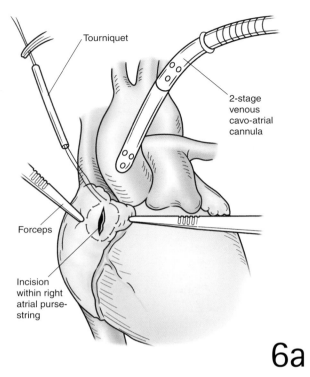

Tourniquet

2-stage
venous
cavo-atrial
cannula

Forceps

Incision
within right
atrial purse-
string

6a

Venous cannulation

6a, b Venous cannulation is performed by opening the atrial appendage within the pursestring with scissors and dividing any obstructing trabeculations within. The cannula is inserted caudally, posteriorly, and slightly laterally and passes into the inferior vena cava (IVC). The pursestring is snugged and the cannula secured with a heavy silk tie. Insertion of the cannula too far caudally can result in passage of the cannula tip into a hepatic vein, with resultant poor venous drainage.

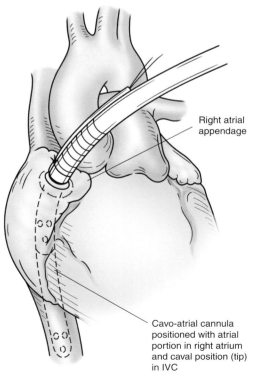

Right atrial
appendage

Cavo-atrial cannula
positioned with atrial
portion in right atrium
and caval position (tip)
in IVC

6b

Coronary sinus cannulation

7 Placement of a retrograde cardioplegic cannula is most easily performed after venous cannulation but before establishment of the bypass. This sequence is recommended because the venous cannula passes in front of the tricuspid valve orifice and into the IVC, so that the only ostium available for the retrograde cannula is the coronary sinus. A gentle curve is created in the cannula, and the balloon is tested before insertion. An incision is made within the pursestring, and the cannula is inserted into the atrium anterior to the venous cavoatrial line. The cannula is then passed into the coronary sinus by advancing the cannula in the line of its curvature with the tip pointing toward the patient's left shoulder. The coronary sinus can be palpated posterior to the IVC to guide its insertion if required. The coronary sinus is a thin-walled structure, and no undue force should be applied on insertion of the cannula. Coronary sinus blood is more deoxygenated than any other venous blood, and effluent of this dark blood from the cannula confirms the position of the cannula. The cannula is deaired, and the cardioplegic and pressure-monitoring lines are connected.

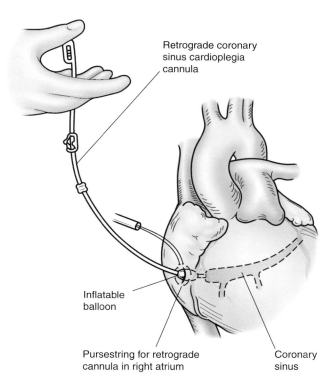

Retrograde coronary sinus cardioplegia cannula

Inflatable balloon

Pursestring for retrograde cannula in right atrium

Coronary sinus

7

Bicaval venous cannulation

8a When entry to the right heart is required, or to optimize exposure in mitral valve surgery, the SVC and IVC are cannulated separately. Right-angled cannulae attach via a Y-connector to the venous line. The pursestring for superior caval cannulation is usually placed in the right atrial appendage; however, it must be placed more posteriorly if the transseptal approach to the mitral valve is used. The inferior caval pursestring is placed in the inferior aspect of the right atrium approximately 2 cm above the cavoatrial junction.

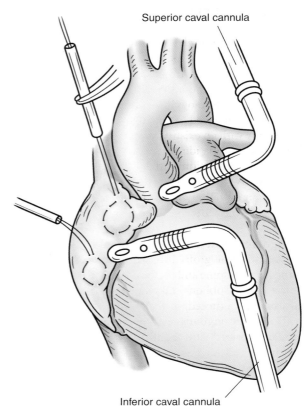

Superior caval cannula

Inferior caval cannula

8a

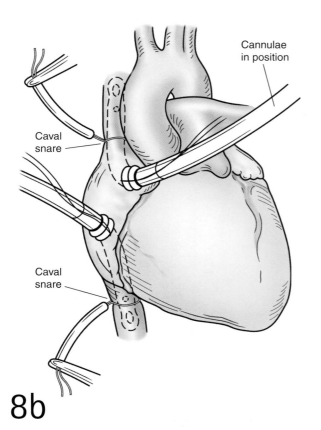

Cannulae in position

Caval snare

Caval snare

8b

8b The superior caval cannula is placed first, as this causes less hemodynamic effect. With retraction on the acute margin of the heart for exposure, the inferior caval cannula can usually be placed without problem; however, if hemodynamic compromise precludes this, the upper cannula can be positioned in the atrium and bypass can be established, allowing safe cannulation of the IVC. The upper cannula is then repositioned into the SVC to provide bicaval drainage.

Caval snares are required if the right atrium is to be opened. The SVC is mobilized by dividing the pericardial reflection superiorly and laterally. Electrocautery should be avoided laterally to prevent injury to the adjacent right phrenic nerve. The medial side of the SVC is mobilized until the right pulmonary artery is visualized. Mobilization of the IVC is performed easily by dividing the thin pericardial reflection between the right inferior pulmonary vein and the IVC.

Femoral vessel cannulation

Arterial flow via the femoral artery can be used when cannulation of the aorta is not possible (e.g. ascending aortic aneurysm or dissection), when the operative incision does not allow exposure to the aorta (e.g. left thoracotomy for descending aortic pathology), or when cardiopulmonary bypass is to be commenced before high-risk sternotomy (e.g. redo sternotomy with an existing ascending aortic graft). The femoral artery is not the ideal site when the aorta cannot be used because of calcification. These patients frequently have associated extensive descending aortic atheroma with the risk of retrograde embolization to the arch vessels.

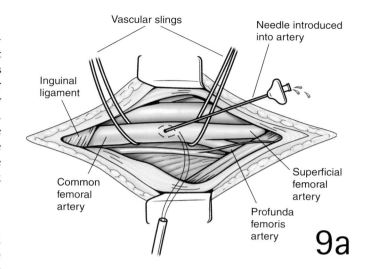

9a Exposure of the common femoral artery is achieved via a vertical groin incision midway between the anterosuperior iliac spine and the symphysis pubis. The lower fibers of the external oblique muscle that form the roof of the inguinal canal are exposed, and the artery is exposed as it emerges below the inguinal ligament. The superficial and deep femoral arteries do not usually require exposure.

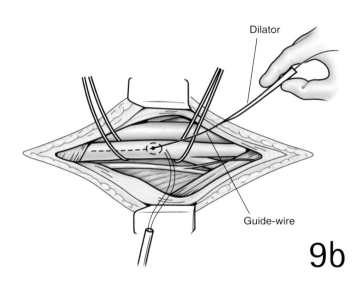

9b, c Tapered arterial cannulae are available, which can be inserted using an 'over-wire' Seldinger technique. A diamond-shaped pursestring is placed in the anterior aspect of the common femoral artery. The artery is cannulated with a needle through which is passed a guide-wire. The needle and dilators are removed and eventually the cannula are inserted over the wire. In adults, an 18-Fr or 20-Fr cannulae can usually be placed that can provide adequate flow. This technique allows for easy removal of the cannula without the need for formal repair of the arteriotomy after decannulation. However, in patients with aortic dissection that extends into the femoral vessels, it is important to perform a transverse arteriotomy with direct visualization and cannulation of the true lumen to prevent malperfusion from inadvertent false lumen cannulation.

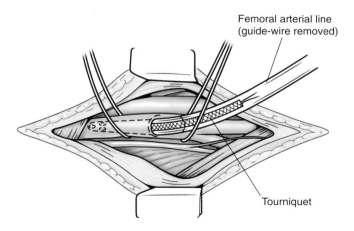

9d The femoral vein can be used for venous cannulation to establish bypass in the setting of right ventricular injury during redo sternotomy or when the right atrium and cavae are not in the operating field (e.g. left thoracotomy). The cannula is placed using a Seldinger technique and is passed via femoral access into the right atrium under transesophageal echocardiographic guidance. The right femoral vein is used preferentially if possible, as it facilitates easier advancement of the cannula through the pelvic vessels into the IVC.

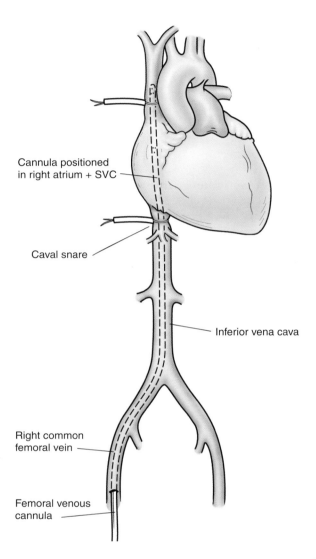

Cannula positioned in right atrium + SVC

Caval snare

Inferior vena cava

Right common femoral vein

Femoral venous cannula

9d

Axillary artery cannulation

10a–d The axillary artery can be accessed via an infraclavicular incision for cannulation. It is usually free of atheromatous disease and, therefore, is used when calcification precludes aortic cannulation. In patients in whom this is suspected, the infraclavicular region should be included in the operative field. A transverse incision is made 2 cm inferior to the middle third of the clavicle. The clavicular and sternal heads of pectoralis major are separated and the clavipectoral fascia divided. The axillary vein is encountered first and is retracted superiorly to expose the first part of the axillary artery, which is mobilized and can be cannulated by the Seldinger technique. The operative approach to the patient with extensive ascending aortic calcification may involve a combination of axillary cannulation and either hypothermic fibrillatory arrest or deep hypothermic circulatory arrest to avoid cross-clamping the aorta.

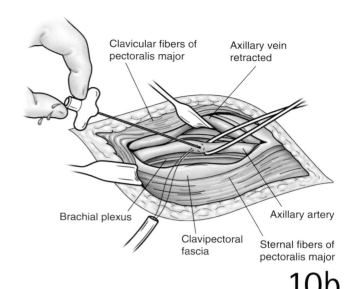

10b

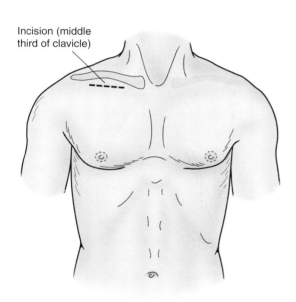

10a

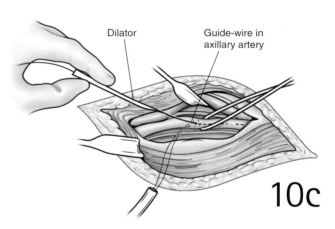

10c

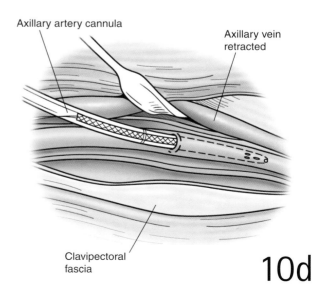

10d

Cannulation via right anterolateral thoracotomy

11a–c In selected, high-risk, redo mitral or tricuspid valve operations, access may be achieved via a right anterolateral thoracotomy. Double-lumen endotracheal intubation is preferred, and the patient is positioned with the right side elevated 30 degrees. A submammary incision is performed from the lateral aspect of the sternum to the midaxillary line, and the chest is entered through the fifth intercostal space. The pericardium is opened anterior to the phrenic nerve, and pericardial adhesions are divided to allow access to right and left atria and to both cavae for bicaval cannulation. The ascending aorta can be accessed through this incision, or an alternative site (femoral or axillary artery) can be used. Procedures on the tricuspid valve can be performed on bypass without cardiac arrest. Mitral valve procedures require cardioplegic arrest if the aorta is accessible for clamping or fibrillatory arrest if the aorta cannot be clamped.

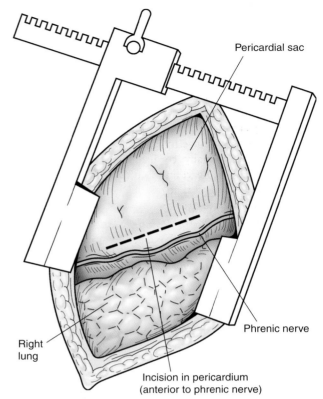

Pericardial sac

Phrenic nerve

Right lung

Incision in pericardium (anterior to phrenic nerve)

11b

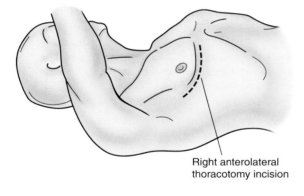

Right anterolateral thoracotomy incision

11a

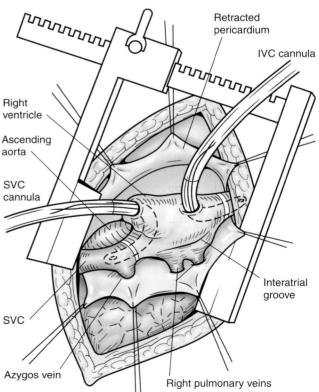

Retracted pericardium

IVC cannula

Right ventricle

Ascending aorta

SVC cannula

SVC

Azygos vein

Interatrial groove

Right pulmonary veins

11c

Initiation of bypass

Cardiopulmonary bypass is commenced at the discretion of the surgeon. The perfusionist begins arterial inflow and ensures satisfactory flow and line pressure. The pressure gradient across the arterial cannula should not exceed 100 mm Hg. Gradients above this suggest malposition, aortic dissection, or inadequate cannula size. If the flow and pressure are satisfactory, the clamp on the venous line is released to allow venous drainage into the circuit by siphonage. The surgeon should visually confirm that dark deoxygenated blood is leaving the heart and oxygenated blood is returning to the arterial line and that the heart rapidly decompresses. Initial perfusion pressures are frequently low due to hemodilution and the vasoactive response to exposure of blood to foreign surfaces. If pressures are low, administration of a vasopressor may be required. Peripheral resistance usually increases gradually as bypass progresses as a result of catecholamine release.

Separation from bypass

Once the requirement for cardiopulmonary bypass is completed, the aim is to allow the transition from supported circulation to native circulation. Before weaning from bypass, the following requirements must be ensured: normothermia, a satisfactory electrocardiographic trace with a stable rhythm and adequate heart rate, adequate myocardial function for weaning, surgical anastomotic hemostasis, normal acid-base and electrolyte status, and satisfactory deairing of the heart and aortic root. If present, the left ventricular vent and retrograde cannula are removed. The lungs are reinflated with valsalva and full ventilation is commenced. Inotropes, if required, are commenced at the determined dose. An intravenous calcium bolus is an excellent inotropic agent in this setting and is administered immediately before separation.

Partial occlusion of the venous line with resultant filling of the right atrium allows the heart to begin ejecting. It is imperative that distention of the heart be avoided at this time. On instruction of the surgeon, the venous line is clamped, and bypass is ceased. The venous line is removed and the pursestring tightened but not tied in the event that bypass needs to be recommenced. The surgeon observes myocardial contractility and volume status of the heart. Frequently, judicious increments of volume are required via the arterial line to optimize preload. The diastolic pulmonary artery pressure and transesophageal echocardiography also provide a guide to ventricular preload. Once hemodynamic stability is confirmed, a test dose of protamine is administered before the arterial cannula is removed. Protamine is continued to the required dose once decannulation has been performed.

POSTOPERATIVE CARE

Initial postoperative care is in an intensive care setting, and monitoring includes continuous electrocardiography, invasive arterial pressure, urine output, drain losses, blood gas measurement, pulmonary artery pressures, and cardiac indices. Most patients return to the postoperative unit intubated until they have demonstrated a period of hemodynamic stability, normothermia, hemostasis, and return of adequate neuromuscular function. Several postoperative issues are unique to patients who are undergoing cardiovascular procedures with the use of cardiopulmonary bypass. Extracorporeal circulation causes activation of platelets, the coagulation pathway, and the fibrinolytic cascade, with resultant coagulopathy. Hypothermia contributes further to the bleeding diathesis. Drain tube losses are monitored, and coagulopathic bleeding is treated as required with administration of platelets, fresh frozen plasma, and cryoprecipitate. External heating lights and blankets and warmed inspired gases are used to achieve normothermia. Cardiac tamponade should be suspected in the patient with features of low cardiac output, raised venous pressures, and high drain losses. Of particular concern is the patient who has large drain losses followed by a dramatic decrease in drainage (due to clot obstruction of the drain tubes). Oliguria is frequently an early sign of developing tamponade. Treatment is by surgical evacuation of pericardial blood and correction of the cause of bleeding.

Patients require a varying degree of cardiovascular support in the early postoperative period, ranging from inotrope infusions to intra-aortic balloon counterpulsation to mechanical ventricular assist devices on occasion. Cardiopulmonary bypass also stimulates the inflammatory pathway, and a systemic inflammatory response is seen to a variable degree. This may require peripheral vasopressor support. Rhythm disturbances are frequently seen in the early postoperative period. Patients who are at risk of bradyarrhythmias have epicardial pacing wires placed intraoperatively. Serum electrolytes, particularly potassium and magnesium, are monitored and replaced accordingly. Tachyarrhythmias are treated pharmacologically or with electrical cardioversion, depending on their morphology and hemodynamic effects.

FURTHER READING

Gravlee, G.P., Davis, R.F., Utley, J.R. (eds.). 1993: *Cardiopulmonary bypass – principles and practice*. Baltimore: Williams & Wilkins.

Mora, C.T. (ed.). 1995: *Cardiopulmonary bypass – principles and techniques of extracorporeal circulation*. New York: Springer-Verlag.

Nolan, S.P., Zacour, R. 1998: Cardiopulmonary bypass. In Kaiser, L.R., Kron, I.L., Spray, T.L. (eds.), *Mastery of cardiothoracic surgery*. Philadelphia: Lippincott–Raven, 277–86.

In addition to the effects of the plasma defense proteins and cytokines that circulate in the blood, the physical forces of the blood flow can have an impact on endothelial function. In many circumstances, blood that circulates during CPB is delivered at a constant pressure, with little pulsatile variation. Because this situation is nonphysiological, investigators have questioned the effects of pulseless perfusion on end-organ function. A growing body of literature implicates the endothelium in the pathological response to pulseless blood flow. Endothelial cells are uniquely situated to serve as the primary transducer of hemodynamically imposed mechanical events. In particular, evidence suggests that endothelial cells serve as mechanoreceptors, by which changes in blood flow or shear stress are recognized by the endothelial cellular membranes and signals are transmitted to intracellular organelles. At the cellular level, when endothelial cells are exposed to varying degrees of shear, they undergo changes. These changes include shape redistribution of the cytoskeleton and organelles, proliferation, expression of adhesion molecules, as well as the production of matrix proteins, release of growth factors, and vasoactive substances. All of these factors can contribute to a dysfunctional, activated endothelial cell layer that promotes vasoconstriction, neutrophil adhesion, and increased microvascular thrombogenicity.

Neutrophil-mediated end-organ destruction

2 Once the endothelium is activated, neutrophils are recruited from the circulation. Activated neutrophils have the ability to impair microcirculatory function by altering endothelial permeability, by causing leukocyte capillary plugging, by releasing vasoactive products, and by causing capillary deformation and compression due to oxygen radical-mediated interstitial edema and cell dysfunction. The process of neutrophil-mediated injury of endothelial cells involves a complex sequence of adhesive events in which products from both cell types affect the cytotoxic outcome. Understanding this sequence of events is necessary to assess potential therapeutic strategies to block this response.

When the endothelial cells become activated by circulating C5a, bradykinin, thrombin, hypoxia, or cytokines, the normally quiescent endothelium expresses neutrophil adhesion molecules, such as the selectins and the integrins. When this process occurs, circulating neutrophils are initially tethered by the selectins, then become firmly adherent to the endothelium by attaching to endothelial-based adhesion molecules such as ICAM. P-selectin, which is expressed in response to hypoxia, C5a, or thrombin, mediates this response in the early immediate phase. E-selectin, which requires transcriptional up-regulation and *de novo* protein synthesis, mediates this response over the subsequent 24 hours. The integrin PECAM, which is found on neutrophils and between the endothelial cells, facilitates passage of the neutrophils between the cell gaps and into the tissue. PECAM is involved in diapedesis and in the subsequent step of migration across the basal lamina. Once neutrophils adhere to and ultimately pass through the endothelium, they are poised to release damaging proteases, elastases, and oxygen-derived free radicals. Assays for byproducts of lipid peroxidation and phospholipid-esterified diene conjugation demonstrate the effects of neutrophil-mediated cell injury in CPB patients. This process is in part regulated by the chemotactic factors, such as C5a, PAF, and interleukin-8, which activate neutrophils to release free radicals and proteases. This process further disrupts endothelial cell barrier function, leading to interstitial fluid accumulation and vasomotor changes. The combination of the inappropriate release of neutrophil proteases and oxygen-derived free radicals damages cell membranes and ultimately has an impact on end-organ function. Furthermore, free radicals play a role in a variety of normal molecular regulatory systems, the dysregulation of which can contribute further to tissue damage.

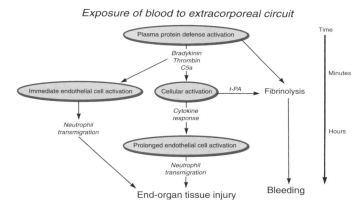

Exposure of blood to extracorporeal circuit

2

CLINICAL MANIFESTATIONS OF THE WHOLE BODY INFLAMMATORY RESPONSE

3 Ultimately, this generalized activation of the plasma protein defense systems and the subsequent endothelial and neutrophil responses with exposure to CPB may result in substantial tissue injury. The inflammatory response to CPB often occurs at subclinical levels. Because of the heterogeneity of individual responses to injury, and the varying degree of chronic organ dysfunction before heart surgery, major organ dysfunction and failure may occur. The extent of injury can be impacted by a number of related features, such as the length of the bypass run, the type of circuitry used, the ischemic time, and especially the use of deep hypothermic circulatory arrest. In most patients, the extent of the inflammatory response to CPB increases significantly as the perfusion time extends beyond 3 hours, and it sharply increases further after 4 hours on CPB. Additionally, patients who come to surgery in shock or experience significant periods of hypoperfusion during and after CPB experience greater injury. Although a few patients may demonstrate a predominant impairment of a single organ system, some degree of impaired organ function can be found in nearly all the body's physiological systems when hypoperfusion and its attendant responses occur.

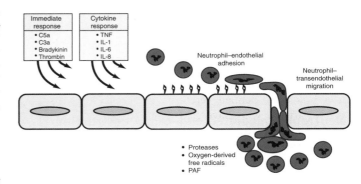

3

Interstitial edema

At the whole body level, one of the most immediate indicators that a patient has experienced the inflammatory consequences of CPB is reflected in the degree of whole body edema and weight gain in the early perioperative period. Interstitial fluid loss results from the development of intercellular gap formation and vascular permeability, both cardinal features of inflammation. The hallmark of this syndrome is peripheral vasodilatation, which is associated with a breakdown of capillary membranes and the accumulation of excess interstitial fluid. This situation results in increased vascular leakage. As capillary permeability increases, interstitial fluid is retained, and function of essentially every organ is temporarily impaired.

Pulmonary dysfunction

Acute postoperative pulmonary dysfunction is one of the most noticeable common effects of CPB. Acute lung injury after CPB can be documented by measuring the alveolar-arterial oxygenation gradient, intrapulmonary shunt, degree of pulmonary edema, pulmonary compliance, and pulmonary vascular resistance. Pulmonary hypertension and lung injury secondary to CPB are worsened by this generalized inflammatory response and may be exacerbated by lung ischemia, which can occur when the lungs are not ventilated during full

CPB. Investigators have examined pulmonary injury in the setting of full CPB, with and without interruption of pulmonary artery blood flow, and found that, although exposure to CPB alone is enough to cause pulmonary injury, cessation of pulmonary blood flow during CPB contributes significantly to this pulmonary dysfunction.

Clinically, this problem is manifested as increased time to extubation early after surgery. Prolonged mechanical ventilation early after surgery increases the incidence of pulmonary complications such as pneumonia. If significant pulmonary dysfunction develops and the patient remains ventilated for more than a few days, expected mortality increases significantly.

Renal dysfunction

In addition to pulmonary dysfunction, a measurable reduction in renal function occurs in a number of patients after CPB. *Renal dysfunction* can be defined as a peak postoperative serum creatinine value that exceeds the preoperative value by 50 per cent or more or a need for dialysis. Acute renal insufficiency or renal failure complicates up to 15 per cent of CPB procedures, with roughly 2 per cent of patients requiring dialysis. Acute renal failure recently has been independently associated with postoperative mortality. In addition to the generalized inflammatory changes that result from CPB, and that may affect the kidneys, the generation of free hemoglobin during CPB can result in increased delivery of toxic-free iron to the renal endothelium and tubular epithelium, providing a major pathway for the induction of post-CPB renal failure.

Neurological injury

Neurological complications can be the most devastating consequences of CPB, in the short and the long term. The reported frequency of stroke ranges from 0.8 per cent to 5.0 per cent in various series. When a stroke does occur, predicted mortality may be as high as 20 per cent. In addition to clearly defined cerebrovascular events or strokes, some patients who have had heart surgery experience a spectrum of neurocognitive changes in the early postoperative period that can have a significant impact on recovery times and even mortality. The incidence of cognitive impairment or delirium is as great as 50 per cent in the first week. Among the reported neurocognitive deficits is memory loss, which may persist and be manifested as difficulty with following directions or performing calculations. Another common finding is depression, especially in the intermediate post-CPB period.

The mechanisms for brain injury with CPB include reduced cerebral blood flow, embolic events, and the systemic inflammatory response to CPB. Although most overt neurological events after CPB, such as emboli, can be attributed to mechanical causes, the effect of intracerebral swelling within the closed cranial vault may be responsible for many of the more subtle neurological events.

Bleeding complications

Abnormal coagulation function is one of the most common hallmarks of heart surgery performed with CPB. An overall tendency to bleed excessively occurs immediately postoperatively, with a later tendency for abnormal thrombosis.

The complexity of the coagulation dysfunction after CPB results from the technical variations in the operative procedures and the many uncontrolled variables that are associated with CPB, including the effects of anesthetic or pharmacological agents, the nature of the priming solution, hemodilution, hypothermia, the type of oxygenator, and the use of transfused blood products. Considerable overlap exists in the inflammatory cascades, coagulation, and fibrinolysis, all of which are activated on CPB and contribute to bleeding in the perioperative period. The impact of bleeding on the overall inflammatory response is most recognizable in the patients who require reoperation for bleeding. In a retrospective analysis of 6 000 patients who require CPB, re-exploration for bleeding was examined as a risk factor for death and complications. The overall incidence of re-exploration was 4.2 per cent and was identified as a strong independent risk factor for operative mortality, renal failure, prolonged mechanical ventilation, adult respiratory distress syndrome, sepsis, and atrial arrhythmias.

THERAPEUTIC APPROACHES

A number of strategies have been developed to limit the generalized inflammatory and systemic effects of CPB. These can be divided into the mechanical, pharmacological, and now computer-aided solutions. Determining the optimal ways to incorporate such strategies into clinical practice may be one of the principal challenges that face heart surgeons in the coming years.

Hypothermia

Active cooling is a strategy that has long been used with apparent success for protecting the patient from systemic injury during CPB. Hypothermic CPB attenuates the intensity of the inflammatory response, as demonstrated by reduced cytokine and elastase production and delayed expression of neutrophil adhesion molecules when compared to normothermic CPB. Most of the protective anti-inflammatory effects of hypothermia are lost, however, during rewarming in the post-CPB period. Hypothermia appears to delay, but does not prevent, endothelial cell activation.

Furthermore, systemic hypothermia can be detrimental. Hypothermia has been shown to impair the activity of the enzymes that are involved in the platelet activation pathways and to reduce the enzymatic activity of clotting factors upon coagulation activation.

Alternative filtering methods

Methods of ultrafiltration and modified ultrafiltration are currently being evaluated in a number of centers as a means of hemoconcentrating patients and potentially removing water from the tissues. Hemofiltration uses the convection process to remove water and some low-molecular-weight substances from plasma under a hydrostatic pressure gradient. Initially, hemofiltration was intended to correct the accumulation of extravascular water during or immediately after CPB; however, several of its side effects appeared to be useful, such as the reduction of postoperative blood loss and immediate improvement in hemodynamics. Conventional methods proved inconsistent; thus, the technique was modified to ultrafilter the patients immediately after cessation of bypass. Additionally, modified ultrafiltration has been found to remove inflammatory mediators such as cytokines from the circulation after CPB. Currently, the effects of modified hemofiltration on mediators of tissue injury are still unclear.

The mechanical removal of leukocytes is possible with the aid of specialized filters that are placed in the CPB circuit.

Experimentally, the mechanical removal of circulating neutrophils from the perfusate by filtration produces a leukopenia that can persist for 8–12 hours after bypass. Leukocyte-depleted animals have less leukocyte sequestration in the lung than do control animals. Less evidence of white cell activation has been found. These differences result in significantly improved pulmonary gas exchange in the post-bypass period.

Heparin–bonded circuits

Heparin coating of the CPB circuitry has been proposed as a technique to reduce the need for heparin as well as the bleeding and the inflammatory complications of CPB. Heparin coating of the extracorporeal circuit not only reduces heparin requirements during cardiac operations but also may reduce organ injury that is associated with CPB. Investigators have demonstrated that heparin-bonded CPB circuits combined with a lower anticoagulation protocol as an adjunct to an integrated blood conservation strategy decrease the incidence and magnitude of transfusion and improve clinical outcomes by reducing the duration of assisted ventilation and surgical intensive care unit and hospital stays. In most such studies, the benefits correlate with a reduction in plasma protein defense activation, monocyte TF expression, and cytokine responses.

Minimally invasive techniques

Recently, considerable effort has been made to avoid the effects of CPB altogether by performing heart surgery without the use of CPB. Mounting evidence suggests that this approach can significantly reduce the inflammatory effects. To date, however, a randomized trial with comparable groups has not been performed; and thus, it is difficult to determine what effect patient selection has on the observed differences in inflammatory response.

Pharmacological methods

STEROIDS

In addition to the mechanical methods of reducing CPB-induced inflammation, a number of pharmacological approaches exist. The classic approach to blunt the inflammatory reaction to CPB is to administer steroids before or during the procedure. This approach derives from the hypothesis that, because CPB has systemic inflammatory effects and steroids are an anti-inflammatory, they must be useful in preventing some of the harmful effects of CPB. In the last decade, however, this logic has been complicated by the finding that steroids have not been shown to benefit patients in a number of carefully designed, large, multi-institutional randomized prospective studies that evaluate the systemic inflammatory response to injury, acute respiratory distress syndrome, and sepsis. Because steroids may not be

beneficial in these disease states in which similar cytokine-mediated whole body injury patterns are present, these drugs may not be of benefit in the milder post-CPB setting. Also unanswered is the question of whether steroids can be harmful when administered in the setting of CPB. Therefore, even though steroids have been evaluated in heart surgery patients in a number of studies, to date the putative benefits from the use of steroids in the setting of CPB are still unproven.

APROTININ

Aprotinin is a polypeptide serine protease inhibitor isolated from bovine lung that inhibits multiple proteases, including trypsin, chymotrypsin, plasmin, tissue plasminogen activator, serum urokinase plasminogen activator, and tissue and plasma kallikreins. Aprotinin has been shown to reduce blood loss and transfusion requirements in patients who have undergone heart surgery. Full-dose aprotinin significantly reduces postoperative blood loss compared with amino caproic acid and desmopressin and decreases transfusion requirements compared with desmopressin.

Additionally, aprotinin may have a significant impact on the degree of inflammation that is seen in CPB patients. Multiple mechanisms appear to be responsible for this observed effect. Experimentally, during simulated CPB, aprotinin immediately inhibits kallikrein and thrombin formation via the intrinsic coagulation pathway. Later, aprotinin inhibits monocyte expression of TF and the extrinsic coagulation pathway. With aprotinin the cytokine response is blunted. Aprotinin-treated patients also have a significant reduction in markers of neutrophil activation. The usual increases of soluble P-selectin in the plasma, platelet surface P-selectin, and leukocyte-platelet conjugates are less in aprotinin-treated patients. In other studies, complement expression is significantly increased on neutrophils after the onset of CPB in the placebo groups but not in the aprotinin-treated patients. Using intravital microscopy, aprotinin does not affect the adhesion of activated neutrophils to the endothelium but significantly inhibits extravasation of leukocytes into surrounding tissues. Aprotinin-treated patients have a significantly reduced elastase level, suggesting that they may have reduced neutrophil-mediated injury. Anti-inflammatory cytokines, such as interleukin-10, appear to be increased in aprotinin-treated patients.

ANTICOMPLEMENT STRATEGIES

An area of great interest recently has been pharmacological prevention of complement activation. Attempts to inhibit complement efficiently include the application of endogenous soluble complement inhibitors (C1 inhibitor, recombinant soluble complement receptor 1 - rsCR1) and the administration of antibodies, either blocking key proteins of the cascade reaction (e.g., C3, C5), neutralizing the action of the complement-derived anaphylatoxin C5a, or interfering with complement receptor 3-mediated adhesion of inflammatory cells to the vascular endothelium.

ANTINEUTROPHIL STRATEGIES

Inhibiting neutrophil adhesive function is an additional technique that may limit the detrimental effects of CPB. The use of monoclonal antibodies to prevent or to interfere with neutrophil adherence to the activated endothelium has been investigated. The effect of a specific monoclonal antibody that affects neutrophil adherence was evaluated in a primate model of CPB and deep hypothermic arrest, using fluid retention as the test parameter. Significantly less fluid was required by animals that were treated with the monoclonal antibody, and correspondingly less weight gain occurred in treated animals. These findings indicate that some manifestations of the systemic inflammatory response may be prevented by blocking the ability of neutrophils to bind to activated endothelium. This approach may be particularly helpful in the setting of heart surgery, where the inflammatory response to CPB is often accompanied by significant ischemia-reperfusion injury.

Other studies have demonstrated that inhibition of neutrophil–endothelial cell binding preserves pulmonary function in animals after CPB. A number of agents that inhibit neutrophil adhesion are now being evaluated in clinical trials in patients with myocardial infarction and adult respiratory distress syndrome and perhaps soon may be used in clinical trials of patients who are undergoing CPB.

Preventing endothelial cell activation

In the future methods may be developed for the prospective prevention of endothelial cell activation pharmacologically. A basic paradigm in endothelial cell biology is that there are genomic responses to specific extracellular signals that result in the transcriptional activation of genes that are not transcribed under normal conditions. In the case of endothelial cell activation, these are the genes that encode for the proteins and that contribute to cytokine release, neutrophil recruitment, and ultimately organ dysfunction in the setting of CPB. In the past decade, much has been published detailing the biology of signal transduction cascades in response to stressful stimuli. In general, extracellular signals bind highly specific receptors on the cell plasma membrane, and this ligand-receptor interaction triggers a cascade of kinases and sequential phosphorylation events that transduces the signal to the nucleus. Depending on the signal and the signaling pathways that are activated, an array of transcription factors are induced that bind to unique DNA sequences and promote transcription.

Computer solutions

Traditionally, determining the flow rates and oxygen content during extracorporeal circulation was more of an art than a science, with the perfusionists making adjustments based on a number of changing variables. For example, to determine the blood gas content and the venous saturation of the returning venous blood, the perfusionist must withdraw blood from the circuit (usually 3–5 mL at a time), place the blood sample on ice, and send it to the laboratory for analysis. The sample is run; then a report is generated and brought back to the perfusionist, who reads and interprets it and makes a decision. This process can take 5–15 minutes even in the best systems. Occasionally, conditions have changed by the time that the test data are available, and subsequent samples must be sent again for analysis. This current system, characterized by inadequate or delayed data access, makes it at times difficult for the perfusionist to achieve a steady state.

A number of groups are working on the provision of continuous availability of physiological data, using on-line and off-line sensing, as well as the computer-assisted closed-loop control of flow rates and oxygen content. Refining this loop by using emerging sensing devices and computer applications may allow the more precise control of extracorporeal circulation and thus a reduced inflammatory impact on the patient.

CONCLUSION

Despite numerous advances in the techniques, technology, and understanding of extracorporeal cardiopulmonary support, the potential for morbidity and mortality still exists when the patient's circulation is artificially supported by CPB. In the last decade, a great deal has been done to characterize the specific inflammatory responses that occur when a patient is placed on CPB. Understanding this response will lead to new techniques and approaches to control it, ultimately making CPB safer and more efficacious.

FURTHER READING

Edmunds, L.H. Jr. 1993. Blood-surface interactions during cardiopulmonary bypass. *Journal of Cardiac Surgery* 8, 404–10.

Hill, C.S., Treisman, R. 1994. Transcriptional regulation by extracellular signals: mechanisms and specificity. *Cell* 80, 199–211.

Pober, J.S., Cotran, R.S. 1990. Cytokines and endothelial cell biology. *Immunological Reviews* 76, 427–48.

Pohlman, T.H., Boyle, E.M. 1996. The host response to injury and infection. In Civetta, J.M., Taylor, R.W., Kirby, R.R. (eds), *Critical care* 3rd edition. Philadelphia: J.B. Lippincott Company, 291–301.

Royston, D. 1996. Preventing the inflammatory response to open-heart surgery: the role of aprotinin and other protease inhibitors. *International Journal of Cardiology* 53(Suppl.), S11–37.

Taylor, K.M. 1998. Brain damage during cardiopulmonary bypass. *Annals of Thoracic Surgery* 65(4 Suppl.), S20–6; discussion: S27–8.

Circulatory arrest

ROBERT STUART BONSER FRCP, FRCS
Honorary Senior Lecturer of Surgery, University of Birmingham School of Medicine; Consultant Surgeon, Cardiothoracic Surgical Unit, Queen Elizabeth Hospital, Birmingham, UK

HISTORY

Work by Bigelow in 1950 introduced the concept that whole-body hypothermia could be used to facilitate cardiac surgery. Cooling would slow metabolism and increase ischemic tolerance, thereby allowing the brain to withstand increasing periods of interrupted blood supply while intracardiac repairs were performed. Early experience with surface cooling was encouraging and was later supplemented by the use of cardiopulmonary bypass to core-cool patients to profoundly hypothermic temperatures before initiating a period of circulatory arrest. In the 1960s, Barnard, Borst, and Lillehei each reported clinical cases in which the technique had been used for the management of aortic arch pathology. In 1975, Griepp demonstrated that the technique offered a simple and relatively safe approach for aortic arch repair. Since that time, profound hypothermia and circulatory arrest have been the main technique used to afford brain protection in aortic arch surgery. Other techniques are also available which may supplement or substitute for circulatory arrest. These include retrograde cerebral perfusion (RCP) and selective arterial cerebral perfusion (SACP). The relative efficacy of these techniques in the clinical situation is now being evaluated.

PRINCIPLES AND JUSTIFICATION

Profound hypothermia and circulatory arrest with or without RCP is a method of brain protection during operations on the aortic arch for aneurysm or dissection. This technique avoids the need for extensive manipulation and clamping of the innominate and carotid arteries, reducing the risk of vessel injury and embolism from atheromatous plaques. This method also allows meticulous operative repair in a blood-free field. Hypothermia and circulatory arrest is specifically useful in the management of acute proximal aortic dissection when reapposition of the dissected layers of the aortic arch is necessary with construction of an open distal anastomosis.

SACP is an alternative technique of brain protection in these cases and has the theoretical advantages of improving brain protection by avoiding the period of cold ischemia of the circulatory arrest period and producing less whole-body hypothermia, which may facilitate recovery.

Circulatory arrest is also commonly used in infants undergoing surgery for complex congenital heart disease. In adults, it has been used in the management of certain intracranial aneurysms and other vascular lesions as well as in the management of renal tumors with extensive invasion of the inferior vena cava.

As circulatory arrest is a period of global central nervous system ischemia, it is not surprising that the principal complication in operations using this technique is neurological injury. The incidence of stroke is approximately two-and-a-half times higher than conventional cardiopulmonary bypass procedures, and more subtle injury, manifest by transient disturbances of consciousness perioperatively or later neuropsychological change, is disturbingly common. The use of profound hypothermia also increases the coagulopathy associated with cardiopulmonary bypass, and the rate of bleeding complications and other morbid sequelae is relatively high. Although circulatory arrest is most commonly used in emergency life-saving surgery, the risk/benefit analysis of its elective use must take into account the higher risks.

PREOPERATIVE ASSESSMENT

Assessment is similar to other cases requiring major cardiac surgery. If carotid artery manipulation or cannulation for SACP is to be considered, preoperative assessment should include ultrasound investigation of the carotid arteries to identify atheromatous plaques and hemodynamically significant stenoses. The cerebral arterial circulation should also be interrogated by transcranial Doppler studies to ensure that the Circle of Willis is intact and to predict that transient occlusion of the vertebrobasilar system is likely to be tolerated.

ANESTHESIA AND SPECIAL CONSIDERATIONS

Monitoring

1 Standard arterial, central venous, and pulmonary artery catheter access and monitoring are required for circulatory arrest procedures. Venous lines are placed from the right side to anticipate the possible division of the innominate vein to improve surgical access. In the presence of aortic dissection, arterial pressure monitoring should be at two sites, proximal and distal to the aortic arch so that the surgeon can observe any pressure differential occurring when bypass is initiated, when the aorta is clamped, or when bypass is reinstituted post-arrest. Such pressure differentials may be an indication of arch malperfusion, and detection may allow corrective action.

A further venous monitoring line advanced from the neck to the jugular bulb is also useful for cerebral venous saturation monitoring and inflow pressure measurement during retrograde venous perfusion. Transcranial Doppler monitoring of middle cerebral artery velocity and near-infrared spectroscopy may give additional information but are optional. Temperature monitoring lines are placed in the esophagus and nasopharynx. Where available, continuous electro-encephalography should be used. After line insertion, autologous blood drawn from the indwelling lines is predonated to facilitate hemodilution during cardiopulmonary bypass and to aid post-bypass hemostasis.

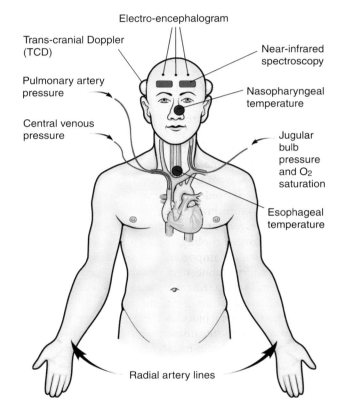

Electro-encephalogram

Trans-cranial Doppler (TCD)

Near-infrared spectroscopy

Pulmonary artery pressure

Nasopharyngeal temperature

Central venous pressure

Jugular bulb pressure and O$_2$ saturation

Esophageal temperature

Radial artery lines

1

ANESTHETIC TECHNIQUES

Anesthetic technique is not materially different than other major heart surgery, and we routinely use a combination of opiate- and propofol-based sedation after induction. Such agents reduce cerebral metabolism, but do not uncouple flow-metabolism relationships and, thereby, reduce cerebral blood flow. We do not routinely use volatile anesthetics. Drug dosages are halved at 22°C. Before circulatory arrest, patients are pretreated with 1 g/kg mannitol. We also administer dexamethasone, but we no longer use thiopentone. Anesthetic drug infusions are discontinued during the arrest period.

Acid–base management

During cooling, a number of metabolic and physicochemical changes occur that affect patient management. The dissociation constant of water rises, leading to a reduction in H$^+$ concentration and increasing pH. Simultaneously, the dissociation constant of the imidazole moiety of histidine in hemoglobin also rises in parallel. The net effect is that blood becomes more alkaline, and the affinity of hemoglobin for oxygen increases. If pH is to be maintained, additional acid in the form of CO_2 is needed. This manipulation of blood pH to combat the alkalinizing effect of cooling is termed *pH-stat acid–base management*. The alternative strategy of allowing pH to rise during cooling represents *α-stat management*. These strategies are important, as they may affect cerebral blood flow and metabolism during cooling and rewarming. During α-stat management, cerebral blood flow remains coupled to metabolism by autoregulation. With pH-stat management, cerebral blood flow becomes dependent mainly on perfusion pressure, uncoupled from metabolism. At a given temperature, brain metabolism may be greater with α-stat management. Increased cerebral blood flow with pH management may improve the rate and homogeneity of cooling, but may conversely expose the brain to a greater embolic load. Nevertheless, there is some evidence of advantage with the pH-stat regime in infant cardiac surgery. Currently, α-stat pH management is used in most adult centers.

OPERATION

Operative details are described in chapters 30–32, but certain points are relevant.

- In cases of acute type A dissection, initial femoral arterial cannulation is necessary. Arterial return is transferred to the prosthetic graft after circulatory arrest to ensure orthograde true luminal flow and prevent pressurization of the false lumen via re-entry tears during persistent distal arterial perfusion.
- In degenerative aneurysms, femoral cannulation, if possible, should be avoided to reduce the risk of athero-embolism during this reversal of arterial flow direction. Our preference is to cannulate the mid- to distal aortic arch with a long cannula, directing flow away from the brachiocephalic arteries. Axillary artery cannulation also has been advocated.
- The venous drainage site is at the surgeon's discretion and will depend on access. Bicaval venous drainage is necessary if venous RCP is contemplated. When renal tumors are being removed from the inferior vena cava, a right atrial drainage basket is used. This bucket can be withdrawn during the arrest period to allow full visualization of the intrathoracic cava.
- When circulatory arrest is contemplated for procedures on the distal aorta with access via a left thoracotomy, arterial inflow and venous drainage is more problematic. If femoral return is used, this must be transposed after the arrest period to the proximal circulation. Right atrial access may be possible with an extensive thoracotomy, particularly if the incision traverses the sternum. In other cases, femoral venous drainage with long catheters passing directly to the right atrium are used, supplemented by drainage of the main pulmonary artery or vacuum assist.

Cardiopulmonary bypass

COOLING

2 Cardiopulmonary bypass is instituted with linear flow at rates of 2.4 L/minute per m², maintaining a perfusion pressure of 55–65 mm Hg using nitrates or α-agonists as necessary. The author persists with this flow throughout the procedure except for during the arrest period. Cooling using the heart-lung machines integrated heat exchanger is commenced immediately, ensuring a maximum gradient between blood and water temperature of 10°C. During the cooling period, the aorta is often clamped while surgery on the aortic root is performed. Throughout the core-cooling and arrest period, the head is packed with ice to prevent environmental warming. During cooling and rewarming, a poor correlation exists between temperature measured in the bladder, esophagus, nasopharynx, and brain. Brain temperature is probably best predicted by esophageal or arterial inflow temperature during these phases. Our practice is to continue cooling until complete equilibration occurs between esophageal and nasopharyngeal temperature for several minutes at 15°C before commencing the arrest period. This goal requires a minimum of 45 minutes of cooling. Other centers use detection of electrocerebral silence on electroencephalogram or suppression of evoked potentials as a guide to the start point of circulatory arrest. If available, jugular bulb saturation monitoring is helpful. Circulatory arrest should not be contemplated until the jugular bulb saturation exceeds 95 per cent. In the context of enhanced hemoglobin oxygen affinity, lower saturations infer continued brain oxygen extraction and metabolic rate. Hemodilution, commenced by prebypass autologous blood predonation, is continued during the bypass period to achieve hematocrits of 20–30 per cent. Hyperoxia is avoided, particularly, to reduce the risk of gaseous embolism formation during rewarming. The use of steroids exacerbates the hyperglycemia and insulin resistance associated with hypothermia. Sliding scale insulin regimes are commenced to combat this situation, but some degree of hyperglycemia is present until postoperative normothermia is achieved.

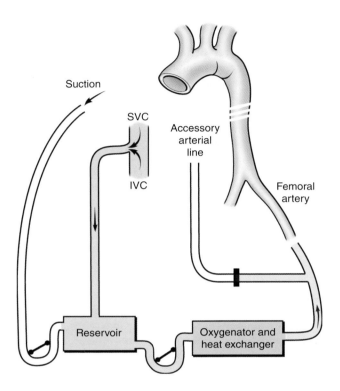

2

Arrest period

The circulatory arrest period is conducted with the patient in the Trendelenburg position to avoid air embolism. All preparation to reduce the ischemic period is undertaken prearrest, including prosthetic graft selection and trimming, preparation of sutures and suture buttress materials, and lighting adjustment. Pump flow is stopped, the patient is partially exsanguinated into the venous reservoir, and any cross-clamp in use is removed. Although suction is required to visualize the aortic arch, excessive aspiration of blood from the innominate, left carotid, and left subclavian arteries is avoided. Surgical reconstruction is performed, bearing in mind that access for placement of additional sutures will be difficult later in the operation. Although prosthetic grafts are relatively impervious at this point due to protein impregnation, suture hole bleeding can be a nuisance. For these reasons, we buttress anastomoses using Teflon on the outside of the native vessel and autologous or bovine pericardium on the graft. After each anastomosis, the graft is pressurized using arterial pump flow via a side arm, allowing detailed hemostatic inspection.

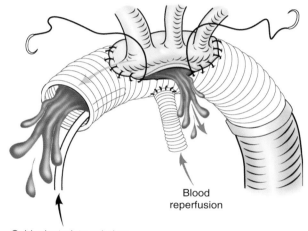

Blood reperfusion

Cold, electrolyte solution

3 At the end of the arrest period, evacuation of air and debris from the aortic arch is necessary. Retrograde arterial perfusion from the femoral artery should be avoided, and the prosthetic graft should be cannulated via a side arm or directly. Displacement of air and fatty debris can be achieved by infusing cold electrolyte solution into the graft during the latter stages of repair. The clear solution allows continued vision while suturing is completed. Pump flow via the graft is gradually restored during this air-drill process, which includes gentle milking of the epiaortic vessels and agitation of the graft to displace pockets of air. Once deairing is complete, cardiopulmonary bypass can be recommenced.

3

Retrograde cerebral perfusion

RCP (i.e. reversing the direction of blood flow in the superior vena cava) has been advocated to improve brain protection during the arrest period by providing substrates, removing catabolites, improving brain cooling, and reducing embolization of debris. These benefits are unproven in humans.

4a If RCP is to be used, a jugular bulb monitoring line is an essential prerequisite. After sternotomy, venous drainage is achieved by bicaval cannulation with snaring of both cavae (some advocate snaring distal to the azygos vein). The bypass circuit includes a 3/8-in. shunt connecting the arterial inflow with the venous drainage tubing that is occluded during the cooling period. At the selected temperature nadir, the patient is positioned with a 15 degree head-down tilt, circulatory arrest is commenced, and the pressure transducers are rezeroed at the level of the angle of the jaw in line with the jugular bulb.

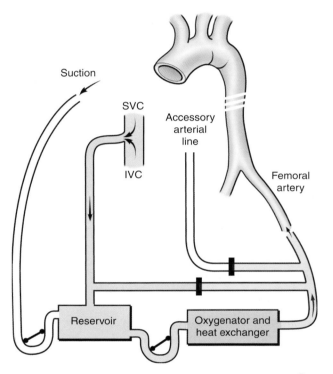

4a

4b Pump flow is gently recommenced, clamping the venous line proximal to the inflow shunt, thus directing flow retrogradely. Pump flows of 150–700 mL/minute are generated, adjusting flow to maintain a jugular bulb pressure of 25 mm Hg or less. Venous drainage from the inferior cava should be occluded during RCP. RCP continues during the arrest period, and throughout this time, desaturated blood may issue from the epiaortic arteries.

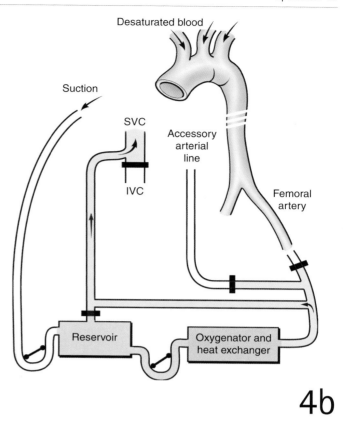

4b

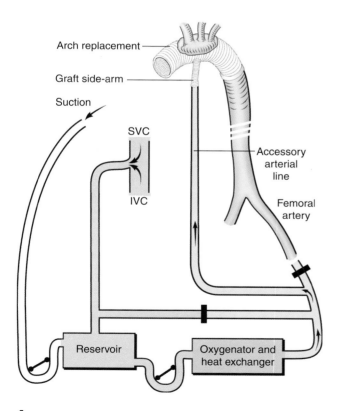

4c

4c RCP can be temporarily halted if vision is obscured during anastomotic construction. At the end of the arrest period, RCP assists in deairing maneuvers. Before reinstitution of bypass, normal superior caval venous drainage should be restored.

Selective arterial cerebral perfusion

5 This technique permits a lesser degree of whole-body hypothermia, as other vital organs have a greater ischemic tolerance. Initial anesthesia, monitoring, and cardiopulmonary bypass are identical in SACP. Right radial artery monitoring is essential. The bypass circuit includes an additional bifurcated line with attached flow probes. For SACP, greater mobilization of the epiaortic vessels is necessary to allow for either snaring or occlusion. Division of the innominate vein is commonly required. At 22°–25°C, the circulation is arrested, the aortic arch is opened, and the innominate and left carotid ostia are identified. Retrograde cardioplegia balloon cannulae are primed from the accessory pump circuit and advanced into the proximal innominate and left common carotid arteries, which are then gently snared around the cannulae. The left subclavian artery is occluded, and arterial perfusion is commenced at a flow rate of 10 mL/kg per minute adjusted to maintain a monitored right radial artery pressure of 50–70 mm Hg. Arch reconstruction is performed with moderate corporeal hypothermic circulatory arrest while brain perfusion continues. As reconstruction of the arch is completed, the cannulae are removed and rigorous deairing is performed. The remainder of the procedure is similar.

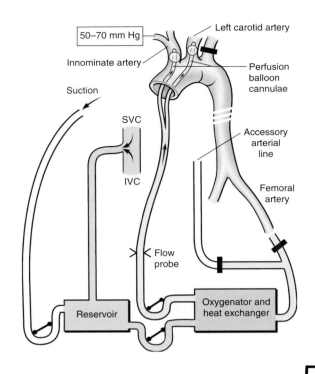

5

6

Rewarming

6 Orthograde perfusion is recommended using an accessory arterial line via a cannula within the arch graft or a sidearm. Perfusate temperature is kept low for the first few minutes after circulatory arrest in an attempt to avoid reflex cerebral vasoconstriction. Suture lines are inspected during this period, after which the patient is rewarmed and any additional proximal surgical procedures are performed. This maneuver is conducted with the same thermal gradient restrictions as mentioned previously together with continued pH, glycemia, and hematocrit management.

Cerebral hyperthermia during rewarming should be avoided as this may exacerbate any ischemic injury. During warming, blood leaving the pump on route to the patient should not exceed 37°C. Complete corporeal rewarming is not possible with this restriction, and bypass is generally discontinued with a core temperature of 35.5°–36.5°C. A significant temperature after-drop inevitably occurs, and patients commonly return to the Intensive Care Unit with temperatures of 32°–33°C.

Hemostasis

Prolonged cardiopulmonary bypass and profound hypothermia conspire to produce a coagulopathy that is further exacerbated by postoperative falls in temperature. The most important hemostatic adjunct is meticulous surgical technique with inspection of each anastomosis immediately after construction using either pressurized cardioplegia or pump flow. Hemostasis is also facilitated by predonation and later transfusion of autologous blood and by empirical supplementation of the coagulation cascade with fresh frozen plasma during the rewarming period. Administration of aprotinin, the antifibrinolytic serine protease inhibitor, after the circulatory arrest period also seems to be helpful. At the end of bypass, after protamine administration, platelet and cryoprecipitate infusion are commonly necessary to obtain satisfactory hemostasis for safe chest closure.

POSTOPERATIVE CARE

Postoperative care is similar to that required for most open heart surgery. Immediately postoperatively, gentle but active attempts should be made to facilitate warming, including infusion of warmed fluids and the use of convective warm air devices. Cardiac output, resistances, and filling pressures should be checked frequently, and significant colloid transfusion may be necessary to accommodate the appearance of an increased vascular space as the patient rewarms. For several hours postoperatively, the brain should be assumed to be exquisitely vulnerable to secondary ischemic insults; thus, hypoxemia, hypoperfusion, and hypotension should be carefully avoided. Once central normothermia is achieved, sedation can be reduced and the patient weaned from the ventilator. During the convalescent phase, an echocardiogram is necessary to exclude a pericardial effusion secondary to permeation of fluid through the prosthetic graft as the protein impregnation is absorbed.

OUTCOME

The outcomes of surgery are primarily dependent on the pathology being treated. Nevertheless, surgery requiring hypothermic circulatory arrest carries an inherent danger of neurological injury. Svensson *et al.* reported outcomes of 656 patients undergoing surgery using circulatory arrest with an overall stroke rate of 7 per cent. Similar risks were reported by Ergin *et al.*, who also found a 20 per cent incidence of transient neurological disturbance. Circulatory arrest durations in excess of 40 minutes are associated with a markedly increased risk of neurological deficit. This risk increases with advancing patient age and the presence of aortic arch atheroma. Even patients with shorter arrest times are at risk of transient neurological dysfunction, and it is now evident that this is a forerunner of later neurocognitive impairment that has a disturbingly high incidence after surgery requiring circulating arrest. Evidence of brain injury demonstrates a similar pattern in children.

RCP has become a popular adjunct to circulatory arrest, but it cannot be used under circumstances other than profound hypothermia. Certainly, evidence exists of some brain blood flow during RCP, but the amount appears small and probably insufficient to provide substrate delivery and catabolite removal. Studies comparing RCP with historical HCA controls suggest clinical benefit, but this must be clarified by prospective studies. Despite the inability of RCP to effect significant true reverse-brain perfusion, the transfer of blood to the epiaortic vessels via venous collaterals may provide some protection against embolic phenomena.

Recent clinical series describing results of SACP report similar outcomes to contemporary reports of circulatory arrest with or without RCP. Continued antegrade perfusion, compared to techniques using circulatory arrest, unequivocally provides superior neuroprotection in the experimental laboratory. No prospective comparative data are available, and all the techniques described have their protagonists.

FURTHER READING

Bonser, R., Wong, C. 2000: Retrograde cerebral perfusion. In Newman, S.P., Harrison, M.J.G., Stump, D.A., Smith, P., Taylor, K. (eds.), *The brain and cardiac surgery: causes of neurological complications and their prevention*, 1st edition. Amsterdam: Harwood Academic Publishers, 199–208.

Ergin, M.A, Griepp, E.B., Lansman, S.L., Galla, J.D., Levy, M., Griepp, R.B. 1994. Hypothermic circulatory arrest and other methods of cerebral protection during operations on the thoracic aorta. *Journal of Cardiac Surgery* 9(5), 525–37.

Griepp, E., Griepp, R. 1997: Use of hypothermic circulatory arrest for cerebral protection during aortic aneurysm repair. In Kawashima, Y., Takamoto, S. (eds.), *Brain protection in aortic surgery*. Amsterdam: Elsevier, 15–36.

Jonas, R. 2000: In Newman, S.P., Harrison, M.J.G., Stump, D.A., Smith, P., Taylor, K. (eds.), *The brain and cardiac surgery: causes of neurological complications and their prevention*, 1st edition. Amsterdam: Harwood Academic Publishers, 319–44.

Kazui, T. 1997: Surgical results of ascending and aortic arch replacement using selective cerebral perfusion. In Kawashima, Y., Takamoto, S. (eds.), *Brain protection in aortic surgery*. Amsterdam: Elsevier, 151–6.

Svensson, L.G., Crawford, E.S., Hess, K.R., *et al.* 1993. Deep hypothermia with circulatory arrest. Determinants of stroke and early mortality in 656 patients. *Journal of Thoracic and Cardiovascular Surgery* 106(1),19–28; discussion 28–31.

Intraoperative myocardial protection: current perspectives and future trends

GIDEON COHEN, MD, MSC, PHD
Assistant Professor, Division of Cardiac Surgery, University of Toronto, Faculty of Medicine; Staff Surgeon, Division of Cardiovascular Surgery,
The Schulich Heart Centre, Toronto, Ontario, Canada

RICHARD D. WEISEL, MD
Professor and Chair, Division of Cardiac Surgery, University of Toronto, Faculty of Medicine; Staff Surgeon, Division of Cardiovascular Surgery,
University Health Network, Toronto General Hospital, Toronto, Ontario, Canada

HISTORY

The advent of direct open heart surgery was made possible by the development of safe and effective cardiopulmonary bypass pumps and oxygenators in the late 1950s. Although enabling the repair of complex intracardiac defects and valvular lesions, such operations were plagued by the predictable occurrence of cardiac failure resulting from the intraoperative interruption of coronary blood flow.

Early interest in the protective effects of induced hypothermia was sparked by the treatment of wartime frostbite injuries in the 1940s. Wilfred G. Bigelow applied such knowledge to the study of hibernating ground hogs, known to reduce their body temperature and physiological activity to a minimum without detriment to the animal. By 1954, surgeons in Toronto successfully employed deep hypothermia and circulatory arrest for the repair of complex congenital cardiac defects in pediatric patients.

Despite such promising results, the requirement for prolonged periods of coronary blood flow interruption during complicated operative procedures proved to be beyond the protective scope of simple systemic hypothermia. Thus, 'cardioplegia', or induced arrest of the heart, was introduced as an adjunctive method of myocardial protection in 1955. Melrose first described the use of potassium citrate to achieve electro-mechanical diastolic arrest of the heart during cardiac surgery. This technique reduced myocardial metabolic demands while enabling brief interruptions in coronary flow to facilitate visualization of the operative field. Unfortunately, myocardial necrosis, presumed to be secondary to potassium concentrations in excess of 240 mmol/L, led to an early abandonment of induced cardioplegic arrest, and a return to previous methods.

Although direct coronary artery perfusion would prove to be useful during simple aortic procedures, the use of induced ventricular fibrillation and mild systemic hypothermia for coronary procedures was limited by poor visualization as well as ongoing evidence of peri-procedural myocardial injury. Intermittent normothermic anoxic arrest with sequential cross-clamping of the aorta during construction of distal coronary anastomoses was employed during some early procedures, but low cardiac output states or fatal cardiac events quickly ensued when ischemic intervals were prolonged.

This chapter reviews current concepts in myocardial protection and the metabolic and physiological rationale behind them. The advantages and disadvantages of differing cardioplegia delivery methods are discussed and the relative merits of various cardioplegic additives are reviewed. In addition to conventional cardioplegia, some less commonly employed alternative techniques are discussed.

CARDIOPLEGIA

Evolution of potassium cardioplegia

Potassium cardioplegia was first introduced by Melrose and colleagues in 1955 for the purpose of achieving mechanical diastolic arrest, thereby minimizing cellular oxygen consumption during interruption of myocardial perfusion. In 1957, Donald Effler used potassium citrate to induce cardioplegic arrest in a clinical scenario. Unfortunately, this technique was soon abandoned when pathological evidence of severe myocardial injury was demonstrated. In 1973, Gay and Ebert reintroduced hyperkalemic cardioplegic arrest using concentrations of potassium which were one-tenth of the doses used by Melrose and Effler. Not surprisingly, the focal myocardial inflammatory lesions noted with earlier cases were eliminated. Thereafter, low-dose potassium cardioplegia administered via a crystalloid solution became the most commonly used clinical method of achieving mechanical arrest during cardiac surgical procedures.

Blood versus crystalloid cardioplegia

Initial approaches to the optimization of myocardial protection during cardioplegic arrest included attempts at oxygenation of the crystalloid delivery solution. This approach was soon followed by the introduction of blood as the primary cardioplegic vehicle. In addition to functioning as an efficient oxygen carrier, whole blood offered the added benefits of an intrinsic buffering capacity, a reduction in myocardial edema (due to its oncotic properties), a minimization of hemodilution, and an improvement in microcirculatory flow. Furthermore, whole blood contains a number of endogenous free-radical scavengers which may aid in the attenuation of ischemia-reperfusion injury.

Such properties led many surgeons to adopt blood-based cardioplegia in the early 1980s. One of the first supportive studies was a randomized clinical trial of blood versus crystalloid cardioplegia performed by Fremes and colleagues in Toronto. In patients undergoing elective coronary bypass surgery, blood cardioplegia was associated with a maintenance of aerobic myocardial metabolism during the cross-clamp period and a decrease in lactate production during reperfusion. Although such metabolic enhancements did not translate into significantly improved clinical outcomes in low-risk patients, higher risk patients with unstable angina who received blood cardioplegia demonstrated a decreased incidence of perioperative myocardial infarction, low output syndrome, and death.

Using separate rolling pumps and heat exchangers, original blood cardioplegic preparations combined cold oxygenated blood from the bypass circuit with a crystalloid solution at a 2:1 or 4:1 ratio, diluted to avoid microvascular sludging. Since the early 1990s, blood cardioplegic solutions with even higher concentrations of blood have been used as hyperkalemia levels have been minimized. Indeed, some surgeons currently use a blood-only cardioplegic solution supplemented with essential electrolytes, including potassium and magnesium (Table 6.1). Menasche demonstrated that this technique of undiluted blood cardioplegia effectively reduced the volume of crystalloid administration from 750 mL to less than 100 mL. Moreover, the intrinsic buffering capacity of blood-only cardioplegia precluded the need for additional buffering agents. Since Menasche's early results, the crystalloid component of our cardioplegia has been simplified, now consisting of only potassium, magnesium, and dextrose.

Table 6.1 *Toronto General Hospital cardioplegic crystalloid solution composition*

Component	High K+ solution	Low K+ solution
KCl	30 mEq/L	8 mEq/L
MgSO$_4$	6 mEq/L	6 mEq/L
Dextrose	50 mmol/L	50 mmol/L

Metabolic substrate enhancement of cardioplegia

Various investigators have demonstrated a depletion in Krebs-cycle intermediates (i.e. glutamate, aspartate, etc.) occurs during prolonged induced ischemic arrest. This metabolic depletion may be partly responsible for the delay in recovery of postoperative myocardial metabolism and function. In a trial by Rosenkranz and colleagues, hearts arrested with glutamate-supplemented cardioplegia achieved earlier metabolic recovery. In a similar trial, patients undergoing elective coronary revascularization were administered an exogenous infusion of Ringer's lactate prior to cardioplegic arrest. Because the myocardial oxidation of fatty acids and glucose (the predominant substrates for aerobic metabolism) is impaired after cardioplegic arrest, lactate, which is readily metabolized to pyruvate, could be a preferred substrate for aerobic metabolism during reperfusion. Indeed, patients who received lactate experienced improved cardiac metabolic and functional recovery and demonstrated a reduction in perioperative ischemic injury in comparison to controls. Although many such additives have been investigated over the years with varying results, metabolic additives, in general, have not been widely adopted due to a lack of observed clinical benefit.

CARDIOPLEGIC TEMPERATURE

Normothermic cardioplegia

Traditional cardioplegic methods employed intermittent infusions of hypothermic (less than 10°C) blood or crystalloid cardioplegic solutions during induced ischemia. Cold cardioplegia, in addition to minimizing myocardial metabolic requirements, enabled an immediate assessment of cardioplegic delivery based on the degree of regional cooling. Some surgeons preferred to further augment myocardial cooling via direct application of topical saline slush or with the use of a cooling jacket apparatus. However, although providing added protection, such topical cooling techniques were occasionally found to be associated with postoperative phrenic nerve palsy and an increased incidence of respiratory compromise.

Although hypothermia provides excellent protection to the arrested heart, functional recovery with reperfusion is often delayed, presumably due to the hypothermic inhibition of myocardial enzymes that may remain inactive for hours following cardioplegic arrest. In 1982, Rozenkranz demonstrated that initial warm induction of cardioplegic arrest prior to administration of hypothermic cardioplegia improved myocardial metabolic and functional recovery. Similarly, Teoh demonstrated that a terminal infusion of warm blood cardioplegia just prior to cross-clamp removal (the so-called cardioplegic 'hot shot') facilitated early myocardial metabolic recovery while maintaining electromechanical arrest. Presumably, normothermic reperfusion enables an early resumption of temperature-dependent mitochondrial enzymatic function and a quick return to aerobic metabolism with resultant adenosine triphosphate (ATP) generation. Moreover, the persistent noncontractile state of the heart enables the use of available ATP for the repair of cellular injury and the repletion of energy stores rather than the maintenance of unnecessary contractile activity. By the late 1980s, the standard technique of myocardial protection in Toronto consisted of intermittent cold blood cardioplegia with a terminal hot shot. In cases of severe preoperative ischemia, warm induction with a substrate-enhanced cardioplegic solution was used.

Warm heart surgery

As early as 1978, Behrendt demonstrated that the basic cardioprotective effects of cardioplegia were independent of hypothermia. Lowering the heart temperature did not reduce myocardial oxygen requirements much beyond that observed with hyperkalemic arrest alone. In 1991, Lichtenstein and colleagues in Toronto extrapolated the benefits of initial and terminal warm cardioplegia to introduce the concept of warm heart surgery. Citing the well-documented deleterious effects of hypothermic cardioplegia (including impairment of mitochondrial energy generation, poor substrate use, and membrane injury), Lichtenstein suggested that the heart be maintained at a temperature of 37°C throughout the cross-clamp period to facilitate the recovery of myocardial metabolism and function following cross-clamp removal. In turn, the metabolic needs of the heart would be met by near-continuous infusions of blood cardioplegia. Buckberg and colleagues would demonstrate the feasibility of such a

method using a canine heart model, where myocardial oxygen consumption was reduced from 5.6 to 1.1 mL × 100 g^{-1} × minute^{-1} when the heart was arrested at 37°C. Lowering the heart temperature to 18°C provided little additional benefit, with a reduction in myocardial oxygen consumption from 1.1 to 0.31 mL × 100 g^{-1} × minute^{-1}.

In 1991, in an attempt to confirm such findings within the clinical setting, Lichtenstein and colleagues described the results of surgery in 121 consecutive patients receiving normothermic antegrade blood cardioplegia during coronary artery bypass graft surgery (CABG). In comparison to a historical cohort of 133 patients receiving hypothermic antegrade blood cardioplegia, warm heart patients demonstrated a lower incidence of perioperative myocardial infarction and intra-aortic balloon pump requirement. Although mortality was also lower in the normothermic group (0.9 per cent versus 2.2 per cent in the hypothermic group), this difference did not reach statistical significance. A spontaneous return to sinus rhythm after cross-clamp removal was observed in 99 per cent of normothermic patients versus only 11 per cent of hypothermic patients. Morbidity and mortality remained low in the normothermic group despite interruptions of the cardioplegic infusion for up to 15 minutes when necessary to facilitate visualization of distal anastomoses. In 1994, Naylor reported the results of a prospective trial involving nearly 2000 CABG patients randomized to receive either normothermic or hypothermic cardioplegia. Although no difference in mortality or myocardial infarction was found between groups, patients in the normothermic group revealed a significantly lower incidence of postoperative low cardiac output syndrome. Similarly, Yau and colleagues demonstrated improved early postoperative myocardial end-systolic elastance, preload recruitable stroke work, and postoperative early diastolic relaxation in patients receiving normothermic versus hypothermic cardioplegia.

Optimal cardioplegic temperature

Normothermic cardioplegia offered the promise of resuscitating the ischemic heart while facilitating early postoperative recovery of myocardial metabolism and function. Unfortunately, inadequate distribution of cardioplegia along with interruption of the cardioplegic infusion during distal anastomoses resulted in substantial anaerobic metabolic activity and warm ischemic injury. To avoid such detrimental effects, we compared the results of tepid (29°C) blood cardioplegia to those of warm (37°C) and cold (4°C) cardioplegia (producing myocardial temperatures of 37°C or 18°C, respectively) in 72 patients undergoing isolated CABG. Myocardial oxygen consumption and anaerobic lactate release were found to be greatest during warm, intermediate during tepid, and least during cold cardioplegic arrest. Warm retrograde and tepid retrograde techniques resulted in greater lactic acid washout during reperfusion. Left ventricular stroke work indices were best after warm antegrade and tepid antegrade in comparison to cold antegrade cardioplegia, and right ventricular stroke work indices were greatest after warm antegrade cardioplegia. Thus, both warm and tepid techniques were beneficial. However, unlike warm cardioplegia, tepid antegrade cardioplegia offered additional protection during cardioplegic interruptions. Moreover, by preventing cold-related injury, myocardial functional recovery with tepid infusions was immediate. Based on these studies, current practice at our institution involves the use of mild-to-moderate hypothermic cardioplegia (myocardial temperatures of 18°C to 29°C) in combination with mild systemic cooling on cardiopulmonary bypass (systemic temperatures of 32°C to 34°C). This strategy may simultaneously optimize both cerebral and myocardial protection.

CARDIOPLEGIC DELIVERY

Antegrade cardioplegic delivery

Standard cardioplegic delivery involves the administration of antegrade infusions via the aortic root at perfusion pressures of 70–100 mm Hg. Delivery is accomplished through a 12-Gauge cardioplegia cannula positioned in the mid ascending aorta. The same cannula can be used for aortic venting between cardioplegic infusions. To achieve electromechanical arrest, initial doses of 500–1 000 mL are usually required (more if left ventricular hypertrophy is present). Thereafter, arrest is maintained by intermittent antegrade infusions into the aortic root as well as via each completed vein graft at the completion of each distal or proximal anastomosis. During valvular surgery, maintenance doses are generally administered every 15 to 20 minutes.

The concern with isolated antegrade cardioplegia, however, is the possibility of hypoperfusion of distal vascular beds due to proximal disease of native coronary arteries (when vein grafts have yet to be completed or when pedicled internal mammary arterial grafts are utilized). Moreover, antegrade cardioplegia may be detrimental in reoperative coronary bypass surgery due to the risk of saphenous vein graft embolization when cardioplegia is delivered via the aortic root. Additional limitations may exist during valvular operations. In patients with significant aortic regurgitation, antegrade cardioplegic delivery via the aortic root may be ineffective, leading to ventricular distention. As such, the aorta must be opened soon after cross-clamp application to enable direct cardioplegic administration via the coronary ostia. Subsequent ostial infusions, however, may obscure the operative field and be cumbersome during valve implantation.

Retrograde coronary sinus cardioplegia

Retrograde cardioplegic delivery via the coronary sinus was first introduced in the early 1980s. Experimental studies demonstrated the feasibility of this approach, which has since been widely adopted, especially for patients undergoing valve replacement or reoperative CABG surgery. In aortic valve surgery, retrograde cardioplegia may obviate the need for antegrade cardioplegic delivery via the coronary ostia. In mitral valve surgery, retrograde cardioplegia is not impeded by mitral retraction, as is often the case with antegrade cardioplegic delivery. For reoperative CABG surgery, retrograde cardioplegia is believed to be beneficial due to the prevention of embolization from old vein grafts.

For effective retrograde coronary sinus cardioplegia, a catheter is introduced through a right atrial purse-string and directed into the coronary sinus. Catheter position is confirmed by palpation and by direct measurement of coronary sinus pressures. Maintenance of acceptable perfusion pressures (40 mm Hg or less) is achieved with a soft self-inflating occlusive balloon designed to maintain adequate myocardial perfusion while preventing perivascular hemorrhage, edema, coronary sinus rupture. If the right atrium is opened and the coronary sinus directly cannulated, placement of a purse-string suture at the base of the coronary sinus prevents catheter dislodgement and minimizes reflux into the right atrium.

Combined antegrade and retrograde cardioplegia

Although delivery of antegrade cardioplegia may be limited by native coronary stenoses, distribution of retrograde cardioplegia may be unreliable to the right ventricle and inhomogeneous to the left ventricle. To overcome such inherent limitations, a combined antegrade and retrograde approach was evaluated at our institution in 1994. Among 75 patients undergoing primary isolated coronary bypass surgery, those receiving a continuous infusion of tepid retrograde blood cardioplegia with intermittent antegrade infusions demonstrated a reduction in myocardial lactate production, a preservation of myocardial high energy phosphates, and improved postoperative myocardial function, suggesting superior overall perfusion of the heart in comparison to antegrade or retrograde techniques alone.

Alternate versus simultaneous combination cardioplegia

Two methods are currently employed for combined antegrade and retrograde cardioplegic delivery. One method involves the use of alternate infusions, the direction of which is controlled by a stopcock on the main cardioplegia line. This method is especially useful in CABG surgery where distal and proximal anastomoses are performed in an alternating fashion. Retrograde cardioplegia can be administered continuously throughout the cross-clamp period or stopped when necessary to facilitate visualization. At the completion of each proximal anastomosis, the stopcock is positioned to provide antegrade perfusion into the native coronary circulation as well as all completed vein grafts. The only disadvantage is the requirement for aortic root deairing before initiation of each antegrade bolus, an added step that can be time consuming and potentially hazardous due to the possibility of air embolism.

Another useful approach for the application of combined cardioplegia eliminates the requirement for repeated deairing of the aortic root. On completion of each distal anastomosis, the proximal aspect of the vein graft is connected to a manifold system that runs in parallel to the retrograde delivery port. This technique results in simultaneous delivery of antegrade cardioplegia through the completed vein grafts as well as retrograde cardioplegia via the coronary sinus. Because the aortic root is vented, this technique does not result in venous congestion or myocardial edema. If a 'two-clamp' technique is used whereby proximal vein grafts are anastomosed to the ascending aorta using a partial occluding clamp, the manifold can be attached directly to the aortic line for simultaneous antegrade perfusion until all proximal anastomoses are completed.

To evaluate the relative merits of these techniques, 60 patients undergoing isolated coronary bypass surgery were randomized to receive near continuous tepid retrograde cardioplegia in combination with either intermittent antegrade cardioplegia through the aortic root (alternate approach) or antegrade cardioplegia delivered concurrently through each completed vein graft (simultaneous approach). Myocardial lactate extraction after cross-clamp release was found to be greater in the simultaneous group compared to the alternate group. Postoperative ventricular function, however, was better in the alternate group. Although both techniques of cardioplegic delivery permitted rapid postoperative recovery of myocardial metabolism and function, the simultaneous delivery method was simple to apply and did not require aortic root deairing between antegrade infusions.

Additional assessments of alternate versus simultaneous cardioplegia have enlisted novel imaging techniques to better assess coronary perfusion. One such study employed sonicated albumin administered with cardioplegia in patients undergoing coronary bypass surgery. With the help of intraoperative transesophageal echocardiography, real-time assessment and quantification of myocardial perfusion was possible. Using such methods, antegrade cardioplegic delivery was found to offer superior perfusion to the left ventricle in comparison to retrograde delivery at similar flow rates. Right ventricular perfusion was poor regardless of the direction of cardioplegic administration. Overall, simultaneous delivery provided the most consistent results and offered the best perfusion of the anterior left ventricle and right ventricle in comparison to antegrade or retrograde routes alone.

Optimal flow rates for integrated myocardial protection

In 1997, we performed a prospective randomized trial to determine the optimal flow rate for simultaneous tepid cardioplegia. Twenty patients undergoing elective CABG were randomized to receive either high (200 mL/minute) or low (100 mL/minute) flow cardioplegic delivery. Tepid retrograde cardioplegia resulted in an accumulation of lactate and hydrogen ions during construction of the first two bypass grafts. The addition of antegrade vein graft infusions at a flow rate of 100 mL/minute resulted in a washout of these accumulated metabolites. A flow rate of 200 mL/minute further improved the washout of metabolic end products. Although postoperative clinical outcomes and hemodynamic parameters were similar between groups in these low-risk patients, such subtle metabolic differences may translate into significant benefit in high-risk patients undergoing coronary bypass surgery.

TECHNICAL ASPECTS OF CARDIOPLEGIA ADMINISTRATION

Following aortic and venous cannulation, a simple 4/0 polypropylene purse-string suture is placed either at the midlevel of the right atrium (2–3 cm lateral to the atrioventricular groove) or at the base of the right atrial appendage to anchor the retrograde cardioplegia cannula. Another 4/0 polypropylene mattress or figure of eight suture is placed on the anterior aspect of the mid-ascending aorta to secure the antegrade cardioplegia cannula. The typical antegrade cannula is a 12-Gauge device with a two-limbed connector enabling both cardioplegic delivery and aortic root venting. The aortic root vent provides for effective decompression of the left heart in CABG procedures, either in between antegrade infusions or during retrograde infusions. As shown in Figure 3, the cardioplegia delivery system can be arranged in such a way as to combine all three delivery routes (antegrade via the aortic root, antegrade via completed vein grafts, and retrograde via the coronary sinus). The surgeon can easily control and isolate cardioplegia delivery through one of three infusion lines while maintaining aortic root decompression through the vent line when necessary.

1 After insertion of the antegrade cannula and preferably prior to initiation of cardiopulmonary bypass, the retrograde cardioplegia cannula is inserted through the atrial pursestring.

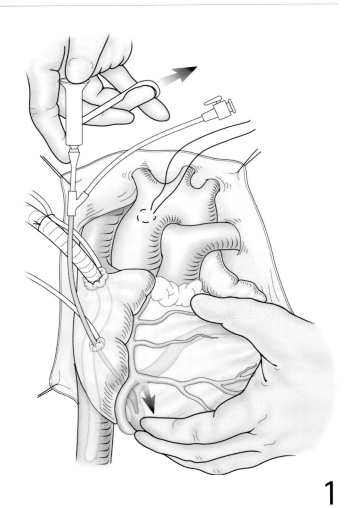

1

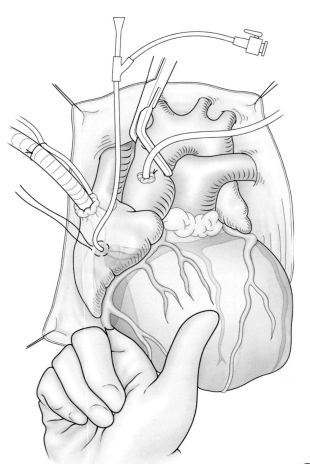

2 The catheter is advanced carefully into the coronary sinus orifice with the position of the cannula tip verified by digital palpation behind the heart. Elevating the heart slightly anteriorly (with the inferior vena cava fixed in place by the previously positioned venous cannula) can facilitate this catheter-positioning maneuver.

2

3 Once the catheter is positioned appropriately, irrigation of the pressure lumen expands the self-inflating balloon near the tip of the catheter. The central catheter lumen is then aspirated, flushed, and zeroed in preparation for subsequent use. When the catheter is properly deployed, coronary sinus pressures range between 20 and 30 cm H_2O.

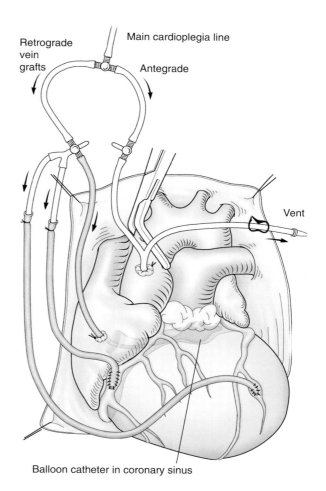

Balloon catheter in coronary sinus

3

ADJUNCTIVE STRATEGIES IN MYOCARDIAL PROTECTION

Early methods aimed at minimizing the risks associated with coronary bypass surgery primarily involved the manipulation of ischemia and reperfusion conditions. Parameters such as cardioplegic composition, temperature, flow direction, and flow rate have been extensively evaluated resulting in near-optimal conditions for current myocardial protection. Not surprisingly, healthy patients presenting for elective coronary bypass surgery face a very low risk of perioperative cardiac morbidity and mortality. Despite such advances, however, conventional cardioplegic techniques may be insufficient in high-risk patients undergoing cardiac surgery. Improvements in the management of such patients may require preoperative pharmacologic manipulation or the application of cardioplegic additives to further improve cardiac protection.

Myocardial preconditioning

Ischemic preconditioning describes the phenomenon whereby a brief episode of myocardial ischemia affords protection against the adverse effects of a subsequent, more prolonged episode of ischemia. Ischemic preconditioning is a powerful endogenously mediated form of myocardial protection and may account for the heart's inherent ability to tolerate brief episodes of induced ischemia during percutaneous catheter interventions and during coronary bypass surgery. Several pharmacological agents have been shown to mimic the beneficial effects of preconditioning without the need for an ischemic stimulus. Such agents include adrenergic agonists, bradykinin, amiloride, and opioids. Unfortunately, many of these agents are either toxic or produce unwanted side effects. Adenosine, believed to be an intermediary in the ischemic preconditioning phenomenon, may prevent such side effects while affording significant myocardial protection during ischemia and reperfusion. Indeed, various studies have suggested a possible role for adenosine in clinical preconditioning. In one such study, administration of intravenous adenosine to patients undergoing elective coronary bypass surgery immediately prior to the initiation of cardiopulmonary bypass resulted in improved cardiac indices and a reduction in postoperative creatine kinase MB isoenzyme release in comparison to nonrandomized controls.

Insulin cardioplegia

Aortic cross-clamping induces anaerobic metabolism during cardioplegic arrest. Persistent lactate release during reperfusion suggests a delay in the recovery of aerobic metabolism and has been shown to be predictive of postoperative ventricular dysfunction. By stimulating the rate-limiting enzyme pyruvate dehydrogenase, insulin may facilitate the early conversion from anaerobic to aerobic metabolism, thus enabling rapid postischemic myocardial recovery of ATP-synthetic capacity. We performed a prospective randomized trial to evaluate the effects of insulin as a cardioplegic additive. Fifty-six patients undergoing isolated coronary bypass surgery were randomized to one of four cardioplegic groups containing either 42 or 84 mmol/L of glucose with or without 10 IU/L of insulin. Although cardioplegic arrest induced anaerobic lactate release in both groups, following cross-clamp removal, patients in the insulin group converted to aerobic lactate extraction compared to persistent lactate release in the placebo group. Insulin increased myocardial pyruvate dehydrogenase activity, but the difference was not significant. Two hours postoperatively, cardiac index and left ventricular stroke work index were higher in the insulin cardioplegia patients versus the placebo group at similar filling pressures.

Nitric oxide/L-arginine supplemented cardioplegia

Nitric oxide (NO) has been shown to reduce ischemia reperfusion damage in experimental animal models. NO is produced from the amino acid L-arginine by the enzyme nitric oxide synthetase (NOS) and has a variety of biological activities. Although cardiomyocytes express a constitutive calcium-sensitive form of NOS, the physiological role of this NOS remains unknown. We examined the effects of L-arginine in a human ventricular myocyte model of simulated ischemia and reperfusion. L-arginine applied during reperfusion afforded significant protection against the adverse effects of ischemia and increased extracellular nitrite concentrations, reflecting NO production. The vasoactive properties of NO may provide additional benefits. We have demonstrated that the vasoconstrictor endothelin impairs the recovery of cardiac function after cardioplegic arrest and that the NOS cofactor tetrahydrobiopterin reverses such adverse effects, possibly by optimizing the delivery of cardioplegia. Thus, the myocardial and vasoactive effects of NO may act in concert to restore normal metabolism and function to energy-depleted hearts undergoing CABG surgery.

Unfortunately, despite such promising laboratory findings, early clinical results have failed to show a significant benefit of L-arginine supplemented cardioplegia. A pilot study performed by Carrier and colleagues from Montreal randomized 50 patients undergoing CABG to receive 1 gram of L-arginine or placebo during the first 30 minutes of cardioplegia. The administration of L-arginine in this manner did not afford a clinical benefit and did not influence the release of postoperative cardiac enzymes. Additional clinical studies are required to further elucidate the optimal dose and timing of L-arginine administration in patients undergoing cardiac surgery.

Additional cardioplegic additives which have been proposed for the purpose of myocardial protection include sodium/hydrogen exchange inhibitors, catecholamine inhibitors, potassium channel openers, opioids and endothelin receptor antagonists. Future applications may involve the simultaneous use of multiple agents for a multi-modal approach to the prevention of ischemia-reperfusion injury.

ALTERNATIVE METHODS OF MYOCARDIAL PROTECTION

The evolution of myocardial protection over the past two decades has focused primarily on the optimization of cardioplegia-induced electromechanical arrest. Despite remarkable advances, however, alternative, more traditional techniques are still used by some surgeons and have merit under certain circumstances in which cardioplegic arrest may not be feasible.

Intermittent ischemic arrest

This method involves intermittent cross-clamping of the aorta for short periods without the use of cardioplegia. Although a relatively dry operative field may result, complete mechanical arrest is seldom achieved. During coronary bypass surgery, the cross-clamp is applied for construction of distal anastomoses. On completion of each distal anastomosis, the cross-clamp is removed and reperfusion is undertaken for a period equal to that of the cross-clamp time. Such a practice facilitates repayment of the oxygen debt. Systemic hypothermia may also be used under such circumstances as an adjunctive measure to further reduce myocardial oxygen demands. Proximal anastomoses are usually constructed during periods of reperfusion with the help of a partial occluding clamp applied to the anterior ascending aorta.

Although this technique may also afford ischemic preconditioning by virtue of the multiple brief ischemic episodes, some disadvantages do exist. Despite the use of systemic hypothermia, ventricular fibrillation may ensue during cross-clamping, resulting in increased myocardial oxygen demands and exacerbation of ischemia in non-bypassed distributions. Moreover, exposure of the heart to repeated episodes of ischemia-reperfusion injury may be detrimental. The requirement for repeated aortic cross-clamping may also be hazardous in patients with atherosclerotic disease of the aorta, due to the risk of cerebral atheroemboli. Finally, the inability to achieve mechanical arrest may result in incomplete revascularization. Nonetheless, despite such potential drawbacks, some surgeons report results in high- and low-risk patients which are quite comparable to those observed with cardioplegic arrest.

Hypothermic fibrillatory arrest

Experimental evidence suggests that subendocardial ischemia can be minimized if a hypothermic, vented, spontaneously fibrillating heart is perfused at pressures of 80–100 mm Hg. Under such circumstances, coronary bypass surgery could be performed with local vessel control thus avoiding the potential complications of global arrest. A study by Akins and colleagues reported the results of hypothermic fibrillatory arrest in 3 085 patients who underwent cardiac operations between 1980 and 1993. The overall mortality in this series was 1.6 per cent, with a 2.5 per cent incidence of perioperative myocardial infarction, and a requirement for intra-aortic balloon pump support in 2.5 per cent of patients. Of note, this series also included 371 patients (12 per cent) who underwent emergent surgery for complications of cardiac catheterization. Hypothermic fibrillatory arrest has also been shown to be safe in high-risk patients and provides a viable option for those patients in whom the risk of aortic cross-clamping is high due to severe atherosclerotic disease. Distal anastomoses can be performed during fibrillatory arrest, whereas proximal anastomoses can be constructed of pedicled mammary arterial grafts off the innominate artery, aortic arch, or subclavian artery.

Atrial protection during cardioplegic arrest

Atrial arrhythmias may occur in up to 60 per cent of patients after cardiac surgery, and represent a significant cause of postoperative morbidity and prolonged hospital stay. In studies employing hypothermic antegrade cardioplegia, a temperature gradient can be demonstrated between the right atrium and right ventricle which may lead to persistent atrial activity during cardioplegic arrest. Although a relationship between persistent atrial activity and postoperative arrhythmias has not been consistently demonstrated, studies have shown a positive correlation between improved myocardial protection and a reduced incidence of postoperative supraventricular arrhythmias, suggestive of a link to intra-operative ischemic injury.

CONCLUSIONS

Current techniques of intraoperative myocardial protection are constantly evolving. To date, changes in cardioplegic composition, temperature and delivery have been successful in optimizing intraoperative myocardial protection, such that stable patients presenting for elective cardiac surgery face a remarkably low risk of perioperative morbidity or mortality. Although such patients likely have little to gain from additional intraoperative protective measures, future improvements may be crucial in reducing the morbidity and mortality in high-risk patients presenting with poor ventricular function and preoperative ischemia.

FURTHER READING

Barner, H.B. 1991. Blood cardioplegia: a review and comparison with crystalloid cardioplegia. *Annals of Thoracic Surgery* **52**, 1354–67.

Cohen, G., Shirai, T., Weisel, R.D., *et al.* 1999. Optimal myocardial preconditioning in humans. *Annals of the New York Academy of Sciences* **874**, 306–19.

Ihnken, K., Morita, K., Buckberg, G.D., *et al.* 1994. The safety of simultaneous arterial and coronary sinus perfusion: experimental background and initial clinical results. *Journal of Cardiac Surgery* **9**, 15–25.

Menasche, P., Subayi, J., Piwnica, A. 1990. Retrograde coronary sinus cardioplegia for aortic valve operations: a clinical report on 500 patients. *Annals of Thoracic Surgery* **49**, 556–64.

Mentzer, R.M., Birjiniuk, V., Khuri, S., *et al.* 1999. Adenosine myocardial protection: preliminary results of a phase II clinical trial. *Annals of Thoracic Surgery* **229**, 643–9.

Teoh, K.H., Mickle, D.A.G., Weisel, R.D., *et al.* 1988. Improving myocardial metabolic and functional recovery after cardioplegic arrest. *Journal of Thoracic and Cardiovascular Surgery* **95**, 788–98.

SECTION II

Surgery for Ischemic Heart Disease

Conventional coronary artery bypass grafting

TIMOTHY J. GARDNER MD
William Maul Measey Professor of Surgery, University of Pennsylvania School of Medicine; Division of Cardiothoracic Surgery, Hospital of the University of Pennsylvania, Philadelphia, Pennsylvania, USA

HISTORY

A variety of surgical procedures have been developed over the last 50 years to treat the symptoms of obstructive coronary artery disease, specifically the chest pain that is such a prevalent and disabling symptom. Beck and others abraded the exposed pericardial surface to induce inflammatory adhesions between the epicardium and the parietal pericardium. More than 50 years ago, an operation was developed by Vineberg in which the transected internal mammary artery (IMA) was implanted in the myocardium. Even thoracic sympathectomy was attempted, with variable degrees of success. In the late 1950s and early 1960s, a few attempts at direct coronary endarterectomy were made.

Coronary artery bypass grafting (CABG) began in earnest, however, in the late 1960s along two parallel paths that included bypassing coronary artery obstructions using either the IMA as the bypass conduit or reversed saphenous vein grafts from the leg. Each approach had early proponents, but the use of saphenous vein grafts became the dominant approach by the majority of cardiac surgeons in the 1970s. This preference was based on the perceived ease of use with the larger and technically less demanding saphenous vein graft, as well as the greater versatility of the vein graft. Saphenous veins could be used to graft any coronary artery site, including arteries on the lateral and inferior wall of the heart. The IMA graft, however, especially the pedicled graft, was limited to anterior and proximal coronary artery sites.

Although many of the earliest CABG procedures were limited to one or two distal coronary artery targets, multi-artery grafting was performed increasingly more often as the procedure grew in popularity and effectiveness. By the late 1970s, just 10 years after the initiation of direct CABG, most patients were receiving multiple bypass grafts with anastomoses to the distal right and circumflex systems in addition to the left anterior descending and proximal right coronary arteries. Some early proponents of the IMA graft persisted in the use of this conduit as a pedicled graft to the left anterior descending coronary artery (LAD).

By the mid-1980s, with CABG being done increasingly often throughout the world and with 10- to 15-year follow-up experience available from the early group of bypass recipients, two extremely important observations were made. Many of the earliest patients to receive bypass grafts were returning 5–10 or 12 years after their operation, with recurrent angina and symptoms similar or even worse than the original complaints that had led to their initial bypass operation. On repeat catheterizations, many were found to have marked progression of atherosclerosis in their native coronary arteries and, even more alarming, had severe obstructive atherosclerosis in the vein grafts that were used in the original procedure. A second unexpected observation was that in patients who had IMA bypass grafts performed previously, graft atherosclerosis and premature graft occlusion were rarely encountered. This observation was even true in patients whose accompanying saphenous vein grafts were severely diseased and/or obstructed.

These surprising findings led to changes in the approach that was taken to CABG in the mid- to late 1980s, which has resulted in the current standard approach to coronary artery bypass surgery. The majority of patients who undergo CABG surgery today receive a pedicled left IMA (LIMA) graft to the LAD. Other required bypasses are constructed using reversed saphenous vein grafts, with proximal aortic anastomoses. This combination of LIMA plus two or more saphenous vein grafts can be described as the traditional, and most common, configuration for patients who have multiple coronary bypass grafting today.

A key feature in current therapeutic approach to patients who undergo coronary bypass is the initiation of specific medications postoperatively to reduce progression of native artery and especially vein graft atherosclerosis. This secondary preventive approach includes the use of aspirin and other antiplatelet agents, lipid-lowering medications, and a variety of other possible drugs that affect baseline coronary artery tone and degree of vasodilation, heart rate, blood pressure, and even endothelial inflammatory susceptibility. Other important components of secondary prevention for patients who have a coronary bypass grafting procedure are weight and stress reduction, dietary compliance, exercise and activity programs, and smoking cessation, whenever applicable.

PRINCIPLES AND JUSTIFICATION

New technical innovations for CABG are described in detail in chapter 8. These include the expanded use of arterial conduits in an attempt to eliminate the need for atherosclerosis-susceptible saphenous vein grafts. In addition, techniques to perform CABG through smaller incisions and without the use of cardiopulmonary bypass are presented. This recent trend to perform 'beating heart' CABG (so-called off-pump CABG) is explored in chapters 9 and 10.

The current standard of including a LIMA pedicled graft in virtually every CABG procedure is based on several reports from the mid-1980s that demonstrated remarkable patency of the LIMA grafts at follow-up of 5–15 years. The majority of these grafts are to the LAD or a major anterior wall branch. Although there has been interest in using arterial conduits for other coronary obstructions, the availability and concern about reliability of arterial grafts other than the pedicled LIMA have persisted. The traditional combined IMA–saphenous vein graft coronary bypass grafting procedure remains the standard well into the new century.

Even when considering possible therapy for a patient with limited coronary artery disease but with involvement of the proximal LAD, many believe that a low-risk, definitive coronary bypass grafting procedure, which uses a pedicled IMA bypass to the LAD and is followed by compulsive secondary preventive techniques, will prove to be superior to multiple, incremental, catheter-based therapies over time, even with the current success associated with intracoronary stenting.

PREOPERATIVE ASSESSMENT AND PREPARATION

All patients who are referred to a surgeon for consideration of CABG will have had a coronary angiogram performed. Often, however, the patient who is referred for CABG should have one or more additional studies. Assessment of global left ventricular function with calculation of the ejection fraction as well as assessment of regional ventricular function, using a perfusion study or two-dimensional echocardiogram, may be helpful. Regional wall motion assessment may be especially important in situations in which coronary arterial branches are completely occluded and not visualized on coronary angiography. The presence of retained regional contractile function, as well as other signs of viability, should prompt an attempt at coronary artery identification and grafting in these areas. The surgeon should assess these studies and discuss his or her plans for bypass grafting with the patient before the procedure. Requests by cardiologists for consideration of bypass grafting should be seen as actual consultations for assessment of suitability for surgery, not prescriptions to perform specific operations according to the judgments made exclusively by the cardiologists or other physicians.

Another important component of preoperative assessment that requires the input of the surgeon is the availability of suitable conduits. Few CABG candidates have such severe peripheral vascular disease that the IMA is not suitable for use as a bypass conduit. A complete occlusion of the proximal left subclavian artery, however, such that a subclavian 'steal' might occur, can be determined by the absence or marked reduction of blood pressure in the left arm. The diagnostic cardiologist should be expected to visualize the LIMA during coronary artery studies in patients with severe brachiocephalic arterial obstructive disease. A commoner problem that causes unsuitability of the LIMA for grafting is seen in patients who have had prior anterior thoracic irradiation, especially those who have been radiated for mediastinal lymphoma. In some instances, the LIMA is encased in dense fibrous scarring from postirradiation inflammation. This situation may also occur in some female patients after mastectomy with postresection chest wall irradiation. The commonest problem that is overlooked by cardiologists when referring patients for multi-vessel coronary artery grafting, however, is the absence of saphenous veins in those who have had saphenous vein stripping because of severe varicosities. In addition, varicosed saphenous veins may pose problems. In either situation, physical examination and ultrasonic venous mapping, especially if lesser saphenous veins might be used, should be undertaken preoperatively.

The surgeon must also assess the patient for comorbid conditions that can be expected to increase operative risk or the degree of difficulty with the operation. The presence of common coexisting states, such as chronic obstructive pulmonary disease, diabetes mellitus, severe peripheral vascular disease, renal insufficiency, bleeding and coagulation disorders, liver disease, autoimmune conditions, and any condition that results in the possible compromise of the patient's immune status, such as HIV-AIDS, should be noted. The presence of concurrent infection, be it cutaneous, respiratory, upper airway, or urinary tract, also should be noted. Not only is such assessment essential for ensuring appropriate comprehensive care of the patient during the surgery, but it also is necessary to provide the patient with a risk-benefit assessment for the proposed surgery. Furthermore, the patient should be expected to understand and participate in the treatment plan to the extent that he or she is committed to postoperative risk modification and secondary prevention measures, as well as immediate postoperative rehabilitation.

OPERATION

Incision

1 Although the entire sternum must be divided for the traditional multi-vessel CABG operation, the anterior chest incision need not extend up to or above the suprasternal notch into the neck. The cephalad extent of the median sternotomy incision can be limited to produce a more acceptable incisional scar for patients who uniformly dislike excessively long or obvious upper chest wall incision scars. The cephalad extent of the incision should be initiated approximately two fingerbreadths below the suprasternal notch and carried down to a point just below the xiphoid process. The sternal saw should be inserted from the top, with the saw guard facing the patient's neck and the saw blade on the caudal side. This maneuver avoids inadvertent cervical extension of the skin incision. After the sternum is divided and retracted, it is occasionally necessary to extend the incision cephalad to avoid undue tension on the midline skin and subcutaneous tissue when the sternum is fully retracted. It is easy to extend the incision at this time, but it is rarely necessary, and a cosmetically acceptable incision usually can be achieved.

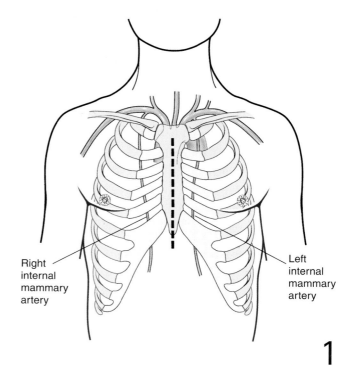

Right internal mammary artery

Left internal mammary artery

1

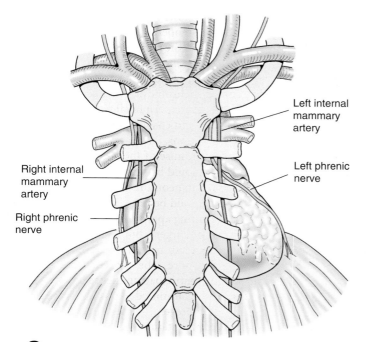

Right internal mammary artery

Right phrenic nerve

Left internal mammary artery

Left phrenic nerve

2

Isolation of the internal mammary artery

2 The mammary artery arises from the left subclavian artery close to the thyrocervical trunk and under the sternal end of the clavicle. It extends on the inside of the anterior chest wall just lateral to the sternum and costosternal cartilages from the clavicle down to the costochondral junction. The IMA branches to form the intercostal arteries, and at the fifth or sixth interspace, the mammary artery divides into its major distal branches. The artery is accompanied by two veins with tributaries from the intercostal vascular pedicle and adjacent chest wall. These veins enter the left subclavian vein just below the origin of the mammary artery from the subclavian artery. The phrenic nerve enters the thorax close to the origin of the IMA and traverses behind the subclavian vein. This nerve can be injured by electrocautery energy near the origin of the IMA.

3 Before heparinization, the left side of the sternum is elevated using a self-retaining retractor that is stabilized by independent fixation to the operating table. Two individual, mobile retractor handles are placed under the sternal edge to elevate the left chest wall upward and laterally. A 1-cm-wide pedicle that includes the mammary artery and accompanying veins is isolated using the electrocautery probe. With the left chest wall elevated, parallel cuts are made in the inner chest wall fascia medial and lateral to the visualized or palpated mammary artery. This dissection plane can be started at approximately the level of the third rib.

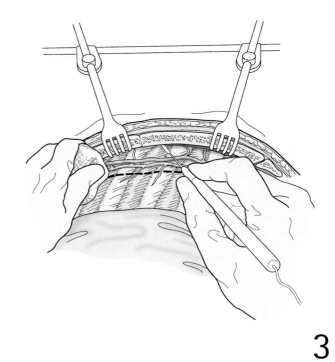

3

4 Once the first portion of the pedicle, including the artery and vein, is gently separated from the chest wall, traction placed on the pedicle allows visualization of the venous tributaries and arterial branches that go to the intercostal vascular pedicle and chest wall. Ideally, the larger branches and tributaries should be occluded on the vessel side with small hemaclips and either clipped or cauterized on the chest wall side. After the first segment of the mammary artery pedicle is isolated from the chest wall, the fascial dissection can be extended down toward the xiphoid process and up to the origin of the IMA from the subclavian, with care taken to identify, clip, and/or cauterize the major venous tributaries and arterial branches. The left parietal pleura is encountered close to where the lateral fascial incision is made to free the mammary artery pedicle from the chest wall. The pleural space often is entered, but pleural continuity can be maintained. It may be theoretically preferable to stay out of the left pleural space whenever possible and to avoid subsequent adhesion formation and/or a reactive pleuritis. In most cases, however, the pleural space is entered to free up the IMA pedicle sufficiently.

Once the mammary dissection is completed, and after systemic heparinization, the artery should be occluded with a soft jaw vascular clamp and ligated distally. Once the artery is divided, the chest wall retractor is removed and the sternotomy retractor positioned. The mammary artery then can be tested for flow, wrapped in a papaverine-soaked sponge, and placed in the lateral mediastinal space or left pleural cavity. Some surgeons occlude the pedicled graft at its cut end with a hemaclip, remove the vascular clamp, and allow flow throughout the length of the mammary artery to avoid distal arterial vasospasm.

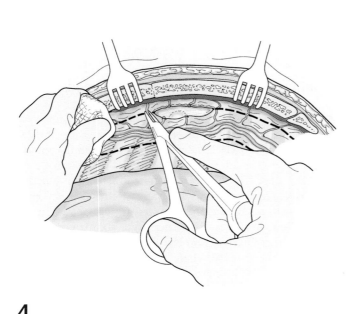

4

Saphenous vein harvest

5 With the patient already positioned with the lower extremities fully prepped and draped into the sterile field, and with the legs partially elevated and bent at the knees, the greater saphenous vein itself is identified or its expected course noted. The vein is then directly harvested through incisions over the vein as it joins the common femoral vein in the medial aspect of the upper thigh. The greater saphenous vein courses along the medial thigh and leg in a sufficiently constant pattern that once the vein is identified either distally or proximally, skip incisions can be made to avoid a long and deforming scar down the entire course of the lower extremity. If multiple incisions and tunneling are used, care should be taken to avoid excessive traction on the vein so that no damage occurs to the vein wall and endothelium. The vein must be handled gently at all times and should not be allowed to dry.

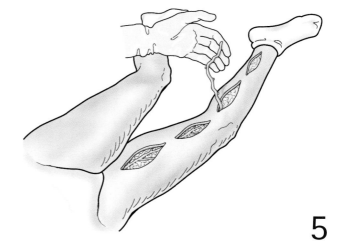

5

Endoscopic vein harvest

6a–c A recent technical innovation in greater saphenous vein harvest has been the use of endoscopic and video-assisted techniques. A variety of devices, retractors, and maneuvers have been described and used. In many patients, it is possible to make two small incisions, one above the knee on the medial aspect of the thigh and the second the standard upper thigh infrainguinal incision. A long tubular scope with a light source at the tip is inserted from the lower incision, and the saphenous vein is followed up its course in the thigh. Visualization is facilitated with subcutaneous insufflation with carbon dioxide. Through the use of a combination of blunt dissection and gentle traction, the tributaries of the vein can be identified, cauterized, and divided. Larger tributaries can be directly clipped. It may be necessary to add a midthigh incision to facilitate vein isolation and branch division at points that are remote from the two initial incisions.

If additional saphenous vein length is required, the endoscopically aided blunt subcutaneous dissection can be continued into the leg, with a midcalf counterincision usually required for adequate visualization. If the entire saphenous vein must be removed, a distal lower leg skin incision near the medial malleolus is made, and direct or tunneled dissection of the distalmost segment of the vein can be accomplished relatively easily. As is the case with other endoscopically performed surgical procedures, successful endoscopic vein harvest requires the acquisition of specific technical skills to achieve successful results. Early errors include avulsion of vein tributaries and subcutaneous hematomas from the division of unrecognized minor arteries and veins. When performed successfully, endoscopic vein harvest results in a marked reduction in wound morbidity and discomfort for the patient.

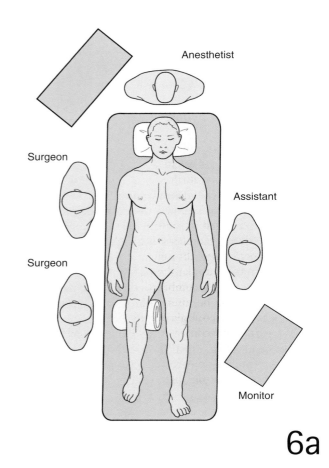

6a

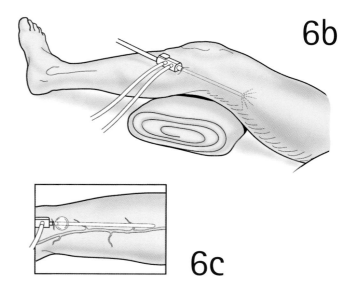

6b

6c

Cardiopulmonary bypass

7 After the distal ascending aorta is assessed for evidence of wall thickening or calcification, pursestring sutures are placed in the proximal aortic arch at the level of the innominate artery. The arterial cannulation site can be moved out onto the aortic arch if there is evidence of localized disease, which can be detected by simple digital palpation or by the use of a directly applied ultrasonic probe. Single venous cannulation is performed through the right atrial appendage using a two-stage cannula, the tip of which is placed in the inferior vena cava. A combined cardioplegic cannula and aortic root vent can be inserted in the midascending aorta. Coronary sinus cardioplegia is not used routinely for initial bypass grafting procedures in patients with well-compensated left ventricular function but can be added easily. A temperature-monitoring probe can be inserted once bypass is initiated into the septum, just to the right of the LAD.

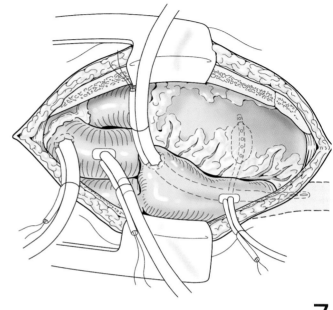

7

Distal anastomoses

VEIN GRAFT ANASTOMOSIS

In conventional CABG procedures in which a pedicled LIMA bypass is placed to the LAD, construction of the distal venous anastomoses should be performed first to avoid possible traction on the mammary artery pedicled graft. In addition, placing the distal vein grafts sequentially allows for direct cardioplegia administration into areas of obstructed arterial flow. For visualization of the distal right coronary artery or the right posterior descending and distal right posterolateral branches, the patient can be placed in a slight Trendelenburg's position with traction applied to the acute margin of the heart.

8a–c Either with gentle manual traction by an assistant or with the use of Silastic tapes placed under the artery, the anastomotic area is stabilized, the epicardium overlying the artery is incised, and the artery is entered. The arteriotomy is then extended with fine scissors for a distance of approximately 6–8 mm. The reversed saphenous vein is slightly beveled and can be anastomosed to the coronary artery with a single 7/0 polypropylene suture.

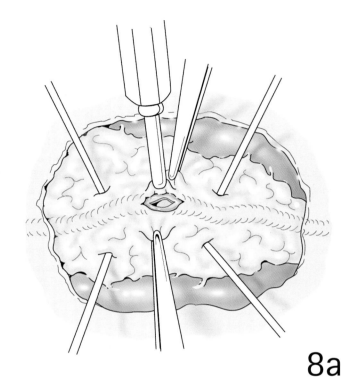

8a

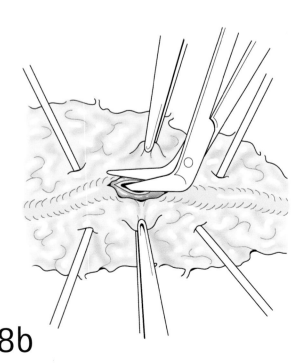

8b

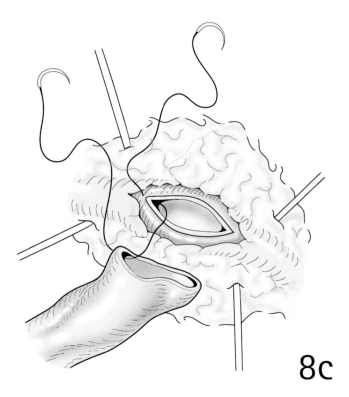

8c

8d, e

With the distal end of the vein held open by the assistant with two fine forceps, a continuous anastomosis is constructed beginning either at the toe or the heel. Three or four suture throws are placed through the vein and the coronary artery, after which the vein is lowered into place and the anastomosis completed with approximately 12–15 continuous sutures. A fine nerve hook can be used to snug up the continuous suture to avoid looseness or gapping of the anastomosis. After the anastomosis is completed, the vein graft should be gently filled with blood from the cardioplegic line and approximately 50 mL instilled into the coronary artery. Any identified sites of anastomotic leakage can then be repaired with single 7/0 sutures. Next, the vein graft should be occluded with a soft-tipped vascular clamp filled with heparinized saline and sized appropriately for a tension-free graft. If a retrograde cardioplegic catheter is in place, additional cardioplegic solution or blood can be administered at this point while the heart is repositioned for additional inferior wall or lateral wall anastomoses.

For lateral wall grafts, it is possible to place a cold lap pad behind the heart and to retract the apex of the left ventricle gently to the right, exposing the vessels of the lateral wall. Exact positioning is dependent on the sites that are chosen for distal anastomoses, and either using gentle manual traction or Silastic tapes, the portion of the obtuse marginal or other lateral arterial branches are stabilized and incised. For open vein graft-to-artery anastomoses and the left lateral aspect of the heart, three or four throws of the continuous 7/0 polypropylene suture are placed, with the vein held open by the assistant. The suturing is begun from outside-in on the vein heel, and the subsequent stitch is placed from the inside of the coronary artery to one side of the apex of the arteriotomy. Suturing is then continued around the heel of the vein graft and the apex of the arteriotomy, after which the vein is lowered into place and the anastomosis completed, with more continuous suture bites brought around the toe of the vein graft. Again, the anastomosis can be assessed for patency and intactness with the administration of 50 mL or more of cold blood cardioplegic solution.

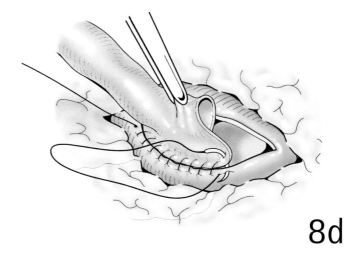

8d

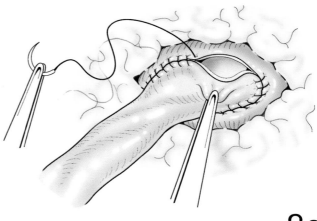

8e

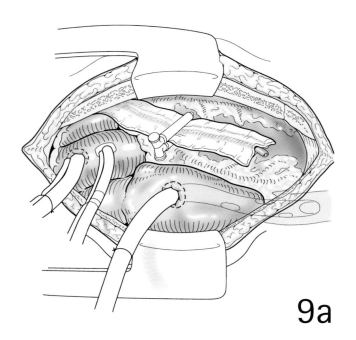

9a

INTERNAL MAMMARY ARTERY ANASTOMOSIS TO THE LEFT ANTERIOR DESCENDING CORONARY ARTERY

9a, b After all of the distal vein graft anastomoses are completed, the IMA is retrieved from the lateral pericardial space or the left pleural cavity and brought up into the surgical field. An appropriate anastomotic site on the left anterior descending artery is identified and can be stabilized with the use of Silastic tapes. Before the artery is incised, the length of the mammary artery pedicle is assessed for adequacy. Should the pedicle graft appear to be too short to reach the intended site, the fascia and muscle tissue of the pedicle can be incised carefully to avoid injury to the artery itself. One or more such transverse fascial incisions can be made with pedicle graft lengthening of up to 5–10 mm for each fascial incision.

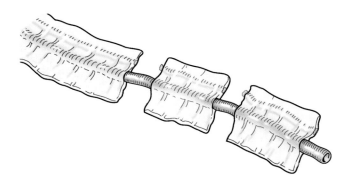

9b

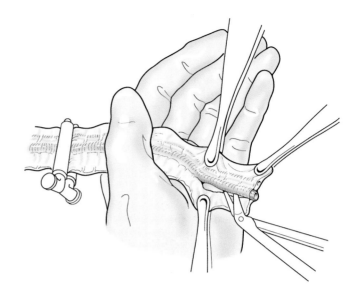

10a–c Once an adequate pedicle length is determined, the LAD is incised and the mammary artery incised on an angle at an appropriate distal site. Because of distal branching of the mammary artery, the artery caliber may be quite small. Every attempt should be made to transect the mammary artery as proximal as possible.

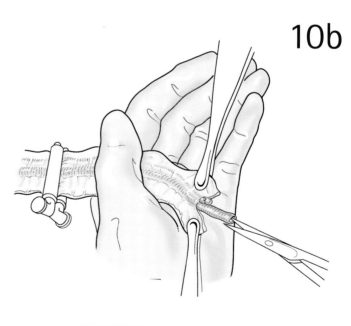

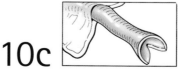

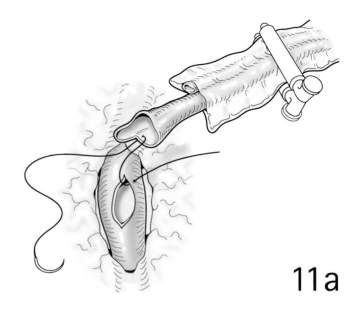

11a

11a, b Avoiding any direct contact with the endothelial surface of the mammary artery itself, and with the assistant holding the mammary artery pedicle in such a way as to expose the distal beveled cut, a 7/0 or 8/0 polypropylene suture is used to construct an anastomosis of approximately 3–4 mm in length beginning near the heel of the mammary artery, with a continuous suture brought around the apex of the LAD arteriotomy. After three or four suture throws are placed between the mammary and LAD, the pedicle graft is lowered onto the surface of the heart, the suture is gently snugged up, and the anastomosis is completed with several additional throws of the polypropylene suture. After the anastomosis is completed and the LAD securely tied in place, the soft vascular clip is removed from the mammary artery pedicle and assessment of flow into the distal LAD is made. In addition, the intactness of the anastomosis is examined. If necessary, an additional suture is placed at any site of anastomotic leakage or bleeding. It may be helpful to use a fine nerve hook to tighten the continuous suture gently before tying the two ends, to avoid anastomotic gapping.

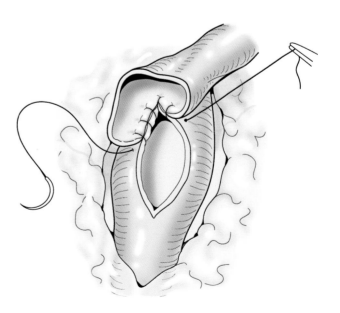

11b

12 Many surgeons secure the IMA pedicle to the epicardial surface to avoid tension on the IMA-to-LAD anastomosis as well as the possibility of pedicle twisting once the heart is filled and contracting. 6/0 Polypropylene can be used, with interrupted sutures placed superficially in the epicardium and through the lateral fascial tissue of the pedicle. Systemic cooling is reversed during construction of the IMA-to-LAD anastomosis, and the aortic cross-clamp is removed once the distal anastomosis is completed. Having an open pedicled LIMA graft provides the obvious benefit of immediate reperfusion past any proximal left anterior descending coronary obstructions while the vein grafts are anastomosed sequentially to the ascending aorta. An alternate strategy is to perform the proximal vein graft-to-aortic anastomoses with the aortic cross-clamp still in place so that all regions of the heart are reperfused once the cross-clamp is removed.

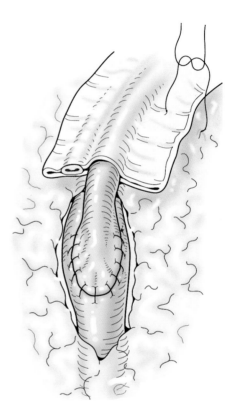

12

Sequential distal vein graft anastomoses

13a–d

In instances in which available vein for grafting is limited or when there is concern about multiple anastomoses on the ascending aorta, one can construct two or more distal touchdown sites with a single vein graft. The optimal spatial relationships of vein graft to artery may be difficult to assess in the decompressed arrested heart. One should avoid tension and excessive length between the end vein segment to the distal coronary artery anastomosis site and the side-to-side vein graft coronary artery anastomotic site that creates the second or third touchdown point for a single vein graft. The easiest orientation for the side-to-side anastomosis is with the vein parallel to the artery. Because the proximal anastomosis is not yet constructed, it is possible to perform the incontinuity side-to-side anastomosis in a similar fashion with the continuous 7/0 polypropylene, placing the initial sutures through the distal end of the venotomy and the distal extent of the arteriotomy. After several sutures are placed with the vein held in the air, traction is applied on the suture, the vein graft is approximated to the artery, and the anastomosis is completed. The precise orientation of the vein graft to the artery can be varied, and the principle remains the same, namely, to place the vein graft onto the artery in such a way that the side-to-side anastomosis is neither under tension nor distorting either artery or vein graft.

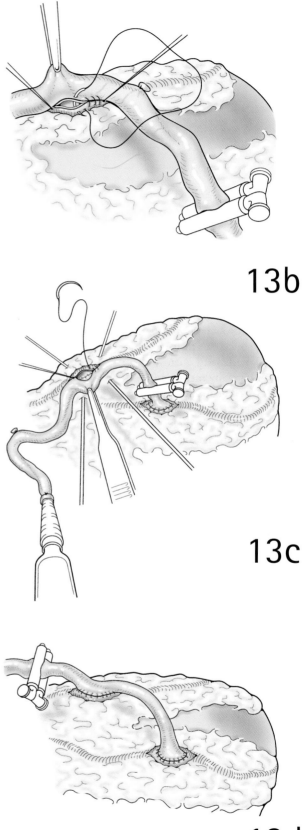

13b

13c

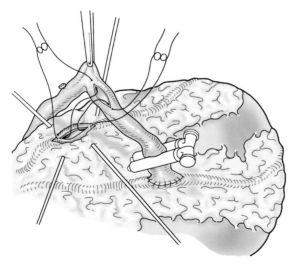

13a

13d

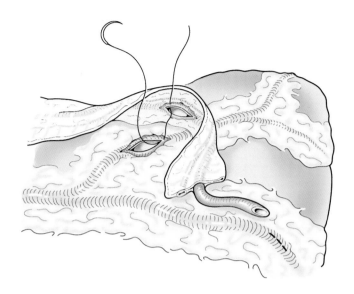

14a

14a, b In the somewhat uncommon situation in which it is necessary to construct more than one distal touchdown site with the pedicled IMA, the order of grafting is reversed and the side-to-side anastomosis is done first, so that the mammary artery pedicle that remains attached to its origin can be freely manipulated. Again, the artery is carefully measured, the overlying fascia at the site of the side-to-side anastomosis is carefully dissected free, a 2- to 3-mm parallel longitudinal incision is made on the under-surface of the IMA, and the anastomosis is begun with the pedicle held in the air. A common problem that can occur when an incontinuity IMA anastomosis is performed is that insufficient length of distal IMA segment is retained, with the result that the end-to-side IMA-to-coronary artery anastomosis is constructed under tension. Many surgeons avoid making multiple distal anastomoses with a single pedicled mammary graft when it is intended for the LAD. This strategy is based on the superior long-term function of the well-constructed LIMA-to-LAD graft.

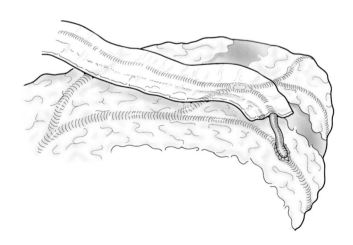

14b

Coronary endarterectomy

Occasionally, one encounters such a diffusely diseased coronary artery that coronary endarterectomy appears to be the only option for a satisfactory distal anastomosis. In general, coronary endarterectomy should be reserved for those rare situations in which an adequate touchdown site for the distal anastomosis cannot be identified. In addition, the smaller the residual arterial size is after the endarterectomy, the more likely that an early graft failure will occur. For this reason, endarterectomy of the right coronary artery is more commonly performed than is endarterectomy of the LAD or lateral wall vessels.

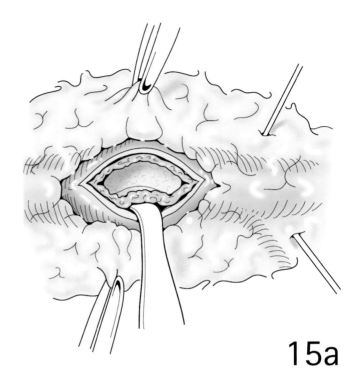

15a

15a–e The endarterectomy technique is begun by establishing a dissection plane between the hard luminal plaque and the outer wall of the coronary artery. A fine tissue elevator can be used to initiate the plaque dissection, with care being taken to avoid disrupting the outer arterial wall. Once the atheromatous luminal plaque is encircled bluntly, the core is grasped firmly and peanut dissectors placed lateral to the coronary artery to provide counter traction as the plaque is gently retracted. On the proximal end, once a reasonable portion of core plaque is retracted or resistance is met, the core should be transected and the proximal plaque allowed to retract back up into the artery. Distally, the same process of counter traction with peanut dissectors and traction on the plaque is applied, with the hope for removal of a tapered distal cast of the artery. After the endarterectomy core is removed, the arterial wall is carefully inspected for residual plaque, which can be gently removed, and the anastomosis is now constructed into a relatively plaque-free area of the artery.

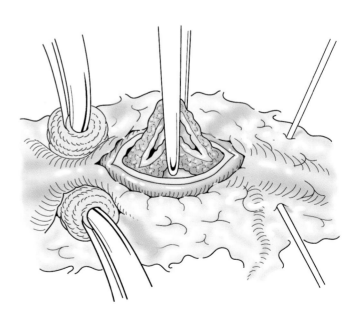

15b

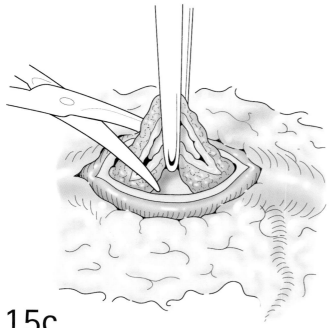

15c

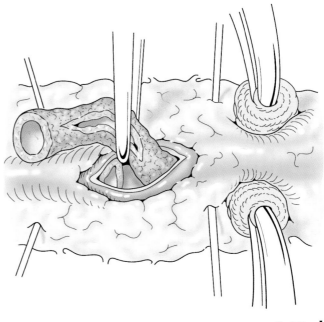

15d

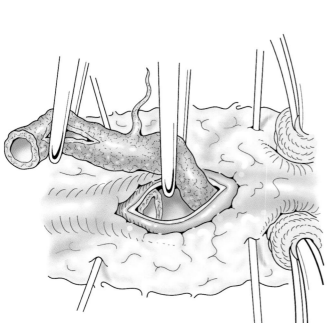

15e

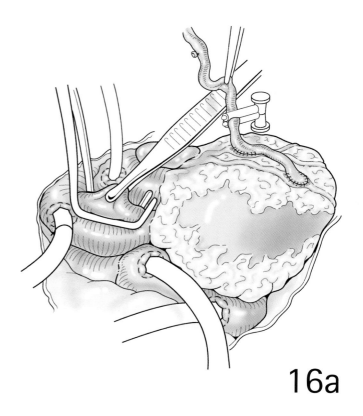

16a

Proximal vein graft anastomoses

16a, b Once the aortic cross-clamp is removed and reflow to the heart is initiated, a vascular occlusion clamp is placed partially across the ascending aorta. This clamp should be positioned with a sufficient portion of the anterior aspect of the ascending aorta excluded in the clamp to allow for two or more aortotomies for vein graft anastomoses. The aortotomy is created by incising the excluded aorta wall with a pointed scalpel tip for a distance of approximately 4 mm, after which an aorta wall punch of variable size, usually 4 mm in diameter, is used to create the aortotomy. The sites for the aortotomies should be carefully chosen to avoid areas of atheromatous or plaque buildup. If an aortic incision and an attempted aortotomy are made in a region of significant wall thickening and obvious atheromatous debris, the site should be closed with a 4/0 or 5/0 Prolene suture and another site chosen for the proximal aortotomy.

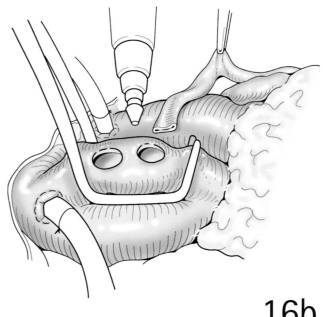

16b

17a–c Once the aortotomy is performed, the assistant should position the beveled proximal end of the vein graft in such a way as to allow for suturing from the outside of the vein at the heel to the inside of the aorta. It is important to construct the anastomosis from inside the aorta out to avoid disrupting atheromatous material in the ascending aorta.

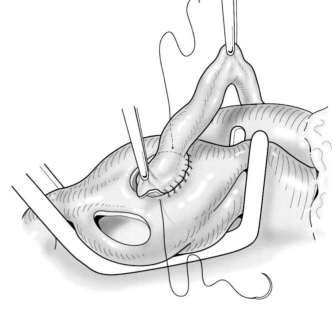

17b

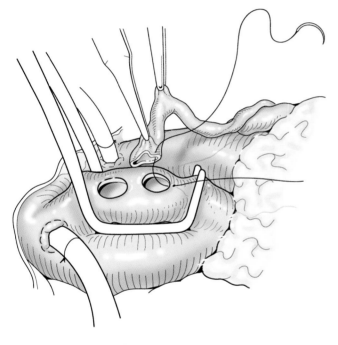

17a

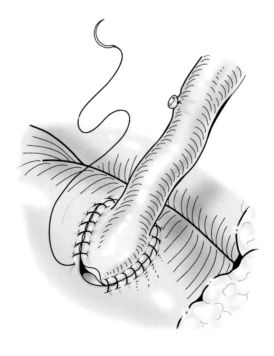

17c

18 After the vein graft to the aorta is secured and all of the proximal anastomoses that are intended within the area of partial occlusion of the ascending aorta are completed, the pump flow should be reduced as the clamp is removed. Next, the vein grafts, which should be temporarily occluded distally, are deaired by fine needle puncture to avoid entrapped air. Blood flow is then established into the distal coronary arteries.

In situations in which significant ascending aortic thickening or atheromatous buildup is apparent or suspected, the use of the side-biting clamp can be avoided by constructing the proximal anastomoses with the cross-clamp still in place. After the distal anastomoses are completed, and with flow through the LIMA graft to the LAD temporarily suspended, appropriate sites on the anterolateral aspect of the ascending aorta can be identified and small aortotomies constructed in the same fashion as described previously. Care must be taken to avoid placing the proximal anastomoses either too close to the aortic root or too lateral, especially on the right aspect of the aorta. With the heart arrested, the pulmonary artery, right atrium, and left ventricular outflow tract are quite decompressed. It is easy to choose inappropriate aortotomy sites that are too proximal or lateral on the ascending aorta under this circumstance.

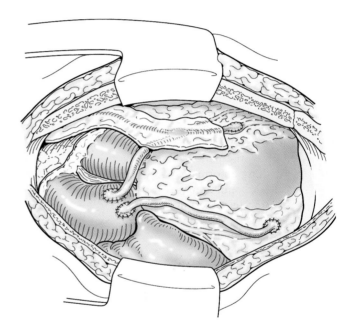

18

POSTOPERATIVE CARE

Separation from cardiopulmonary bypass, reversal of heparinization, wound closure, and general physiological management should be expeditiously and simply managed. In some situations, the patient's hemodynamic stability is sluggish, especially if the ischemic period was protracted because of the construction of multiple grafts. Low-dose inotropic stimulation may be helpful, but excessive inotropic administration may inappropriately increase the energy demands on the postischemic heart and may contribute to a low cardiac output state several hours after surgery. In patients with extensive and diffuse coronary artery disease, especially older patients, maintenance of an adequate perfusion pressure may also be an important component of early postoperative management, particularly because vasodilatation may develop from hemodilution, rewarming, or other postcardiotomy changes. Such pathological vasodilatation may be easily reversed with low-dose alpha-adrenergic stimulation.

Complete systemic rewarming should be achieved to avoid hypothermia-induced myocardial depression or excessive vasoconstriction. After systemic cooling during cardiopulmonary bypass, the patient's extremities may remain cold. Despite attaining a normal core body temperature near the end of the cardiopulmonary bypass run, the patient may quickly become hypothermic in the immediate postbypass period. In this case, topical rewarming should be carried out once the patient is in the ICU.

Adequate drainage of the mediastinal space is enhanced with a posterior pericardial drainage tube, along with an anterior tube placed just to the right of the heart. If the left pleural cavity has been entered for harvest of the LIMA, an infero-posterior drainage tube should be placed, as well as in the left pleural space.

OUTCOMES

From the mid-1980s until recently, patients who underwent CABG were warned by their physicians and surgeons that late failure of vein grafts should be expected. Various estimates of the scope of graft failure have been that 50 per cent or more of grafts would occlude between 5 and 10 years after surgery. On the other hand, most estimates of late functioning of the LIMA graft to the LAD were for a 90 per cent or greater probability.

The LIMA graft is now being constructed to the LAD in the great majority of patients who have a CABG procedure. The use of this graft approaches 100 per cent in patients younger than 65 or 70 years old who undergo CABG and have disease present in the LAD system. As a result of this shift to continue mammary artery grafting over the last 10 or 15 years, and in recognition of the fact that this particular graft configuration remains functional for many years in more than 90 per cent

of patients and conveys clear survival benefit for most patients because of sustained patency and flow to the LAD system, the number of patients who present for reoperation and repeat CABG has declined somewhat in the last few years. When a patient has had the traditional operation and is referred for repeat CABG today, frequently the LIMA-to-LAD graft is found to be functioning, whereas one or more of the vein grafts have occluded.

Even this finding, however, is occurring less frequently, because intensive secondary preventive measures have been applied to patients who present with severe coronary artery disease that requires bypass grafting. Strong evidence that antiplatelet agents such as aspirin and lipid-lowering medications enhance the resistance of native arteries and bypass conduits to progressive atherosclerosis has fostered the long-term pharmacological treatment of post-CABG patients.

To what extent the expanded use of arterial conduits in younger patients who require bypass grafting enhances the durability of the coronary bypass procedure remains to be established. For the majority of patients who present in need of bypass grafting, especially those in the older age range, and particularly those who can be expected to follow secondary preventive protocols carefully, this traditional procedure of a LIMA graft to LAD and saphenous vein grafts to the remaining obstructed coronary arteries is believed to be quite reliable. This improvement in durability of benefit from the traditional CABG procedure should be conveyed to the prospective patient, who may have been subjected to faulty information about excessively frequent coronary artery bypass graft failures based on outdated follow-up information.

FURTHER READING

Barner, H.B., Standeven, J., Reece, J. 1985. Twelve year experience with the internal mammary artery for coronary bypass. *Journal of Thoracic and Cardiovascular Surgery* 90, 668–75.

Campeau, L., Enjalbert, M., Lesperance, J., *et al.* 1984. The relation of risk factors to the development of atherosclerosis in saphenous vein bypass grafts and the progression of disease in the native circulation: a study of 10 years after aortocoronary bypass surgery. *New England Journal of Medicine* 311, 1329–32.

Edwards, F.E., Clark, R.E., Schwartz, M. 1994. Impact of internal mammary artery conduit on operative mortality in coronary revascularization. *Annals of Thoracic Surgery* 57, 27–32.

Gotto, A.M. Jr. 1998 Risk factor modification: rationale for management of dyslipidemia. *American Journal of Medicine* 104, 6S–8S.

Loop, F.D., Lytle, B.W., Cosgrove, D.M., *et al.* 1986. Influence of the internal-mammary-artery graft on 10-year survival and other cardiac events. *New England Journal of Medicine* 314, 1–6.

Lytle, B.W., Loop, F.D., Cosgrove, D.M., *et al.* 1985. Long-term (5–12 years) serial studies of internal mammary artery and saphenous vein coronary bypass grafts. *Journal of Thoracic and Cardiovascular Surgery* 89, 248–58.

Expanded use of arterial conduits

BRIAN F. BUXTON MB, MS, FRACS, FRCS
Professor of Cardiac Surgery, University of Melbourne School of Medicine, Melbourne, Victoria, Australia; Director of Cardiac Surgery, Austin Hospital, Heidelberg, Victoria, Australia

HISTORY

Most of the techniques for the correction of coronary artery disease were developed in the latter part of the twentieth century. The extensive modification, evaluation, and refinement of procedures; the development of angioplasty and stenting; and an improved understanding of basic pathological mechanisms (in grafts and in native coronary arteries) have led to the current multidisciplinary approach to the management of coronary artery disease. These changes have been associated with an improvement in the quality of life and survival rates for patients who are undergoing coronary artery bypass grafting.

The use of the internal thoracic artery (ITA) as a graft to revascularize the myocardium originated with the work of Vineberg in 1946, when he ligated the ITA distally and implanted it into a tunnel in the left ventricle. Arterial interposition grafts were pioneered for clinical use by the Canadian surgeon, Gordon Murray, in 1954. Direct arterial revascularization followed. The early use of the human autologous saphenous vein by Sabiston in 1962 and Garrett in 1964 predated the widespread use of firstly interposition and then aortocoronary vein grafts by Favaloro and Johnson. The first series of ITA grafts was reported by Green and colleagues in 1966. Following the report from the Cleveland Clinic by Floyd Loop and others in 1986, the use of single and subsequently bilateral ITA grafts became routine.

The expanded use of arterial grafts using *in situ* ITAs and gastroepiploic or splenic arteries was advocated by Sterling Edwards. However, initially this approach did not prove popular. Carpentier also attempted to use the radial artery (RA) as a free graft, but the early results were disappointing. Since then, the gastroepiploic, inferior epigastric, subscapular, radial, and ulnar arteries have all been used in clinical practice. However, except for the RA, none of these vessels has had wide acceptance.

In 1992, Acar and colleagues reintroduced the RA graft after discovering that many of Carpentier's initial RA grafts had remained patent and free from disease. The ability to achieve extensive arterial revascularization of patients with multi-vessel coronary artery disease was further enhanced by the introduction of techniques of sequential, T- or Y-grafting and extension grafting. Therefore, extended arterial grafting is now possible in the majority of patients using combinations of the proximal and distal grafting techniques and a variety of conduits.

PRINCIPLES AND JUSTIFICATION

The fundamental principle behind using arterial grafts is to provide durable conduits that can be deployed, with low morbidity and mortality, to bypass obstructive lesions in the coronary arteries. The *in situ* left or right ITA, when grafted to the left anterior descending coronary artery (LAD), has a patency of 90–95 per cent at 10 years. Although no direct comparisons of the late patency of arterial free grafts (AFGs) compared with saphenous vein grafts exist, the evidence suggests that the late patency of arterial grafts is superior. The choice of the target artery may also affect the outcome.

Despite the increase in surgical complexity, the early morbidity or mortality using arterial grafts compared with vein grafts is not different. Indeed, current survival data suggest that a benefit is associated with bilateral versus single ITA grafting. So far, no documented survival benefit has been demonstrated when using additional AFGs.

PREOPERATIVE ASSESSMENT AND PREPARATION

General

Patients who present for coronary artery bypass surgery are frequently elderly. They often experience other manifestations of atherosclerosis and frequently have single- or multi-organ dysfunction. Thus, the preliminary assessment should evaluate not only their coronary arteries but also their peripheral vascular and cerebrovascular circulation and general organ function.

High-quality coronary angiography is required in all patients, usually within 12 months of surgery, or less if a recent ischemic event has occurred. If valve disease or poor left ventricular function with an intracardiac thrombus is suspected, a preoperative echocardiogram is mandatory. In elective cases, cardiac catheterization and left ventriculography are performed. In patients with a low ejection fraction due to stunning or hibernation, stress echocardiography, thallium scintigraphy, positron emission tomography, or magnetic resonance imaging may be required to evaluate myocardium perfusion or viability.

A systematic review of the pulmonary, renal, and hepatic function is routinely performed. A coagulation profile and assessment of platelet function may be required in patients with a history of bleeding or use of antiplatelet therapy. Particular attention should be paid to the chest x-ray to exclude chronic obstructive airways disease or other pulmonary pathology. If any doubt exists about lung function, pulmonary function tests should be performed. This test is of particular importance in patients undergoing bilateral ITA harvest.

Assessment of conduits

INTERNAL THORACIC ARTERY

The ITA is rarely affected by atherosclerosis, although mild intimal hyperplasia is common. Therefore the ITA is rarely discarded. In our experience the ITA can be used in 99 per cent of patients. A major contraindication is the presence of an aortic arch or subclavian artery atheroma, which can be detected, respectively, by a bruit in the neck or a reduction in the radial pulse. Patients who present for reoperation usually have their ITAs angiographed to exclude the possibility of injury from previous surgery.

RADIAL ARTERY

The RA has a relatively high prevalence of intimal disease compared with the ITA. Ultrasound examination of the RA is therefore desirable to identify arteries that have intimal plaques and calcification. Intimal disease and calcification are particular problems in older patients, patients with diabetes, and those with peripheral vascular disease. Ultrasound exam-

ination of the forearm arteries identifies disease in the ulnar artery and also any anatomical variations of the RA, such as a high origin from the brachial artery.

A modified Allen's test is used for screening all patients who are undergoing RA harvesting; a recovery time of less than 10 seconds is considered normal. However, the RA can be removed safely in some patients with a recovery time that is longer than normal if the Doppler ultrasound assessment of hand collateral circulation is normal. The main concern is a false-negative test, which may result in the removal of a dominant RA in a patient with an absent, hypoplastic, or damaged ulnar artery. This situation may occur in the presence of a persisting median (interosseous) artery or a proximal origin of the palmar branch of the RA.

SAPHENOUS VEIN

Although arterial grafting is preferred, all patients should have at least one leg prepared for saphenous vein harvesting in case suitable arterial grafts are not available. Evaluation of the peripheral pulses is essential if saphenous vein grafts are to be used in addition to arterial conduits. A glossary of techniques that are used for arterial graft harvesting is presented in Table 8.1.

Table 8.1 *Glossary of techniques for arterial harvest*

Skeletonized	The artery is removed without any surrounding tissue.
Semiskeletonized	The artery is left with collateral veins. An example of this technique is when the radial artery is harvested with the venae comitantes.
Pedicled	The arterial graft is surrounded by collateral veins and other tissues. For example, an ITA pedicle contains the transversus thoracis muscle and fascia, extrapleural tissue, pleura, nerves, and lymphatic drainage channels.
In situ	The two types of *in situ* grafts are the ITA, which retains its connection to the first part of the subclavian artery, and the gastroepiploic artery, which remains joined to the gastroduodenal artery.
Arterial free graft	All anatomic attachments are disconnected.

Grafting strategy

Removal of a major artery for use as a graft subjects the patient to the risk of ischemia and sepsis. Harvesting arterial grafts is time consuming; and once on bypass, it is difficult to access additional arterial conduits is difficult. Therefore, a grafting strategy needs to be formulated before cardiopulmonary bypass. Our preference for treating patients younger than 70 years who have multi-vessel coronary artery disease is to use both ITAs and one RA; in older patients, we use a single ITA and one or both radial arteries. Patients with unstable symptoms who require emergent or salvage procedures usually receive one ITA supplemented with saphenous vein grafts to reduce the harvesting time and, thus, the period of myocardial ischemia. In patients who have a severely diseased or calcified aorta, off-pump coronary bypass surgery to minimize the risk of cerebral atheroembolism is preferred using one or both *in situ* ITA grafts and an RA graft. Other options include choosing alternative cannulation sites (e.g. the femoral or axillary artery) or, in extreme situations, using deep hypothermia with replacement of the ascending aorta.

The decision about the sites for the distal anastomoses and the routing of *in situ* ITA grafts is usually made during the surgical procedure because it is often difficult to predict the best configuration. Where possible, we direct both *in situ* ITA grafts to the left system. The RA is grafted to the remaining vessels and is either attached proximally to the aorta or to the left ITA (LITA) as a Y-graft. When additional length is required, the RA can be anastomosed to the distal ITA as a graft extension. Using sequential anastomoses can increase the number of distal anastomoses.

When a single LITA is used, this artery is usually grafted to the LAD. When using both *in situ* ITAs, the RITA is anastomosed to the LAD or diagonal branch after passing anterior to the aorta. This strategy leaves the LITA for grafting the circumflex system. Less commonly, the transverse sinus route is chosen for grafting the RITA to the intermediate or proximal circumflex marginal; the LITA is then sutured to the LAD.

ANESTHESIA

A number of different anesthetic techniques can be used in patients who are being treated for coronary artery disease. The basic principles are to provide a narcotic-based relaxant anesthesia, with an inhalation agent supplemented as required.

Our preference is to introduce lines for invasive monitoring before induction. Arterial blood pressure is monitored through an RA line; when bilateral RA grafts are planned, a femoral or brachial arterial line is used. The RA pressure may be inaccurate during cardiopulmonary bypass, particularly in the presence of hypothermia or subclavian arteriosclerosis.

Although the central venous pressure frequently correlates with the left atrial filling pressure, this correlation is not always the case. We advocate the use of routine pulmonary artery catheterization and monitoring in all patients who have arterial coronary artery bypass grafting so that cardiac output and the response to pharmacological manipulation can be assessed precisely. Monitoring arterial and mixed venous blood gases is essential during cardiopulmonary bypass. Serum potassium also needs to be monitored regularly and kept within a range of 4–5 mmol/L.

Transesophageal echocardiography is being used perioperatively with increasing frequency to provide qualitative and quantitative information about cardiac filling and regional contractility and to detect the presence of an intracardiac thrombus and associated valve disease. Myocardial ischemia can be detected by a segmental wall motion abnormality. Echocardiography can also detect unexpected problems such as the presence of a left atrial or left ventricular thrombus or ischemic mitral regurgitation. Transesophageal echocardiography and epiaortic ultrasound have proved valuable in the assessment of aortic atheroma, which is often not palpable and, if left unchecked, is a potential source of atheroembolism.

OPERATION

Techniques for harvesting arteries

INTERNAL THORACIC ARTERY

Anatomy

1a, b

The ITA arises from the first part of the subclavian artery in the root of the neck just above and behind the sternal end of the clavicle and descends anteromedially behind the internal thoracic jugular and brachiocephalic veins. The phrenic nerve crosses the ITA obliquely from its medial to its lateral side, the nerve usually passing in front of the artery. The artery descends vertically 1 cm lateral to the sternal border, behind the first six costal cartilages, between the anterior intercostal membranes and internal intercostal muscles. Down to the level of the second or third costal cartilage, the ITA is separated from the pleura by a strong layer of endothoracic fascia and inferiorly by the transversus thoracis muscle. The ITA is accompanied by venae comitantes, which join to form a single vein at the level of the third costal cartilage; the internal thoracic vein ascends medial to the artery and terminates in the brachiocephalic vein; note that the right internal thoracic vein terminates at a lower level than the left internal thoracic vein. At the level of the sixth intercostal space, the ITA divides into terminal branches: the musculophrenic artery and the superior epigastric artery.

The pericardiacophrenic artery is the first branch of the ITA and usually divides near the upper limit of the mobilization of the ITA. This branch lies immediately behind the lateral or inferior border of the subclavian vein, where it accompanies and supplies the phrenic nerve. Several other branches arise from the upper ITA to supply the manubrium, the sternothyroid muscle, and the mediastinum.

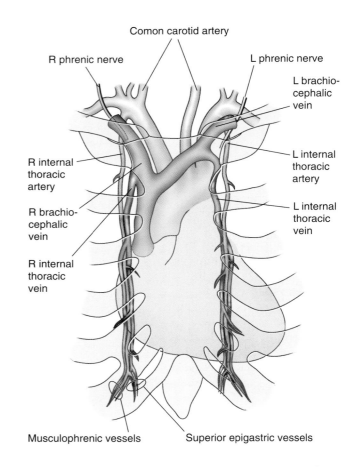

1a

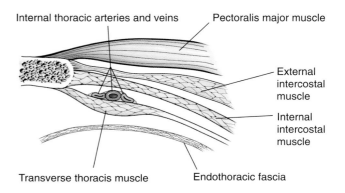

1b

2 In the anterior intercostal spaces, the perforating, sternal, and intercostal branches of the ITA form a rich anastomosis that supplies the sternum. The ITA branches are connected with the posterior intercostal arteries and terminal branches of the superior, epigastric, and musculophrenic arteries. In addition to the classic anterior branches, the anatomic variants consist of sternal/perforating, sternal/intercostal, and persisting/posterior intercostal branches. These branches should be divided near the ITA to preserve the collateral supply of the sternum and minimize the risk of sternal ischemia. This figure has been modified with permission from de Jesus RA, Acland RD. Anatomic study of the collateral blood supply of the sternum. *Ann Thorac Surg* 1996;59(1):163–168.

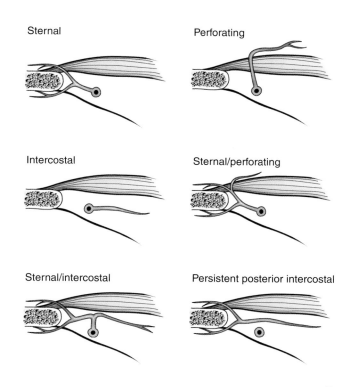

Sternal   Perforating

Intercostal   Sternal/perforating

Sternal/intercostal   Persistent posterior intercostal

2

Surgical technique

3a–d
The RITA is normally mobilized after the left side has been completed (see Chapter 7). Harvesting the RITA with a pedicle has the advantage of simplicity, and the surrounding tissue provides protection for the ITA. The disadvantages are greater disruption of the chest wall and the graft length is shorter than when the skeletonized technique is used. The technique proceeds in a similar fashion to that of the left; however, at the proximal end, additional dissection is required to obtain maximal length. After the second and first perforating branches are divided, the ITA dissection is continued proximally until it disappears beneath the inferior border of the right brachiocephalic vein. Division of the pericardiacophrenic, manubrial, sternothyroid, and mediastinal branches in the triangle formed by the ITA and internal thoracic vein and the phrenic nerve is important. Division of these branches and mobilization of the ITA above and behind the lower border of the brachiocephalic vein provides an additional 1 cm in length.

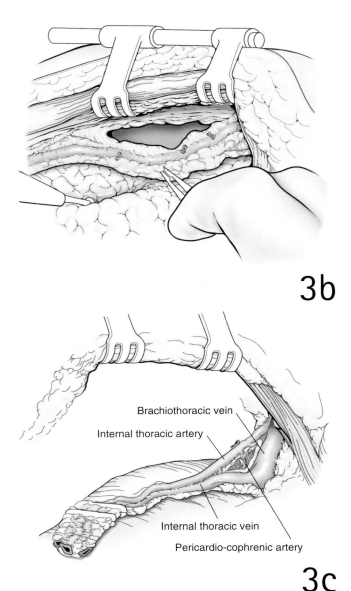

3b

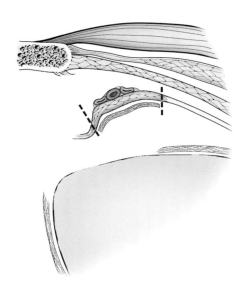

3a

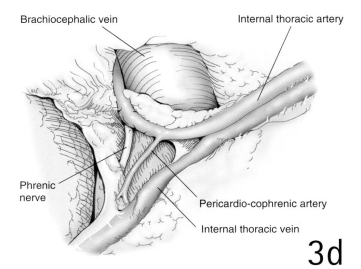

3c

Brachiothoracic vein

Internal thoracic artery

Internal thoracic vein

Pericardio-cophrenic artery

Brachiocephalic vein

Internal thoracic artery

Phrenic nerve

Pericardio-cophrenic artery

Internal thoracic vein

3d

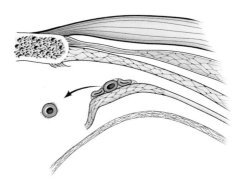

4a

4a, b
Because of the asymmetry of the heart, achieving the maximum length of the RITA is desirable so that left-sided coronary arteries or distal right coronary artery (RCA) branches can be anastomosed directly. Skeletonization or semiskeletonization techniques provide additional length and have the added advantage of preserving the collateral blood supply of the chest wall. Our preference is semiskeletonization, which is particularly important in elderly and diabetic patients, in whom sternal ischemia is more likely to cause infection.

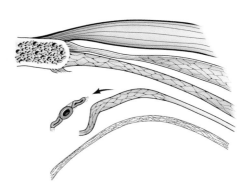

4b

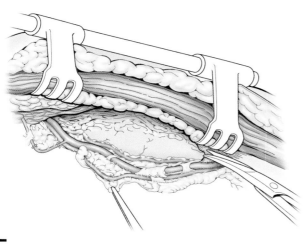

5

5
After elevation of the chest wall, the RITA and collateral veins are exposed through one of the upper anterior intercostal spaces by separation of the attachment of the transversus thoracis muscle and fascia from the sternum. The ITA and veins are mobilized by separation from the transversus muscle and fascia. The dissection is extended distally to include a length of the musculophrenic or superior epigastric artery. The proximal dissection continues superiorly beneath the lower border of the brachiocephalic vein. In the upper two intercostal spaces the ITA is separated from the pleura only by endothoracic fascia; and if the ITA is harvested carefully, the technique can be performed entirely extrapleurally. The RITA is passed posterior and lateral to the thymus and then medially to enter the pericardium through a small window created with the angle between the superior vena cava and the left brachiocephalic vein. The location, deep in the mediastinum, separates the RITA from the posterior aspect of the sternum, thus preventing injury at reoperation.

RADIAL ARTERY

Anatomy

6 The RA arises from the bifurcation of the brachial artery in the cubital fossa and terminates by forming the deep palmar arch in the hand. The RA lies immediately beneath the deep fascia, surrounded by collateral veins. The brachioradialis muscle and the lateral cutaneous nerve of the forearm cover its proximal portion. The terminal sensory branch of the radial nerve lies immediately lateral to the proximal third of the RA.

The RA has a number of anatomical variations. The most common and important variation is the high origin of the RA, which occurs in 14 per cent of upper limbs. In these patients, the RA is found to originate in the proximal half of the brachial artery in 11 per cent, with 2 per cent arising from the axillary artery and 1 per cent from the distal and upper brachial artery above the cubital fossa. In the forearm, the position of the artery is usually constant.

Anastomoses at the wrist and hand vary. In a recent anatomical study, the superficial palmar arch of the ulnar artery was found to provide the blood supply to all fingers in 67 per cent of hands. The 'classic' type of superficial palmar arch, in which the superficial branch of the RA joins the superficial palmar arch of the ulnar artery, was found to be relatively uncommon (12.5 per cent). The complete deep palmar arch, in which continuity exists between the deep palmar branches of the radial and ulnar arteries, was found in 87.5 per cent of hands. However, every hand had at least one major branch connecting the radial and the ulnar arteries.

Three structures may be damaged during harvesting, the lateral cutaneous nerves of the forearm, the superficial branch of the radial nerve, and the deep branch of the radial nerve. Damage to this latter structure, although rare, can cause serious complications, as it provides the motor supply to the extensor muscles of the forearm. Care should be taken when dissecting the proximal part of the RA to avoid deep retraction proximally toward the brachial artery.

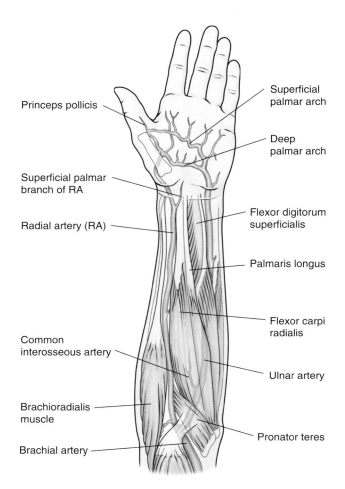

Princeps pollicis

Superficial palmar branch of RA

Radial artery (RA)

Common interosseous artery

Brachioradialis muscle

Brachial artery

Superficial palmar arch

Deep palmar arch

Flexor digitorum superficialis

Palmaris longus

Flexor carpi radialis

Ulnar artery

Pronator teres

6

Surgical technique

7a, b The artery is exposed through an incision overlying and slightly medial to the RA. After the deep fascia is divided, the RA can be seen with its paired venae comitantes. To mobilize the RA, the deep fascia should be divided just lateral to the tendon of the flexor carpi radialis muscle. A few small branches pass vertically and supply the brachioradialis muscle. These branches may cause a hematoma if damaged. The RA is semiskeletonized and is mobilized with its venae comitantes. Side branches are divided between metal clips and clipped close to the artery, whereas smaller branches can be cauterized. We have used an ultrasonic probe and found this technique to be satisfactory, although somewhat slower than the clipping technique.

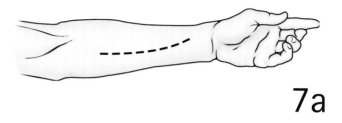

7a

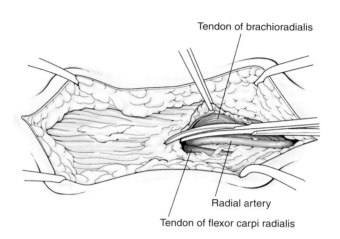

Tendon of brachioradialis

Radial artery

Tendon of flexor carpi radialis

7b

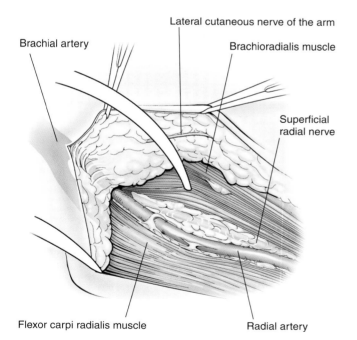

Lateral cutaneous nerve of the arm

Brachial artery

Brachioradialis muscle

Superficial radial nerve

Flexor carpi radialis muscle

Radial artery

8 The distal end of the RA is divided approximately 2 cm above the wrist, after the distal end of the wound is elevated. The proximal end of the RA can be followed to the bifurcation of the brachial artery. The bifurcation is heralded by the presence of the radial recurrent artery and a complex of large veins. Once the distal end has been divided, a solution of papaverine, 1 mmol/L (40 mg/100 mL), mixed with an equal amount of blood or Ringer's lactate is injected into the distal end of the artery. The distal end is then clipped and allowed to dilate under arterial pressure while the upper end of the dissection is completed. The RA is usually divided approximately 1 cm distal to the bifurcation of the brachial artery; if extra length is required, the recurrent RA can be divided.

8

ULNAR ARTERY

Occasionally, when we have had no other choice, we have used the ulnar artery as a bypass conduit. Patients who have a dominant RA, as judged by an abnormal Allen's test, are unable to have this vessel harvested. The ulnar artery has been found to be a satisfactory alternative in many of these patients. The major concern with removing the ulnar artery is its proximity to the ulnar nerve, which supplies the intrinsic muscles of the hand. Direct trauma or ischemia may cause an ulnar nerve palsy.

Anatomy

The ulnar artery arises in the cubital fossa as the larger of the two terminal branches of the brachial artery. The ulnar artery (UA) passes along the medial aspect of the flexor compartment of the forearm and terminates at the flexor retinaculum. In the cubital fossa, the ulnar artery lies on the brachialis muscle lateral to the median nerve. The UA leaves the cubital fossa deep to the pronator teres muscle and is crossed by the median nerve. In the flexor compartment of the forearm, the ulnar artery lies on the flexor digitorum profundus. Before it meets the ulnar nerve, the artery passes deep to the flexor digitorum superficialis, underneath the fibrous arch between its humeroulnar and radial origins. In the distal two thirds of the forearm, the UA lies lateral to the ulnar nerve and is surrounded by a pair of collateral veins, which have numerous interconnecting crossover branches. Numerous arterial branches called arteriae nervorum supply the ulnar nerve.

The ulnar artery has three named branches, the anterior and posterior ulnar recurrent arteries, which arise in the cubital fossa, and the common interosseous artery, which is seen at the upper end of the dissection where it arises just within the flexor compartment of the forearm. Anterior and posterior carpal arteries lie near the pisiform bone and are not normally seen.

Surgical technique

9 The arm is abducted, the forearm externally rotated, and the ulnar artery exposed through an incision along the line of the artery. The incision commences 2–3 cm above the wrist, extending vertically to the midpoint of the forearm, then curves in a forward direction toward the bicipital tendon and ends approximately 5 cm below the elbow joint.

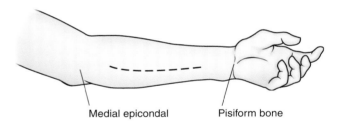

Medial epicondal   Pisiform bone

9

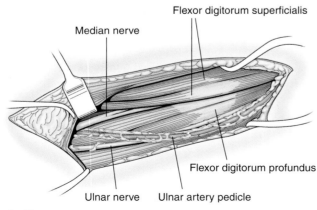

Flexor digitorum superficialis
Median nerve
Flexor digitorum profundus
Ulnar nerve   Ulnar artery pedicle

10

10 The artery is exposed after the division of the deep fascia lateral to the flexor carpi ulnaris tendon and is removed in the lower two thirds of the forearm. Great care is required to avoid handling the ulnar nerve during the division of the arteriae nervorum. When the lower part of the ulnar artery has been mobilized, the 1-mmol/L papaverine solution is injected distally and the artery allowed to dilate. The ulnar artery is mobilized in the upper third of the forearm, where it passes beneath the flexor digitorum superficialis and the overlying palmaris longus and flexor carpi radialis. At the apex of the muscular tunnel, formed by the superficial flexor group anteriorly and the flexor digitorum profundus muscle posteriorly, the median nerve crosses the ulnar artery. Retraction of the median nerve must be avoided. The ulnar artery is transected below the point of origin of the common interosseous artery.

GASTROEPIPLOIC ARTERY

The gastroepiploic artery is sometimes used as a third *in situ* arterial graft when the ITA cannot reach the posterior surface of the heart or when other conduits are not available.

Anatomy

11 The right gastroepiploic artery (RGEA) is the largest terminal branch of the gastroduodenal artery. The RGEA lies between the posterior surface of the duodenum and the anterior surface of the pancreas and travels along the greater curvature of the stomach between the two layers of the greater omentum, along with the gastroepiploic veins. The RGEA terminates by anastomosing with the left gastroepiploic artery, which arises from the splenic artery near the hilum of the spleen.

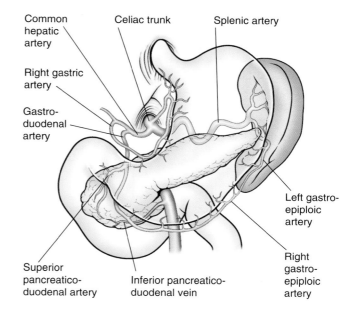

11

Surgical technique

12a, b

The median sternotomy incision is extended inferiorly for a further 5 cm. Following ITA harvesting, the peritoneum is opened to expose the stomach. The right gastroepiploic artery is seen along the greater curvature of the stomach. A nasogastric tube is used to empty the stomach. The gastroepiploic artery is palpated so that its size can be evaluated. The right gastroepiploic artery and pedicle, including the veins, are detached from the omentum, and the branches are ligated with silk or a metal clip. Usually, the gastroepiploic artery is removed from the lower two thirds of the greater curvature of the stomach, extending distally but not beyond the pylorus. Further dissection may cause injury to the superior pancreaticoduodenal artery.

The right gastroepiploic pedicle can be introduced into the pericardial cavity anteriorly or by a posterior route through a 2- to 3-cm hole in the diaphragm. The posterior or retrogastric approach has been advocated to reduce the risk of graft injury at reoperation for a cardiac or abdominal procedure. The right gastroepiploic artery is usually grafted to an artery on the inferior wall of the heart.

INFERIOR EPIGASTRIC ARTERY

The size and length of the inferior epigastric artery (IEA) vary; and in many patients, when it is used alone, the length is not sufficient for an independent graft. The IEA is probably best used as a composite graft with the LITA, either as a Y- or extension graft.

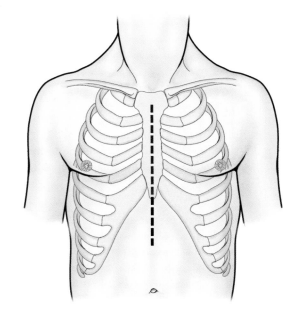

12a

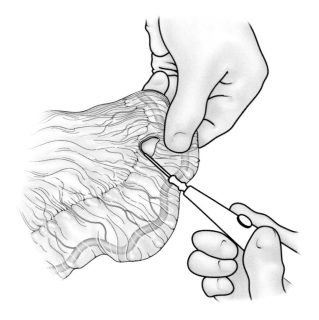

12b

Anatomy

13 The IEA arises from the medial aspect of the external iliac artery, opposite the origin of the deep circumflex iliac artery, and gives branches to the spermatic cord, pubis, abdominal muscles, and skin. Traveling anterior to the peritoneum, it pierces the transversalis fascia and the extension of the rectus sheath. Above the arcuate line, it continues between the rectus muscle and the posterior rectus sheath. IEA terminates by anastomosing with small branches from the superior epigastric artery.

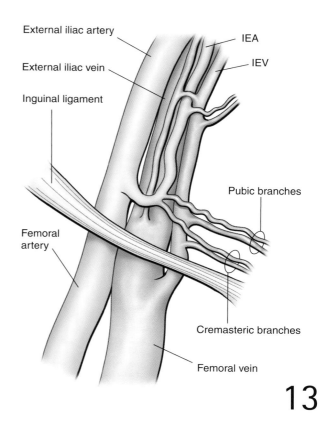

13

Surgical technique

14 Bilateral IEA harvesting can be carried out through a midline or paramedian subumbilical incision. Exposing the lower end of the epigastric artery at its origin using a midline incision is difficult, as the artery lies beneath the rectus muscle. In the midline approach, a separate oblique incision in the groin may be required to approach the lower end (or origin) of the IEA.

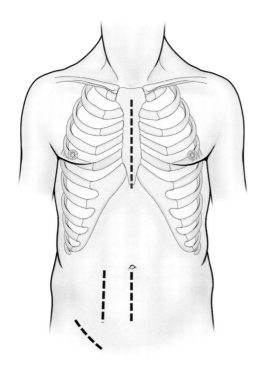

14

15 A lateral or paramedian incision gives more access and is used if a longer length of artery is required, particularly at the lower end. The rectus muscle can be retracted medially to expose the IEA up to the level of the umbilicus. This approach, however, results in denervation of the rectus muscle. The lower margin of the rectus muscle and the surrounding tissues that contain the spermatic cord are lifted to expose the IEA, where it arises from the external iliac artery.

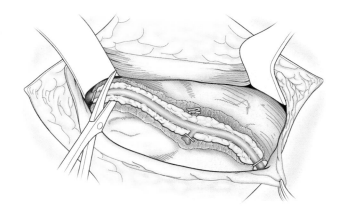

Grafting procedure

16a–f The final plan of how best to deploy the arterial grafts is made after harvesting, following exposure of the heart and the institution of coronary-pulmonary bypass. The LITA is readily anastomosed to the left-sided vessels. The LITA is passed anterior to the phrenic nerve through a window or a slit in the pericardium to reach the LAD or diagonal artery. When passed behind the phrenic nerve, the LITA normally reaches the distal marginal branches of the circumflex system. The RITA, when fully mobilized, can be attached to the LAD, intermediate or anterior circumflex marginal branches, passing either anterior to the aorta, or through the transverse sinus.

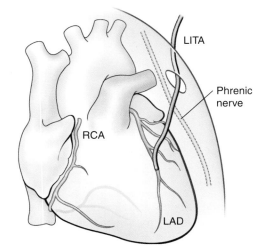

16a

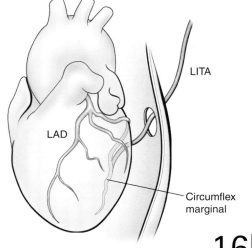

16b

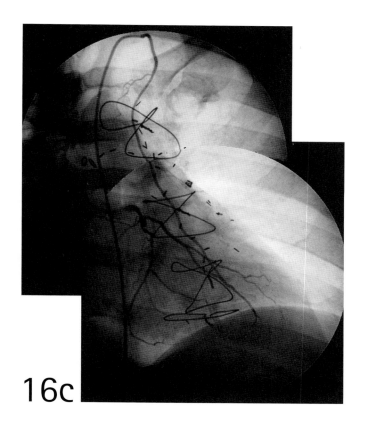

16c

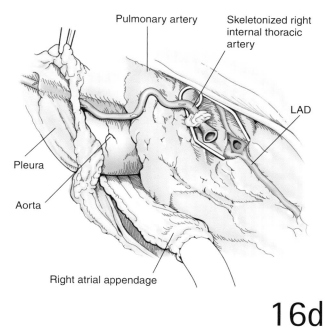

16d

Pulmonary artery

Skeletonized right internal thoracic artery

LAD

Pleura

Aorta

Right atrial appendage

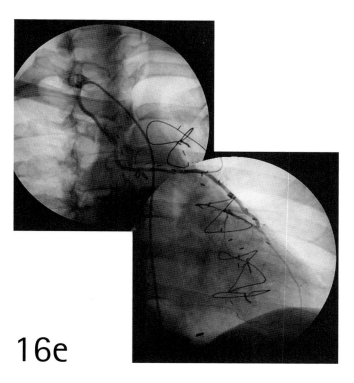

16e

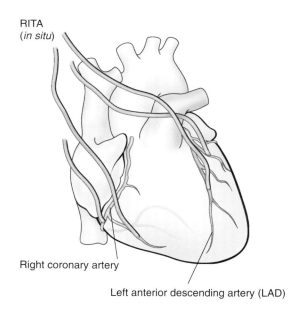

16f

RITA (*in situ*)

Right coronary artery

Left anterior descending artery (LAD)

17 The *in situ* RITA is usually not long enough to reach the distal RCA or its branches. In some patients, however, the RITA can be sutured to the posterior descending or even the posterolateral branch of the RCA by passing it behind the vena cava.

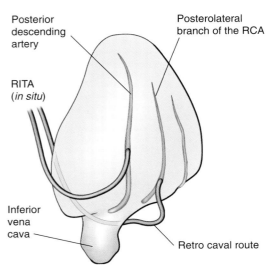

17

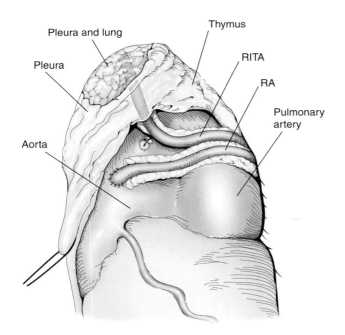

18

18 In planning a bilateral ITA procedure, the target site for the RITA should be assessed before the LITA. Contrary to what is commonly believed, reoperation even with an anteriorly placed RITA graft which is passed posterior to the thymus, and anterior to the aorta, is not a difficult procedure. However, before closure, the pericardium and the thymus should be approximated over the RITA. At reoperation, the arterial pedicle is readily identified and controlled, either inside the pericardium or the pleural space. The course across the ascending thoracic aorta lies distally near the aortic cannulation site and well above the site of an arteriotomy for a subsequent aortic valve replacement.

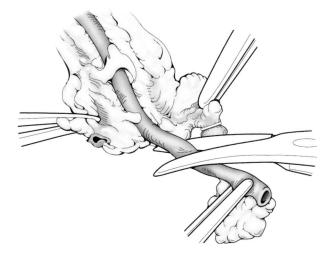

19a

Anastomotic techniques

DISTAL ANASTOMOSIS (END-TO-SIDE TECHNIQUE)

19a–c
A 4- to 5-mm coronary arteriotomy (two or three times the diameter of the native coronary artery) is placed at the point that is free from disease. The end of the arterial graft is fashioned so that the circumference of the graft just exceeds that of the native coronary artery.

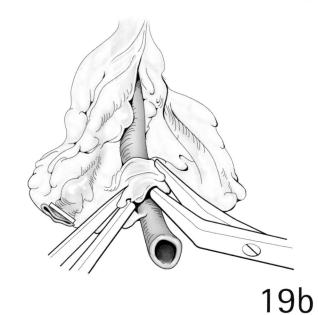

19b

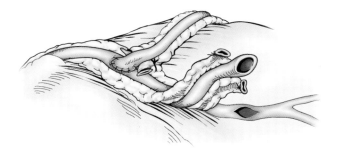

19c

20a–e

The native coronary artery is orientated away from the surgeon. Through the use of a two-arm suture, the anastomosis is commenced at the proximal end of the coronary arteriotomy at the point furthest from the surgeon. One suture is passed from the lumen to the exterior of the coronary artery and clipped; the other arm is placed through the heel of the arterial graft. After two or three sutures have been inserted, the graft is then approximated to the native vessel. Suturing, using a forehand technique, is then continued from outside to inside the lumen of the coronary artery until the distal end of the arteriotomy is reached. The apex of the graft is rotated to expose the distal end of the arteriotomy. Commencing proximally, the surgeon sews the second suture from outside the graft through the anastomosis to the outside of the coronary artery. This suture is continued to the distal end of the anastomosis. Placement of the apical sutures at the distal end is facilitated by traction on the last loop of the first suture.

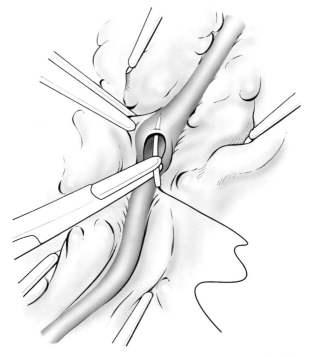

20a

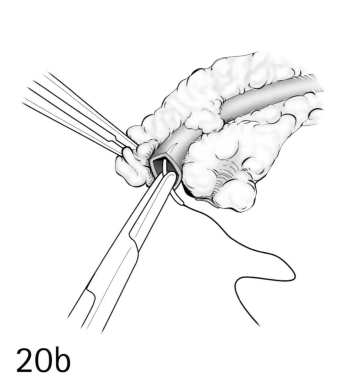

20b

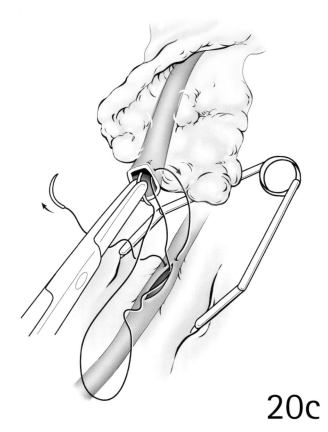

20c

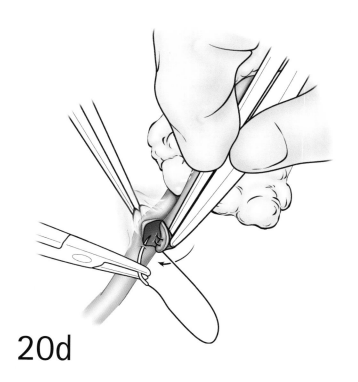

20d

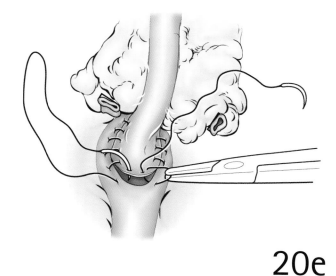

20e

SEQUENTIAL ANASTOMOSIS (SIDE-TO-SIDE TECHNIQUES)

Parallel technique

21 Sequential anastomoses conserve the length of arterial conduits by increasing the number of distal anastomoses. The technique of a parallel anastomosis is almost identical to the standard technique used for an end-to-side anastomosis. A parallel anastomosis may require an additional length of conduit to avoid tension between the anastomotic points by grafting, for example, the circumflex marginal branches. This technique is suited to anastomosing the LAD with its diagonal branch, when the latter is closely aligned to the LAD. This technique is not suitable for proximal or laterally placed diagonal branches where angulation may occur at the site of the side-to-side anastomosis. In these cases Y-grafting is preferable.

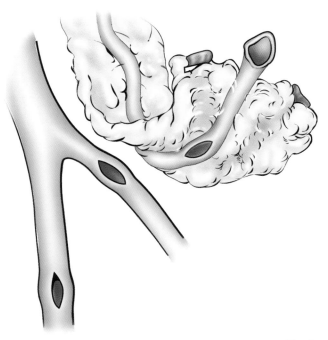

21

22a–c The site for anastomosis of the LITA with the diagonal branch is chosen with the heart distended and lying in its normal position. A marking clip is placed on the ITA pedicle at the site of the proposed anastomosis. Sufficient length of ITA proximal to the side-to-side anastomosis should be left so that the heart can be elevated without putting tension on the graft. The first sutures are placed from within the native vessel and graft and are continued using a forehand technique down the left side of the anastomosis to the heel. The distal (free) end of the ITA graft is elevated to facilitate placement of the heel sutures. The second suture is then continued down the medial side of the anastomosis to the heel, where the two ends are tied. A stay suture is placed distal to the side-to-side anastomosis to maintain the alignment of the LITA graft. The end-to-side anastomosis between the distal LITA and the LAD completes the sequential graft.

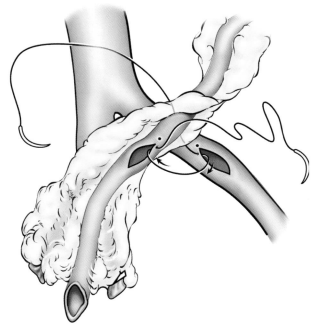

22a

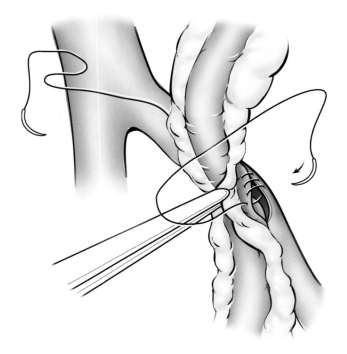

22b

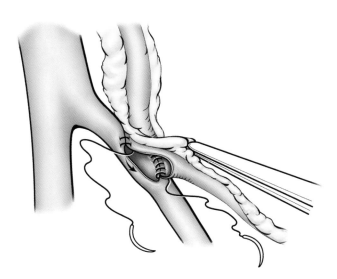

22c

Diamond technique

The diamond technique is useful for grafting the circumflex marginal coronary artery branches, which lie parallel and often close to one another, and also for grafting the postero-lateral and posterior descending branches of the RCA. Diamond-shaped anastomoses are necessary when graft length is insufficient to create the loops that are required for the parallel technique. The distance between the end-to-side and end-to-end anastomoses is judged by either distending the heart or grasping the pericardium with forceps and stretching it to its natural limit. A few extra millimeters of length in the graft allow space for inspecting the end-to-end and the end-to-side anastomoses and provide additional length if the left ventricle becomes overdistended.

23a–d
The arteriotomies should be small to avoid distortion of the native artery or the graft at the site of the anastomosis. In general, the length of the arteriotomies should be similar to, or only marginally greater than, the diameter of the native coronary artery or conduit. The side-to-side anastomosis can be performed before or after the end-to-side technique. Our preference when grafting the marginal branches is to perform the distal anastomosis first and then to allow the graft to rotate away from the surgeon to expose the site for the side-to-side anastomosis. The proximal anastomosis is performed last. When the Y-graft technique is used, the sequence is reversed, with the side-to-side anastomosis being performed first. Suturing is commenced at a point farthest from the surgeon, at the apex of the native coronary artery. Three or four sutures are placed before the graft and native vessels are approximated. The lateral side of the anastomosis is sutured to the distal end of the native arteriotomy. Elevation of the graft as the suture is continued around the right-hand side of the anastomosis, finishing at the point nearest the surgeon, facilitates this maneuver. The other suture is used to complete the anastomosis. The suture is tied after the graft is distended with blood to minimize the risk of stricture or narrowing of the anastomosis. Occluding the vessel beyond the anastomosis checks hemostasis. Additional tacking sutures are not usually required with a diamond technique.

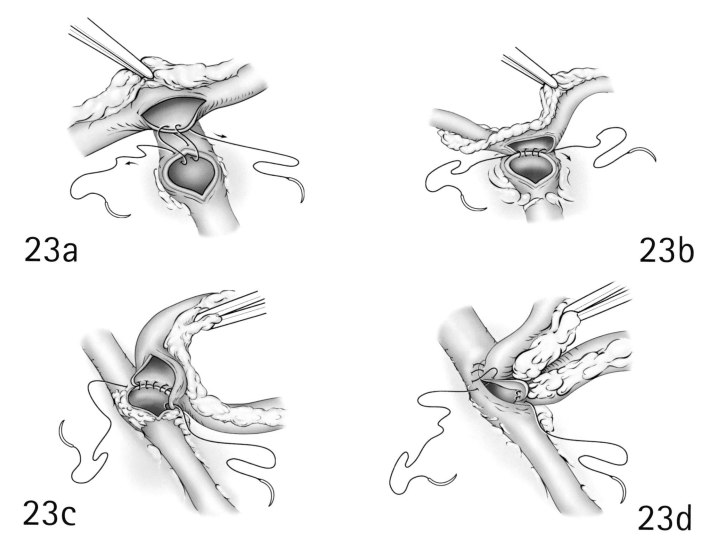

23a

23b

23c

23d

PROXIMAL ANASTOMOSIS

Aortic anastomosis

The anastomosis is commenced on the aorta at a point furthest from the surgeon, using a monofilament suture and a forehand technique. The heel sutures are placed through the aorta and the graft. The right side of the anastomosis is completed using a forehand technique. The left side is then completed and the anastomosis tied at its apex.

Left internal thoracic artery: Y-graft

24a–d
The anastomosis is performed on the chest wall side of the LITA, immediately after it enters the pericardial cavity. The LITA and the arterial free graft (AFG) (e.g. RA or a segment of distal ITA) are dilated with the papaverine mixture to dilate the arteries maximally and facilitate the anastomosis. The anastomosis is normally performed before bypass. With the heart decompressed, a 4- to 5-mm incision is made in the ITA. The AFG is then cut obliquely and the arteriotomy matched to that of the ITA. Suturing is usually commenced at the proximal end of the ITA and the apex of the free graft and continued distally using a forehand technique. The distal sutures are placed more accurately if the free graft is elevated to expose the heel. The suture line is completed using a forehand technique down the opposite side of the anastomosis to the heel, where the sutures are tied. Usually, a support suture is placed in the acute angle of the 'Y'. When the AFG is to be anastomosed more distally with the LITA, it may be better to start at the heel of the AFG and the distal end in the left internal thoracic arteriotomy.

In the situation in which a circumflex marginal branch has already been grafted and the graft is of insufficient length to reach the aorta, the LITA can be used for the site of the proximal anastomosis via the Y-graft technique. The LITA usually measures 2–3 mm in diameter near the point of entry into the pericardial cavity. In some patients, however, the LITA is small, even after dilatation. Under these circumstances, a Y-graft is probably best avoided in case flow into the lower end of the LITA is obstructed.

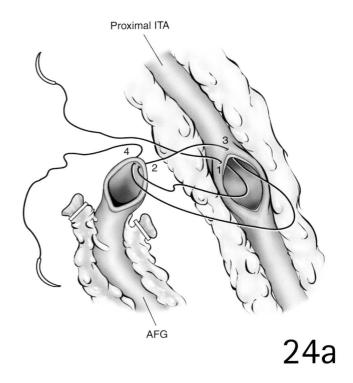

Proximal ITA

AFG

24a

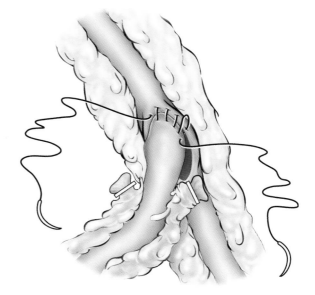

24b

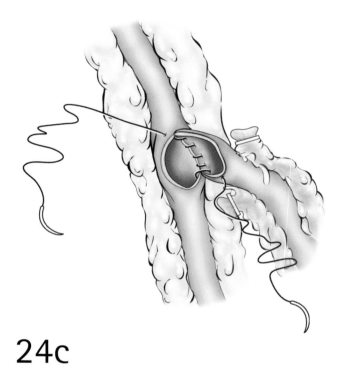

24c

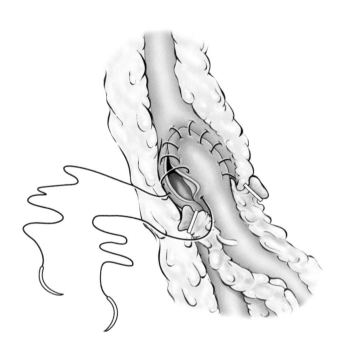

24d

Graft extension

If the length of the RITA is insufficient to reach the terminal branches of the RCA, a segment of AFG can be used to extend the RITA graft to the distal target artery. The technique of extension grafting often only requires a short length of an AFG to reach either the posterior descending or posterolateral branch of the RCA without tension.

25a–c The distal end of the RITA and proximal end of the AFG are transected at an approximately 45-degree angle after having been dilated previously with the papaverine solution. Suturing is usually commenced at the apex of the AFG, which is joined to the heel of the *in situ* ITA graft. Sutures continue around the left side of the anastomosis to the apex. Rotating the anastomosis through 180° exposes the sutures in the heel of the free graft. The second suture is placed along the opposite side of the anastomosis, and the sutures are tied after release of the clamp to distend the pedicle. Additional stay sutures are placed on either side of the anastomosis to prevent rotation at the anastomotic site. Distal flow is checked before the terminal end-to-side anastomosis is commenced.

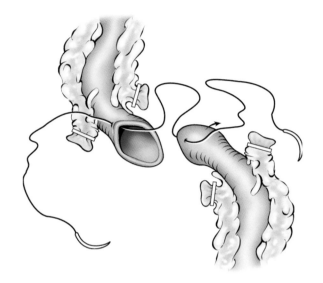

25a

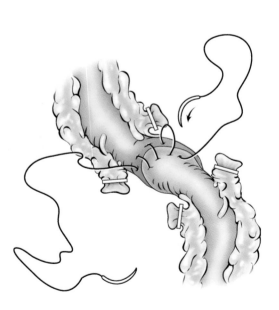

25b

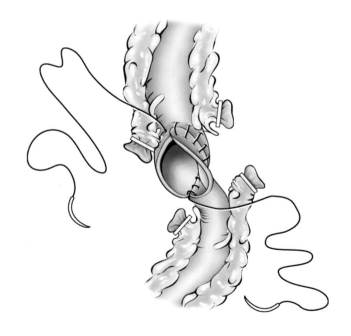

25c

POSTOPERATIVE CARE

In patients who have arterial grafts, it is important to maintain a mean blood pressure of greater than 70 mm Hg (or preferably greater than 80 mm Hg), with a cardiac index in excess of 2.5 L/m². In those patients in whom the cardiac index is low (less than 2.5 L/m²), our preference, particularly when grafting with an RA graft, is to use a low-dose 'inodilator' (phosphodiesterase III inhibitor) such as milrinone. This drug enhances myocardial contractility and arterial dilatation by increasing the intracellular concentration of cyclic guanosine monophosphate, thereby raising the level of intracellular calcium. Alternatively, nitroglycerin, which also relaxes the vascular muscle via the nitric oxide–cyclic guanosine monophosphate pathway, can be used. The aim is to optimize the cardiac index (to greater than 2.5 L/m²) and to produce a vascular resistance of between 1 000 and 1 500 dynes/second per cm⁻⁵. We have not observed any graft spasm in patients who have been given topical as well as systemic vasodilators. Diltiazem is not used because of the potential for myocardial depression. Patients with multiple arterial grafts appear to tolerate or even benefit from a high mean arterial pressure. However, hypotension should be avoided. In patients who are excessively dilated and have a high cardiac index, or cannot increase their cardiac output sufficiently to compensate, noradrenaline (norepinephrine) may be required to achieve a mean arterial pressure of 70–80 mm Hg and a normal systemic vascular resistance.

Arterial grafts have a large number of branches, and meticulous hemostasis is necessary to avoid postoperative bleeding, particularly in patients who are receiving antiplatelet agents. Protamine sulfate, an infusion of platelets and coagulation factors, and the use of antifibrinolytic agents may reduce bleeding in this latter group of patients.

Another complication to guard against is ischemia. Sternal ischemia occurs more frequently in patients with insulin-dependent diabetes. Bilateral ITA grafting is to be avoided in very elderly, obese, and diabetic patients. If the ITA must be used in such a patient, a skeletonized technique may minimize the risk of sternal ischemia and subsequent infection. RA harvesting offers a potential risk of hand ischemia. In a recent study of 2 417 patients who underwent RA removal, however, fingertip ischemia developed in only 2 individuals, both of whom suffered from scleroderma.

OUTCOME

We have performed extended arterial grafting in more than 5 500 patients with multi-vessel disease since 1985. However, the majority of these procedures have been performed over the last 5 years. Table 8.2 shows the graft vessels used from 1985 to 2000. The early complication rates are shown in Table 8.3.

In relation to survival rates for extended arterial grafting, the most definitive survival analysis of bilateral compared

Table 8.2 *Grafts used for extended arterial grafting from 1985 to 2000 (5 529 patients)*

Graft	n (%)
Left internal thoracic artery	5450 (99)
Right internal thoracic artery	2546 (46)
Radial Artery Single	3909 (70)
Radial Artery Bilateral	1603 (29)
Ulnar Artery	24 (0.4)
Inferior epigastric artery	30 (0.5)
Gastroepiploic artery	5 (0.1)

Table 8.3 *Early complications of complete arterial grafting (5 529 patients)*

Complication	n (%)
Death	61 (1.1)
Myocardial infarction	46 (0.8)
Stroke	57 (1.0)
Sternal infection	122 (2.2)

with single internal artery grafting confirms that two ITA grafts are superior to a single ITA graft and are associated with a decreased risk of death, reoperation, and angioplasty. In patients with multiple risk factors, the difference between receiving bilateral versus single grafts is evident in the first 10 years after operation and a longer period in patients with few risk factors. Grafting bilateral ITAs to the left coronary system appears to offer an advantage over grafting the RITA to the right side.

In relation to the patency of arterial grafts, the landmark paper by Loop *et al.* in 1986, indicating that the patency of the *in situ* LITA when anastomosed to the LAD exceeds that of saphenous vein grafts, set the stage for the introduction and acceptance of arterial grafts. The patency of the LITA when anastomosed to the LAD is approximately 90–95 per cent at 10 years. Furthermore, the patency of the RITA when anastomosed as an *in situ* graft to the LAD has an identical patency at 10 years. The same study also demonstrated a fourfold increase in graft failure when a native coronary artery with a stenosis of less than 60 per cent compared with 80–100 per cent is grafted and a twofold increase in graft failure when a free compared with an *in situ* RITA graft is used. A similar increase in failure occurred when the RCA was grafted. The late results of other arterial grafts, however, are less well known. The RA has a 5-year patency of approximately 87 per cent. Few late results are available for the gastroepiploic or inferior epigastric arteries.

The *in situ* ITA is the conduit of choice in coronary artery bypass surgery. In patients with multi-vessel coronary artery disease, bilateral ITA grafting is now the procedure against which all other grafting techniques are measured. Extending the use of other arterial grafts and surgical techniques is the next logical development for patients with multi-vessel coronary artery disease, particularly in view of the poor late results using saphenous vein grafts. In terms of future developments, pharmacological interventions, in combination with the knowledge gained from the Human Genome Project, are likely to provide us with the ability to slow the rate of progress of disease in the native circulation, as well as to improve the patency of all types of bypass grafts.

ACKNOWLEDGMENTS

The author gratefully acknowledges Dr. Permyos Ruengsakulrach, Senior Cardiac Fellow at the Austin Hospital, for his contribution to this chapter; Beth Croce for her illustrations; and Dr. Tania Lewis for her editorial assistance.

FURTHER READING

Buxton, B.F., Komeda, M., Fuller, J.A., Gordon, I. 1998. Bilateral internal thoracic artery grafting may improve outcome of coronary artery surgery. Risk-adjusted survival. Circulation 98(19 Suppl.) II1–6.

Loop, F.D., Lytle, B.W., Cosgrove, D.M., et al. 1986. Free (aorta-coronary) internal mammary artery graft. Late results. Journal of Thoracic and Cardiovascular Surgery 92, 827–31.

Lytle, B.W., Blackstone, E.H., Loop, F.D., et al. 1999. Two internal thoracic artery grafts are better than one. Journal of Thoracic and Cardiovascular Surgery 117, 855–72.

Possati, G., Gaudino, M., Alessandrini, F., et al. 1998. Midterm clinical and angiographic results of radial artery grafts used for myocardial revascularization. Journal of Thoracic and Cardiovascular Surgery 116, 1015–21.

Ruengsakulrach, P., Sinclair, R., Komeda, M., et al. 1999. Comparative histology of radial artery versus internal thoracic artery and risk factors for development of intimal hyperplasia and atherosclerosis. Circulation 100(Suppl. II), II 139–44.

Schmidt, S.E., Jones, J.W., Thornby, J.I., Miller, C.C. 3rd, Beall, A.C. Jr. 1997. Improved survival with multiple left-sided bilateral internal thoracic artery grafts. Annals of Thoracic Surgery 64, 9–14.

Options for off-pump coronary revascularization

ERIK W. JANSEN MD, PHD
Department of Cardiothoracic Surgery, Utrecht University, University Medical Center, Heart-Lung Institute, Utrecht, The Netherlands

HISTORY

Kolessov pioneered off-pump, beating heart coronary artery bypass grafting (CABG) in St. Petersburg in 1964. He used simple epicardial stay sutures for stabilization to graft the left internal mammary artery (IMA) to the left anterior descending artery (LAD). He also pioneered facilitated anastomosis techniques using a one-shot stapling device with alignment of the artery rims by suction.

Off-pump CABG hibernated almost completely for three decades, although Drs. Benetti and Buffolo continued to perform a low volume of beating heart coronary surgery in South America. The advent of the heart-lung machine changed the scene, allowing a noncompromised, well-controlled revascularization. Based on the work of the Cleveland Clinic group, a worldwide expansion of CABG occurred in the 1970s. The introduction of specific local cardiac wall stabilizers at the end of the last century changed the scene again. Recent reports suggest that CABG can be performed safely without a heart-lung machine. Thus, in selected patients coronary surgery became 'less invasive.' Present estimates suggest that 20 per cent of isolated CABG procedures are performed off-pump.

PRINCIPLES AND JUSTIFICATION

The challenge of off-pump CABG is to construct a coronary anastomosis on a 1.25- to 2.5-mm internal diameter–moving vessel. The accuracy of off-pump CABG is based on three-dimensional stabilization of the target site segment without affecting the myocardial function. The motion of the target is complex and consists of slow and fast components, the latter particularly in the end-diastolic filling phase of the heart. This motion makes accurate microvascular suturing without mechanical stabilization impossible. Therefore, proper local cardiac wall stabilization to minimize myocardial movement and to optimize presentation of the target coronary artery is the cornerstone of beating heart surgery.

Currently, three methods of tissue stabilization exist: (1) suction fixation, (2) pressure fixation, and (3) vessel loop-plate fixation. The stabilizer may be retractor based or operation table rail based.

1a The suction-based 'Octopus' was developed at Utrecht University Medical Center. Suction fixation allows tissue stabilization and presentation in a neutral plane so as not to compress the myocardium. The Octopus I two-pod stabilizer (Medtronic, Minneapolis, MN) is mounted on the operation table rail and has the advantage of being able to be used in all access routes including port access. The Octopus I also enables unlimited spreading of the epicardial fatty tissue and, thus, further immobilization in the z-direction, as most coronaries are embedded in a discrete groove in the fatty tissue. The Octopus II one-arm stabilizer (Medtronic, Minneapolis, MN) is (sternal) retractor based, like most current stabilizers today, and is easier to use. Spreading of the tip of the pods is still possible. Suction fixation requires additional measures such as management of tubing and suction, separate for left and right in the Octopus I and combined in the Octopus II.

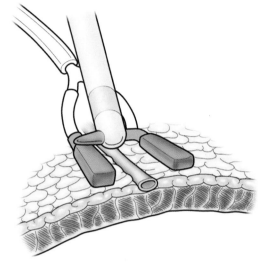

1a

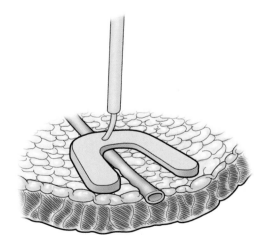

1b Tissue stabilization by pressure is easier to apply but exerts more pressure on the heart. However, compared to suction fixation, the technique has less grip on the heart, and slipping may occur.

1b

1c Vessel loop-plate fixation uses a combination of simultaneous foot plate stabilization and a vessel loop under the target vessel for stabilization, leading to segmental occlusion simultaneously. The foot plate, however, is more difficult to use in sequential grafting because of its size.

'Off-pump,' beating heart surgery is a striking renovation in the history of CABG. This technique enables bypass grafting without the disadvantages of cardiopulmonary bypass. The latter involves many issues, such as cannulation of the ascending aorta, hemodilution, foreign surface activation of the blood, coagulation disorders, temperature changes, cross-clamping of the aorta, and global myocardial ischemia. By omitting cardiopulmonary bypass itself, the systemic inflammatory response and organ damage, particularly to blood, brain, lung, kidney, and bowel, can be reduced.

'Less invasive CABG' should be performed whenever feasible. In some patients, avoidance of touching the ascending aorta is crucial to avoid embolization of atherosclerotic debris, particularly to the brain. In others (1) harvesting the IMA in a skeletonized way to preserve the donor site and for longer conduits, (2) keeping both pleurae closed in sternotomy cases to prevent atelectasis (the IMAs are extrapleural structures), (3) using arterial grafts for longevity of revascularization, or (4) avoiding additional leg wounds (particularly in patients with diabetes) is important.

In off-pump CABG, special skills are required. The surgeon should be familiar with stabilization techniques and should know how to handle hemodynamic changes during displacement and how to deal with the ischemic sequelae of temporary coronary occlusion to prevent bailout situations. Considerable experience with traditional cardiac surgery is required. Nevertheless, off-pump CABG is only justified if graft patency rates of bypasses are comparable to those of the traditional arrested heart surgery and full revascularization is achieved. Exceptions to these rules may exist in special conditions, such as in myocardial salvage and the treatment of angina in patients who have a short life expectancy. Off-pump CABG carries a number of theoretical limitations compared to on-pump CABG, including compromised exposure, critical immobilization, compromised visualization due to bleeding from the arteriotomy, and less freedom in dissection and extension of the length of the arteriotomy.

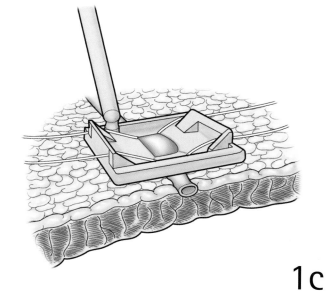

1c

PREOPERATIVE ASSESSMENT AND PREPARATION

Proper patient selection is crucial to a successful beating heart coronary artery bypass program. Traditional on-pump CABG undoubtedly offers the most freedom of revascularization with respect to the number and quality of vessels. Local tortuosity, local intramyocardial or even a subepicardial course, or a local plaque may limit this freedom, as does a crossing vein.

Basically, patients with isolated proximal coronary artery disease with well-visualized more distal segments are good candidates for off-pump surgery. Diffuse coronary artery disease is the most important exclusion criterion. A collaterally filled vessel may be of poor quality and small size leading to unpredictable results. The inclusion criteria tend to be stricter in less accessible areas of the myocardium, such as the posterolateral wall, where vessel size and myocardial function are even more crucial. On the anterior wall even vessels of 1-mm internal diameter can be accepted.

2 An example of a good candidate for four-vessel revascularization is given in Figure 2. Limited access bypass grafting raises additional issues such as accessibility for harvesting of the arterial conduit and that of the target coronary artery. In this respect body posture and orientation of the heart in the chest may be important determinants. Paradoxically, in some obese patients full sternotomy may lead to more limited dissection than small incision surgery. In addition, sternotomy offers a superior view, which is an important issue in early experience.

Poor left ventricular function (left ventricular ejection fraction less than 30 per cent) and cardiomegaly are not absolute contraindications. Instability based on hibernation and/or stunning and critical left main disease are probably best treated by unloading of the ventricle using on-pump techniques.

Preoperatively, the operative strategy is explained to the patient. In experienced hands, bailout situations due to critical ischemia rarely occur (less than 1 per cent), and conversion to cardiopulmonary bypass for technical reasons is rare (less than 3 per cent). Thus, the nature of the procedure can be anticipated with reasonable certainty.

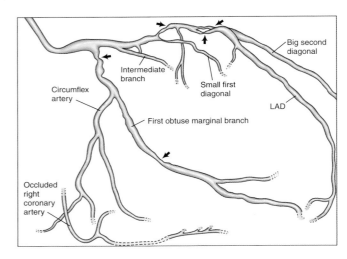

2

OPERATIVE PLANNING

Anesthesia

Particularly in the elderly, the mode of anesthesia has become increasingly important now that 'tailoring of anesthesia to the patient' in off-pump CABG has become available. Recently, a ('light') general anesthesia (induction pancuronium, 0.1 mg/kg; propofol, 2 mg/kg; and sufentanil, 0.25–0.5 µg/kg, followed by propofol, 2–3 mg/kg per hour) and regional thoracic epidural analgesia (bupivacaine 0.5 per cent, 0.05–0.1 mL/kg and 2–3 mL/hour) have been used in our institution. The latter has potential advantages. Including attenuated general anesthesia, blockage of the sympathetic reflexes, and opening myocardial collateral circulation, thus making the myocardium less susceptible to temporary segmental occlusion. Furthermore, this technique dilates the arterial (IMA) conduits, reduces the stress response (which may hyperactivate the clotting mechanism), and, finally, facilitates postoperative pain and thus pulmonary toilet.

Preferably, the epidural catheter is positioned the day before surgery, allowing testing with the patient awake and avoiding bleeding complications. Paradoxically, this 'more invasive anesthesia' may lead to 'facilitated recovery' during the first 48 hours. More traditional types of anesthesia also can be used. The main objective is early awakening, but not necessarily in the operating room.

Monitoring is achieved by arterial line, central venous catheter, oximetry, mixed venous saturation, cardiac output (by Swan-Ganz catheter or transit-time ultrasound probe on the ascending aorta), transesophageal echocardiography, and electroencephalography or transcranial Doppler. Continuous on-line ST-segment analysis is a sensitive parameter to detect early ischemia and is recommended.

Single lung ventilation in thoracotomy access procedures is an important modality. This technique facilitates harvesting. Keeping the patient warm is most important. Therefore, all infusions should be warmed, warming blankets are recommended, and the operating room temperature should be higher than that needed for on-pump procedures.

Anticoagulation

During the off-pump CABG, heparin is given before the conduits are cut distally. A moderate dose of heparin (1.5 mg/kg) is administered. During the procedure, activated clotting time is kept at greater than 250 seconds. At the end heparin is either not reversed or only 25 mg of protamine is given, as platelet function is preserved in off-pump surgery. Antithrombosis prophylaxis is continued during admission, with high molecular heparin given subcutaneously. After the patient awakens from anesthesia, acetylsalicylic acid is started.

Management of arterial conduits

To prevent spasm of arterial conduits, intravenous amlodipine is started intraoperatively and continued for 3 weeks orally.

OPERATION

Access

3 Currently, the sternotomy access is most commonly used because it offers wide access to all major coronary artery segments. In addition, better understanding of the pump function of the displaced heart and particularly the advent of new 'tricks' to subluxate the beating heart without compromising the pump function favor this approach. Currently, the anterior thoracotomy, the subxiphoid laparotomy (median), and the posterior thoracotomy are used for subsets of patients with limited one vessel disease. In favorable topography, the anterior thoracotomy, the distal sternotomy, the transverse curved laparotomy and the left posterior thoracotomy allow multiple grafting, provided that the vessels are nearby and, in the case of the anterior thoracotomy, no wide-angled diagonal-LAD fork is present.

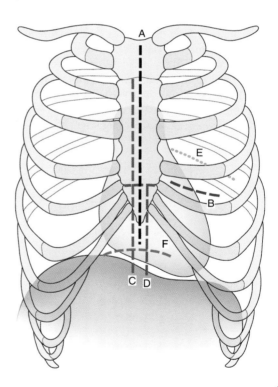

3

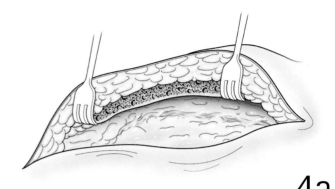

4a

4a, b, c A second, major advantage of the sternotomy is that the IMAs can be harvested in the usual familiar way using a table based retractor (Rultract, Cleveland, OH). They are harvested in the skeletonized way and, after the pericardium is opened, routed behind the thymus ventral to the phrenic nerve through a separate stab wound in the pericardium. Endoscopic harvesting can be used in combination with non-sternotomy access and in port-access CABG. The pedicled gastroepiploic artery (GEA) is routed through a 2-cm cut in the diaphragm immediately to the left of the falciform ligament.

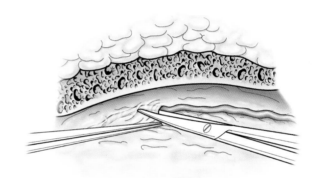

4b

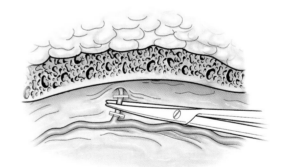

4c

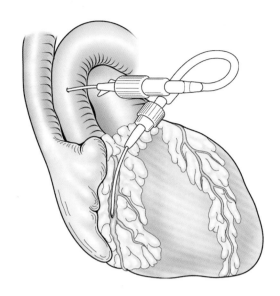

9a

9a, b We found that in almost all vessels the 'clamp and sew' technique is warranted. Critical ischemia only occurred on temporary occlusion of the distal RCA at the level of the crux, and temporary shunting was necessary only at this site. At this location an aorto-coronary shunt that is made of components available in every operating room (16-gauge catheters; Figure 9a) should be used, and at other sites a very soft intraluminal shunt is used (Figure 9b). We found that 20 mL/minute was sufficient to treat ischemia and normalize ST-segment elevations within 30 seconds.

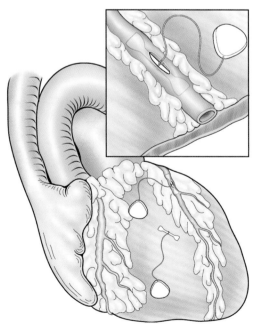

9b

9c–g Temporary occlusion can be performed in several ways: an atraumatic microvascular clamp (Acland [Landmark Surgical Instrumentation and Equipment, Merseyside, UK]; Figure 9c), Silastic snare (Figure 9d), buttressed suture (Figure 9e), or disposable clip (Figure 9f). Occluding the vessel also distally using atraumatic microvascular clamps (Acland) produces a dry anastomosis site and imitates clean globally arrested heart surgery. Preferably, the clamps should be positioned from aside in order not to compromise the suture-loop handling. This has an additional advantage of preserving the collateral flow to the distal myocardium. Alternatively, a blower/mister should be used to maintain a clear view (Figure 9g).

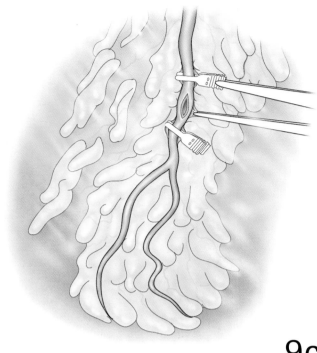

9c

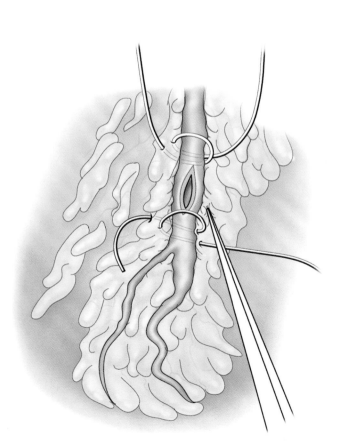

9d

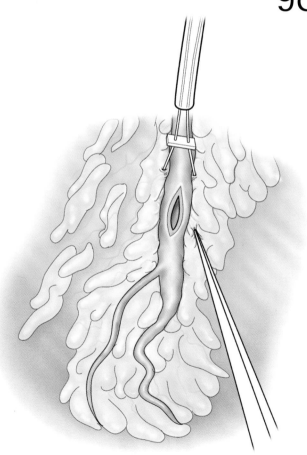

9e

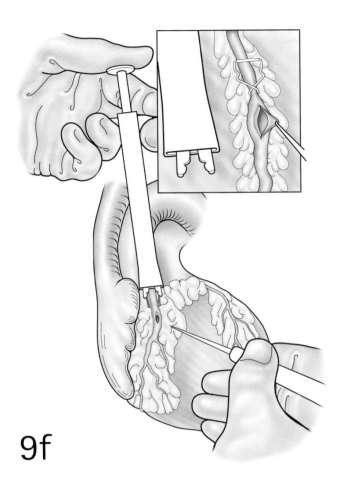

9f

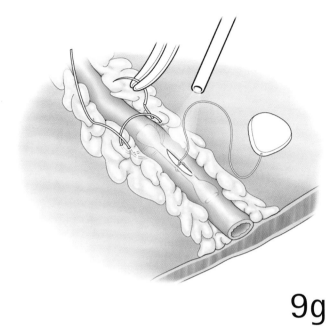

9g

Anastomosis

9h A single, running 8/0 or 7/0 suture is used, usually with a one-needle technique. In grafting of the diagonal sequential to the LAD, the side anastomosis is performed using a two-needle technique, starting with the back wall first, suturing the coronary artery from outside to inside. This method is used because of the orientation of the vessel to the surgeon. In the distal RCA anastomosis, the toe is most distal and therefore is done first, using the two-needle technique.

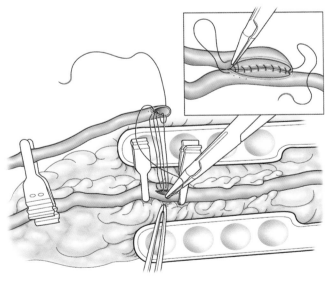

9h

Quality assessment

Intraoperative quality assessment can be performed by angiography or, more practically, transit-time ultrasound graft flow measurement. In combination with simultaneous assessment of additional parameters, such as the qualitative flow pattern, the ratio flow-mean arterial blood pressure, and – before tying the knot – assessment of free graft flow, native coronary flow, and distal stump pressure, transit-time ultrasound graft flow measurement has additional value.

Alternative access routes

LEFT ANTERIOR THORACOTOMY

10a–d Isolated revascularization of the most important coronary artery, the LAD, is most suitable via a small left anterior thoracotomy in the fourth or fifth intercostal space. The patient is intubated using a double-lumen tube. Through this incision the left IMA can be harvested either directly or video assisted. Usually, the pleura is opened, and the left lung is deflated. In the incision the left IMA is identified carefully. The left accompanying vein is clipped and cut. More length is gained caudally and craniad by meticulous dissection while the wound is gradually opened with a small retractor. Harvesting in the skeletonized way using fine DeBakey forceps and the cautery spatula is preferred. The endothoracic fascia is gradually opened, and small strands are cauterized using low energy coagulation ('coagulation/fulgurate'). All branches are clipped and cut in between to avoid thermal damage. Desiccation is prevented by a small pad with diluted papaverine. By hoisting the craniad ribs by a retractor attached to the table rail or by a thoracic wall tilting device which in turn is attached to the wound retractor, dissection can be completed up to the level of the first intercostal space. High dissection is particularly necessary in planned jump grafts to the diagonal branch and LAD. If additional length is necessary distally, the cartilage of the caudal rib is cut with a knife from the inside to enable easy healing and to avoid damaging the IMA. The cartilage is sutured at closure. The least invasive technique is the Cohn 'H-graft' preparation. In this technique a graft is used as an interposition graft without dissection of the IMA (Figure 10c). Resection of cartilage may be necessary in this H-graft. Careful wound closure is important to prevent lung herniation.

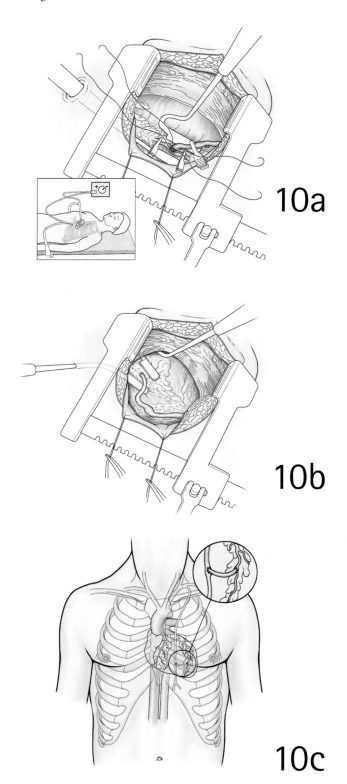

10a

10b

10c

After heparinization, the IMA is distally cut between clips. The pericardium is opened longitudinally, and the lateral rim is suspended, after which two-lung ventilation can usually be resumed. The LAD is identified. A peanut swab may help to identify its position by assessing the right ventricle transition to the more solid septum from right to left. Then a retractor or table rail based stabilizer is positioned. When the Octopus I suction paddles are used, the paddle to the left side of the LAD (straight right paddle) is positioned through a separate stab wound, and the paddle to the right side of the LAD (left preformed paddle) is positioned aside in the wound. Suction (−400 mm Hg) is activated, and dissection is started, followed by spreading of the pods. Microvascular clamps are used for local segmental occlusion. A short, 1-minute 'wait and see' for ST-segment changes is used before arteriotomy, which is preferably performed with a diamond knife. The already prepared IMA is then grafted to the LAD. Before and after tying, quality assessment is performed.

In sequential grafting, which is only feasible in a narrow-angled diagonal-LAD fork, the diagonal side-to-side anastomosis is always performed first. Exposure is feasible with suction fixation by median displacement of the anterolateral myocardium. In this anastomosis, a two-needle technique is performed, whereas in end-to-side anastomosis, the parachute down the heel technique is preferred (see the section "Anastomosis").

The Cohn graft may be particularly suitable to perform a salvage revascularization of the LAD in a poor-risk patient. This graft is a short interposition between the IMA and the LAD with radial artery or saphenous vein graft (Cohn H-graft; Figure 10c). Therefore, cartilage is resected to expose only a short segment of the LAD. The anastomosis is usually performed first on the LAD and then to the IMA. Competition or steal phenomenon seems not to be an issue, as little diastolic flow augmentation may relieve angina (Figure 10c).

Alternatively, for off-pump single LAD grafting in redo cases or in the absence of an IMA, the subclavian artery or preferably the proximal axillary artery can be used as the inflow conduit, utilizing a saphenous vein graft or radial artery (Figure 10d). The artery is exposed via an infraclavicular incision, retracting the pectoralis major muscle and pectoralis minor muscle, median to the deltoid muscle. The artery is identified above the vein, encircled, and segmentally clamped. After the proximal anastomosis at the caudal-dorsal aspect (to prevent kinking) has been completed, the left lung is deflated. The adjacent intercostal space is opened with a curved forceps for 2–3 cm (in case of a narrow space through the bed of the locally resected second or third rib). Using a long-grasping forceps, the surgeon passes the graft to the small left anterior thoracotomy. A light cable may help, also to check for hemostasis of the intercostal space. Then the LAD anastomosis is performed as described (Figure 10a).

Graft flow is measured, preferably with the stabilizer removed, as this may affect distal myocardial tissue perfusion. Protamine is given, starting with 25 mg. The pericardium is closed, leaving 4 cm IMA intrapericardially to facilitate redo surgery. The thoracotomy wound is closed, leaving a pleuradrain via the stab wound.

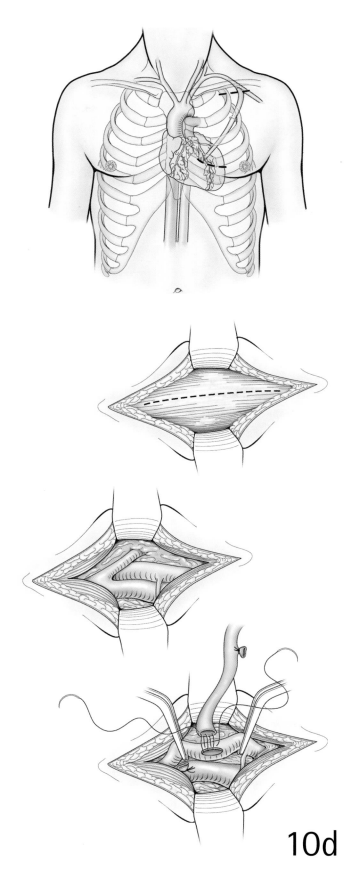

10d

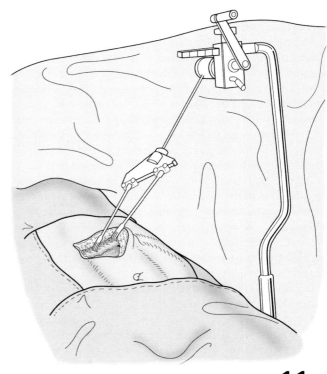

11a

PARTIAL T-STERNOTOMY–SUBXIPHOID APPROACH

11a, b, c
The thoracic integrity may be preserved by distal T-sternotomy in the second intercostal space up to the xyphoid, for grafting of LAD, diagonal and RCA (Figure 3c). An ITA retractor (Rultract, Cleveland, OH) is used for bilateral IMA harvesting (Figure 11a, b, c). By caudal extension of the 12 cm incision with 3 cm, the GEA can be harvested. This access can be used for the more distal target coronary segments of these coronary arteries. Exposure and stabilization is similar to full sternotomy using the woundretractor based stabilizer and the ITA retractor in addition.

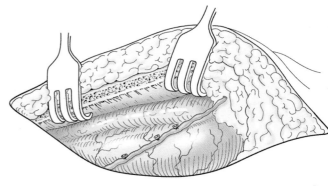

11b

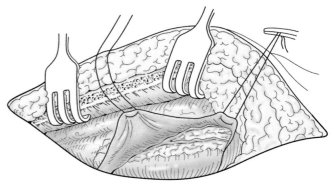

11c

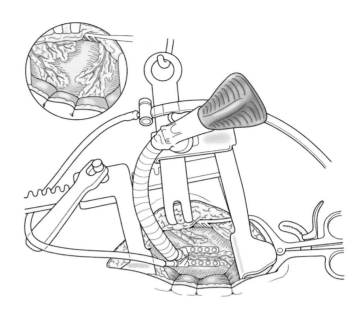

12a

12a, b To preserve the thoracic integrity alternatively, a transverse curved laparotomy (3f) can be used. When both rectus abdomini muscles are released of the lower costal margin, and the pericardium is opened, the GEA is harvested directly and the IMA is harvested as described previously or endoscopically. The lower edge of the thoracic cage is lifted with a table rail mounted ITA retractor hook attached to the distal sternum (after removal of the xiphoid), giving a good exposure of the antero-inferior wall of the heart. It gives access to distal LAD and RCA. The Octopus II stabilizer can be mounted on this retractor to stabilize the coronary artery. Suturing of the caudal (diaphragm) pericardial rim to the skin elevates the pericardial sac ventrally. In addition, the apical suction device can help in exposure of the target artery.

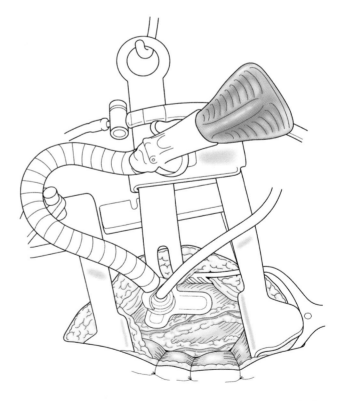

12b

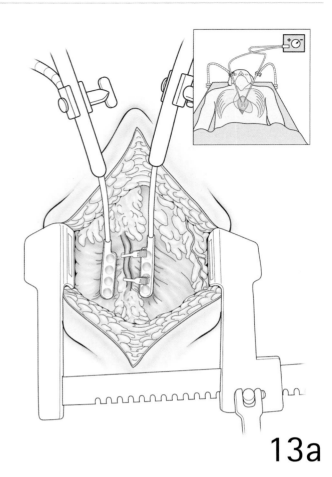

13a

A more distal small T-sternotomy with subxiphoid extension is usually reserved for isolated distal RCA, including the PDA. This approach saves the thoracic cage and allows use of the right GEA. Only patients with a (sub)totally occluded RCA with demonstrated collateral circulation should be included, as the early flow capacity of the GEA may be insufficient, and ischemic hemodynamic deterioration may occur.

13b

For this single-vessel grafting, the distal sternotomy has to be extended toward the umbilicus for only 5 cm (3d). The assistant presents the greater curvature manually by grabbing the stomach around the gastric tube or with a Duval clamp. The GEA is harvested in the pedicled way using multiple clips or the harmonic scalpel, starting with the gastric side and then the omental side guided by tactile feedback of the pulsating GEA between index finger and thumb, and down to its origin to obtain full length. By utilizing small bites, length is optimized. After assessment of the required length, the patient is heparinized. The conduit is ligated distally (sparing the gastric wall) and routed intrapericardially anterior to the liver, directly adjacent to the falciform ligament so that the GEA can be routed to the distal RCA or PDA without kinking. Alternatively, the GEA can be routed retrogastric, behind the left lobe of the liver and through the omental bursa and through a 3 cm hole in the diaphragm.

Using only a soft tissue retractor, the table rail–based Octopus I with two straight paddles may be used. It immobilizes the target vessel well and may present the target site ventrally by hoisting the myocardium. The anastomosis is performed with an 8/0 running suture, starting with the toe and using the two-needle technique.

Quality control is by Doppler signal. The transit-time probe should not be used, as the vessel may become spastic.

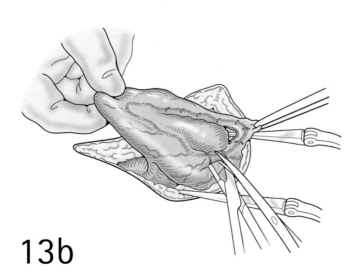

LEFT POSTERIOR THORACOTOMY

14 Left posterior thoracotomy is useful for redo surgery. The patient is in the right lateral position. Double-lumen intubation is recommended. A 15-cm posterior thoracotomy in the fifth or sixth intercostal space exposes the circumflex artery branches well (14). The pericardium is opened posterior to the phrenic nerve. For the diagonal branch and the LAD grafting, the thoracotomy incision should be extended anteriorly and the pericardium also opened ventrally to the phrenic nerve. The quality of the descending aorta as the inflow conduit is sometimes disappointing. Alternative inflow conduits have been discussed previously. The radial artery and saphenous vein can be used. Tissue stabilization can be retractor based (thoracotomy retractor) or table rail based.

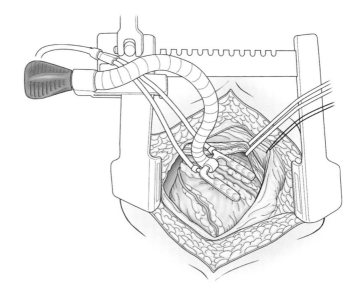

14

POSTOPERATIVE CARE

In off-pump CABG, treatment is directed to early awakening and extubation, sometimes in the operating room. Thoracic epidural anesthesia and normothermia facilitate early recovery. The mental recovery after off-pump surgery is usually striking, especially after light combined anesthesia. Patients are soon alert.

The circulation is stable. Inotrope use, if necessary during surgery, is rarely needed postoperatively. The blood loss is generally less than is seen with traditional bypass surgery. This situation may be explained by the absence of hemodilution and no damage to the blood constituents, particularly the platelets. As less protamine is given, it is recommended that an activated clotting time level should be checked early when unexpected blood loss occurs. The drain can be removed after 24 hours (in more recent experience only the pericardial cavity is drained).

Low-dose acetylsalicylic acid (80 mg) is started as soon as the patient is awake. Thrombosis prophylaxis (nadroparine) is continued during admission, as well as amlodipine (for 6 weeks). Sotalol is given prophylactically for 6 weeks to prevent atrial fibrillation. Early mobilization is encouraged on day 1. Discharge is on day 5–6. Diuretics are given only once or twice during admission, less than in traditional on-pump CABG.

OUTCOME

Based on the observational and randomized evidence so far, the outcome of off-pump coronary surgery is promising. The mortality of off-pump CABG approaches zero in a selected group of patients with reasonable coronary arteries and ventricles. In this group, off-pump CABG is safe and more cost effective. Furthermore, conversions due to ischemia rarely occur when an experienced team of surgeon and anesthesiologist perform the operation; and as a consequence, a standby heart-lung machine is not needed. Underrated coronary pathology or poor left ventricular function may still require incidental conversion to cardiopulmonary bypass. Patency rates almost equal those that are seen in on-pump CABG. In several reports, patency rates of up to 95 per cent have been cited using arterial grafts. Thus, arterial grafting for longevity also seems feasible in off-pump grafting.

By avoiding the instrumentation of and the use of extracorporeal circulation, the morbidity of coronary bypass surgery has diminished. Water damage is less, the inflammatory response is less, the blood loss is less, infections are less, postoperative paroxysmal atrial fibrillation is less frequent, renal function is better preserved, and the neuropsychological outcome is expected to be better than after traditional surgery. Recovery is accelerated, although hospital stay is only reduced by 1 day, as patients feel more secure after heart surgery in the hospital. The results in patients with associated risk factors, such as advanced age, poor lung function, poor renal function, peripheral vascular disease, and diabetes, who might benefit particularly from off-pump CABG, have to be awaited from randomized trials.

Certainly, a learning curve exists for off-pump CABG compared to traditional on-pump CABG. Details are important. In a fair percentage of patients, off-pump bypass is technically more demanding and time consuming than on-pump CABG. Currently, it is anticipated that off-pump isolated coronary surgery may double to 40 per cent of patients.

FURTHER READING

Borst, C., Jansen, E.W.L, Tulleken, C., *et al.* 1996. Coronary artery bypass grafting without cardiopulmonary bypass and without interruption of native coronary flow using a novel anastomosis site-restraining device ('Octopus'). *Journal of the American College of Cardiology* **27(6)**, 1356–64.

Calafiore, A.M., Teodori, G., DiGiammarco, G., *et al.* 1999. Multiple arterial conduits without cardiopulmonary bypass: early angiographic results. *Annals of Thoracic Surgery* **67**, 450–6.

Gründeman, P.F., Borst, C., van Herwaarden, J., Mansvelt Beck, H.J., Jansen E.W.L. 1997. Hemodynamic changes during displacement of the beating heart by the Utrecht Octopus method. *Annals of Thoracic Surgery* **63**, S88–92.

Jansen, E.W.L, Borst, C., Lahpor, J.L., *et al.* 1998. Coronary artery bypass grafting without cardiopulmonary bypass using the 'Octopus' method: results in the first 100 patients. *Journal of Thoracic and Cardiovascular Surgery* **116**, 60–7.

Kolessov, V.I. 1967. Mammary artery–coronary artery anastomosis as method of treatment for angina pectoris. *Journal of Thoracic and Cardiovascular Surgery* **54**, 535–44.

Nierich, A., Diephuis, J., Jansen, E.W., *et al.* 1999. Embracing the heart: perioperative management of patients undergoing off-pump coronary artery bypass grafting using the Octopus tissue stabilizer. *Journal of Cardiothoracic and Vascular Anesthesia* **13(2)**, 123–9.

10

Multi-vessel coronary revascularization on the beating heart

EREZ SHARONI MD
Cardiothoracic Surgery, Rabin Medical Center, Bielinson Campus, Petach Tikva, Sackler School of Medicine, Tel Aviv, Israel

JOHN D. PUSKAS MD, MS
Associate Professor of Surgery, Division of Cardiothoracic Surgery, Emory University School of Medicine; Attending Cardiothoracic Surgeon, Department of Surgery, Crawford Long Hospital of Emory University, Atlanta, Georgia, USA

HISTORY

Coronary artery bypass grafting (CABG) was born in the 1960s as surgery on the beating heart. However, improvements in cardiopulmonary bypass (CPB) and the introduction of cardioplegia caused a huge expansion in arrested heart surgery. Despite the advantages offered by these techniques (e.g. a bloodless and motionless environment), a few surgeons continued to perform coronary revascularization on the beating heart, usually motivated by cost containment. More recently, off-pump coronary artery bypass grafting (OPCAB) has been repopularized in an effort to avoid the diffuse inflammatory response, multi-organ dysfunction, and neurological complications associated with CPB. The authors and others have recently shown excellent graft patency, improved outcomes, and lower costs with OPCAB.

PRINCIPLES AND JUSTIFICATION

OPCAB must be performed in such a way that complete revascularization is not compromised by the surgeon's decision to avoid CPB. Multiple reports have documented the vital importance of complete revascularization for long-term cardiac event-free survival after CABG. To be considered a viable or attractive alternative to CABG on CPB, OPCAB must provide the same revascularization with less morbidity. If OPCAB is to be a safe and reliable procedure, hemodynamic stability must be maintained throughout.

The OPCAB procedure differs from conventional CABG on CPB in several very important ways. The most fundamental difference is that the patient's heart must support his or her circulation during OPCAB, whereas the heart-lung machine provides that function during CABG on CPB. This fact requires the OPCAB surgeon to manipulate the heart to expose each coronary artery target in such a way that ventricular filling and function are not impaired. Although the heart may be grossly compressed to expose coronary targets on CPB, it must be displaced without being compressed to maintain hemodynamic stability during OPCAB. Once the techniques for safe cardiac displacement and coronary exposure are mastered, the construction of coronary anastomoses during OPCAB proceeds in much the same fashion as for CABG on CPB; therein lies the 'secret' of OPCAB.

With a clear understanding of the exposure techniques described in this chapter, a surgeon skilled in CABG on CPB may approach virtually all primary, isolated, elective coronary patients off-pump. Redo and emergency cases introduce a more complex set of considerations and should be approached selectively and with caution. Patients for whom OPCAB may be inappropriate are patients in cardiogenic shock, suffering ischemic arrhythmias, or with physical conditions that profoundly limit rotation of the heart (e.g. pectus excavation or previous left pneumonectomy). Intramyocardial or unusually small or calcified coronary arteries may be safely bypassed off-pump only with the benefit of considerable experience.

The patient risks entailed in OPCAB procedures are similar to those for CABG on CPB and include, among others, a finite risk of death, myocardial infarction, stroke, bleeding, and infection. Numerous retrospective reports have shown a reduction in these risks for patients having OPCAB compared to those having CABG on CPB, but prospective randomized trials to date have had limited statistical power and have confirmed some, but not all, of these claims

PREOPERATIVE ASSESSMENT AND PREPARATION

Indications for OPCAB are identical to those established for CABG. Contraindications to CPB that may disqualify some very high-risk patients from conventional CABG do not apply to the same degree to OPCAB. Coronary revascularization candidates must undergo a complete history and physical examination. If the Allen's test is inconclusive, radial and ulnar artery duplex examinations are performed before radial arteries are harvested. Pulmonary function tests are performed only in patients with severe chronic obstructive pulmonary disease (COPD) or active pulmonary disease. Criteria for preoperative carotid duplex examination include left main disease, peripheral vascular disease, carotid bruits, history of CVA or transient ischemic attack, heavy tobacco use, or age older than 65 years. A thorough informed consent is obtained.

ANESTHESIA

All patients undergoing OPCAB require at least an arterial line and central venous line for monitoring. Significantly depressed left ventricular (LV) function mandates a Swan-Ganz catheter. Those patients with severe ventricular dysfunction may benefit from preoperative placement of an intra-aortic balloon pump. General endotracheal anesthesia with low-dose narcotic and inhalational agents allows for rapid awakening with adequate pain control. Fluid resuscitation is accomplished with lactated Ringer's solution rather than saline or colloid. Blood pressure is maintained with low-dose norepinephrine instead of phenylephrine, when needed. Good communication between the surgeon and the anesthesiologist throughout the procedure is essential. Multiple displacements of the heart during OPCAB subject the patient to repeated hemodynamic changes and require an attentive anesthesiologist.

OPERATIVE PROCEDURE

Experience with OPCAB over 5 years has allowed an evolution in surgical technique. Early in the experience, inotropic support for hemodynamic instability was commonly required during OPCAB. Since the refinement of techniques for cardiac positioning and stabilization, the use of inotropics is infrequent.

The OPCAB procedure differs in many ways from on-pump CABG, but the skin entry and sternotomy are identical. A number 10 blade knife is used through the skin and fat, down to the fascia. Electrocautery is then used only selectively for bleeding and to divide the muscles and fascia at the middle of the sternum. Standard sternotomy is performed with a sternal saw. An upward-lifting Favaloro mammary retractor is used to harvest the left internal mammary artery (LIMA) and/or the right internal mammary artery (RIMA). This retractor aids in exposure of the arteries and minimizes chest wall trauma. Heparin is given (1.5 mg/kg) with a target activated coagulation time (ACT) of more than 300 seconds. Heparin (3 000 units) is reinfused every 30 minutes to maintain an ACT of more than 300 seconds. This regimen is prompted by the recognition that heparin metabolism is more rapid in warm OPCAB patients than in those cooled on CPB.

After heparin is given, the mammary is divided, and a mixture of papaverine and lidocaine is injected into the lumen of the mammary artery and allowed to reside there for 15–30 minutes. The OctoBase sternal retractor (Medtronic, Minneapolis, MN) is placed. This retractor is specifically designed for the Octopus III stabilizer (Medtronic, Minneapolis, MN), which can be secured to any aspect of the retractor.

1 **T-shaped pericardiotomy** A wide T-shaped pericardiotomy is performed, dividing the pericardium from the diaphragm down towards – but not into – the left and right phrenic nerves. The left and right pericardiophrenic artery and vein branches are carefully clipped and divided to avoid postoperative bleeding. Both pleural spaces are opened widely whenever access to the left lateral wall is required. Care is taken during the dissection to clip any large vessels encountered and to avoid the phrenic nerves. Division of the diaphragmatic muscle slips that insert on the right side of the xiphoid is important to allow elevation of the right sternal border, creating space for rightward cardiac displacement. Similarly, excision of a large right-sided pericardial fat pad will provide additional room.

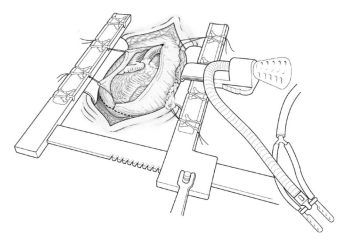

1

2 **Epiaortic ultrasound** All patients undergo epiaortic ultrasound early in the case, which may add only 1 or 2 minutes to the procedure. Epiaortic ultrasound guides the surgeon in individualized placement of aortic clamps and proximal anastomoses to reduce the risk of embolism of atherosclerotic debris from the ascending aorta. Grade IV or V atherosclerosis of the ascending aorta anastomoses mandates avoidance of aortic manipulation. Other possible sites for proximal anastomoses include the innominate artery, LIMA, and RIMA. Alternatively, the new automatic proximal connector devices (i.e. Symmetry Bypass System, St. Jude Medical, Minneapolis, MN) may be used if a soft spot can be identified on the ascending aorta, as these devices are deployed without an aortic clamp.

Rolled towels elevating right sternal border (optional). Placement of two rolled towels under the right limb of the sternal retractor elevates the right sternal edge, allowing the heart to be repositioned towards the right without compression against the sternum or retractor. One or two heavy pericardial sutures are placed on the left pericardium above the phrenic nerve. Division of the left side of the pericardium off the diaphragm towards the phrenic nerve is important, so that traction on this left pericardium may assist in rotating and displacing the heart toward the right to visualize the left lateral wall.

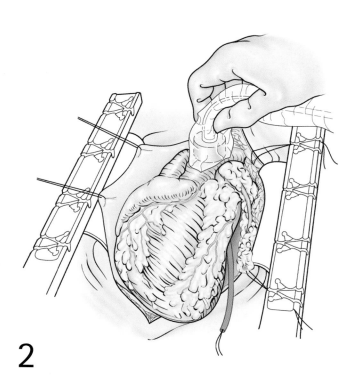

2

3 Placement of deep pericardial traction suture   The most important traction suture is a deep posterior pericardial suture placed approximately two-thirds of the way between the inferior vena cava and the left pulmonary vein at the point where the pericardium reflects over the left atrium. Care should be taken with placement of this suture to avoid the aorta, esophagus, left lung, and pulmonary veins. The suture is covered with a rubber catheter to prevent trauma to the epicardium.

The heart is allowed to roll with gravity into the left or right chest, facilitated by table rotation, traction suture(s), and, occasionally, a cotton sling. The heart should never be compressed against the sternum or pericardium. The right pericardial traction sutures are released when exposing the left side of the heart; similarly, the left traction sutures are released when exposing the right coronary artery (RCA). Pericardial sutures on both the right and left sides are never under tension simultaneously when displacing the heart to expose coronary targets. Gentle application of these techniques maintains stable hemodynamics while providing excellent exposure.

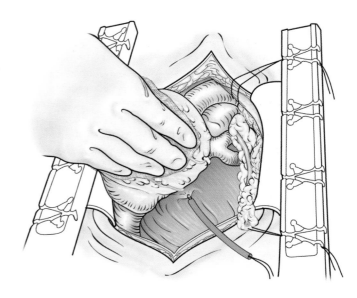

3

Cardiac displacement and presentation of coronary targets

Cardiac displacement techniques for exposure of the inferior and lateral vessels are different.

Exposure of inferior wall   For the RCA and inferior wall vessels such as the posterior descending artery and LV branch or posterolateral obtuse marginal coronary artery (PLOM), the deep stitch is pulled toward the feet and clamped to the drapes. The Octopus III stabilizer is attached to the left limb of the off-pump coronary artery bypass grafting sternal retractor (OctoBase, Medtronic, Minneapolis, MN). The patient is placed in the Trendelenburg position with the theater table tilted to the right. The base of the heart is elevated. The apex is oriented vertically.

The lateral vessels are approached by allowing the base of the heart to descend and rolling the apex of the heart under the right sternal border.

4 Exposure of lateral wall without starfish   As mentioned, the right pleural cavity is opened, and the traction sutures on the right pericardium are released. The left-sided traction sutures are pulled up taut on the retractor, and the table is rotated sharply to the right to aid in rolling the heart into the right chest. The deep stitch is pulled towards the patient's left shoulder and secured to the drapes. The Octopus III stabilizer is mounted on the right side of the retractor, and its arm reaches across the heart, both aiding in presentation and accomplishing stabilization of the obtuse marginal coronary arteries. A cotton sling may facilitate exposure of the marginal vessel in cases of cardiomegaly.

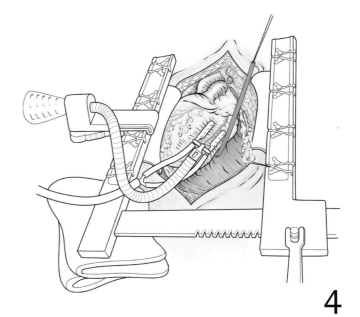

4

5 **Exposure of lateral wall with starfish** At least two corporations have recently introduced cardiac positioning devices (i.e. Axius Xpose Device, Guidant, Indianapolis, IN; and Starfish, Medtronic, Minneapolis, MN) that use suction to attach to the apex of the heart and can elevate and displace the heart to provide exposure of coronary targets with little hemodynamic compromise. These devices are aids in exposure/presentation and are not designed for coronary stabilization. They are used in conjunction with coronary stabilizers, such as the Octopus III stabilizer, and they may facilitate OPCAB exposure, particularly in cases of cardiomegaly and depressed LV function.

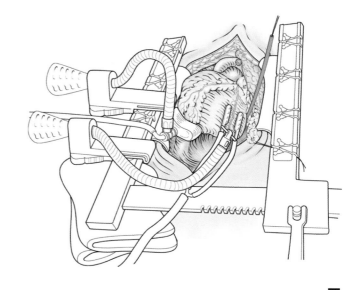

5

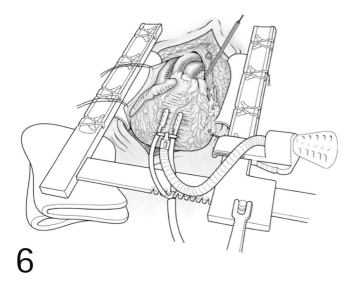

6

6 **Exposure of anterior wall** In contrast to targets on the inferior and lateral walls, the anterior vessels [left anterior descending (LAD) and diagonals] are exposed with very little manipulation of the heart. The deep stitch is secured to the left drapes, and the Octopus III stabilizer is brought onto the heart from the caudal aspect or left limb of the retractor. Care is taken to divide the pericardium to allow the mammary pedicle to fall posteriorly in the apex of the left chest.

Coronary stabilization and grafting

The Octopus III stabilizer is a suction device, not a compression device. Therefore, good tissue capture can be achieved while applying the device at the mechanical median of the cardiac cycle, rather than vigorously compressing the cardiac chambers. Thus, stabilization is optimized, and mechanical interference with ventricular function is minimized. Once the device is applied, a few seconds may be needed for the heart to recover. If hemodynamics are compromised, the degree of compression should be reduced, and the mechanical median of the cardiac cycle should be more clearly identified by releas-

ing the knob of the Octopus III arm while maintaining suction. The suction is maintained to avoid losing tissue capture. After the appropriate position for the limb is determined, the Octopus III arm is tightened once more. The malleable pods on the Octopus III allow one to spread the epicardium adjacent to the coronary targets, significantly improving visualization of the vessel. The malleable pods may be bent up, down, or in a curve. They may be bent or rotated independent of each other to accommodate irregular epicardial surfaces.

After optimal exposure is obtained, a soft silastic vessel loop (Quest Medical, Allen, TX) is placed around the target vessel for occlusion. The loop is placed proximal to the chosen anastomotic site, never distally. Avoiding entrance into the ventricle and trauma to the epicardial veins with the vessel loops is wise. When this problem occurs, a superficial epicardial suture will reliably stop bleeding. The vessel loop may be directed out of the surgeon's field of view with the aid of a loose pericardial suture serving as a pulley.

Once the distal anastomosis is underway, the anesthesia team must continuously communicate with the surgical team. Any changes in hemodynamics should be quickly addressed. Bradyarrhythmias may be promptly and easily treated with atrial and/or ventricular pacing. Occlusion of the RCA proximal to the atrioventricular nodal artery may cause bradycardia, which reliably responds to epicardial pacing.

The target vessel is opened with a coronary knife and the arteriotomy is extended with coronary scissors. The field is kept free of blood by dispersing the retrograde bleeding with a humidified ClearView Blower/Mister (Medtronic, Minneapolis, MN). The blower/mister uses warm, humidified, pH-balanced fluid and carbon dioxide to clear the target site of blood and help expose the intima of the coronary artery. Blowing on the target should only be done when placing the needle through the tissue to minimize intimal trauma. Good visualization is critical for a precise anastomosis. The intima of both the conduit and coronary artery is visualized with each stitch. Optical magnification (3.5 × loupes), a headlight, and Castroviejo needle drivers are used on all anastomoses. Each distal anastomosis is constructed with 8/0 monofilament suture to optimize precision, unless severe calcification requires a larger, stronger needle.

An intracoronary (or aortocoronary) shunt may be placed if significant hemodynamic compromise occurs due to ischemia after target vessel occlusion. The shunts (Medtronic, Minneapolis, MN) range in size from 1.5 mm to 3.0 mm, in 0.25 mm increments. These shunts are easily placed and removed. They are used infrequently, but are kept available in the room for all cases. Intracoronary shunts may be particularly helpful with large right coronary arteries (where bradyarrhythmias may occur), intramyocardial vessels (where placement of an occlusive vessel loop may be hazardous), and critical anatomy (where occlusion of a key collateralizing vessel may be poorly tolerated). The coronary shunt is removed before tying the suture on the distal side and re-establishing flow. Air is allowed to expel from the anastomosis before tying the suture. The conduit should be occluded with an atraumatic bulldog clamp until the proximal anastomosis is performed to prevent retrograde bleeding and loss of coronary perfusion.

Sequence of grafting in off-pump coronary artery bypass grafting

In off-pump coronary surgery, the chosen sequence of grafting is important to maintain hemodynamic stability and avoid critical ischemia. As a general rule, the collateralized vessel(s) are grafted first and then reperfused by performing the proximal anastomosis(es), unclamping the internal mammary flow, or connecting the perfusion-assisted direct coronary artery bypass (PADCAB) apparatus. The last coronary target grafted is the collateralizing vessel(s). This strategy obviates interrupting vital flow from the collateralizing vessel(s) to the collateralized vessels until after the collateralized vessel(s) have been grafted.

Performing the proximal anastomoses first makes estimation of graft length difficult. At times, the proximal anastomoses may be performed early in the operative sequence to aid in early reperfusion of a collateralized vessel. If the LIMA→LAD graft must be performed first, a long mammary pedicle may be necessary to avoid tension on the LIMA anastomosis during subsequent cardiac displacement to expose lateral wall targets.

Suggestions concerning the sequence of grafting follow:

- Perform the anastomosis to the completely occluded, collateralized vessel(s) first. The collateralizing vessel may then be safely grafted. This strategy will minimize myocardial ischemia.
- The LIMA→LAD anastomosis should be performed first if the LAD is collateralized or in cases of tight left main stenosis. This anastomosis is performed last when the LAD is the collateralizing vessel.
- The proximal anastomosis can be performed first or early after the distal anastomosis if the target is a critical, collateralized vessel. This strategy allows simultaneous perfusion during the occlusion of the collateralizing vessel and minimizes overall myocardial ischemia.
- Beware the large RCA. The RCA, particularly if large and dominant, can cause significant problems when occluded during OPCAB. Acute occlusion of a moderately stenotic RCA may lead to severe hemodynamic compromise due to bradycardia. The surgeon must be prepared to use an intracoronary shunt or epicardial pacing to promptly correct bradyarrhythmias.
- Beware mitral regurgitation in OPCAB. Prolonged cardiac displacement combined with mitral regurgitation may contribute to a downward hemodynamic spiral. Ischemic mitral regurgitation should be addressed early in the procedure; this goal can be accomplished by grafting and perfusing the culprit vessel responsible for papillary muscle dysfunction.
- Graft sequence should be individualized, depending on anatomic patterns of coronary occlusion and collateralization, myocardial contractility, atherosclerosis of the ascending aorta, conduit availability, and graft geometry.

Perfusion–assisted off-pump coronary artery bypass grafting

With experience and gentle application of the principles described previously, virtually all coronary vessels can be safely exposed, stabilized, and grafted during OPCAB. However, the cumulative effect of sequential coronary occlusions can occasionally lead to a downward spiral of hemo-dynamic stability. At times, accessory perfusion to the myocardium may be helpful while other vessels are occluded. PADCAB allows for direct perfusion of myocardium subtended by a coronary bypass target artery – either during performance of the distal anastomosis, by means of an olive-tipped intracoronary catheter, or after completion of the distal anastomosis – by providing controlled flow down the conduit.

7 PADCAB Inflow to the PADCAB circuit and pump is provided by a catheter placed in the ascending aorta or femoral artery. The Quest MPS system (Quest Medical, Allen, TX) allows for exact control of coronary perfusion pressure. Pharmacological additives and temperature control may accentuate its protective effects. The coronary perfusion pressure during PADCAB is independent of systemic pressure. This technique is especially helpful in collateralized targets, as coronary flow may be driven through collaterals to supply adjacent myocardium. One can also measure and document graft patency and flows with the circuit. Multiple grafts may be perfused simultaneously, by use of a multi-limbed perfusion set. Discontinuation of flow through all the grafts simultaneously must not be done when the proximal anastomoses are performed. Each graft should be disconnected from the multi-limb perfusion set separately to perform its proximal anastomosis. PADCAB is used selectively by the authors to minimize regional ischemia and improve myocardial protection in cases of critical coronary anastomosis and profound cardiac dysfunction. Some practitioners use PADCAB routinely to optimize myocardial perfusion and hemodynamic stability for all OPCAB cases.

Proximal anastomoses to the aorta are performed with an aortic partial occlusion clamp. The systolic pressure is brought down to approximately 90–95 mm Hg before application of the clamp. Once the clamp is applied, the aortotomies are created with a 4.0-mm aortic punch. The application of the aortic clamp is guided by the results of epiaortic ultrasound scanning as previously discussed. Vein graft anastomoses are constructed with 5/0 or 6/0 monofilament suture and arterial grafts with 7/0 monofilament suture. Any graft taken as a 'T' off the IMA is anastomosed with 8/0 monofilament. Air is expelled by tying the final suture after removing the cross-clamp. The vein grafts are kept occluded until punctured with a 25-gauge needle to expel air. Arterial grafts are not punctured, but are allowed to backbleed before cross-clamp removal.

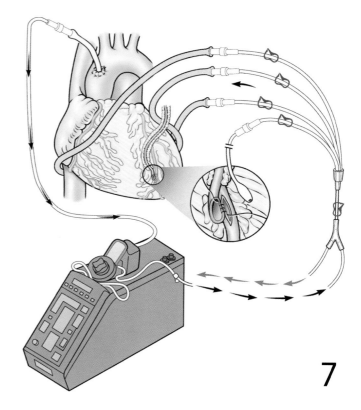

7

After completion and reperfusion of all grafts, protamine is administered (0.75–1.0 mg/kg) to correct the ACT to approximately 150 seconds. As hemostasis is being achieved, three chest tubes are routinely placed, one in each pleural space and one in the mediastinum. Temporary pacing wires are used only if the patient requires epicardial pacing immediately before chest closure. The chest is closed in standard fashion. Nine sternal wires are routinely used to facilitate a tight sternal closure. Interrupted fascial sutures below the xyphoid assure a tight fascial closure. The subdermis and skin are closed with running absorbable sutures.

OUTCOMES

As with other new techniques, a learning curve is associated with OPCAB. With persistence and patient attention to detail, this technique can be mastered and performed reproducibly and reliably. OPCAB may show improved outcomes compared with conventional CABG, especially in patients for whom CPB has elevated risks. Thus, all cardiac surgeons should be comfortable with this technique.

FURTHER READING

Ascione, R., Williams, S., Lloyd, C.T., Sundaramoorthi, T., Pitsis, A.A., Angelini, G.D. 2001. Reduced postoperative blood loss and transfusion requirement after beating-heart coronary operations: a prospective randomized study. *Journal of Thoracic and Cardiovascular Surgery* 121(4), 689–96.

Buffolo, E., de Andrade, C.S., Branco, J.N., Teles, C.A., Aguiar, L.F., Gomes, W.J. 1996. Coronary artery bypass surgery without cardiopulmonary bypass. *Annals of Thoracic Surgery* 61, 63–6.

Guyton, R.A., Thourani, V.H., Puskas, J.D., *et al.* 2000. Perfusion-assisted direct coronary artery bypass: selective graft perfusion in off-pump cases. *Annals of Thoracic Surgery* 69(1), 171–5.

Puskas, J.D., Vinten-Johansen, J., Muraki, S., Guyton, R.A. 2001. Myocardial protection for off-pump coronary artery bypass surgery. *Seminars in Thoracic and Cardiovascular Surgery* 13(1), 82–8.

Puskas, J.D., Thourani, V.H., Marshall, J.J., *et al.* 2001. Clinical outcomes, angiographic patency, and resource utilization in 200 consecutive off-pump coronary bypass patients. *Annals of Thoracic Surgery* 71(5), 1477–84.

Puskas, J.D., Williams, W.M., Duke, P.G., *et al.* 2003. Off-pump coronary artery bypass grafting provides complete revascularisation with reduced myocardial injury, transfusion requirements and length of stay: a prospective randomised comparison of two hundred unselected patients undergoing off-pump versus conventional coronary bypass grafting. *Journal of Thoracic and Cardiovascular Surgery* 125, 797–808.

van Dijk, D., Nierich, A.P., Jansen, E.W., Nathoe, H.M., Suyker, W.J., Diephuis, J.C. 2001. Early outcome after off-pump versus on-pump coronary bypass surgery: results from a randomized study. *Circulation* 104, 1761–6.

Reoperative coronary artery bypass grafting

PATRICK G. MAGEE MB, CHB, FRCS
Consultant Surgeon, Department of Cardiothoracic Surgery, London Chest Hospital, London, UK

PRINCIPLES AND JUSTIFICATION

Reoperative coronary artery bypass grafting (redo CABG) is challenging and dangerous. Most reported series describe increased mortality and complications after redo CABG. Although previous reports had suggested a progressive increase in the occurrence of reoperative CABG, more recently this increase appears to be plateauing. This decline may be related to more common use of arterial grafts, in particular, the left internal mammary artery (LIMA); the benefits of secondary prevention, especially the use of lipid lowering drugs and aspirin; and the increased use of percutaneous transluminal coronary angioplasty and stenting to treat stenosed vein grafts. The need for repeat coronary surgery results from vein graft disease, progression of native coronary atherosclerosis, or a combination of these factors. Approximately 40 per cent of saphenous vein grafts are occluded 10 years after CABG, and a further 30 per cent are stenotic, primarily due to vein graft atherosclerosis. Graft atherosclerosis is much less common when arterial grafts are used. The left internal mammary graft appears to be especially resistant to atherosclerotic deterioration. Problems associated with redo CABG include the need for resternotomy and establishing cardiopulmonary bypass in a scarred or distorted pericardial space, the presence of stenotic but patent grafts, the difficulty of locating coronary arteries, and the availability of a conduit for additional graft construction.

Indications for redo coronary surgery are essentially those for first-time CABG. Although the benefits are similar, however, the risks tend to be higher; therefore, reoperation should be reserved for those at greater risk or those with more disabling symptoms. In particular, patent grafts and, especially, patent arterial grafts may be damaged at reoperation, and this risk should be considered in the decision-making process. If the left internal mammary has been properly positioned laterally at the primary operation, then a patent LIMA to the left anterior descending artery should not complicate reoperation.

Emergency reoperative coronary surgery carries a significantly increased risk; therefore, all efforts should be made to settle unstable patients before undertaking surgery.

PREOPERATIVE ASSESSMENT AND PREPARATION

The patient's need for revascularization will have been assessed in the normal way, and angiography will have demonstrated the native coronary anatomy and the condition of the existing bypass grafts. Review of the angiogram, however, may reveal contrast washing in and out of a native vessel, indicating that a portion of a bypass graft is patent, even if it had not been selectively demonstrated.

Previous angiograms, whenever available, should be reviewed — a good distal vessel that was visualized on a previous angiogram but is not seen on the current film is likely to still be present and represents a good target. As a general principle, coronary arteries do not disappear. Previous operative notes also often provide useful information. A vessel described in a previous operative report by an experienced surgeon as being small and of poor quality will likely remain the same later.

Assessment of left ventricular function by angiography, multiple gated acquisition scan, or echocardiogram also will be useful in determining whether there are likely to be graftable targets. A normally contracting region of the left ventricle is likely to contain suitable vessels and graftable arteries.

It may also be helpful to demonstrate viability in regions with nonvisualized arterial target vessels. This possibility can be assessed using thallium scanning, positron emission tomography scanning, or stress echocardiography.

OPERATION

Sternotomy

Before painting and draping, external defibrillator plates should be attached to the patient's back. Should the patient unexpectedly develop ventricular fibrillation before the heart is dissected out, these may allow normal rhythm to be re-established and, thus, avoid the need for rapid and possibly inaccurate dissection.

Damage to underlying structures during sternal opening and subsequent mobilization is a real risk. This risk is enhanced if, for example, aortic dilatation is present, or a patent graft crosses or approaches the midline [e.g. a right internal mammary artery (IMA) to a left coronary or a patent LIMA]. The proximity of the LIMA to the midline and sternum should have been determined by the preoperative studies, especially the angiogram and the chest x-ray, which should include a high-quality true lateral view.

1 In situations in which the risk of injury is felt to be increased, the groin vessels or the axillary artery should be dissected out and possibly even cannulated. If the risk is particularly high, cardiopulmonary bypass can be established before opening the chest. This strategy produces an obvious advantage in terms of safety, with decompression of the aorta and other vascular structures. A significant disadvantage may be increased postoperative bleeding, as the dissection of the scarred pericardial structures is carried out with the patient fully heparinized.

Regardless, in all resternotomies, the groin should be at least painted and draped, and a cannula suitable for femoral cannulation should be readily available. In addition, the perfusionist should be in the operating theater, and the lines for the bypass circuit should be on the operating table. Blood should be available in the theater suite.

Many surgeons use aprotinin from the outset. There have been fears expressed about its use in coronary surgery because of possible procoagulant effects. Although these concerns are disputed, it is not our practice to use aprotinin during redo coronary surgery.

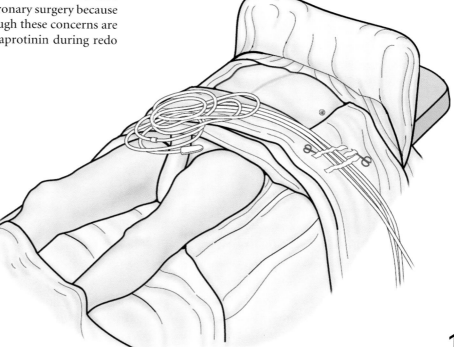

1

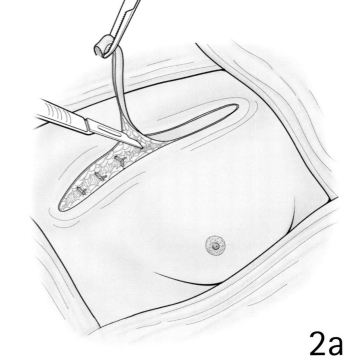

2a

2a, b The previous scar may be excised, and the incision is then deepened down to the sternal wires. These are divided anteriorly and bent back, but not removed.

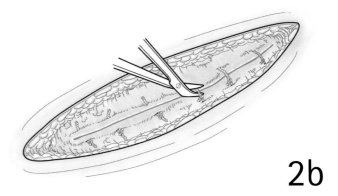

2b

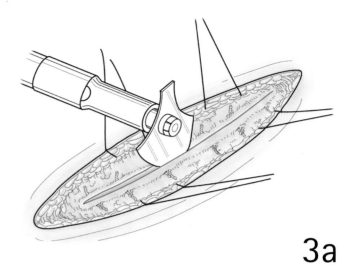

3a

3a, b The sternum is then divided down to the wires with an oscillating saw. The outer layers of the sternum are distracted, usually using the key to the retractor inserted sideways, and the inner table is then divided using heavy scissors while the sternum is elevated by stay sutures.

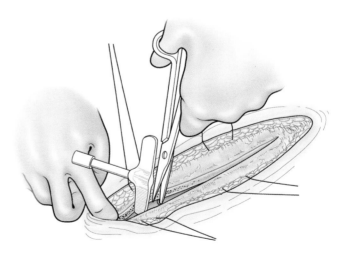

3b

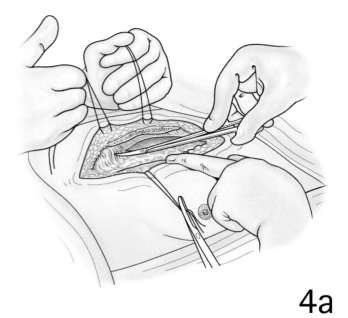

4a

Mobilization and cannulation

4a, b Once the sternum has been divided, sharp dissection should be used to separate each side of the sternum from the underlying structures. A sternal retractor may then be inserted, but should only be opened slowly and gradually as dissection progresses to avoid injury, especially to the right ventricle and innominate vein, both of which are at particular risk of stretch injury.

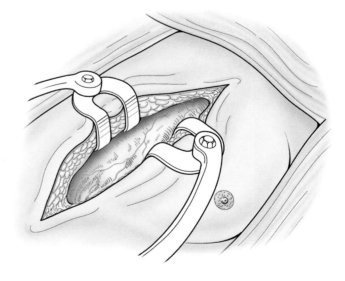

4b

5 Subsequent dissection should start at the level of the diaphragm, where the correct plane is usually easy to identify. Dissection should then proceed up to the right side, around the right atrium, and on to the aorta. Dissection should at all times be sharp, as blunt finger dissection is liable to cause tearing and subsequent bleeding. It is important to remain in the correct plane, particularly when dissecting out the aorta, as a 'bald' aorta (i.e. one denuded of its adventitia) will cause subsequent problems, especially when clamped or when a proximal vein graft anastomosis is being constructed.

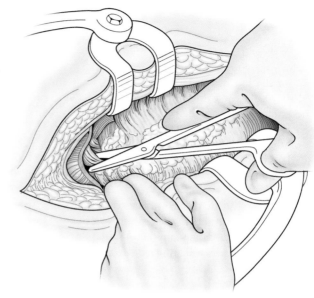

5

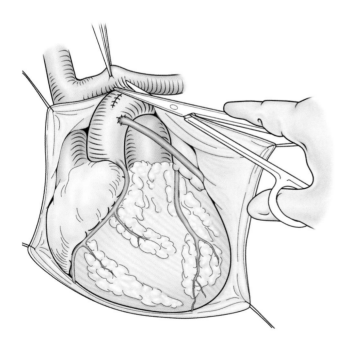

6

6 If difficulty is encountered in identifying the correct plane on the aorta, it is helpful to commence dissection on the caudal margin of the innominate vein. If all tissue posterior to the vein is left on the aorta, the correct plane will be entered, and the aorta then can be dissected out to allow cannulation and cross-clamping. Because of the presence of old proximal anastomoses and a previous cannulation site, it may be necessary to mobilize distally onto the arch below the innominate vein to provide sufficient space on the aorta for recannulation.

7 Care should be taken to avoid manipulation of old grafts, which might result in embolization of the atheromatous debris on the luminal aspect of the graft. It should also be noted that a patent LIMA may encroach on the midline at approximately the level of the angle of Louis and may be adherent to the back of the sternum or aorta. This configuration of the LIMA graft and subsequent problems can be avoided at the first operation by cutting a deep **V** in the pericardium and thus allowing the lung to be anterior in relationship to the IMA.

At this stage, but before cannulation, the IMA(s), if they have not been used at the first operation, can be dissected out in the normal way. Obviously, before preparing the IMA, the left anterior chest wall must be freed from underlying structures.

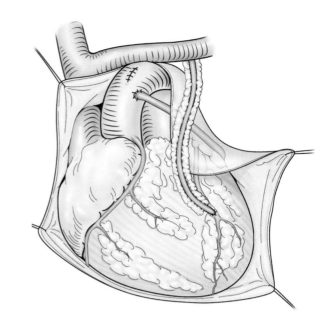

7

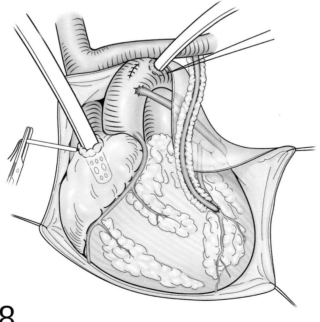

8

8 Cannulation can then proceed in the normal way, although insertion of the aortic cannulation may be more difficult than normal because of the thickening and rigidity of the aortic wall as a result of previous cannulation. If the aorta is quite atherosclerotic or if there is insufficient space, the femoral (or axillary) artery can be cannulated. Venous cannulation is usually made via a pursestring directly on to the right atrial wall, and a single basket-tip cannula gives satisfactory drainage, although many surgeons now prefer a two-stage venous cannula.

Further mobilization of the heart is best carried out on bypass. Only that part of the heart needed to do the operation should be mobilized (e.g. in the rare event of reoperation requiring only right coronary grafting, the left side of the heart need not be mobilized). It is preferable, in general, to complete mobilization with the heart arrested, and this approach is clearly safer in the presence of diseased vein grafts. Regardless, every effort should be made to avoid manipulation of atherosclerotic vein grafts, using, as much as possible, a 'no-touch' approach.

Myocardial protection

9 Although similar techniques of myocardial protection used in first-time operations can be used successfully in reoperation, particular problems should be considered in reoperation. These are related to adequate delivery to all areas of the myocardium and the avoidance of atheroembolism from diseased grafts. For these reasons, most surgeons now use a combination of antegrade and retrograde cardioplegia. This maneuver is most commonly accomplished with cold blood cardioplegia. Antegrade cardioplegia can be delivered using a dual lumen cannula which allows for subsequent aortic root venting. The retrograde cardioplegic solution is delivered by a transatrial coronary sinus catheter with a self-inflating balloon tip. The retrograde route not only allows delivery of the cardioplegic solution, but may also cause accumulated atherosclerotic debris to float out of the coronary arteries and remaining patent vein grafts. It is worth collecting some of the blood cardioplegia mixture before connecting up the antegrade, and then using this to inject completed vein grafts as an additional means of delivery of the antegrade cardioplegia.

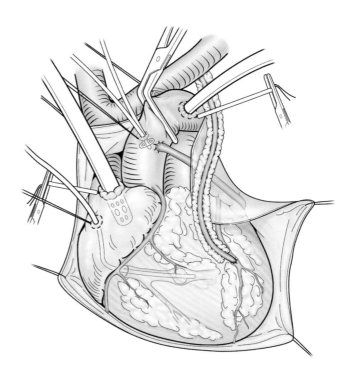

9

Revascularization

DISTAL ANASTOMOSES

10a Once the heart is arrested and dissection completed, revascularization can commence. As in all revascularizations, it is important to have an operative plan. However, in redo surgery, this plan must be flexible and may change depending on location of the vessels, the state of the existing grafts, and the availability of conduit. Old vein grafts provide a useful marker to locate the sites for regrafting.

No consensus exists about what should be done with old grafts, both patent and stenotic. If the vein graft appears totally normal, angiographically and at reoperation, our practice is now to leave this alone. Formerly, any graft older than approximately 5 years would have been replaced, but there is now increasing recognition that these grafts may be 'protected' in some way, and there is no proven benefit in replacing them.

If a graft is totally occluded with no flow and does not impede the lie of a new graft, it can be safely left in place, as there is no risk of embolism. If an old vein graft is significantly diseased, however, and the native coronary artery requires regrafting, then it is best to remove the original graft. In this situation, it is preferable to transect and oversew the vein graft rather than just ligating it, which risks dislodging atheroemboli into the distal coronary artery or retrograde into the ascending aorta. The native coronary artery is then grafted distal to the previous anastomosis.

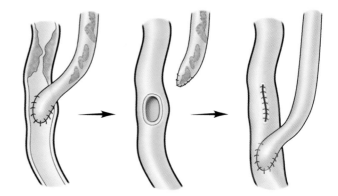

10a

10b Alternatively, the new graft may be anastomosed to the previous anastomotic site, which has been trimmed to leave only a small rim *in situ*. This technique is particularly useful where a native vessel is buried or there is diffuse disease. It also ensures that removal of the old graft does not devascularize any subtended myocardial territory. This approach, however, cannot be used if further significant disease has developed in the native vessel beyond the site of the anastomosis. In this situation, it may be necessary to place a new second graft distally to ensure adequate regional revascularization.

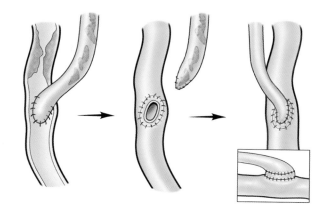

10b

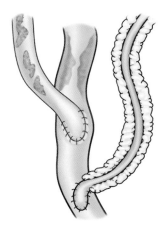

10c

10c However, if the stenosed vein graft is going to be replaced with an arterial graft, in particular with a mammary artery, the vein graft should be left *in situ* because of the risk of initial hypoperfusion. Alternatively, the stenosed graft could be replaced with a new segment of vein in addition to the new arterial graft.

PROXIMAL ANASTOMOSES

11 Adhesions and scarring may render the aorta thickened and rigid, making new proximal anastomoses more difficult. A partial occlusion clamp may be difficult to place for this reason. If this is the case, all proximal anastomoses can be constructed during a single period of ischemia before removal of the aortic cross-clamp. Although this strategy does result in an increased cross-clamp time, it has the advantage of reducing aortic trauma and providing good visualization for all proximal anastomoses.

Sites for anastomosis are often at a premium on the aorta, and it is common and acceptable to use the vein hoods at previous proximal anastomosis sites, which are usually free from atheroma. Alternatively, end-to-side anastomoses can be constructed from one graft to another. The cap, or hood, of either new or existing vein grafts often is the best site for the proximal aortic anastomosis of free arterial grafts.

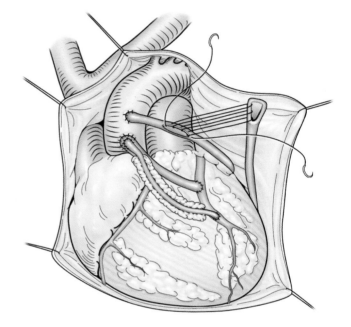

11

ALTERNATIVE TECHNIQUES FOR REOPERATION

Off-pump techniques with various stabilizers are being used more frequently for reoperation, and this procedure is referred to in chapter 9. Similarly, some use of both left and right thoracotomy for reoperation for the circumflex and right coronary arteries, respectively, has occurred in recent years.

OUTCOME

Redo CABG carries higher mortality and morbidity than first-time operation carries. In most series, this higher mortality persists despite a falling mortality for first-time operations. Yet, the same factors responsible for the improvement in outcomes in primary operation apply in reoperations. The most likely explanation for this persistently increased risk is an increase in the risk profile of the patients undergoing operation.

For example, elderly patients undergoing reoperation carry an increased risk. This increased risk, in fact, occurs when there are other risk factors, such as an emergency operation or poor left ventricular function. Without these added risk factors, the operation can be carried out in the elderly with satisfactory results.

Patients undergoing reoperation tend to have more advanced coronary atherosclerosis. For this reason, and for reasons potentially related to availability of conduit and location of coronary arteries, it is more difficult to achieve complete revascularization. Accordingly, the long-term results of reoperation, both in terms of initial relief of angina and avoidance of the recurrence of angina, are less favorable than with first-time operation. Despite this, satisfactory outcomes and long-term results can be achieved, although coronary reoperation continues to represent a technical challenge.

FURTHER READING

Awad, W.I., DeSouza, A.C., Magee, P.G., Walesby, R.K., Wright, J.E., Uppal, R. 1997. Re-do cardiac surgery in patients over 70 years old. *European Journal of Cardio-thoracic Surgery* 12, 40–6.

Borger, M.A., Rao, V., Weisel, R.D., *et al.* 2001. Reoperative coronary bypass surgery: effect of patent grafts and retrograde cardioplegia. *Journal of Thoracic and Cardiovascular Surgery* 121, 83–90.

He, G.-W., Acuff, T.E., He, Y.-H., Ryan, W.H., Mack, M.J. 1995. Determination of operative mortality in reoperative coronary bypass grafting. *Journal of Thoracic and Cardiovascular Surgery* 110, 971–8.

Shapira, I., Isakov, A., Heller, J., Topilsky, M., Pines, A. 1999. Long-term follow-up after coronary artery bypass grafting reoperation. *Chest* 115, 1593–7.

Yamamuro, M., Lytle, B.W., Sapp, S.K., Cosgrove, D.M., Loop, F.D., McCarthy, P.M. 2000. Risk factors and outcomes after coronary reoperation in 739 elderly patients. *Annals of Thoracic Surgery* 69, 464–74.

Yau, T.M., Borger, M.A., Weisel, R.D., Ivanov, J. 2000. The changing pattern of reoperative coronary surgery: trends in 1230 consecutive reoperations. *Journal of Thoracic and Cardiovascular Surgery* 120, 156–63.

12

Repair of postinfarction septal rupture

HARTZELL V. SCHAFF MD
Stuart W. Harrington Professor of Surgery, Division of Cardiovascular Surgery, Mayo Clinic; Professor of Surgery, Division of Cardiovascular Surgery, Saint Mary's Hospital, Rochester, Minnesota, USA

ALFREDO J. RODRIGUES MD PHD
Assistant Professor of Cardiothoracic Surgery, School of Medicine of Ribeirão Preto, University of São Paulo, São Paulo, Brazil

HISTORY

Postinfarction rupture of the interventricular septum was recognized in the middle of the nineteenth century, and Cooley *et al.* reported the first surgical repair in 1957. The first long-term survivor of surgical repair of postinfarction ventricular septal defect (VSD) had the operation at the Mayo Clinic in 1963 by Dr. John W. Kirklin. Since these earlier efforts, the surgical management of postmyocardial infarction VSD has changed from an operation reserved for patients who survived several weeks or months after the septal rupture (usually performed through a right ventriculotomy), to an emergency operation in the majority of cases. Although many advances in medical and surgical management have improved operative results, surgical repair of postinfarction septal rupture still is an exigent procedure.

PRINCIPLES AND JUSTIFICATION

Myocardial rupture is an important cause of death after myocardial infarction and is found in approximately 15 per cent of patients in autopsy series. Among patients with myocardial rupture, approximately 85 per cent have rupture of the free wall of the left ventricle, 10 per cent have rupture of the interventricular septum, and 5 per cent have papillary muscle rupture leading to acute mitral valve regurgitation. Myocardial rupture is often associated with a first myocardial infarction and with patients who have poor collateral blood flow to the area of ischemia/infarction. A frequent clinical observation is that patients with myocardial rupture have unusually friable myocardium, even in areas remote from the infarct.

In the prethrombolytic era, the reported incidence of postinfarction rupture was 1–2 per cent, and in-hospital mortality was 90 per cent in those managed medically and 40–50 per cent in patients having urgent repair. In current practice, early reperfusion of acute myocardial infarction with fibrinolytic drugs or percutaneous balloon angioplasty appears to have reduced the incidence of myocardial rupture. In the GUSTO-1 trial, 84 of 41 021 patients treated with thrombolysis had postinfarction septal rupture (0.2 per cent). In these patients, the median time from symptom onset to diagnosis was 1 day (range, 0–47 days), 94 per cent of the cases were identified within 1 week, and the left anterior descending coronary artery was the most common infarct-related vessel. Despite aggressive medical management and the general availability of cardiac surgery, 30-day mortality was 73.8 per cent compared to 6.8 per cent for other patients with acute myocardial infarction. Among patients managed medically, 30-day mortality was 94 per cent compared to 47 per cent for patients selected for surgical repair.

The poor natural history of postinfarction ventricular septal rupture argues against delay in operation for patients who are otherwise fit enough to undergo surgery. Previously, some clinicians advised postponing repair in anticipation of a more stable patient and/or firmer, scarred myocardial tissue that would be better able to hold sutures than the often-friable peri-infarction tissue encountered in the acute setting. This strategy, however, results in a natural selection process that may optimize surgical mortality but results in the death of many patients who deteriorate and are not offered surgical treatment. Nowadays, most experienced surgeons agree that operation for postinfarction VSD should be undertaken promptly.

The primary goal of operation for postinfarction in VSD is correction of intracardiac shunting and the resulting low cardiac output. Forty to fifty per cent of patients will have single-vessel disease or minimal atherosclerosis in other major vessels. For patients with significant associated coronary artery disease, concomitant surgical revascularization may reduce further ischemic damage in the perioperative period and improve quality of life and long-term survival. Although the benefit of concomitant coronary artery bypass is intuitive, the potential advantages are difficult to prove in clinical series. Therefore, although most patients can tolerate the additional time required for angiography and the small risk of contrast dye worsening renal function, operation should not be delayed for catheterization if the patient is hemodynamically unstable, despite appropriate support as described in this chapter.

PREOPERATIVE ASSESSMENT AND PREPARATION

Patients with postinfarction ventricular septal rupture generally manifest systemic hypotension and clinical evidence of poor perfusion. These patients may be comfortable in the supine position in contrast to those with mitral valve regurgitation due to postinfarction papillary muscle rupture; acute mitral regurgitation after myocardial infarction invariably causes breathlessness and orthopnea. Although preoperative use of intra-aortic balloon pump has not been proven to reduce operative mortality, clinical experience suggests that it is useful in most patients, as it reduces left ventricular afterload and left-to-right shunting while improving coronary arterial blood flow.

Often, inotropic drugs are used to support hemodynamics before and during induction of anesthesia. Prolonged effort at pharmacological therapy preoperatively is rarely helpful and may be detrimental if operation is delayed unnecessarily. Systemic vasodilators are an important element in managing patients with left ventricular dysfunction in acute myocardial infarction, especially for patients with mitral valve regurgita-tion. However, vasodilator therapy should be used with caution in patients with acute VSD because of the possibility of worsening hypotension and systemic organ perfusion.

In contemporary practice, diagnosis of postinfarction VSD is confirmed by echocardiography and color flow Doppler mapping. Echocardiography can localize the defect, determine right and left ventricular function, and identify mitral valve dysfunction, free wall rupture, and other abnormalities. If standard transthoracic imaging suggests a VSD (e.g. right ventricular enlargement, pulmonary artery hypertension) but does not identify the location, transesophageal study may be useful.

Right heart catheterization with the Swan-Ganz catheter may be helpful in establishing diagnosis of VSD by the finding of a step-up in oxygen saturation from the right atrium to the pulmonary artery. Hemodynamic monitoring and periodic measurement of oxygen saturation from right atrial and pulmonary artery blood samples are useful in the immediate postoperative period. Some degree of residual shunting occurs in as many as 30 to 40 per cent of patients after repair. Thus, measured 'cardiac' output with the Swan-Ganz catheter in such patients will reflect pulmonary blood flow that will exceed systemic cardiac output. The finding of normal or high 'cardiac' output measured by a pulmonary artery catheter in a postoperative patient who has clinical evidence of poor organ perfusion should raise suspicion of residual shunting, which can be confirmed by measurement of oxygen saturations and by echocardiography.

As mentioned previously, preoperative invasive hemodynamic study is rarely indicated, and cardiac catheterization should be limited to coronary angiography to reduce delay in operation and to minimize nephrotoxicity of contrast medium. During preoperative catheterization, we insert an intra-aortic balloon even in patients who have stable hemodynamics; intra-aortic balloon support stabilizes patients during induction of anesthesia and is an important feature of postoperative care. In addition to augmenting coronary perfusion pressure, intra-aortic balloon support in postoperative patients reduces peak left ventricular pressure and minimizes the risk of patch disruption or further myocardial rupture.

OPERATION

Surgical techniques

We use high-flow (2.4 L/minute per m²) cardiopulmonary bypass with normothermic perfusion or systemic mild hypothermia (32°–34°C). Single or bicaval venous cannulation may be used; the latter is preferred when extensive resection of the inferobasal portions of the ventricle is necessary. The method of repair is dictated by the location of the septal defect and the extent of surrounding myocardial necrosis. For most patients, the VSD is exposed by incision through the area of infarction. In a few patients with small inferobasal septal defects, repair can be accomplished through a right atriotomy working through the tricuspid valve orifice. An important principle is adequate débridement of infarction tissue so that the perimeter of the defect can be identified clearly, and sutures can be anchored to viable myocardial tissue. Frequently, the VSD will appear relatively small, but other serpiginous communications will exist in surrounding tissue.

Anterior septal rupture

1 In rare instances, anterior myocardial infarction can cause a VSD at the apex of the septum. These effects may be amenable to amputation of the distal portions of the left ventricle, septum, and right ventricle. Repair is achieved by direct closure of the right and left ventricles against the septum using large felt strips to buttress the suture line.

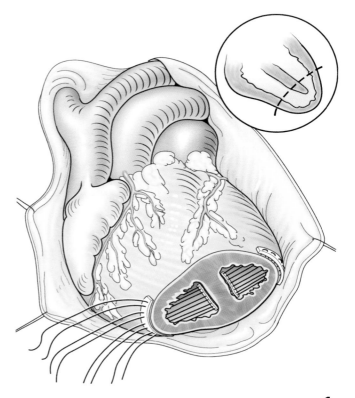

1

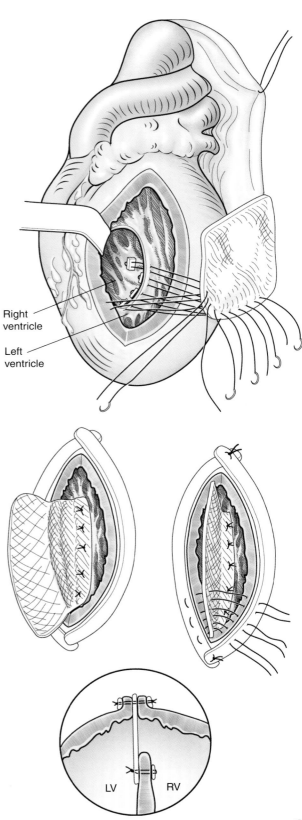

Right ventricle

Left ventricle

LV   RV

2 More commonly, anterior VSDs are approached through an incision in the infarcted portion of the anterior left ventricle. Infarcted myocardium in the left ventricular free wall and septum should be débrided widely to expose the septum adequately and to identify viable muscle that will hold sutures securely. An oversized intracardiac patch of Dacron or Teflon is tailored to the shape of the defect and positioned on the left ventricular side of the septum. We prefer to anchor the patch by passing felt-reinforced mattress sutures of 3/0 or 2/0 polypropylene from the right ventricle, through the septum, and through the patch. Sutures should enter viable myocardium at least 2 cm from the defect and must be tied securely but with care not to pull through muscle.

Anteriorly, the patch is trimmed to the appropriate height, and the left and right ventricular free walls are closed against the patch in a sandwich fashion with felt-reinforced sutures. Most patients with acute VSD will have little or no chronic enlargement of the left ventricle, and care should be taken not to make the patch too small, because doing so will distort the ventricle and create additional tension on the suture lines.

If infarctectomy of the anterior left ventricular free wall is extensive, patch closure of this defect may be necessary to prevent undue tension on the suture line and to maintain adequate ventricular volume. In such cases, the free wall patch is closed against the septal patch and right ventricle.

Another method of closing the septal defect uses patches on either side of the septum. This can be accomplished by folding an oversized patch and closing the free walls of the ventricles against the folded edge or by using two separate patches.

2

Posterior septal rupture

3 Usually occurring near the base of the heart, posterior septal rupture can occasionally be exposed through the right atrium and tricuspid valve. Secure closure of the defect can be awkward with this approach, because the tricuspid valve apparatus interferes with exposure and because it is difficult to situate a large patch on the left ventricular side of the septum.

More commonly, posterior postinfarction VSDs are exposed through an incision in the adjacent infarcted myocardium. The apex of the left ventricle is retracted upward, and an incision is made in the midportion of the posterior ventricular wall, parallel to the descending posterior coronary artery, but close to the septum to avoid injury to the posteromedial papillary muscle.

As in closure of anterior septal rupture, an oversized patch is sutured to the left side of the septum with felt-reinforced mattress sutures that pass through the full thickness of the septum. Often, the infarctectomy extends near the mitral valve annulus and laterally to the posteromedial papillary muscle. To prevent distortion of these structures and to achieve secure closure, patch repair of the free wall of the ventricle is necessary. The ventriculotomy is closed in two layers, buttressed on strips of pericardium or Teflon felt. Again, biological glue may be helpful.

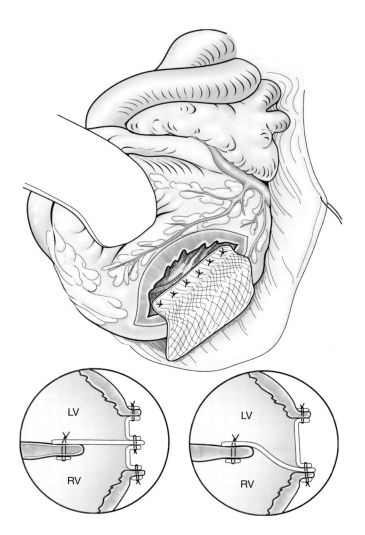

3

4a–c
An alternative approach for repair of post-infarction VSD is the exclusion technique described by David *et al*. With this method, a large glutaraldehyde-fixed bovine pericardial patch or a synthetic patch is anchored to the left side of the septum using a running suture secured to endocardium far away from the area of infarction. Infarct exclusion has the theoretical advantage of minimizing distortion of ventricular geometry and cavity size. Also, the method minimizes manipulation of the right ventricular myocardium that may be friable because of ischemia.

Simultaneous myocardial revascularization

If myocardial revascularization is planned, distal graft-to-coronary anastomoses are performed before VSD repair to minimize retraction on the ventricular suture lines. Bypass of the artery supplying the acute infarct is rarely indicated because of transmural damage and the frequent need to excise portions of the vessel during infarctectomy.

Weaning from cardiopulmonary bypass

Intra-aortic balloon counterpulsation is used in all patients both for hemodynamic support and for afterload reduction to lessen peak left ventricular pressure. Left ventricular dysfunction of a variable degree will be present in all patients, but when ventricular failure is severe, other correctable causes should be evaluated. Transesophageal echocardiography is essential to evaluate right and left ventricular function and detect significant residual shunts and/or mitral valve regurgitation. Also, we routinely draw simultaneous blood samples from the right atrium and pulmonary artery to detect residual intracardiac shunting. A simplified formula for estimating the ratio of pulmonary to systemic blood flow (Qp/Qs) is the following:

$$(Qp/Qs) = \frac{\text{Arterial O}_2 \text{ sat} - \text{mixed venous (right atrial) O}_2 \text{ sat}}{\text{Pulmonary venous O}_2 \text{ sat} - \text{pulmonary artery O}_2 \text{ sat}}$$

Besides the use of inotropic drugs, judicious use of volume loading may be helpful if right ventricular dysfunction exists due to ischemia or infarction.

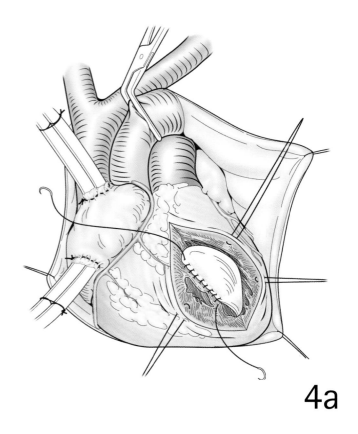

4a

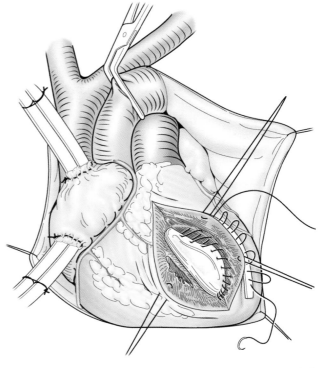

4b

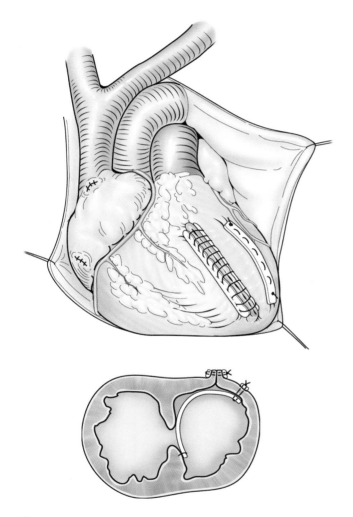

4c

OUTCOME

Even in the current era, in-hospital mortality of patients undergoing repair of postinfarction septal rupture is high, ranging from 19 to 47 per cent. As might be expected, risk of early death is highest in patients with preoperative shock, and in most series, inferior septal rupture is associated with higher mortality than that due to anterior septal rupture. Risk of early death is especially high in patients with inferior VSDs who have associated right ventricular infarction.

Some degree of residual left-to-right intracardiac shunting is not uncommon after repair. Indeed, as many as 40 per cent of patients will have residual defects identified by Doppler echocardiography. In most instances, these leaks will be small (Qp/Qs less than 1.5) and hemodynamically unimportant. However, if the Qp/Qs is greater than 1.5, early reoperation should be considered.

Patients who survive the early postoperative period after repair of postinfarction ventricular septal rupture can be expected to have a good late outcome. In the experience of David and Armstrong, actuarial survival 8 years after VSD repair was 59 per cent, and Dalrymple-Hay *et al.* reported finding 5-year survival of 72 per cent and 10-year survival of 39 per cent. These results and the dismal prognosis of patients not undergoing operation argue for an aggressive surgical approach to postinfarction septal rupture.

FURTHER READING

Cooley, D.A. 1998. Postinfarction ventricular septal rupture. *Seminars in Thoracic and Cardiovascular Surgery* **10**, 100–4.

Dalrymple-Hay, M.J., Langley, S.M., Sami, S.A., *et al.* 1998. Should coronary artery bypass grafting be performed at the same time as repair of a post-infarct ventricular septal defect? *European Journal of Cardio-thoracic Surgery* **13**, 286–92.

Dalrymple-Hay, M.J., Monro, J.L., Livesey, S.A., Lamb, R.K. 1998. Postinfarction ventricular septal rupture: the Wessex experience. *Seminars in Thoracic and Cardiovascular Surgery* **10**, 111–16.

David, T.E., Armstrong, S. 1998. Surgical repair of postinfarction ventricular septal defect by infarct exclusion. *Seminars in Thoracic and Cardiovascular Surgery* **10**, 105–10.

Lemery, R., Smith, H.C., Giuliani, E.R., Gersh, B.J. 1992. Prognosis in rupture of the ventricular septum after acute myocardial infarction and role of early surgical intervention. *American Journal of Cardiology* **70**, 147–51.

Madsen, J.C., Daggett, W.M. Jr. 1998. Repair of postinfarction ventricular septal defects. *Seminars in Thoracic and Cardiovascular Surgery* **10**, 117–27.

13

Surgery for acute myocardial infarction

GERALD D. BUCKBERG, MD
Professor of Surgery, David Geffen School of Medicine at UCLA, Los Angeles, California, USA

FRIEDHELM BEYERSDORF, MD FETCS
Professor of Surgery, Department of Cardiovascular Surgery, Albert-Ludwigs-Universitat Freiburg, Freiburg, Germany

PRINCIPLES

Acute myocardial infarction is caused by acute coronary occlusion and is the major cause of death in Europe and in the United States. Patients are almost always treated by thrombolysis, percutaneous transluminal coronary angioplasty (PTCA), or both to avoid or reduce myocardial necrosis. Nevertheless, in-hospital mortality is due principally to cardiogenic shock because of extensive ischemic muscle damage. Previous surgical results of coronary artery bypass grafting for left ventricular (LV) power failure have been disappointing because intraoperative ischemic injury is superimposed on severe damage already sustained by the myocardium. In general, surgical revascularization has been restricted to patients with acute occlusion after elective PTCA with or without thrombolytic therapy.

During the last several years, new knowledge has been gained in the pathophysiology of acute coronary occlusion on ischemic and nonischemic remote myocardium that has evolved into a new surgical strategy for revascularization of patients with evolving myocardial infarctions and failed PTCA.

Studies of the natural history of acute regional ischemia have shown that acute occlusion of a coronary artery not only affects the ischemic myocardium but causes structural, functional, and metabolic alterations in the remote and adjacent myocardium. These changes in the remote myocardium may be even more severe if the remote myocardium is supplied by a stenotic coronary artery. Furthermore, many experimental and clinical studies have shown that normal blood reperfusion of myocardium, injured previously by ischemia, may lead to reperfusion-induced injury if normal unmodified blood is reperfused. This damage can be reduced or even avoided by therapeutic interventions to control the condi-

tions and composition of new blood supply during the initial reperfusion period.

These observations on the pathophysiology of acutely ischemic myocardium as well as myocardium remote from the ischemic zone have led to the development of operative strategies intended to restore early segmental contractility in the previously ischemic area and to restore or maintain hypercontractility in remote myocardium. These strategies involve use of mechanical cardiac decompression on total vented bypass and use of warm substrate-enriched blood cardioplegia to resuscitate acute ischemic muscle and metabolically depleted remote muscle.

PATHOPHYSIOLOGY OF ACUTE MYOCARDIAL INFARCTION

Studies of the natural history of acute regional ischemia after coronary occlusion show that acute occlusion of a coronary artery not only affects the ischemic myocardium, but causes structural, functional, and metabolic alterations in the remote and adjacent myocardium.

Ischemic myocardium and reperfusion

The regional wall motion abnormalities after acute coronary occlusion are accompanied by progressive ultrastructural and biochemical sequences. However, the myocardial cell remains intact and viable up to after 6 hours of ischemia, as long as the damaged tissue is not exposed to a sudden reperfusion with unmodified blood.

Although blood reperfusion with normal blood successfully reverses the transient damage imposed by a 15 minute coronary occlusion, massive structural, biochemical, and functional changes, which are not seen in the ischemic region before reflow, occur with unmodified reperfusion after as little as 40 minutes of regional ischemia. Normal blood reperfusion after longer periods of ischemia of up to 6 hours has been shown to produce such extensive transmural necrosis that muscle salvage is unlikely. To what extent this myocardial reperfusion injury, which occurs with unmodified blood reperfusion, depends on the length and severity of the ischemic injury, at least when the ischemic interval is not prolonged, is not clear. Brief ischemic intervals or longer periods of ischemia in regions with high collateral blood flow might result in preserved cellular regulatory mechanisms and resistance to reperfusion injury, whereas normal blood reperfusion after longer periods of severe ischemia always results in additive myocardial damage.

Our approach to reduce or avoid this additional injury after reperfusion, and thus preserve ventricular function even after prolonged periods of ischemia, is based on very specific management of the ischemic region during the initial reperfusion phase, before normal blood reperfusion is allowed to occur.

The current strategy for controlled reperfusion incorporates modification of each parameter or condition of reperfusion, including total heart decompression, gentle reperfusion pressure, regional cardioplegia, normothermia, prolonged reperfusion duration, as well as optimization of the reperfusate solution, including oxygenation of the perfusate, presence of potassium for cardioplegic effect, addition of metabolic substrates glutamate/aspartate, hypocalcemia, buffering of acidosis, hyperosmolarity, oxygen free-radical scavengers, hyperglycemia, and white cell depletion. All of these myocardial protective strategies evolved from our previous studies of the heart subjected to induced ischemia. This approach allows for early recovery of contractility in the ischemic region after acute coronary occlusion intervals averaging 6 hours (2–3 hour range).

Remote myocardium

1 The function capacity of ventricular myocardium remote from the acute ischemic region is the principal determinant of early survival after an otherwise nonlethal coronary occlusion, with less than 30 per cent of left ventricle at risk. Survival after acute coronary occlusion is determined not only by the size or extent of the infarct, but also by the capacity of remote, nonischemic myocardium to support the systemic circulation. Cardiogenic shock with LV power failure occurs if more than 40 per cent of the LV muscle mass acutely loses its contractile properties, or if ventricular function in the nonischemic or remote myocardium is not adequate to compensate for the acute loss of less than 40 per cent of contractile mass. Failure of remote muscle to hypercontract may be caused by one or more of the following factors:

- Compensatory hypercontractility in the ventricular regions remote from the infarct, which might be present during the initial few hours after the acute coronary occlusion, may decrease progressively to normokinesis and eventually to hypokinesis. Our experimental studies have shown that despite maintenance of normal or increased blood flow, even with an open coronary artery into the infarcted region, mild energy and substrate depletion and subsequent evidence of anaerobic metabolism in the remote muscle often occurs several hours after the acute coronary occlusion. Figure 1 illustrates segmental shortening (ultrasonic crystals) of remote myocardium during simulated single vessel disease (LAD occlusion) and multivessel disease (LAD occlusion and Cx stenosis). Note: (1) compensatory hypercontractility in isolated LAD occlusion and survival of all 11 animals (open circles) and (2)

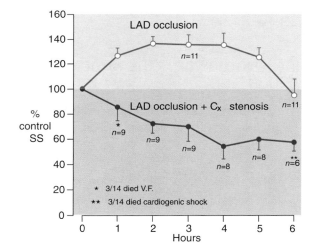

1

progressive remote muscle hypocontractility in simulated multivessel disease (solid circles) and high mortality from cardiogenic shock. This figure has been reproduced with permission from Beyersdorf, F., Acar, C., Buckberg, G.D., *et al.* 1989. Studies on prolonged acute regional ischemia. III. Early natural history of simulated single and multivessel disease with emphasis on remote myocardium. *Journal of Thoracic and Cardiovascular Surgery* **98**: 368–80.

- Remote myocardium may become relatively ischemic if it is supplied by stenotic coronary arteries. When called on to increase contractile function, compensatory hypercontractility may not occur or be sustained because of inadequate coronary artery flow reserve. The result is cardiogenic shock, intractable ventricular fibrillation, or both. We found remote muscle may become progressively hypocontractile, with resultant reduction in stroke work index, even when the remote region is supplied by a non-critical stenotic coronary artery (Figure 1). Such functional deterioration is accompanied by moderate substrate- and energy-depletion and more pronounced evidence of anaerobic metabolism, despite normal blood flow.

- A previous myocardial infarction that reduces the available muscle mass in the remote myocardium (i.e. a patient with an acute left anterior descending (LAD) coronary artery occlusion and a previous inferior infarction secondary to prior occlusion of the right coronary artery) has only a limited capacity to develop compensatory hypercontractility in the now 'nonischemic myocardium.' Such a patient may progress to cardiogenic shock after a brief interval after acute coronary occlusion.

These observations form the basis for our strategy directed at maximizing myocardial protection of ischemic and remote myocardium during operations for acute coronary occlusion and cardiogenic shock.

OPERATION

Surgical technique for patients with acute myocardial infarction

Historically, surgical interventions have been undertaken during or soon after an acute myocardial infarction only for complications of acute cardiac necrosis leading to acute mitral incompetence, ventricular septal rupture, or free wall perforation. Coronary revascularization after acute coronary occlusion generally is only performed after a failed angioplasty when bypass surgery can be initiated almost immediately after the onset of ischemia. In the future, patients with a spontaneously occurring acute coronary occlusion, especially patients with additional coronary stenoses in regions of the heart remote from the site of infarction, may be considered as possible candidates for surgical treatment to reduce the likelihood of progression to a large transmural myocardial infarction and to avoid cardiogenic shock. Surgical treatment for

this patient group should include complete myocardial revascularization using controlled reperfusion for myocardial protection.

If reperfusion with unmodified blood has already been instituted after a prolonged period of ischemia as a result of thrombolysis, perfusion balloons, laser balloons, directional atherectomy, PTCA, stents, or reperfusion catheters, severe reperfusion damage is already present and cannot be expected to be reversed by controlled reperfusion. Therefore, when an acute coronary occlusion occurs in the catheterization laboratory that can be expeditiously traversed with a guide wire, a perfusion catheter or stent should be placed to restore flow and attenuate the ischemic injury. If a complete coronary occlusion has been present for more than 1 or 2 hours, further extended attempts at catheter dilatation should be avoided lest the ischemic damage progress to complete infarction.

Surgical techniques for pre- and intraoperative application

PREOPERATIVE

In unstable patients without peripheral vascular disease and without severe atherosclerosis of the descending and abdominal aorta, intra-aortic balloon pumping is started via a small surgical femoral vessel cutdown. In addition, intravenous metabolic support with an amino acid-enriched glucose-insulin-potassium infusion is begun.

INTRAOPERATIVE

The surgical strategy for acute myocardial infarction can be separated into the phases of (1) total vented bypass, (2) aortic cross-clamping, (3) regional controlled reperfusion, and (4) prolonged beating empty state.

TOTAL VENTED CARDIOPULMONARY BYPASS

Extracorporeal circulation is established as quickly as possible by means of connecting single venous and aortic cannulation to a membrane oxygenator primed with lactated Ringer's solution. The left ventricle is vented routinely by a catheter passed from a right pulmonary vein and through the left atrium. For patients in hemodynamic collapse who require preoperative cardiopulmonary resuscitation, peripheral cannulation is used for extracorporeal bypass. A common femoral vein is cannulated, and the catheter advanced into the right atrium and the common femoral artery or distal iliac artery is cannulated in the usual fashion. Once the patient is established and is stable on cardiopulmonary bypass, antegrade delivery of blood cardioplegia is delivered with a cardioplegic needle inserted into the ascending aorta. For retrograde delivery, the coronary sinus is cannulated transatrially.

PERIOD OF AORTIC CROSS-CLAMPING

The strategies for myocardial protection with blood cardioplegia in patients with acute coronary occlusion during the period of aortic cross-clamping may be separated into the phases of induction, maintenance and distribution, and global reperfusion. The total blood cardioplegic dose is divided equally between antegrade and retrograde delivery for induction, maintenance, and reperfusion.

INDUCTION

Cardioplegia may be induced immediately after extracorporeal circulation has begun and the pulmonary artery is collapsed. Starting the antegrade perfusion before aortic clamping ensures aortic valve competence. The blood cardioplegic solution may be given cold or warm.

MAINTENANCE OF CARDIOPLEGIA

After each distal anastomosis or not later than every 20 minutes, multidose cold blood cardioplegic solution is delivered antegrade into the aorta and into each graft 200 mL/minute over 1 minute after completion of each distal anastomosis. Thereafter, retrograde delivery through the coronary sinus is done for 1 additional minute. Systemic rewarming is begun after the last distal anastomosis has been started.

GLOBAL REPERFUSION

After completion of the last distal anastomosis, leukocyte-filtered, warm (39°C) diltiazem-containing, substrate-enriched blood cardioplegia is given into the aorta and into all accessible grafts for 2 minutes at 150 mL/minute. The composition of the reperfusate solution (mixed 4:1, with four parts blood from the heart-lung machine) is shown in Table 13.1. Thereafter, the aortic clamp is removed. A white blood cell filter is now added to the circuit to ensure maximal leukodepletion during warm reperfusion.

CONTROLLED REGIONAL REPERFUSION

2 After removal of the aortic clamp, leukocyte-filtered, pressure-controlled blood cardioplegia is given at a flow rate of 50 mL/minute and an infusion line pressure of less than 50 mm Hg into the graft supplying the region revascularized for acute coronary occlusion. This regional reperfusion is continued for an additional 18 minutes. In patients with acute occlusion of the left main coronary artery or with acute occlusion of two coronary arteries, flow is increased to 100 mL/minute and given into both vein grafts. Normal blood is delivered into the remainder of the heart via the aortic segment not included in the tangential clamp (Figure 2). Cannulation of a side branch of the vein graft allows delivery of the controlled blood cardioplegic reperfusate while the proximal anastomosis is performed so that no additional ischemic time is imposed on the previously ischemic region. The proximal anastomosis of the vein graft supplying the ischemic region is always constructed first. Immediately after this 18-minute regional reperfusion period, the tangential clamp is removed, and normal blood flow is restored.

Table 13.1 *Composition of the concentrated crystalloid solution to allow for a 4:1 (blood/cardioplegic solution) mixture for BCP induction (high-potassium), maintenance (low-potassium), and controlled regional reperfusion*

	BCP induction (ml)	BCP maintenance (ml)	Controlled regional reperfusion (ml)
Glucose 5%	250	250	500
CPD*	50	50	200
THAM (0.3 mol/L)	200	200	200
Glutamate/aspartate (13 mmol each)†	250	250	250
KCl (1 mEq/ml)	60	40	40
Diltiazem‡	–	–	300 µg/kg bw

bw, Body weight of the patient; CPD, citrate phosphate dextrose; THAM, tromethamine.
*Biotest, D-6072 Dreieich, Germany.
†Ajinomoto GmbH, Hamburg, Germany, prepared by the pharmacy of the J.W. Goethe-University, Frankfurt, Federal Republic of Germany.
‡Gödecke AG, D-1000 Berlin 10, Federal Republic of Germany.

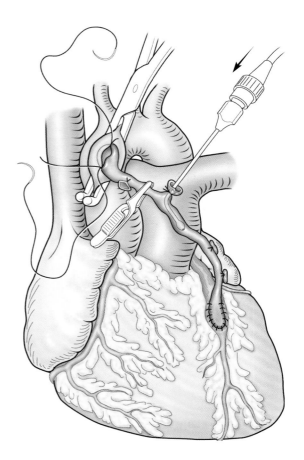

2

BEATING EMPTY STATE

The heart is maintained in the beating and empty state for 30 additional minutes after completion of the controlled regional cardioplegic reperfusion. Reperfusion of jeopardized myocardium is best achieved by lowering oxygen demands and increasing oxygen delivery. The oxygen requirement of nonischemic muscle can be reduced to 50 per cent by converting a beating working heart (9 mL/100 g/minute) into the beating empty state (4.5 mL/100 g/minute). Whereas the oxygen requirements of dyskinetic muscle are almost 55 per cent of beating working needs, decompression by total vented bypass abolishes systolic bulging and produces an immediate fall in regional oxygen uptake to 1 mL/100 g/minute.

Even with a large, two-stage right atrial drainage cannula in place or with bicaval cannulation and caval tapes, continuous left heart decompression may not be assured without the presence of a cardiac chamber vent. Some coronary sinus return, bronchial flow, or both will enter the left ventricle, distend it, and create an increase in LV wall tension. Under such circumstances, occasional LV ejection may occur despite apparent right heart decompression. Therefore, effective left heart decompression requires a ventricular vent, usually placed through the mitral valve and left atrium. Extracorporeal circulation is slowly discontinued after 30 minutes of beating empty state. Bypass is resumed for an additional period if cardiac output is not satisfactory.

OUTCOME

The results of this surgical strategy have been evaluated in several single- and multicenter trials. Patients were included in these studies even with prolonged periods of ischemia of up to 24 hours, and a high percentage of patients went to the operating room in cardiogenic shock. The diagnosis of cardiogenic shock was confirmed by the accepted clinical criteria of hypotension, oliguria, evidence of inadequate peripheral perfusion, elevated left atrial filling pressures, and the need for inotropes, intra-aortic balloon pump assistance, or both. Regional contractility was assessed in all patients during the immediate postoperative period by echocardiography, radionuclide ventriculography, or both. The wall motion score was graded from 0 (normal) to 4 (dyskinesia).

Early recovery of substantial regional contractility occurred in 70–80 percent of patients treated by controlled reperfusion; the majority of patients showed normokinesis or only mild to moderate hypokinesis by the seventh postoperative day. Reperfusion arrhythmias were infrequent. Despite the fact that hemodynamic instability was present preoperatively in 49 of 89 patients (55 per cent), this situation was usually reversed in 18–24 hours postoperatively, and hospitalization averaged only 9 days despite delay of treatment for up to 23 hours. Hospital mortality was 5.6 per cent (5 of 89 patients).

These clinical results together with our recent reports comparing controlled reperfusion to patients undergoing standard coronary artery bypass grafting techniques as well as studies from other authors provide confirmation of our belief that the fate of jeopardized myocardium is determined by how the reperfusion strategy is managed, rather than by how quickly the blood supply is restored.

The most recent report of controlled regional blood cardioplegic reperfusion is a multicenter clinical trial applying these concepts to patients with acute evolving infarction. A total of 156 patients with acute coronary occlusions were treated in five different institutions according to the principles of controlled reperfusion. The results of this study showed that despite long ischemic intervals (6.3 hours), high incidence of LAD occlusion (61 per cent), multi-vessel disease (42 per cent), and cardiogenic shock (41 per cent), surgical mortality was only 3.9 per cent and regional wall motion recovered significantly in 140 of 156 patients (90 per cent) patients. The only deaths (6 out of 66 patients) occurred in patients presenting in severe cardiogenic shock. No mortality occurred in the 90 patients that were hemodynamically compensated at the time of controlled reperfusion.

Furthermore, a review of PTCA for acute myocardial infarction in recent reported series that included more than 1 200 patients showed overall mortality of 9.2 per cent despite successful PTCA in 93 per cent of patients after only 3.6 hours of ischemia. In these PTCA series, subgroup mortality was highest if there was LAD occlusion, multi-vessel disease, age older than 70 years, cardiogenic shock, or unsuccessful PTCA. Additionally, mortality in the GISSI trial was 9 per cent in unselected patients treated by thrombolysis within 2 hours of chest pain and increased to 13 per cent in patients treated after a longer time interval. The recent ISIS-3 preliminary results in 44 000 patients showed 35-day mortality rates of approximately 10.5 per cent in the patients receiving streptokinase, antistreptase, and duteplase. These clinical results of reperfusion with unmodified blood in beating-working or bypassed hearts suggest that the validity of conventional reperfusion must be reassessed, because early return of contractile function is marginal. These clinical findings are consistent with the many experimental studies examining unmodified reperfusion.

Late outcome results after normal blood reperfusion of myocardial infarcts and with resultant akinesia or dyskinesia of the acutely ischemic region reveal progression to congestive heart failure and can be predicted by measurement of LV end-systolic volume (ESVI) within 90 minutes of reperfusion. Despite successful thrombolysis or mechanical dilatation of an acute coronary occlusion, the incidence of delayed congestive heart failure and mortality at 1 year rises progressively if ESVI is greater than 40 mL/m^2 and increases to 30 per cent or higher late mortality if ESVI is greater than 60 mL/m^2. This severe cardiac failure develops despite the absence of angina or inducible ischemia in the previously ischemic zone revascularized or reperfused, or both, with unmodified blood.

These findings, coupled with the benefits of controlled reperfusion at the time of acute coronary occlusion, suggest that surgically modified reperfusion after acute myocardial infarction reduces the early mortality and limits the late development of congestive heart failure.

FURTHER READING

Allen, B.S., Buckberg, G.D., Fontan, F.M. 1993. Superiority of surgical reperfusion versus PTCA in acute coronary occlusion. *Journal of Thoracic and Cardiovascular Surgery* **105**, 864–84.

Beyersdorf, F., Sarai, K., Maul, F.D., *et al.* 1991. Immediate functional benefits after controlled reperfusion during surgical revascularization for acute coronary occlusion. *Journal of Thoracic and Cardiovascular Surgery* **102**, 856–66.

Beyersdorf, F., Mitrev, Z., Sarai, K., *et al.* 1993.Changing patterns of patients undergoing emergency surgical revascularization for acute coronary occlusion. Importance of myocardial protection techniques. *Journal of Thoracic and Cardiovascular Surgery* **106**, 137–48.

O'Keefe, J.H. Jr., Rutherford, B.D., McConahay, D.R., *et al.* 1989. Early and late results of coronary angioplasty without antecedent thrombolytic therapy for acute myocardial infarction. *American Journal of Cardiology* **64**, 1221–30.

Migrino, R.Q., Young, J.B., Ellis, S.G., *et al.* 1997. End-systolic volume index at 90 to 180 minutes into reperfusion therapy for acute myocardial infarction is a strong predictor of early and late mortality. *Circulation* **96(1)**, 116–21.

Rogers, W.J. 1991. Update on recent clinical trials of thrombolytic therapy in myocardial infarction. *Journal of Invasive Cardiology* **3**, 11A–19A.

14

Synchronous carotid endarterectomy and coronary revascularization

CLIFFORD FREDERICK HUGHES AO, MBBS, FRACS, FACC, FACS
Clinical Associate Professor, Division of Surgery, University of Sydney Faculty of Medicine; Head, Cardiothoracic Surgical Unit, Royal Prince Alfred Hospital, and the Baird Institute for Applied Heart and Lung Surgical Research, Sydney, New South Wales, Australia

BRUCE G. FRENCH FRACS
Head and Cardiothoracic Surgeon, Department of Cardiothoracic Surgery, Liverpool Hospital, Liverpool, New South Wales, Australia; Cardiothoracic Surgeon, Royal Prince Alfred Hospital, Camperdown, New South Wales, Australia

PRINCIPLES AND JUSTIFICATION

Cerebrovascular events are among the more common (5.5–50.0 per cent) noncardiac complications that are associated with cardiac surgery. A well-recognized and increasing incidence of stroke or transient ischemic events occurs with the increasing age of cardiac patients. The incidence of hemodynamically significant carotid lesions is as high as 20 per cent and is a powerful predictor of stroke after coronary revascularization. Furthermore, patients who are undergoing surgery for extracranial cerebrovascular disease are at increased risk of perioperative coronary events, particularly if they have symptomatic coronary artery disease. More than 50 per cent of patients who have carotid endarterectomy have overt ischemic heart disease.

It is not surprising, therefore, that many approaches to the management of combined coronary and carotid artery disease have been promulgated. Although some authors recommend independent surgery based on the presenting clinical signs and symptoms alone, others have advocated staged but separate procedures, some recommending that the carotid artery problem be approached first and others prioritizing the coronary obstructions. Either of these latter approaches involves the potential complications of two anesthetics and procedures as well as the risk of a complication in the non-operated territory before it is revascularized.

In 1984, we began a policy of synchronous combined procedures for patients with significant coronary artery disease and significant carotid disease. *Significant* is defined in our unit as coronary artery disease that requires surgery for symptomatic or prognostic indications and a symptomatic carotid stenosis of greater than 75 per cent or an asymptomatic carotid stenosis of greater than 90 per cent. Recognizing that it was unlikely that prospective randomized trials would occur, we believed it important that surgeons refine their preferred technique and measure the outcomes. We describe one such method, which, in our hands, appears to produce satisfactory outcomes in this controversial area of surgery.

PREOPERATIVE ASSESSMENT AND PREPARATION

All patients who present for coronary artery surgery should have a complete vascular evaluation. Any symptoms or signs that suggest cerebrovascular events, regardless of their severity, that could be attributed to a carotid territory lesion should be thoroughly investigated. All patients with a proven neurological history or a bruit should have carotid ultrasonic duplex examination. Although we do not yet advocate routine carotid duplex scanning for all younger patients, we have a low threshold for obtaining this study. The older the patient, the more likely we are to obtain a carotid artery duplex scan. Patients with a history of other vascular disease (aortic aneurysms, femoropopliteal disease, etc.) are screened preoperatively as well for the presence of carotid artery disease. Whenever carotid endarterectomy is planned, we obtain a digital subtraction angiogram. Although this study is not essential, it provides very useful anatomical information for the surgeon.

Conversely, patients who are about to undergo carotid surgery should have a thorough cardiac evaluation. A history or symptoms of ischemic heart disease mandate a thorough investigation, including, when appropriate, stress testing (electrocardiographic or radionuclide) and, if necessary, angiography.

The risks, benefits, and indications for the recommended procedure should be discussed thoroughly with the patient and family. Because many of these patients are receiving anticoagulants, preoperative medications must be reviewed thoroughly and, when appropriate, aspirin, antiplatelet agents, nonsteroidal anti-inflammatory agents, and warfarin (Coumadin) derivatives ceased before the planned surgery. For unstable patients, intravenous heparin is continued until the morning of surgery.

ANESTHESIA AND PERFUSION

The anesthetic approach to patients who are undergoing combined carotid artery and coronary surgery needs careful planning. Venous access sites in the neck must be positioned so that they do not interfere with the sterile field or incisions. For unilateral carotid surgery, central lines are placed in the contralateral internal jugular vein. If bilateral carotid surgery is necessary, subclavian veins can be used. Early in our experience, we did not use pulmonary artery catheters but placed a left atrial catheter via the right superior pulmonary vein immediately before discontinuing cardiopulmonary bypass. A pulmonary artery catheter, however, can be inserted through a subclavian vein. The left radial artery is used for arterial monitoring unless it is needed as a conduit, in which case the right radial or, rarely, a femoral artery is cannulated.

The usual cardiac anesthesia techniques are used, but particular care is taken to avoid swings in blood pressure before cardiopulmonary bypass and to maintain adequate perfusion pressures while on cardiopulmonary bypass. Continuous EEG or other forms of cerebral monitoring have been used occasionally, but not routinely. We regularly use intermittent, anterograde, cold blood cardioplegic solution to provide myocardial protection. We do not inject the carotid sinus nerve with local anesthetic in a combined procedure but insist on careful pharmacological blood pressure control throughout the operation.

OPERATION

The aim of the combined procedure is to minimize the duration of risk to either vascular territory before and during the operation. The procedure is planned to provide optimal exposure, the most rapid revascularization of both vascular territories, and adequate protection of the brain and the myocardium. All members of the surgical, nursing, anesthetic, and perfusion teams must be aware of the proposed sequence of dissections. The teams should rehearse the positioning of the patient, instrument trays, and lines and the surgical sequences for each part of the procedure. Headlights and magnification are essential.

Sequence of surgical incisions

1 The patient is positioned with the neck hyperextended and the head tilted away from the side of planned surgery. After the skin is prepared, drapes are positioned so that the entire side of the neck can be seen. Drapes can be readily fixed to the skin with a stapler. The entire operative field is then covered with an adhesive (iodine-impregnated) drape. Depending on operative circumstances, the incisions are then carried out in the following order:

1 Right carotid endarterectomy and left internal mammary artery (LIMA in Figure 1) conduit: The median sternotomy is performed, the internal mammary artery harvested, and then the carotid artery exposed.
2 Left carotid endarterectomy and left internal mammary artery conduit: If two surgeons are available, the incisions can be carried out simultaneously.
3 Bilateral carotid endarterectomy and left internal mammary artery conduit: The left internal mammary artery can be harvested while the left carotid artery is exposed. The right carotid artery can then be exposed.

The order of incisions varies, depending on the availability of experienced surgeons and whether a radial artery is also harvested. In our unit, one surgeon with vascular and cardiac training performs the carotid and the coronary revascularization, working with two assistants. However, the technique also allows independent cardiac and vascular teams to work together.

Sternal incision

A standard median sternotomy incision is performed, commencing 1 cm below the suprasternal notch. The sternum is divided and periosteal hemostasis assured. The internal mammary artery is then harvested and prepared for use as a conduit. We spray the graft adventitia with papaverine solution, and then gauze, soaked in papaverine, is wrapped around the conduit, which is left *in situ* until required.

The thymic fat pad is then mobilized, double ligated, and divided. The pericardium is opened in the midline and retracted laterally with three 2/0 Ti-cron stay sutures (Davis & Geck, Hamilton, Bermuda) on each side.

During this same period, other conduits are harvested from a leg or arm as required. Aortic and atrial pursestring sutures are placed so as to be prepared to initiate cannulation for cardiopulmonary bypass.

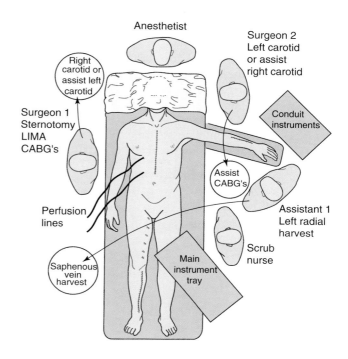

1

Carotid incision

2 The incision begins 1 cm below the ear lobe and posterior to the inferior angle of the mandible, so as to avoid the great auricular nerve and the mandibular branch of the facial nerve. The incision continues inferiorly along the anterior border of the sternocleidomastoid muscle, curving anteriorly toward the midline two thirds of the way down the neck. This anterior extension should follow a skin crease.

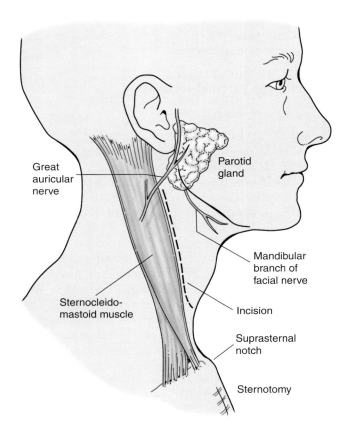

Great auricular nerve

Parotid gland

Mandibular branch of facial nerve

Sternocleido-mastoid muscle

Incision

Suprasternal notch

Sternotomy

2

IDENTIFICATION OF CAROTID ARTERY BIFURCATION

3 Using diathermy, the surgeon cauterizes superficial vessels and incises the platysma in the line of the incision. A small retractor is placed deep to this muscle. The great auricular nerve should be identified posteriorly and preserved. The fatty tissues that overlie the palpable carotid artery are then incised with diathermy. Small vessels should be specifically cauterized or ligated and divided. The common facial vein is then identified and dissected free with scissors. It is doubly ligated or, if necessary, suture ligated and then divided. This vein directly overlies the carotid bifurcation. Occasionally, there may be more than one vein. The retractor is then repositioned to retract the sternocleidomastoid muscle and the internal jugular vein posteriorly. The carotid sheath is incised longitudinally. Starting inferiorly, the common carotid artery is gently mobilized. The surrounding structures are dissected off the carotid vessels, which should be manipulated as little as possible. The plane of the dissection is on the carotid adventitia so as to avoid damage to the vagus nerve. A soft vessel sling is placed around the common carotid artery 1–2 cm below its bifurcation.

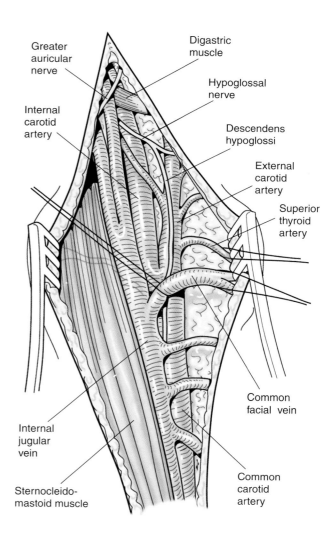

Greater auricular nerve

Internal carotid artery

Digastric muscle

Hypoglossal nerve

Descendens hypoglossi

External carotid artery

Superior thyroid artery

Common facial vein

Internal jugular vein

Sternocleido-mastoid muscle

Common carotid artery

3

4 As the dissection continues superiorly along the external carotid artery, several sizable branches are encountered. The superior thyroid artery, which passes downward and anteriorly, is encircled with a Blalock sling (double throw of a 2/0 Ti-cron suture). This sling can be used as a snare and for retraction. The smaller ascending pharyngeal branch is more posterior and is controlled in a similar fashion. It is rarely necessary to ligate these vessels permanently.

The dissection of the internal carotid artery is completed last. Commencing at the bifurcation, the descendens hypoglossi nerve is identified and mobilized posteriorly. It can be divided if the exposure proves difficult (a rare circumstance). As dissection continues superiorly the hypoglossal nerve must be identified and preserved. It appears below the posterior belly of the digastric muscle, emerging between the internal jugular vein and the internal carotid artery, and passes superficially across the internal and the external carotid arteries. The descendens hypoglossi nerve separates from the main trunk of the hypoglossal nerve and can be traced superiorly to locate the nerve. The hypoglossal nerve is usually identified and preserved without mobilization. If sharp dissection is necessary, the nerve should not be touched, and care should be taken to avoid injury to its accompanying blood supply. The exposure of the internal carotid artery is continued superiorly as far as is necessary to be able to position a small vascular clamp above the palpable atheroma. The posterior belly of the digastric muscle can be divided in the rare situation of a high carotid bifurcation. Soft vessel slings are passed around the internal and external carotid arteries. The tissue between these vessels is quite tough and contains the carotid sinus nerve, which can be safely divided. We use sharp dissection in this area. Hemostats are not applied to any slings at this stage, to avoid inadvertent traction on the vessels. The most appropriate DeBakey–atraumatic ring handle bulldog clamps, usually with bent shanks, are then selected so that they can be positioned without interfering with the proposed arteriotomy. A small moist gauze is placed in the wound while cardiopulmonary bypass is begun. Heparin is given via a central line and adequate anticoagulation confirmed by the activated clotting time.

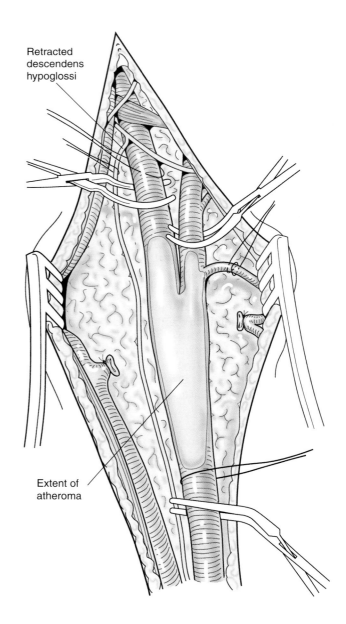

Retracted descendens hypoglossi

Extent of atheroma

4

Cardiopulmonary bypass

5 Routine aortic and two-stage venous cannulations are performed and the cannulae positioned so that they are not in the way of the neck dissection. Cardiopulmonary bypass is begun and cooling commenced to a nasopharyngeal temperature of 25°C. The perfusion pressure is kept above 60 mm Hg.

A left ventricular vent is inserted through a pursestring suture on the anterior surface of the right superior pulmonary vein. This 20-gauge, fenestrated right-angled cannula is usually introduced without difficulty into the left ventricle, with care taken to ensure that it is not inserted too far. The vent is then connected to a side arm of the venous line and passive venting continued throughout the case.

The coronary conduits are then inspected and prepared. The internal mammary artery is divided distally, its flow checked, and the distal end prepared. A soft clip is then applied distally to this conduit. Cold saline (5°C – not iced slush) is poured into the pericardial cavity.

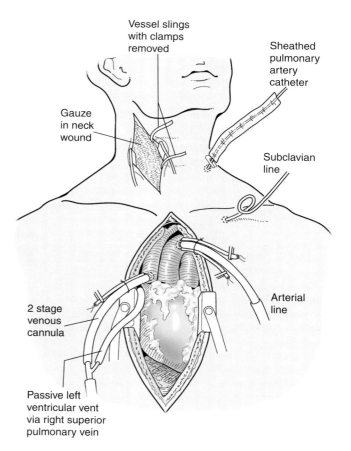

Vessel slings with clamps removed

Sheathed pulmonary artery catheter

Gauze in neck wound

Subclavian line

Arterial line

2 stage venous cannula

Passive left ventricular vent via right superior pulmonary vein

5

Carotid arteriotomy

6 When the heart fibrillates (at approximately 28°C), it is checked to ensure that no ventricular distention exists, after which the carotid endarterectomy is performed. The preselected vascular clamps are applied to the common carotid artery and its two branches. The branches of the external carotid are controlled by gentle traction on the Blalock slings. A longitudinal incision is then made through the adventitia on the anterolateral surface of the carotid bulb. The incision is carried just through the adventitia until a plane between the atherosclerotic plaque and the adventitia can be established. The length of this incision is extended inferiorly into the common carotid artery below any obvious localized plaque or for approximately 1.5 cm below the bifurcation if the entire vessel is diseased. The incision extends superiorly into the internal carotid artery to a point immediately beyond the bifurcation. The incision can be extended superiorly later.

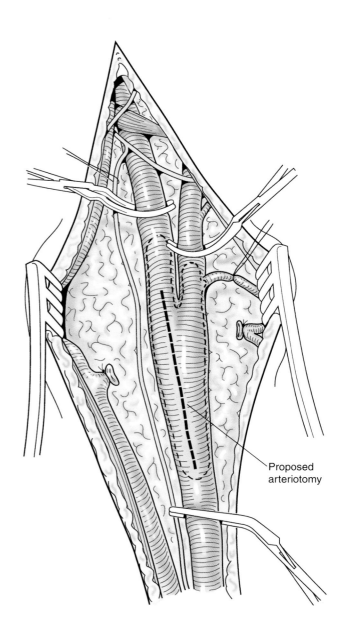

Proposed arteriotomy

6

ENDARTERECTOMY OF THE COMMON CAROTID ARTERY

7 Using a small blunt (Watson-Cheyne) dissector, the plaque is mobilized from within the adventitia. Care is taken not to damage the adventitia particularly posteromedially. The adventitia is gently retracted by the assistant or with 4/0 monofilament traction sutures. When the common carotid artery atheroma is completely mobilized at this level, a fine (Mixter) right-angled clamp is passed around it, inside the adventitia, and, using an 11-scalpel blade, the atheroma is divided.

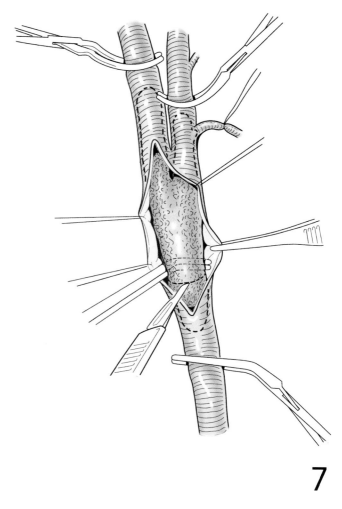

7

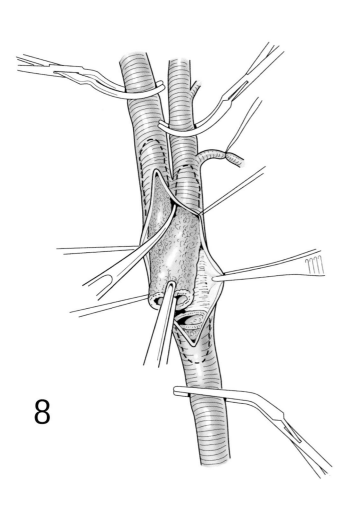

8

ENDARTERECTOMY OF THE EXTERNAL CAROTID ARTERY

8 The specimen is grasped with blunt forceps, because fine forceps may lacerate the plaque, and the dissection is continued superiorly until the external carotid artery is encountered. With gentle retraction laterally, the external carotid plaque is gently teased out of this vessel. Intimal extensions into the superior thyroid and ascending pharyngeal branches are often seen and are usually retracted out without difficulty. While applying gentle traction laterally and inferiorly, the external carotid clamp can be removed momentarily. This maneuver usually enables the specimen to be removed completely from within the external carotid artery.

ENDARTERECTOMY OF THE INTERNAL CAROTID ARTERY

9 The atheromatous plaque is then gently retracted inferiorly and blunt dissection continued into the internal carotid artery. Care is taken around the bifurcation to ensure that the adventitia is not breached. Usually, the plaque thins out as the dissection proceeds superiorly. The vessel wall often partially everts, making the dissection easier. Eventually, the thin normal intima fractures, and the specimen is removed. The author usually completes this portion of the dissection with one hand on the internal carotid clamp, releasing it gently as the specimen is finally removed with the other. The adventitia incision can be extended superiorly, if necessary, to ensure adequate visualization of the distal 'tail' of the dissection. However, if the incision is limited to that portion of the vessel affected by the atheromatous plaque, the risk of stenosis as the arteriotomy is closed is minimized.

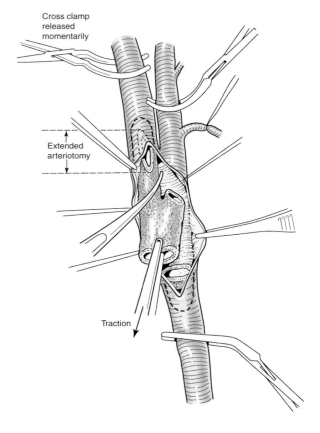

9

DÉBRIDEMENT

10 The vessel wall is then carefully inspected, and any loose strips of atheroma that remain are carefully peeled away. The internal carotid artery is closely inspected to ensure that there is no loose flap superiorly. Retraction with a small right-angled forceps assists visualization.

If there is any concern about a distal intimal flap or the possibility of dissection, this tissue is 'tacked' to the adventitia with 7/0 monofilament suture passed from the internal aspect of the plaque through the adventitia and secured external to the vessel. The internal carotid artery clamp is again momentarily released to provide retrograde flushing of the vessel. Finally, the wall of the dissected artery is dried with a gauze 'peanut' and again inspected to ensure that there is no loose debris.

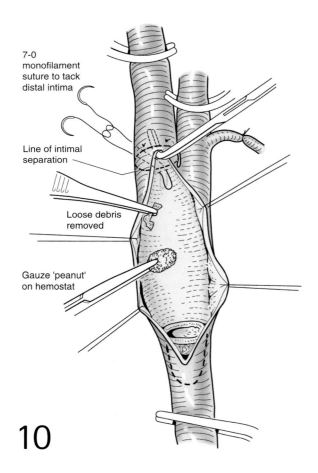

10

CLOSURE OF THE ARTERIOTOMY

11 If the incision has remained on the plaque-containing portion of the vessel, a venous patch is not usually necessary. The arteriotomy is closed with a double 6/0 monofilament suture that commences superiorly. The last two remaining loops of this suture are left loose inferiorly and the clamp on the internal carotid artery again released momentarily to fill and deair the vessel. This clamp is reapplied and the external carotid artery clamp removed. Once deairing is complete, the common carotid artery clamp is released, and the suture is pulled taut. The artery is then gently palpated as the internal carotid clamp is released. Maintaining traction on the first suture, the second arm of the 6/0 monofilament suture is then used to overrun the suture line and tied proximally.

SAPHENOUS VEIN PATCH

If concern exists that direct closure may narrow the lumen of the internal carotid artery, a small patch of saphenous vein can be used. A 6/0 monofilament suture is utilized.

INTRA-ARTERIAL SHUNTS

We do not use intra-arterial shunts. Adequate cerebral protection is provided with the core cooling achieved on cardiopulmonary bypass. The patient's temperature regularly drifts from 28°C to 25°C during the endarterectomy.

The Silastic slings around the common and internal carotid arteries are then removed. The Blalock sling on the superior thyroid artery is loosened but left *in situ* without a hemostat, as is the sling on the external carotid artery. This strategy provides the opportunity for rapid traction on the vessel should urgent access be required during the remainder of the procedure. A gauze square is loosely placed in the wound and the retractor removed.

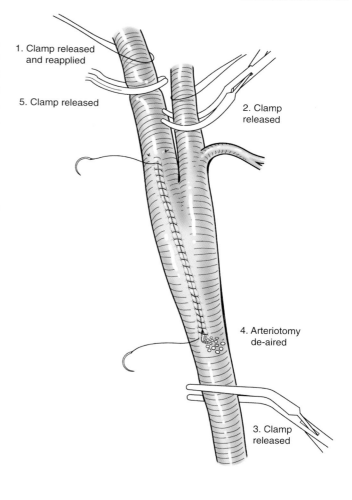

1. Clamp released and reapplied
5. Clamp released
2. Clamp released
4. Arteriotomy de-aired
3. Clamp released

11

Coronary revascularization

After completion of the cervical procedure, the aorta is cross-clamped and cardioplegic solution instilled. For routine coronary artery surgery, anterograde aortic root infusion is used. If a critical left main stem stenosis exists or if concomitant valve surgery is also required, retrograde coronary sinus delivery also is used.

Coronary arteries are then grafted in the routine fashion. No changes in conventional coronary grafting techniques are used. Rewarming is commenced during the last distal anastomosis. Proximal anastomoses are usually completed using a side-occluding clamp on the ascending aorta. If, however, as is often the case in these patients, significant aortic atheroma is present, the proximal anastomoses are completed proximal to the aortic cross-clamp before it is removed.

When the patient is fully rewarmed, all suture lines, including those in the neck, are checked for adequate hemostasis. Once sinus rhythm, or a paced rhythm, if necessary, is estab-

lished, cardiopulmonary bypass is gradually discontinued. The heparin is reversed after all anastomoses have been inspected again and all cannulae have been removed.

Chest drains are inserted and the cervical retractor repositioned. The carotid anastomosis is again checked and a small (10-gauge/3.5-mm), fenestrated suction drain inserted percutaneously. The drain is positioned so that it is not lying against the now soft adventitia of the carotid artery. The wound is again packed with gauze while the sternotomy is inspected, hemostasis assured, and the sternotomy closed. Finally, the cervical incision is again inspected to ensure that no bleeding occurs from the small superficial vessels in the neck. The platysma and subcutaneous tissues are closed with Vicryl sutures (Ethicon J&J, New Jersey), and the skin incision is closed with a running subcuticular Dexon suture (Davis & Geck, Hamilton, Bermuda). Transparent hydrocolloid dressings are then placed over both incisions.

POSTOPERATIVE CARE

Postoperative care centers principally on management of the patient's hemodynamics and ventilation. Sedation is discontinued early to observe the patient's neurological status. Sedation and analgesics can be reinstituted once the patient has responded appropriately. We favor early extubation in stable patients. Nursing and intensive care staff must be aware of the possibility of cervical hemorrhage and respiratory obstruction from a neck hematoma. Protocols for immediate evacuation of the wound and return to the operating room, if respiratory obstruction occurs, should be established. Early central neurological abnormalities should prompt urgent carotid duplex study. If carotid occlusion or obstruction is identified, patients should be returned to the operating room for re-exploration and restoration of carotid artery flow.

Cardiac postoperative care is dictated according to the usual intensive care unit protocols. Hypertension should be managed aggressively and hypotension avoided, especially in patients with cerebrovascular disease and procedure-induced cerebral ischemia.

Facial nerve injuries are rare if the above techniques are followed. Occasionally, a patient may complain of weakness in the lower lip related to traction or compression of segmental branches of the facial nerve. This is almost always temporary.

Long-term follow-up of patients with combined disease who have extensive or premature atherosclerosis, or both, should occur at 6- to 12-month intervals, and both carotid arteries should be assessed with ultrasound surveillance. Daily low-dose aspirin is prescribed for all coronary artery surgery patients. If contralateral carotid disease is present that has not been operated on, dipyridamole (Persantine), 75 mg three times a day, may be a useful therapeutic regimen as well.

OUTCOME

The optimal management of patients with significant coronary and carotid stenoses will remain controversial in the absence of large, multi-center randomized trials of synchronous versus staged approaches. Many authors, however, have described the synchronous operation with excellent results. Our own experience supports these reports. Perioperative stroke rates of between 1.6 and 5.5 per cent are usually associated with the higher-risk patient. We have noted no strokes in patients with asymptomatic carotid lesions that were treated synchronously. Rates of death between 1.7 and 5.5 per cent and a myocardial infarction incidence of 0.8–4.7 per cent are similar or better than those for staged procedures.

Synchronous carotid endarterectomy and coronary artery bypass grafting represent an acceptable and perhaps preferable method for the management of patients with both coronary and carotid stenoses. Not only are there significant clinical benefits to staged procedures but also important economic gains (i.e. reduced operating room time, intensive care stay, and hospital bed days) for patients, hospitals, and health care providers.

FURTHER READING

Akins, C.W., Moncure, A.C., Daggett, W.M., et al. 1995. Safety and efficacy of concomitant carotid and coronary artery operations. Annals of Thoracic Surgery 60, 311–7.

Brenner, B.T., Brief, D.K., Alport, J., Golderkrawl, R.J., Parsonnet, V. 1987. The risk of stroke in patients with asymptomatic carotid stenosis undergoing cardiac surgery: a follow-up study. Journal of Vascular Surgery 5, 269–77.

Gardner, T.J., Horneffer, P.J., Manolio, T.A., Hoff, S.J., Pearson, T.A. 1986. Major stroke after coronary artery bypass surgery: changing magnitude of the problem. Journal of Vascular Surgery 3, 684–7.

Minami, K., Morshuis, M., Mirrow, N., Reiß, N., Körfer, R. 1996. Concomitant carotid artery stenosis in coronary artery bypass candidates: staged or simultaneous revascularization. Annals of Thoracic and Cardiovascular Surgery 2, 247–53.

Ricotta, J.J., Faggioli, G.L., Castlione, A., Hasset, J.M. 1995. Risk factors for stroke after cardiac surgery: Buffalo Cardiac-Cerebral Group. Journal of Vascular Surgery 21, 359–63.

Takach, T.J., Reul, G.J., Cooley, D.A., et al. 1997. Is an integrated approach warranted for concomitant carotid and coronary artery disease? Annals of Thoracic Surgery 64, 16–22.

15

Transmyocardial laser revascularization

KEITH A. HORVATH MD
Associate Professor of Cardiothoracic Surgery, Department of Surgery, Northwestern University Medical School;
Attending Surgeon, Department of Surgery, Northwestern Memorial Hospital, Chicago, Illinois, USA

HISTORY

Transmyocardial laser revascularization (TMR) was developed to treat severe angina in patients with diffuse coronary artery disease that could not be treated by the conventional methods of coronary artery bypass grafting (CABG) or percutaneous transluminal coronary angioplasty (PTCA). TMR was initially performed by Mirhoseini who used TMR in conjunction with CABG in the early 1980s. The use of a laser as sole therapy on the beating heart required advancements in the technology. The carbon dioxide laser was the first to be used clinically, and the results from individual institutions and from multicenter trials from 1995 through 1999 demonstrated a dramatic improvement in the symptomatic relief of angina.

As a result of the success of the procedure, CO_2 TMR obtained U.S. Food and Drug Administration approval in 1998 and has been performed on more than 15 000 patients around the world. Originally used to treat patients as sole therapy for their end-stage coronary disease, TMR has been increasingly used in combination with coronary bypass grafting to provide a more complete revascularization to territories of the heart that could not be grafted.

PRINCIPLES AND JUSTIFICATION

As sole therapy, the procedure is performed on patients with severe, disabling angina, the majority of whom are in Canadian Cardiovascular Society angina class IV. By definition, these patients have recurrent chest pain that significantly alters their quality of life and is refractory to maximal medical therapy. Other surgical options for such patients are limited. For the sole-therapy patient, the possibility of cardiac transplantation exists, although most of these patients have a reasonable ejection fraction and are not suffering from heart failure as much as they are suffering from angina. Due to the scarcity of organs, these patients rarely undergo transplantation. Extensive coronary revascularization and endarterectomies may also be an option, but these procedures carry a higher rate of risk.

Of patients treated with CO_2 TMR as sole therapy, 75 per cent experience a significant reduction in angina postoperatively (i.e. decrease in angina of two or more classes). These results at 1 year have been maintained beyond 5 years. In addition to the symptomatic improvement, objective findings, including the improvement in myocardial perfusion with a CO_2 laser, have also been documented. This improvement in symptoms and perfusion is achieved while the patients typically decrease their medical regimen. All this can be achieved with morbidity and mortality that is typically less than that of a reoperative CABG. Of note, however, is that patients with recent or ongoing episodes of unstable angina requiring intravenous medications to control their chest pain have had a higher mortality rate due to the tenuous nature of their disease and the instability of their condition. Although patients such as these can undergo TMR as sole therapy, their risk can be reduced if they can be stabilized and off of intravenous medications for as short an interval as 2 weeks.

More than one wavelength of light has been used for TMR. In addition to CO_2, holmium:yttrium-aluminum-garnet (Ho:YAG) lasers have been used. Despite achieving a similar reduction of short-term angina relief, the Ho:YAG laser has never been demonstrated to improve perfusion or provide a long-term benefit. The recent failure of the Ho:YAG device to perform myocardial revascularization percutaneously (PMR) casts further doubt on the efficacy of this wavelength of light. These clinical differences stem from a significant difference in the laser–tissue interaction between CO_2 and Ho:YAG lasers.

The exact mechanism whereby CO_2 TMR achieves its clinical benefit is unknown. The original thought that the laser channels remain patent has been broadened to include a stimulation of angiogenesis as a result of the laser energy.

PREOPERATIVE ASSESSMENT AND PREPARATION

Patients who undergo CO_2 TMR as sole therapy present with severe angina that requires frequent use of sublingual nitroglycerine to carry out their activities of daily living and, in fact, often leads to repeat hospital admissions. In at least one study, such patients were admitted, on average, five times in the year before undergoing TMR; as a group, these patients averaged 0.5 admissions in the year post-TMR. These patients are then well known to their internist and cardiologist and are on maximal medical therapy to control their symptoms. In addition to verifying the severity of their symptoms, preoperative assessment includes documentation of severe coronary artery disease, which typically includes a recent cardiac catheterization. The angiogram is worth repeating if it has not been performed in the previous 6 months. Occasionally, progression of disease in vein grafts (as many of these patients have undergone previous bypass surgery) may be amenable to conventional methods of revascularization. Once the diffuse nature of the disease is confirmed, evidence of reversible ischemia should be documented. This situation may be accomplished with myocardial perfusion scanning, rest, and stress echocardiography, or with cine and perfusion magnetic resonance imaging. For patients in whom a very small amount of myocardial ischemia is surrounded by a significant area of myocardium infarction, the procedure should be avoided. The success in such patients is limited. Additionally, severely depressed ejection fraction (less than 20 per cent) was used as a cutoff for the aforementioned clinical trials, and TMR should not be considered a therapy for heart failure unless a significant amount of reversible ischemia or hibernating myocardium is present that may lead to an improvement in myocardial function after revascularization.

Used in combination with CABG, the preoperative evaluation is the same as that of any CABG patient. The decision to use TMR in combination is frequently done intraoperatively. For example, an occluded artery on an angiogram may prove to be graftable in the operating room and may be revascularized by CABG. If not bypassable, then the decision to use TMR would be made at that time. By review of the angiogram, the surgeon may have an idea of whether all territories will be graftable. For patients in whom TMR may be beneficial as an adjunct, its use is discussed preoperatively.

ANESTHESIA

TMR for sole-therapy patients is performed via a left thoracotomy; and therefore, their general anesthetic can be supplemented by a thoracic epidural. This approach is beneficial in managing postoperative pain. Additionally, single-lung ventilation via bronchial blocker or double-lumen endotracheal tube may assist the surgeon in exposure, particularly in patients who have had previous CABG. If an epidural is not used, then analgesia of post-thoracotomy may be obtained via local infiltration of the intercostal muscle with local anesthetic. For patients who undergo TMR plus CABG, the anesthetic is the same as that for those who undergo CABG alone.

OPERATION

1 Transmyocardial laser revascularization performed as an open surgical procedure is typically done through a left anterolateral thoracotomy in the fifth intercostal space. The patient is placed in a supine position with a roll under the left side from the shoulder to the waist to elevate the left hemithorax. Skin preparation includes at least one or both groins, particularly in patients with low ejection fractions or unstable angina, as they may require intraoperative placement of an intra-aortic balloon pump. After the establishment of adequate general endotracheal anesthesia, an 8- to 12-cm skin incision is made as diagrammed. Exposure of the heart through this incision can typically be achieved without division of the ribs or costal cartilages.

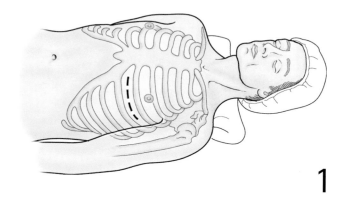

1

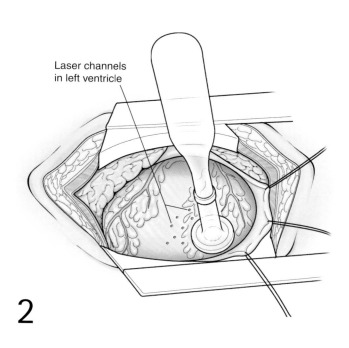

Laser channels in left ventricle

2

2 Once the ribs are spread by a retractor and the lung is deflated, the pericardium is opened to expose the epicardial surface of the heart. Care must be taken to avoid previous bypass grafts. The left anterior descending artery is identified and used as a landmark of the location of the septum. The inferior and posterior lateral portions of the heart can be reached through this incision with a combination manual traction and placement of packing behind the heart, and, as illustrated, the use of a right-angled laser handpiece. Channels are created starting near the base of the heart and then serially in a line approximately 1-cm apart toward the apex, starting inferiorly and then working superiorly to the anterior surface of the heart. As some bleeding from the channels occurs, commencement of the TMR inferiorly keeps the anterior area clear and expedites the procedure. The number of channels created depends on the size of the heart and on the size of the ischemic area. Myocardium that is thinned by scar, particularly when the scar is transmural, should be avoided, as TMR will be of no benefit to these regions, and bleeding from channels in these areas may be problematic. Transesophageal echocardiography should be used to confirm transmural penetration of the laser energy. The vaporization of blood by the laser energy as the laser beam enters the ventricle creates an obvious and characteristic acoustic effect as noted on transesophageal echocardiography.

3 To minimize postoperative incisional pain, particularly in patients who have not had previous bypass surgery, the TMR procedure can be performed with video-assisted thoracoscopy. Again, the patient is positioned supine with the left hemithorax elevated by a roll. The left upper extremity may also be retracted cranially to facilitate placement of the thoracoscope. The thoracoscopic ports may be placed in the fifth or fourth intercostal space. Through the same 10-mm port incision used for the thoracoscope, an endoscopic grasper may be placed to facilitate the dissection. Once the camera has been placed, additional ports can be created under thoracoscopic guidance. As the heart is immediately adjacent to the chest wall, endoscopic instrumentation may not be necessary, and standard instruments may be introduced through these additional incisions. The incisions should be triangulated to provide maximum facility for dissection and exposure.

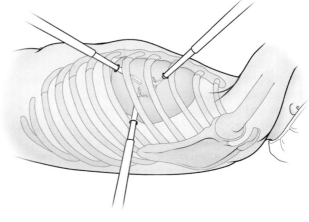

3

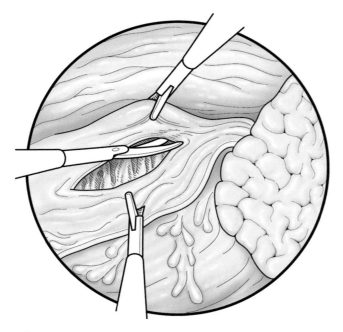

4 This view from the thoracoscope demonstrates the grasper, which is placed through the same thoracoscope incision at 6 o'clock on this picture, and an additional grasper placed through a third intercostal incision port at 1 o'clock. These two graspers are used to elevate and separate the pericardium, which is divided using standard dissecting scissors placed through a more anterior fifth intercostal incision. Care is taken to avoid the left phrenic nerve during this dissection.

4

5 Laser handpieces can be introduced through any of the ports with replacement of the thoracoscope as needed to allow the creation of TMR channels on all areas of the left ventricular surface. A straight handpiece, as demonstrated here, is being introduced through the third intercostal incision. With a combination of the use of the straight and right-angled handpieces, all surfaces can be covered. Bleeding from the channels is controlled either with direct finger pressure or the use of sponge stick placed after removal of the handpiece.

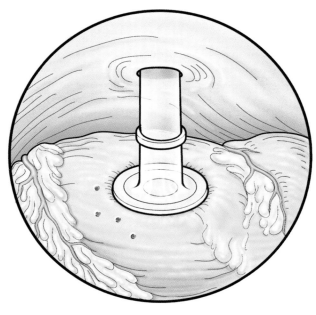

5

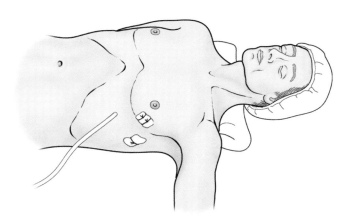

6 The thoracoscopic incisions are closed with three layers of absorbable suture, and a dry sterile dressing is applied. A chest tube is placed through one of the fifth intercostal incision sites to provide adequate evacuation of air and/or fluid from the pleural cavity postoperatively.

6

POSTOPERATIVE CARE

The majority of sole-therapy patients are extubated in the operating room. Their postoperative care is somewhat different from the standard post-CABG patient. Because of the angiogenic effects, the revascularization by TMR improves with time. The postoperative care is therefore different than that of a CABG patient. Care must be taken to avoid myocardial stress, which includes adequate pain control and maintenance of perfusion pressure. Hemodynamic instability or marginal cardiac output should be treated first by insertion of an intra-aortic balloon pump. This procedure may be done intraoperatively before TMR in patients with low ejection fractions or unstable angina. Typically, with a CO_2 laser, prophylaxis for arrhythmias is not required postoperatively. For a combination, TMR plus CABG, the postoperative care is the same as for CABG alone.

OUTCOME

Due to the severity of their disease, sole-therapy–TMR patients experience an early morbidity and mortality rate similar to that of reoperative CABG. Occasionally, chest pain may occur postoperatively, but this pain is typically less frequent than that which the patient experienced preoperatively. Over time, these symptoms decrease. Both randomized and non-randomized data indicate that 75 per cent of the patients have a decrease of two or more angina classes at 1-year follow-up. Longer-term angina relief of over 5 years postoperatively has also been demonstrated with CO_2 TMR. In a recent report, patients had an average angina class of 3.7 preoperatively, and the average was 1.5 at 1 year and 1.6 at 5 years postoperatively.

Anecdotal reports of reoperative TMR for patients who develop a new area of reversible ischemia, typically over a year after the original procedure, have been published. Patients also exist who undergo bypass surgery or angioplasty after TMR due to the progression of their disease. As a result, recurrent chest pain late after TMR should be initially investigated with repeat cardiac catheterization to determine whether conventional methods are feasible.

The outcomes in patients who have TMR in combination with CABG have, not surprisingly, demonstrated a similar improvement in symptoms. Using cine magnetic resonance imaging, we have demonstrated an improvement in wall motion in areas that received the laser treatment alone. Obviously, this improvement may be related to the bypass grafting for these combination patients. Of note, however, is that no evidence of microinfarction in the laser-treated areas exists. Further studies to delineate the benefit of TMR with CABG are underway.

For patients with severe angina due to diffuse coronary disease, CO_2 TMR has provided significant short- and long-term angina relief. In combination with CABG, TMR also provides a method to completely revascularize patients who have graftable and ungraftable vessels.

FURTHER READING

Cooley, D.A., Frazier, O.H., Kadipasaoglu, K.A., et al. 1996. Transmyocardial laser revascularization: clinical experience with 12-month follow-up. *Journal of Thoracic and Cardiovascular Surgery* 111, 791–9.

Frazier, O.H., March, R.J., Horvath, K.A. 1999. Transmyocardial revascularization with a carbon dioxide laser in patients with end-stage coronary artery disease. *New England Journal of Medicine* 341, 1021–8.

Horvath, K.A., Aranki, S.A., Cohn, L.H., et al. 2001. Sustained angina relief five years after transmyocardial revascularization with a CO2 laser. *Circulation* 104(Suppl I), I-81–I-84.

Horvath, K.A., Cohn, L.H., Cooley, D.A., et al. 1997. Transmyocardial laser revascularization: results of a multicenter trial with transmyocardial laser revascularization used as sole therapy for end-stage coronary artery disease. *Journal of Thoracic and Cardiovascular Surgery* 113, 645–54.

Horvath, K.A., Mannting, F., Cummings, N., Shernan, S.K., Cohn, L.H. 1996. Transmyocardial laser revascularization: operative techniques and clinical results at two years. *Journal of Thoracic and Cardiovascular Surgery* 111, 1047–53.

Mirhoseini, M., Cayton, M. 1981. Revascularization of the heart by laser. *Journal of Microsurgery* 2, 253–60.

SECTION III

Surgery for Valvular Heart Disease

16

Mitral valve replacement

LAWRENCE H. COHN MD
Virginia and James Hubbard Professor of Cardiac Surgery, Harvard Medical School; Chief of Cardiac Surgery, Brigham and Women's Hospital, Boston, Massachusetts, USA

HISTORY

This history of mitral valve surgery begins with the first successful operation by Cutler at the Peter Bent Brigham Hospital in 1923, which was developed further there after World War II by Harken *et al*. The first reliable mitral valve replacement device was developed in the late 1950s. In 1959, Nina Braunwald of the National Institutes of Health made the first successful implantable prosthetic valve, but the first universally applied mitral valve replacement device was a ball-and-cage valve developed by Albert Starr and Lowell Edwards. The Starr–Edwards mitral valve, first implanted in 1961, was the gold standard for many years, until the late 1960s, when second- and third-generation valves began to appear with different design features. The Starr–Edwards ball valve, which is still in use today, is an effective device for relieving the obstruction of the mitral orifice, but its usage has decreased because of the relatively high rate of thromboembolism that occurs despite anticoagulation.

The next generation of valves were lower profile, tilting disk valves, which were developed and used in the 1970s and 1980s. Bileaflet valves replaced these single-disk valves, particularly after the St. Jude medical valve was first used in 1977. This valve has been implanted in more than 1 million patients worldwide. Bioprosthetic valves were developed along a parallel track at the same time. The first of these was the Hancock valve, developed in 1970, and the Carpentier–Edwards valve (1976). These tissue valves were used extensively in the 1980s, but it became apparent that their principal shortcomings were limited durability and structural valve degeneration. Valve calcification and leaflet tearing became serious problems and were much worse than with similar bioprostheses in the aortic area. As a result, the bioprosthetic mitral valve substitute now is generally limited to patients who cannot undergo mitral valve repair, are older than age 70 years, and are in sinus rhythm. The Carpentier–Edwards bovine pericardial valve in the mitral position, similar to that used currently worldwide in the aortic area, has been shown to be more durable than the porcine valve in European and Canadian trials and has recently been introduced for use in the United States.

PRINCIPLES AND JUSTIFICATION

Mitral stenosis

For patients with mitral valve stenosis, valve replacement is the ultimate surgical therapy. Valve replacement usually is performed in patients who have calcified valves that cannot be reconstructed. The initial intervention for a noncalcified, fibrotic mitral valve stenosis is percutaneous balloon dilatation. If this procedure is not successful, open mitral commissurotomy with reconstruction of the valve generally is a success. Although aggressive decalcification and reconstructive techniques for patients with advanced mitral valve stenosis can be done, the long-term results, in general, have been poor, and valve replacement is usually carried out for the advanced calcified mitral stenotic valve.

Mitral regurgitation

The majority of patients who undergo surgery for mitral regurgitation today can undergo mitral valve repair, including individuals with degenerative, rheumatic, infectious, and/or ischemic etiologies of mitral valve disease. The myxomatous degenerated valve, the so-called floppy valve, is now reparable in as many as 95 per cent of cases. In ischemic mitral regurgitation, ring annuloplasty can be efficacious, but long-term results depend on coronary artery disease and left ventricular function. The regurgitant rheumatic valve often can be reconstructed, but, as noted in the previous section, if the valve is moderately to severely calcified and stenotic as well, it may require replacement. In mitral valve endocarditis, reconstruction occasionally is possible, but often the valve is extensively infected and requires excision, débridement, and valve replacement, with reconstruction of the annulus with autologous pericardium.

With either stenosis or regurgitation, symptoms of pulmonary congestion and heart failure often are present. In patients with mitral regurgitation, there may be instances in which they are relatively symptom free, but, because of dilatation and/or deterioration of left ventricular function related to chronic volume overload, they are candidates for surgery. The onset of atrial fibrillation and dilatation of the left atrium may be an indication for early surgery.

Indications for bioprosthetic valves

The bioprosthetic porcine valve primarily has been used in older patients (70 years of age or older), although in some specific situations younger patients may request or require bioprosthetic valve replacement. For example, in a young woman who intends to become pregnant, use of a bioprosthesis can avoid warfarin anticoagulation and fetal injury during pregnancy. Patients of any age who are in normal sinus rhythm, or those who wish to avoid anticoagulation, may have a bioprosthetic valve inserted. Additionally, in patients who are younger than 70 years, particularly those with coronary artery disease in sinus rhythm, a bioprosthetic valve may be an excellent choice, as expected longevity in these individuals is reduced.

Indications for mechanical valves

Prosthetic mechanical mitral valve replacement is probably more common than use of a bioprosthetic valve. The current availability of a durable bileaflet valve has resulted in long-term effectiveness and fewer thromboembolic complications. For the patient in chronic atrial fibrillation who requires long-term anticoagulation, and in any patient who wishes to minimize the likelihood of a reoperation, a prosthetic mitral valve is indicated.

PREOPERATIVE PREPARATION

Many patients who undergo mitral valve replacement have had long-standing medical treatment for congestive heart failure, pulmonary congestion, and right-sided congestive failure. Medications include the common cardioactive, vasodilator, and diuretic drugs, and, in general, patients who receive these medications are well compensated hemodynamically before surgery. A cardiac catheterization should be performed in all patients older than 40 years, primarily to identify coronary artery disease. Echocardiography is important diagnostically in all forms of mitral valve disease, and it may be unnecessary to perform cardiac catheterization to establish the diagnosis of mitral stenosis or regurgitation. Most patients in chronic atrial fibrillation have been on long-term anticoagulation, and this should be tapered approximately 2 or 3 days before surgery so as not to interfere with the normal clotting mechanism perioperatively.

An important component of mitral valve involvement that needs to be addressed is the possibility of right-sided heart failure, which may include severe tricuspid regurgitation, a functional abnormality that is determined by the degree of pulmonary hypertension. If tricuspid regurgitation is present, liver and renal function may be impaired. Liver abnormalities are common in patients with extensive tricuspid regurgitation secondary to long-standing mitral valve disease, and coagulation function may be impaired. Renal dysfunction, resulting in salt and water abnormalities in long-standing mitral valve disease, need to be meticulously addressed before surgery. Restorative therapy may require several preoperative days in such extremely ill patients.

ANESTHESIA

Anesthesia management for mitral valve replacement is the standard cardiac narcotic/inhalational anesthesia, which facilitates early postoperative extubation. Additionally, a transesophageal echocardiogram should be placed for all patients who are undergoing mitral valve surgery. The transesophageal echocardiogram is used not only to document the quality of the operative procedure and cardiac function but also to look for intracardiac air when the patient is being weaned from cardiopulmonary bypass. In addition to the transesophageal echocardiogram, an arterial and venous line, a urinary catheter, and usually a prebypass-placed pulmonary artery catheter to measure pulmonary artery pressures and cardiac output are used for monitoring.

OPERATIVE PROCEDURE

Incision

1 The standard incision for mitral valve replacement has been a complete median sternotomy. In our clinic, this technique is used if the patient has concomitant coronary artery disease that requires a coronary artery bypass. Conventional complete median sternotomy for patients who are undergoing combined mitral valve surgery and coronary artery bypass grafting is shown in Figure 1. This drawing demonstrates bicaval cannulation, distal ascending aorta, and anterograde and retrograde blood cardioplegia techniques through ascending aorta and through a retrograde coronary sinus cannula. The retractor shown is the Cosgrove retractor (St. Jude Medical, Inc., St. Paul MN 55117).

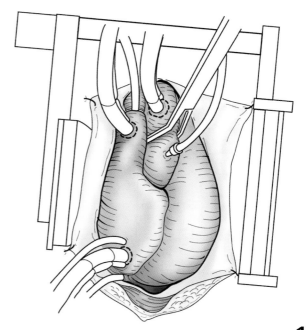

1

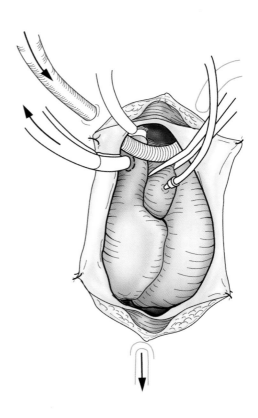

2a

2a, b
The minimally invasive approach can be used in all other patients who require isolated mitral valve surgery. The lower ministernotomy involves a 6- to 8-cm incision that is made over the lower sternum, preserving the xiphoid and then carrying the incision rightward into the second intercostal space. The cannulation and myocardial protection regimen for minimally invasive mitral valve surgery is shown in Figure 2, which demonstrates bicaval cannulation and isolation of the right atrium. The cannulation is performed through a right-angle cannula to the superior vena cava. A percutaneous femoral vein catheter is inserted through the mouth of the inferior vena cava. The right atrium is isolated by tourniquet tapes.

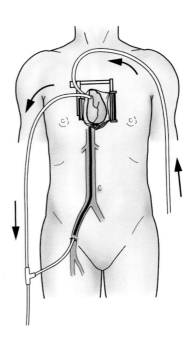

2b

3 Another incision that is utilized is the anterior right thoracotomy, which is primarily used for complicated reoperations, particularly in patients who have had a prior coronary bypass and now present with patent grafts. This incision can also be used in a patient who already has had an aortic valve replacement. The approach for reoperative mitral valve replacement performed through the right anterior thoracotomy approach is demonstrated in Figure 3. Cannulation usually is via the femoral artery/femoral vein, as well as the superior vena cava. The right anterior thoracotomy through the fourth intercostal space provides adequate exposure to the right atrium.

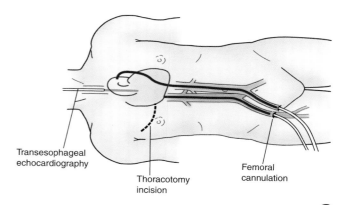

Transesophageal echocardiography

Thoracotomy incision

Femoral cannulation

3

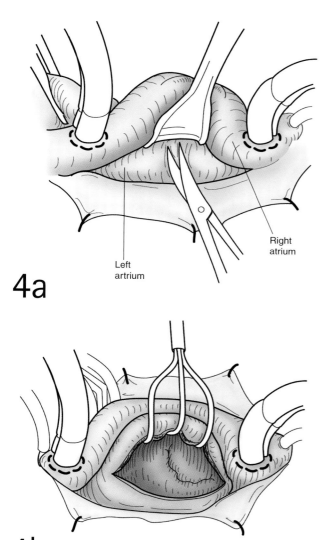

Left artrium

Right atrium

4a

4b

4a, b After the complete median sternotomy, the left atrium is opened after Sondergaard's plane is developed in the intra-atrial area. Dissection of this plane is helpful because it allows the operator to get closer to the mitral valve by dissecting the right atrium off the left atrium, thus allowing the incision to be far more medial.

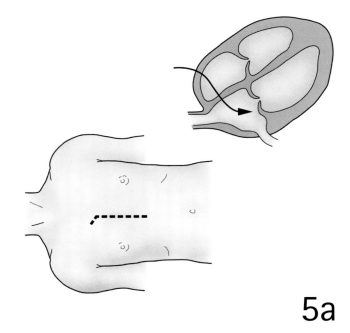

5a

5a–d The steps for exposure for a minimally invasive mitral valve replacement are shown, including the lower hemisternotomy with rightward extension in the second intercostal space (Figure 5a). A posterior right atrial incision is made above the interatrial groove, and the right atrium is entered (Figure 5b).

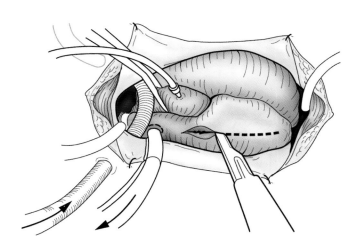

5b

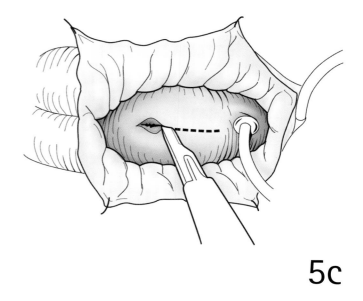

5c

This step is followed by an incision in the atrial septum, beginning at the foramen ovale and extending caudally toward the coronary sinus (Figure 5c). Stay sutures, placed on the incised septum, and gentle retraction allow for excellent exposure of the mitral valve through the limited sternotomy (Figure 5d).

As shown in Figures 3 through 5, small venous cannulae (24 Fr) are inserted directly into the right atrium. Alternately, a technique of percutaneous right femoral vein cannulation with extension of a 21-Fr catheter up to the right atrium can be used, along with assisted venous drainage in all cases to obtain excellent venous return. Arterial cannulation can almost always be achieved in the distal ascending aorta. Once on bypass, the heart is fibrillated electrically, the aorta is cross-clamped, and antegrade blood cardioplegia is given. If the patient is to have concomitant coronary artery bypass, retrograde cardioplegia is also given via a catheter inserted into the coronary sinus via the right atrium. Placing bypass grafts to the left coronary system, however, is difficult via a limited sternotomy.

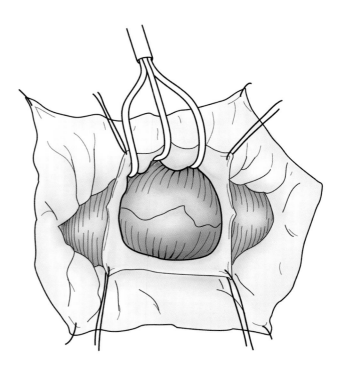

5d

Intracardiac technique

6 Mitral valve replacement requires removal of an appropriate amount of valve tissue to allow insertion of an adequate-sized prosthesis, but at the same time preserving as many of the papillary muscle–chordal–annular attachments as possible to ensure preservation of left ventricular function postoperatively and to prevent cardiac rupture. In addition, valve implantation necessitates awareness of anatomical structures near the mitral valve annulus, in particular, the circumflex coronary artery, which is contiguous and may be injured by deep placement of periannular sutures. Once the incision is made in the left atrium, a self-retaining retractor is currently used. This allows for excellent exposure of the valve without the need for manual assistance. Once the left atrium is opened, a weighted vent is placed in the inferior aspect of the left atrium for drainage of the pulmonary venous effluent, which is derived from bronchial return from the arterial circulation on bypass. The valve then is assessed to determine whether reparative or replacement techniques are required.

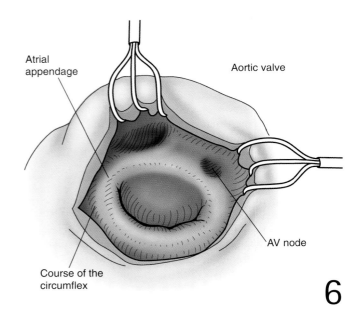

6

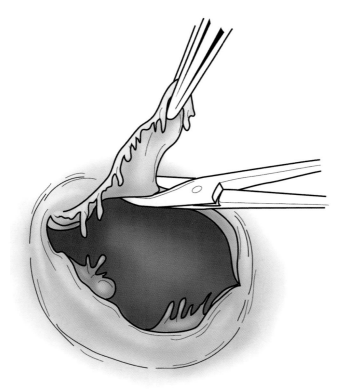

7 Several techniques are available for implantation, depending on the pathology and the type of prosthesis to be inserted. If one is dealing with calcified, rheumatic mitral stenosis, the anterior leaflet is excised with a residual rim of approximately 5 mm. In rheumatic mitral stenosis, the calcified posterior leaflet often cannot be left in place. Because of extensive scarring and chordal shortening, the size of the prosthesis to be inserted may be limited, unless the posterior leaflet is carefully excised.

7

8a, b If myxomatous degeneration is present that is causing regurgitation with a large floppy valve and it is determined that a valve replacement must be performed, and especially if the patient's left ventricular function is impaired, attempts should be made to preserve the anterior as well as the posterior leaflet along with the accompanying papillary muscle, chordal, and annular interaction. Care must be taken, particularly in large floppy valves, to make sure that the tissue is adequately tucked below the annulus correctly and tightened to the annulus to prevent obstruction of a mechanical valve by subannular protrusion of preserved valve tissue. Separate techniques are required for preservation of the anterior and posterior leaflet chordae. Once the valve has been excised, or partially excised, and the chordae have been tightened up to the annulus, valve replacement sutures can be inserted.

The translocation technique involves moving portions of the anterior leaflet that contain the chordae to the posterior leaflet and suturing them at that point. Furling describes incising a portion of the anterior leaflet and then folding the rest of the leaflet back to the anterior annulus, preserving the anterior chordae and papillary muscles.

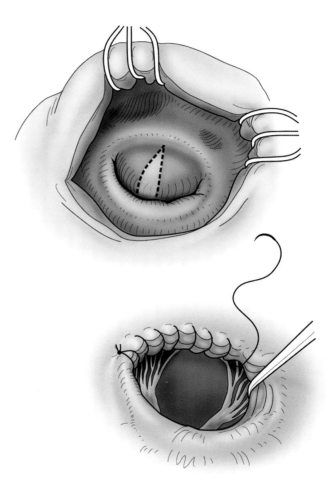

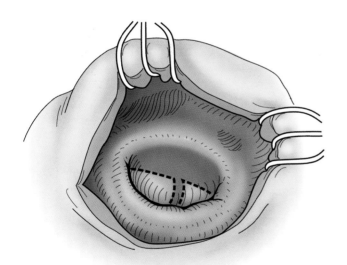

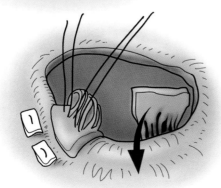

8a

8b

9a Suture techniques vary according to the type of valve inserted. For all mechanical prosthetic valves, we use everting, double-armed mattress sutures with Teflon pledgets to prevent any possibility of subannular obstruction of the valve leaflets by protruding tissue. The sutures are passed from the atrial aspect to the ventricular aspect into the valve sewing ring. Each stitch is tagged sequentially with a small hemostat. The average mitral valve requires approximately 12–14 mattress sutures.

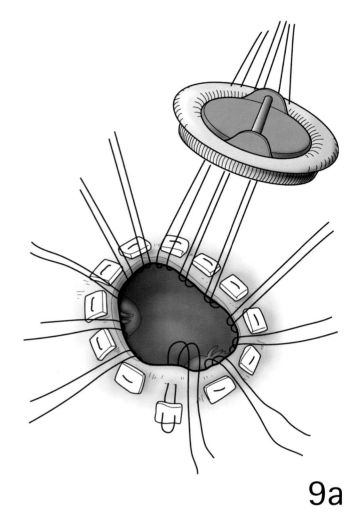

9a

9b With the use of a bileaflet prosthetic valve, the prosthesis is positioned so that the axis of the hinges is perpendicular to the native valve commissures. This placement prevents any obstruction to opening and closing of the disk.

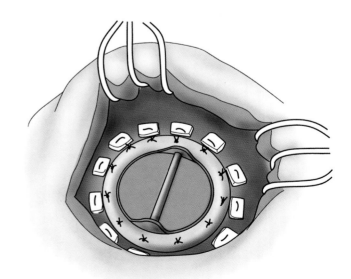

9b

10 If a bioprosthetic valve or Starr-Edwards valve is to be inserted, the valve sutures come from below upward in noneverting fashion, because this approach is more secure and allows for insertion of a slightly larger bioprosthesis. With the large cushioned sewing ring, there is little chance of interference with normal valve function. Once the sutures are placed in the valve sewing ring, the valve is lowered, and the knots are tied and cut.

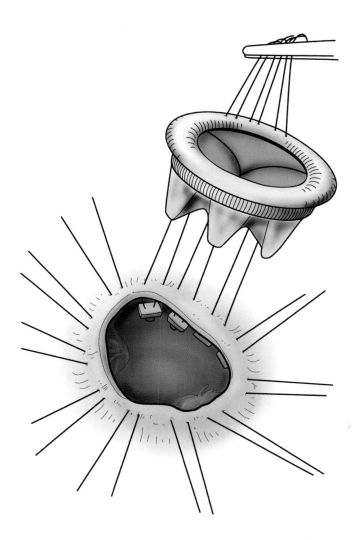

10

11 It is generally our practice to fill the left ventricle gently with saline before removing the cross-clamp so as to displace air into the left atrium. We do not use catheters to keep the valve insufficient while deairing is carried out. The left atrium is then closed with a running 3/0 Prolene suture, and the patient's head is lowered, the pump flow is lowered, and the cross-clamp is removed. Closure of the interatrial septum and right atrium after a minimally invasive mitral valve operation requires two suture lines.

Separation from cardiopulmonary bypass

Before weaning from cardiopulmonary bypass, after the patient is rewarmed, intracardiac air must be removed. The transesophageal echocardiogram is very effective in monitoring this, and it can also provide information related to left ventricular function, valve function, and so forth. When the patient is rewarmed and the air has dissipated from inside the heart, bypass is discontinued by interrupting venous drainage, correlating with a balanced systemic and venous pressure. Mediastinal and right thoracic chest drains are placed, and the standard sternal (either full, lower mini, or right thoracotomy) closure is performed.

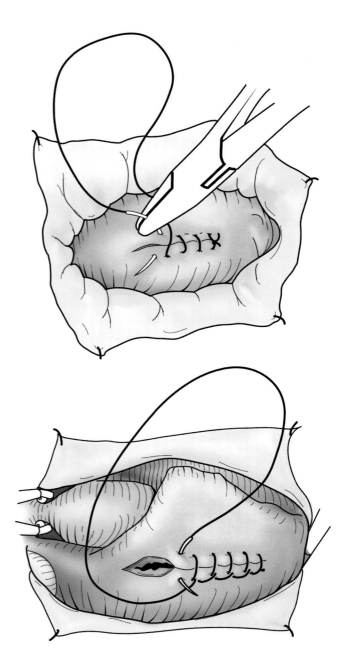

11

POSTOPERATIVE CARE

Postoperative care is directed toward resumption of the normal cardiac output as quickly as possible, reducing lung water so as to improve respiratory function and managing electrolytes, bleeding parameters, and arrhythmias. Postoperative arrhythmias, particularly supraventricular tachycardias such as atrial fibrillation, are very common. Metoprolol, 25 mg twice a day, is given prophylactically. Other drugs, such as amiodarone or calcium channel blockers, can be administered periodically. Emergency cardioversion is occasionally required but is rarely successful in mitral valve patients who have had a long history of atrial fibrillation.

Anticoagulation is prescribed for all patients who are undergoing mitral valve replacement, either mechanical or bioprosthetic valve, and is usually maintained for at least 6 weeks. When the patient is seen postoperatively in the outpatient setting, has remained in sinus rhythm, and has a bioprosthetic valve, anticoagulation can be tapered off over the next 7 days, with one aspirin a day prescribed henceforth. If the patient remains in chronic atrial fibrillation, however, whether it be with a bioprosthetic or prosthetic valve, anticoagulation with warfarin must be continued indefinitely. The ideal therapeutic international normalized ratio after mitral valve replacement is 2.5–3.5. When intra-atrial clots are found during operation, or when the patient has a very enlarged left atrium or chronic low cardiac output, immediate postoperative low-molecular-weight dextran or continuous reduced-dose heparin should be considered until the ideal international normalized ratio is reached.

OUTCOME

The results of current mitral valve replacement surgery are quite good. The operative mortality of this operation is in the range of approximately 5 per cent overall and lower for patients under the age of 70. The risk is increased if there is concomitant coronary artery disease that requires bypass. Reoperative mitral valve surgery carries an approximately 6–10 per cent operative mortality, which also is higher with coronary bypass. In the situation of true emergency that requires mitral valve replacement, such as with a ruptured papillary muscle, operative risk increases to the range of 10–15 per cent, or higher if multiple comorbidities are present. Ninety per cent of the surviving patients improve to at least New York Heart Association class I or II. The probability of survival after mitral valve replacement at 10 years is 50–60 per cent with either a tissue or mechanical heart valve. The occurrence of thromboembolism is approximately 1.5–2.0 per cent per patient year and is much lower in patients with a small left atrium, sinus rhythm, and bioprosthetic valve. Conversely, the incidence of thromboembolism is higher in patients who have a large left atrium and chronic atrial fibrillation and in those who receive a mechanical valve. Anticoagulant-related hemorrhage varies from 1 per cent to 2 per cent per patient year. Freedom from structural valve degeneration with a porcine valve is only 30 per cent at 15 years. The incidence of prosthetic valve endocarditis is similar for both types.

Mitral valve replacement by mechanical or bioprosthetic valve has revolutionized the care of patients with severe mitral valve disease. Although it is performed less commonly than before because of the marked increase in the use of reconstructive procedures, particularly for mitral regurgitation, mitral valve replacement is still a very important and very reliable technique for the treatment of unreconstructable mitral valve disease.

FURTHER READING

Akins, C.W. 1991. Mechanical cardiac valve prosthesis. *Annals of Thoracic Surgery* 52, 161.

Cohn, L.H., Couper, G.S., Aranki, S.F., *et al.* 1994. The long-term results of mitral valve reconstruction for the 'floppy valve' valve. *Journal of Cardiac Surgery* 9, 2 Suppl. 278.

Horskotte, D., Schulte, H.D., Bircks, W., Strauer, B.E. 1993. The effect of chordal preservation on late outcome after mitral valve replacement: a randomized study. *Journal of Heart Valve Disease* 2, 150.

Jamieson, W.R.E., Hayden, R.I., Miyagishima, R.T., *et al.* 1991. The Carpentier-Edwards standard porcine bioprosthesis: clinical performance to 15 years. *Journal of Cardiac Surgery* 5, Suppl. VI: V1-550.

Khan, S., Chaux, A., Matloff, J. 1994. The St. Jude valve: experience with 1000 cases. *Journal of Thoracic and Cardiovascular Surgery* 108, 1010.

Starr, A., Edwards, M.L. 1961. Mitral replacement: clinical experience with a ball valve prosthesis. *Annals of Surgery* 154, 726.

17

Aortic valve repair

TIRONE E. DAVID MD
Professor of Surgery, University of Toronto Faculty of Medicine; Chief, Division of Cardiovascular Surgery, Toronto General Hospital, Toronto, Ontario, Canada

HISTORY

Tuffier is believed to have performed the first aortic valve repair in a patient with aortic stenosis in 1913. The operation consisted of digital invagination of the dilated ascending aorta wall and 'dilatation' of the stenotic valve. Following the popularization of Gibbon's and Lillehei's methods for extracorporeal circulation in the mid-1950s, aortic insufficiency, which had largely defied closed efforts at correction, was somewhat more responsive to open plastic procedures. Since then, a variety of reports have been published on repair of aortic insufficiency by suturing two adjacent cusps together to correct prolapse or by excising the noncoronary cusp and its aortic sinus and narrowing of the aortic root and proximal ascending aorta, thus converting the aortic valve into a bicuspid valve. Because only a few patients could have aortic valve repair, various autologous tissues, such as pericardium, aortic wall segments, full-thickness left atrial wall, central tendon of the diaphragm, peritoneum, and fascia lata, were used for reconstruction of heart valves. With the development of prosthetic heart valves, aortic valve repair became a rare operation and was largely limited to pediatric cases of subaortic ventricular septal defect and aortic insufficiency due to prolapse of the right cusp. With the development of transesophageal Doppler echocardiography and better understanding of the functional anatomy of the aortic valve, interest in aortic valve repair was renewed.

PRINCIPLES AND JUSTIFICATION

The aortic root functions as a unit, and a sound knowledge of its anatomical components and their geometrical relationships is indispensable to repair the aortic valve and reconstruct the aortic root. The aortic root has four anatomical components: aortic annulus, aortic cusps, aortic sinuses, and sinotubular junction. The aortic annulus attaches the aortic root to the left ventricle. The annulus is attached to the interventricular muscle in approximately 45 per cent of the circumference and to fibrous structures in 55 per cent. Histological examination of the aortoventricular junction reveals that the aortic root has a fibrous continuity with the anterior leaflet of the mitral valve and membranous septum, and it is attached to the muscular interventricular septum through fibrous strands. Because the entire circumference of the aortoventricular junction contains a band of connective tissue, it is reasonable to refer to it as *aortic annulus*. The aortic annulus has a scalloped shape.

The aortic cusps have a semilunar shape, and their bases are attached to the aortic annulus in a scalloped fashion. This anatomical arrangement creates three triangles beneath the aortic cusps. These triangles are part of the left ventricle. The triangle beneath the right and left cusps is made of interventricular muscle, whereas the other two triangles are made of fibrous tissue. The highest point of these triangles where two aortic cusps come in contact is called the *commissure*, which is located immediately below the sinotubular junction. The sinotubular junction is where the aortic root ends and the ascending aorta begins. The segments of arterial wall that are delineated by the aortic annulus proximally and by the sinotubular junction distally are called *aortic sinuses* or *sinuses of Valsalva*.

The geometrical relationships and the function of the various components of the aortic root are interrelated. The areas of the aortic cusps probably determine the size of the aortic root. The aortic cusps are attached to the aortic annulus in a scalloped fashion. The length of the base of an aortic cusp is approximately 1.5 times longer than the length of its free margin. The free margin of an aortic cusp extends from one commissure to the other. Thus, the lengths of the free margins of the aortic cusps are related to the diameter of the aortic annulus and sinotubular junction.

1 The transverse diameter of the aortic annulus (AA) at the lowest level of the aortic cusps is 10–20 per cent larger than the diameter of the sinotubular junction (STJ) in children and young adults, but these diameters tend to equalize in older patients. The lengths of the free margins (FM) of the aortic cusp must exceed the diameter of the aortic orifice because when the aortic valve is closed, each cusp extends from one commissure to the center of the aortic root and to the other commissure.

The aortic root is attached to contractile and fibrous components of the left ventricle. During systole, the interventricular septum shortens and moves inward, and the anterior leaflet of the mitral valve is pushed away from the center of the left ventricular outflow tract. Thus, during systole, the area of the aortic root that is attached to the anterior leaflet of the mitral valve is exposed to greater tension than the area attached to the muscular interventricular septum. These dynamic changes in the geometry of the aortic annulus play a role in the function of the aortic valve. Although all three aortic cusps open synchronously during systole, the noncoronary cusp, its annulus, and commissures open more than the left side of the aortic valve and consequently are exposed to greater stress (LaPlace's law). This situation may explain why the noncoronary aortic sinus and its annulus tend to dilate more than the other sinuses in patients with degenerative disease of the aortic root.

The aortic sinuses are important to maintain coronary artery blood flow throughout the cardiac cycle as well as to create eddies to close the aortic cusps during diastole. The aortic root is very elastic in young patients, expanding considerably during systole and shortening during diastole. However, the number of elastic fibers decreases with aging, and the aortic root becomes less compliant in older patients. The root expands minimally in elderly patients.

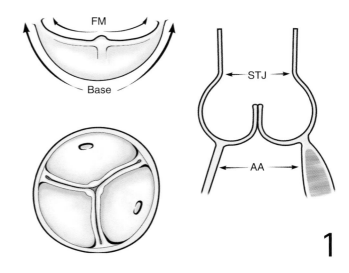

1

2 Aortic insufficiency is caused by anatomical abnormalities of one or more components of the aortic root. Dilation of the sinotubular junction causes outward displacement of the commissures of the aortic cusps and prevents central coaptation, resulting in aortic insufficiency. This is the mechanism of aortic insufficiency in patients with ascending aortic aneurysm, mega-aorta syndrome, and long-standing hypertension causing a dilated and elongated ascending aorta. These patients are usually in their sixth or seventh decade of life.

Dilation of the aortic sinuses does not cause aortic insufficiency if the diameter of the aortic annulus and of the sinotubular junction remain unchanged. However, in patients with degenerative disease of the aortic root, the sinotubular junction eventually dilates, and aortic insufficiency ensues. In patients with more advanced degenerative disease of the media, such as those with Marfan's syndrome or its forme fruste, the aortic annulus may also dilate, creating so-called annuloaortic ectasia. In this condition, the fibrous components of the left ventricular outflow tract become enlarged, and the normal relationship between muscular (45 per cent of the circumference) and fibrous components (55 per cent of the circumference) is altered in favor of the fibrous component. Most of the dilation occurs beneath the commissures of the noncoronary aortic cusp.

Bicuspid aortic valve causes aortic insufficiency because of prolapse of one or both cusps. The free margin of the larger of the two cusps, usually the one that contains a raphe, becomes elongated and prolapses. In addition, these patients often have mild to moderate dilation of the aortic root, particularly of the aortic annulus.

Type A aortic dissection causes aortic insufficiency because of detachment of one or both commissures of the noncoronary cusp of the aortic valve, with resulting prolapse. Most of these patients also have pre-existing dilation of the aortic root, which contributes to the pathophysiology of aortic insufficiency.

Rheumatic valvulitis of the aortic valve can cause cusp thickening, scarring with contraction, and commissural fusion. Some degree of aortic stenosis is often present in these cases. Rheumatic aortic valve disease is commonly associated with rheumatic mitral valve disease.

Ankylosing spondylitis, Reiter's syndrome, osteogenesis imperfecta, rheumatoid arthritis, systemic lupus erythematosus, and idiopathic giant cell aortitis are connective tissue disorders that can be associated with aortic insufficiency, usually because of scarring of the aortic cusps. Subaortic membranous ventricular septal defect causes aortic insufficiency because of down-and-outward displacement of the aortic annulus along the right cusp, which, with time, may become elongated and increase the degree of cusp prolapse.

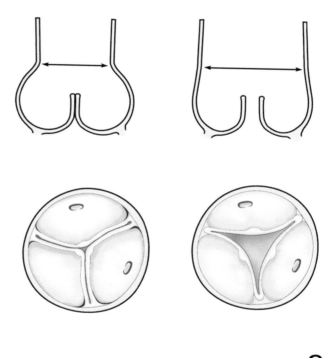

2

SELECTION OF PATIENTS FOR AORTIC VALVE REPAIR

Earlier operation is probably justifiable in patients with severe aortic insufficiency if the aortic valve is reparable. Aortic valve repair can be satisfactorily performed only in a small proportion of patients with aortic valve disease. Repair is seldom useful in patients with aortic stenosis. Open aortic valvotomy for congenital aortic stenosis in children has been largely replaced by percutaneous balloon valvotomy as a palliative procedure. Mechanical débridement of mildly calcified tricuspid aortic valves is sometimes performed in elderly patients in whom the primary indication for cardiac surgery is coronary artery disease. The calcific deposits should be limited to the aortic annulus and base of the cusps and should be removed manually. If the calcium extends into the body of the cusp, the aortic valve should be replaced with a bioprosthetic valve, preferably a stentless porcine valve to minimize transvalvular gradients.

Aortic valve repair is a valuable operative procedure for certain patients with aortic insufficiency due to prolapse of an aortic cusp or due to dilation of the aortic root with normal aortic cusps. Dilation of the aortic root is the most common cause of aortic insufficiency in North America.

Transesophageal echocardiography is currently the best diagnostic tool to study the aortic root and the mechanism of aortic insufficiency. Each component of the aortic root must be carefully assessed to determine the cause of aortic valve dysfunction. Dilation of the aortic root or ascending aorta, or both, and bicuspid aortic valve disease are the most common entities that are suitable for aortic valve repair. In both instances, the number of aortic cusps, their thickness, the appearance of the free margins, and cusp excursion during the cardiac cycle represent the most important information needed to determine reparability of the valve. Information regarding the morphology of the aortic sinuses, sinotubular junction, and ascending aorta is also important. The diameters of the aortic annulus, aortic sinuses, sinotubular junction, and the heights of the cusps should be measured. The lengths of the free margins of the cusps should be estimated if possible. Dilation of the sinotubular junction is easily diagnosed by echocardiography. If the aortic sinuses, cusps, and annulus appear to be normal, and the aortic insufficiency is central, simple adjustment of the sinotubular junction restores valve function. This situation is frequently the case in patients with ascending aortic aneurysm and mega-aorta syndrome. Individuals with dilated sinotubular junction and aortic sinuses but with echocardiographically normal aortic cusps may also have aortic valve repair, although a more complex reconstruction of the aortic root is needed. This case occurs in patients with Marfan's syndrome or its forme fruste. In our experience the probability of aortic valve repair decreases as the diameter of the sinotubular junction increases. When the diameter of the sinotubular junction exceeds 50 mm, the aortic cusps often are thinned, are overstretched, and contain stress fenestrations in the commissural areas. The diameters of the aortic sinuses or of the ascending aorta are less important. We have found patients with normal aortic cusps and ascending aortic aneurysms of 6 cm or greater in diameter. Dilation of the aortic sinuses may be associated with dilation of the aortic annulus and sinotubular junction; for this reason, patients with aortic root aneurysms and echocardiographically normal aortic cusps should be operated on when the diameter of aortic sinuses reaches 50 mm.

Patients with aortic insufficiency due to prolapse of a bicuspid aortic valve are also candidates for aortic valve repair, providing that echocardiography demonstrates pliable, thin, and mobile cusps without calcification and prolapse of only one of the two cusps. Children with subaortic ventricular septal defect and aortic insufficiency are also candidates for aortic valve repair. Rheumatic valvulitis and other nonrheumatic inflammatory diseases of the aortic valve are less suitable for valve repair.

PREOPERATIVE ASSESSMENT AND PREPARATION

Patients younger than 50 years of age and without coronary artery risk factors do not need coronary angiography before surgery, but it should be performed in older patients. It is imperative that candidates for aortic valve repair understand before surgery that repair may not be feasible once the aorta is opened at operation and that aortic valve replacement may be necessary. For this reason, alternative procedures must be discussed with the patient before surgery. As with any valve operation, poor dental hygiene and other potential sources of postoperative bacteremia must be corrected before elective operations.

ANESTHESIA

The anesthetic agents and techniques are the same as for any open heart procedure that uses cardiopulmonary bypass.

OPERATION

Aortic valve repair is usually performed through a median sternotomy, particularly in patients with extensive vascular disease such as those with aneurysm and coronary artery disease. Isolated repair of the aortic valve can also be performed through an 8- to 10-cm skin incision and partial or full midline sternotomy.

Cardiopulmonary bypass is established by cannulating the distal ascending aorta or transverse aortic arch, depending on the extent of the aneurysm. Regardless of the aortic valve or aortic root pathology, the best approach to expose the aortic valve for repair is through a generous transverse aortotomy that is at least 1 cm above the commissures. In cases of aneurysm, the aorta should be transected completely.

Myocardial protection during the aortic cross-clamp is provided by intermittent shots of cold blood cardioplegia that are delivered directly into the coronary artery orifices by inserting soft, self-inflating balloon cannulae and securing them to the adjacent aortic wall. A ventricular vent is inserted through the interatrial groove.

The components of the aortic root are then carefully assessed. The principal determinant of aortic valve repair is the quality of the aortic cusps. The number of cusps, their thickness, their pliability, and the presence of fenestrations are observed. The motion of the cusps is best appreciated by suspending the commissures to a normal position. If there is prolapse of one cusp, it is corrected by one of the methods described below. Next, the lengths of the free margins of the three cusps are measured. The diameters of the aortic annulus and of the sinotubular junction should be smaller than the average length of the free margins of the aortic cusps. If not, surgical reduction should be part of the valve repair.

Repair of cusp prolapse

3 Prolapse of an aortic cusp is corrected by shortening the free margin. This maneuver can be done by plicating the central portion of the cusp with full-thickness sutures. If the cusp is very thin, horizontal mattress sutures with a fine strip of pericardial pledget on each side can be used. The degree of shortening of the length of the free margin depends on the lengths of the free margins of the other cusps.

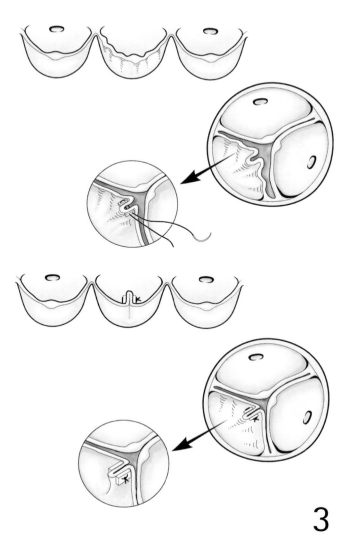

3

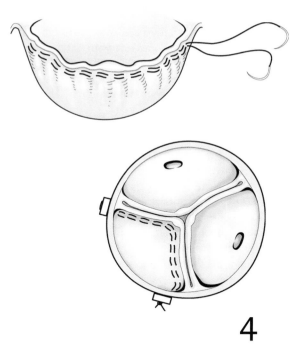

4 Minor prolapse of a thinned-out cusp or of a cusp with a fenestration along its commissural attachment can be corrected by weaving a double layer of a 6-0 expanded polytetrafluoroethylene suture along the free margin from commissure to commissure.

4

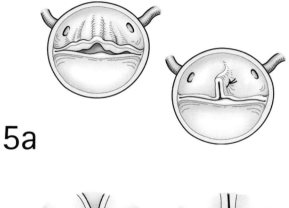

5a

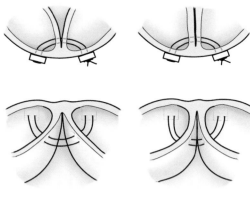

5a, b In bicuspid aortic valve disease, the anterior cusp is usually the one that prolapses. That cusp often contains a raphe, which should be excised. After the length of the free margin of the prolapsing cusp is corrected, the subcommissural triangles can be plicated to increase the coaptation area of the cusps. This plication is accomplished by passing a horizontal mattress suture from the outside of the aortic root to the inside, including the aortic annulus immediately beneath the commissural areas.

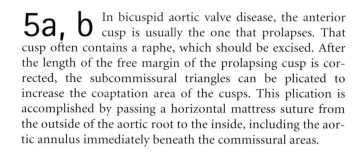

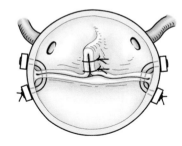

5b

Remodeling of the aortic root

6a–c Most patients with ascending aortic aneurysm and aortic insufficiency have normal or near normal aortic cusps and aortic sinuses. Correction of the aortic insufficiency is accomplished by replacement of the ascending aorta, with adjustment of the diameter of the sinotubular junction. The diameter of the sinotubular junction is estimated by approximating the three commissures to a point where all three cusps coapt centrally. The ascending aorta should be transected 5 mm above the sinotubular junction and a tubular Dacron graft sutured at the level of the sinotubular junction. It is important to space the three commissures in the graft according to the length of the free margin of the cusps. Thus, if one cusp is longer than the others, the distance between its commissures should be proportionally longer. Another important consideration is the diameter of the graft in relation to the size of the patient. Large patients should have proportionally larger grafts because a small graft may increase left ventricular afterload. We avoid grafts that are smaller than 26 mm in large patients. If the sinotubular junction should be smaller than 26 mm, the graft is reduced in diameter only at the anastomotic area.

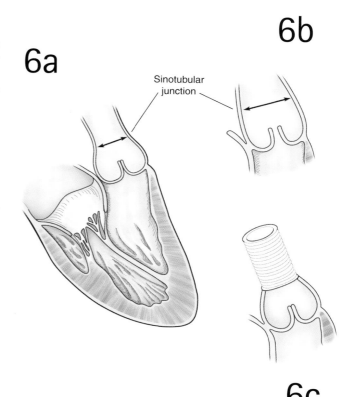

6a

6b

Sinotubular junction

6c

7a–d If one or more aortic sinuses are dilated or involved by dissecting aneurysm, they should be replaced with a properly tailored tubular Dacron graft. The aortic root is dissected circumferentially down to just below the level of the aortic annulus. The coronary arteries are detached from their respective aortic sinuses with a rim of arterial wall around their orifices. The aortic sinuses are excised, leaving 4–8 mm of arterial wall attached to the aortic annulus (4 mm around the commissures and 8 mm on the bottom of the aortic cusps). A tubular Dacron graft of a diameter equal to or slightly smaller than the average length of the free margins of the cusps is tailored to create three neoaortic sinuses. These neoaortic sinuses are tailored in one end of the graft by making three longitudinal incisions in the graft at least as long as the diameter of the graft. The edges are trimmed to make them semicircular in shape. The commissures of the aortic valve are secured on the outside of the upper part of the neosinuses with 4/0 polypropylene sutures that are passed from the inside to the outside of the graft and from the inside to the outside of the commissures of the aortic valve. Before these sutures are tied, they can be passed through a Teflon felt pledget and left on the outside of the aortic wall. The neoaortic sinuses made of Dacron fabric are then sutured to the aortic annulus and remnants of arterial wall, with those sutures used to suspend the commissure. The graft should lie on the inside of the remnants of the arterial wall. Once all three sinuses have been reconstructed, the coronary arteries are reimplanted.

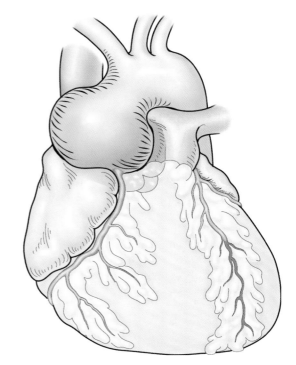

7a

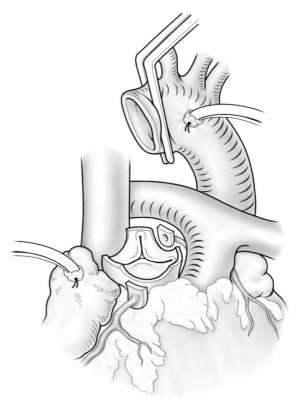

7b

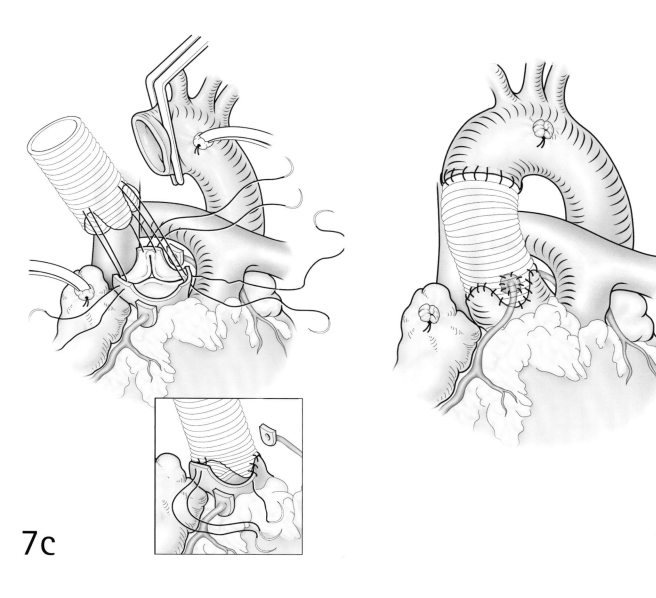

7c

7d

Reimplantation of the aortic valve

8a–c Reimplantation of the aortic valve is an alternative procedure to remodeling of the aortic root for patients with aortic root aneurysm. Reimplantation is particularly useful in patients with annuloaortic ectasia, Marfan's syndrome, or acute type A aortic dissection. It places the entire aortic valve inside a tubular Dacron graft. The aortic sinuses are excised as described for the remodeling procedure. Next, multiple horizontal mattress sutures (3/0 or 4/0 polyester) are placed from the inside to the outside of the left ventricular outflow tract. These sutures should be placed on a single horizontal plane along the fibrous components of the outflow tract and follow the scalloped shape of the aortic annulus along the muscular ventricular septum. Teflon felt pledgets should be used if the fibrous component is thin. A tubular Dacron graft with a diameter of 2–4 mm larger than the average lengths of the free margins of the cusps is chosen. Three equidistant marks are created in one of its ends, and an 8- to 10-mm triangular excision is made in one of the thirds to correspond to the commissure subtended by the interventricular muscle. Three plicating sutures are placed in between the spaces marked to align the commissures to reduce the diameter of the graft by 2 to 4 mm. The sutures that were passed through the left ventricular outflow tract are then passed from the inside to the outside of this tailored end of the graft. It is important to distribute these sutures evenly, particularly along the muscular septum. Most of the reduction in the diameter of the aortic annulus should be accomplished beneath the commisures of the noncoronary aortic cusp. The valve is placed in the inside of the graft, and all sutures are tied on the outside. This suture line stabilizes the aortic annulus and reduces its diameter. The reduction in diameter should be strictly beneath the commissures of the noncoronary aortic cusp. The three commissures are then resuspended inside of the graft and secured to it using horizontal mattress sutures with 4/0 polypropylene with pledgets. These sutures are also used to secure the remnants of the aortic wall and aortic annulus to the graft. The coronary arteries are reimplanted into their respective neoaortic sinuses. Because the diameter of the graft is larger than the average lengths of the aortic cusps, the spaces between the commissures are plicated with polypropylene sutures to create neo-aortic sinuses and reduce the diameter of the sinotubular junction. The coaptation level of the aortic cusps is inspected again and shortening of their free margins is done as needed.

Aortic valve repair must be performed with intraoperative Doppler echocardiography. At the completion of the procedure, no more than trace aortic insufficiency is acceptable. In addition, the morphology of the repaired valve is very important. Persistent prolapse of one cusp may progress with time and causes recurrent aortic insufficiency. It is better to correct the prolapse with a second pump run and further shortening of the free margin of the cusp. Central aortic insufficiency without prolapse is usually due to inadequate coaptation of

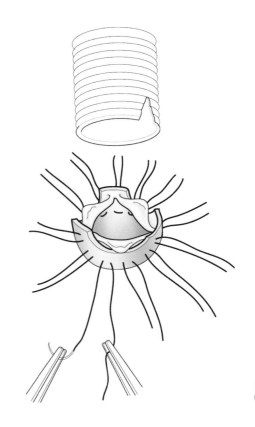

8a

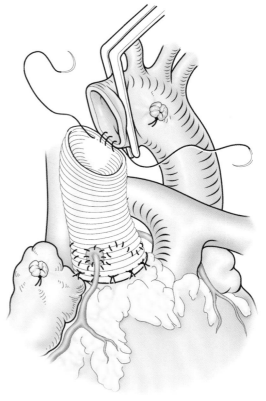

8b

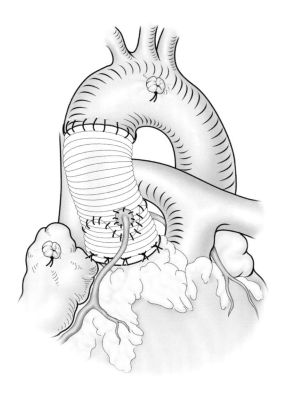

the cusps. This situation can be corrected by further reduction of the diameter of the sinotubular junction without placing the patient back on cardiopulmonary bypass and with echocardiographic guidance. A temporary plication of the graft at the level of the sinotubular junction is done and the valve function assessed by Doppler echocardiography.

8c

POSTOPERATIVE CARE

Patients who had aortic valve repair or aortic valve-sparing procedures receive the same care as any patient who undergoes heart surgery under cardiopulmonary bypass. Our patients are usually extubated for 3–4 hours of observation for hemodynamic stability and hemostasis. Most patients are cared for in an intensive care setting during the first day. They are then discharged to a cardiac surgical ward. They receive analgesic and cardiac medications as needed. We do not anticoagulate these patients, but they all receive aspirin during the first three postoperative months or permanently if they also had coronary artery bypass graft. Most patients are discharged from the hospital within 5–7 days.

OUTCOMES

The outcomes of aortic valve-sparing operations for dilated aortic root or ascending aorta, or both, have been excellent. In a recent review of our experience with the first 161 patients, 103 had an aortic root aneurysm and 58 had an ascending aortic aneurysm. The clinical profiles of these two subgroups were quite different: Patients with an ascending aortic aneurysm were older and had more severe aortic insufficiency and more extensive vascular disease, such as transverse arch aneurysm and coronary artery disease. The incidence of dissecting aneurysms was the same in the two subgroups. Almost one half of those with aortic root aneurysm had Marfan's syndrome. Overall, the operative mortality was 2 per cent, the actuarial survival at 10 years was 80 per cent, and the freedom from aortic valve replacement was 98 per cent. The long-term survival for patients with aortic root aneurysm was significantly higher than for patients with ascending aortic aneurysm, but the difference was likely related to age and associated diseases more than the operative procedure.

The long-term results of aortic valve repair of the bicuspid aortic valve have also been very good. Clinical experience has shown that it is important to leave none or only a trace of aortic insufficiency after the repair of bicuspid aortic valves. Uncorrected prolapse is associated with a high risk of early recurrent aortic insufficiency.

FURTHER READING

Bailey, C.P., Hirose, T., Zimmerman, J. 1977. Valvular heart disease: the reconstructive approach. In Davila, J.C. (ed.), *Second Henry Ford Hospital International Symposium on Cardiac Surgery*. New York: Appleton-Century-Crofts, 7–29.

David, T.E. 1999. Surgery of the aortic valve. *Current Problems in Surgery* **36**, 421–504.

David, T.E., Armstrong, S., Ivanov, J., *et al.* 2001. Results of aortic valve-sparing operations. *Journal of Thoracic and Cardiovascular Surgery* **122**, 39–46.

Kunzelman, K.S., Grande, J., David, T.E., *et al.* 1994. Aortic root and valve relationships: impact on surgical repair. *Journal of Thoracic and Cardiovascular Surgery* **107**, 162–70.

Yacoub, M.H., Gehle, P., Chandrasekaran, V., *et al.* 1998. Late results of a valve-preserving operation in patients with aneurysm of the ascending aorta and root. *Journal of Thoracic and Cardiovascular Surgery* **115**, 1080–90.

18

Aortic valve replacement

JAMES I. FANN MD
Assistant Professor of Cardiothoracic Surgery, Stanford University School of Medicine; Surgeon of Cardiothoracic Surgery, Stanford University Medical Center, Stanford, California, USA

BRUCE A. REITZ MD
Norman E. Shumway Professor and Chairman, Department of Cardiothoracic Surgery, Stanford University School of Medicine, Stanford, California, USA

HISTORY

Aortic valve surgery dates back to 1912, when Tuffier dilated a stenotic valve by invaginating the ascending aortic wall with his finger to access the valve, thereby avoiding a direct opening in the aorta. In the 1940s and 1950s, various attempts were made to dilate a stenotic aortic valve. Brock directed instruments via the right subclavian and innominate arteries, Bailey and colleagues directed a finger through a sleeve sewn to the side of the ascending aorta, and Bailey and colleagues and Ellis and Kirklin used dilators passed through the left ventricle. Because of unpredictable results and limited success, however, these procedures were abandoned. During this time, Hufnagel and Campbell independently developed and experimentally implanted prosthetic valves, constructed of a mobile ball inside a plastic cage, in the descending thoracic aorta to treat aortic regurgitation. In 1954, Hufnagel reported a series of patients who underwent such a descending thoracic aortic operation with acceptable outcomes at relatively short follow-up. Two years later, Murray successfully implanted a homograft aortic valve in the descending thoracic aorta.

Until the advent of cardiopulmonary bypass enabling intracardiac repair, no reliable means of correcting aortic stenosis was available, and placement of a valve prosthesis in the descending thoracic aorta was only partially successful for treating aortic regurgitation. In 1960, Harken et al. performed the first successful subcoronary aortic valve replacement using a caged ball device, and Starr and Edwards reported the first mitral valve replacement, also a caged ball prosthesis. With the clinical success of the Starr-Edwards mechanical mitral and aortic prostheses, they soon became important benchmarks in the history of valve prostheses. Since then, the design and development of mechanical valves have evolved. Currently, the majority of such prostheses are constructed partially or totally of pyrolytic carbon.

Concurrent with the development of mechanical prostheses, tissue valve substitutes (homograft valves as well as heterografts fabricated of such materials as porcine valve, bovine pericardium, and fascia lata) were introduced and evaluated. In 1962, Duran and Gunning described a method of subcoronary implantation of a homograft valve. In the mid 1960s, heterograft bioprostheses were evaluated and clinically implanted in the aortic position. Because early tissue valves used formaldehyde as a fixative, premature tissue degeneration and calcification were particularly problematic. In 1968, Carpentier and associates used glutaraldehyde as a fixative for the stent-mounted porcine valve to enhance the durability of bioprostheses. At present, the spectrum of biological valve substitutes for the diseased aortic valve includes stented and stentless porcine valves, stented pericardial valves, aortic and pulmonary homografts, and pulmonary autografts.

PRINCIPLES AND JUSTIFICATION

Most patients with aortic valvular stenosis have calcific aortic valve sclerosis, bicuspid aortic valve, or rheumatic valve disease. The most common cause is calcific aortic valve sclerosis, which affects older patients and typically becomes clinically significant in the seventh or eighth decade of life. Patients with bicuspid aortic stenosis, which occurs in upward of 1 per cent of the population, come to medical attention between their third and sixth decade. The incidence of rheumatic valve disease has decreased in the United States; patients with this disease may be asymptomatic for years and often have mitral valve involvement as well. Patients with aortic stenosis are at increased risk of sudden death, in particular, those with symptoms such as angina and syncope. Indications for aortic valve surgery include the presence of symptoms in patients with moderate to severe aortic stenosis; surgery is also indicated for the asymptomatic patient with severe aortic stenosis, with or without impaired left ventricular function, because of the increased risk of ventricular arrhythmias and sudden death.

The etiology of pure aortic regurgitation includes degenerative valve disease, annuloaortic ectasia, infective endocarditis, rheumatic heart disease, and various inflammatory and other miscellaneous disorders. Often, patients with aortic stenosis have some degree of associated regurgitation. Those with predominant aortic regurgitation remain asymptomatic for years. When symptoms do become evident, the most common is that of congestive heart failure and less often angina; syncope is unusual in patients with aortic regurgitation. In patients in whom acute or sudden aortic regurgitation develops, urgent valve replacement usually is required because of the rapid onset of congestive heart failure and pulmonary edema. The optimal timing of valve replacement for those with chronic aortic regurgitation, however, remains controversial. Operations are clearly indicated in patients who are symptomatic; in asymptomatic or minimally symptomatic patients, indications for surgery usually are related to the degree of left ventricular enlargement (e.g. left ventricular end-diastolic dimension greater than 6.0 cm). Patients with severely compromised left ventricular function preoperatively have a greater risk of operative mortality and persistent heart failure than those with normal left ventricular function.

Currently, no ideal valve substitute is available. Although mechanical prostheses are associated with greater durability compared with biological valve substitutes, many patients who receive bioprostheses do not require chronic anticoagulation and consequently have fewer anticoagulant-related complications. Although the main disadvantage of biological valves is their limited durability due to fibrocalcification and leaflet disruption, the performance of bioprostheses is perceived to have improved over the years, a finding that has been attributed to more appropriate patient selection and improved valve design and preparation. The choice of valve replacement is thus dependent on a number of patient-related variables, such as the patient's age, medical compliance, contraindications to anticoagulation, expected longevity, and level of comfort. Other important factors in determining the type of valve include expected durability of the prosthesis, the underlying pathological process, and the anatomy of the patient's aortic valve and root. Mechanical prostheses often are recommended for younger adults, provided that they have no contraindications to anticoagulation. In older patients, porcine or pericardial stented bioprostheses are often favored. Compared to the stented bioprostheses, the newer stentless porcine valves are believed to produce less hemodynamic obstruction, although any advantage with respect to long-term durability is still unproven. Homografts or autografts are being used more often, particularly in younger patients, to avoid the need for anticoagulation. In individuals who require replacement of the aortic root, composite valve grafts with a mechanical prosthesis or bioprosthesis, homografts, autografts, or stentless porcine roots all can be used.

PREOPERATIVE ASSESSMENT AND PREPARATION

Patients who require aortic valve replacement for stenotic or regurgitant lesions need a thorough evaluation for potential areas of infection, such as dental status and respiratory or urinary systems. Because aortic stenosis results in increased afterload and impaired left ventricular emptying, preoperative management is focused on maintaining adequate cardiac output and systemic perfusion. Stroke volume and cardiac output are enhanced by increased left ventricular preload. Systemic vascular resistance is maintained to support adequate diastolic and coronary perfusion pressure. Beta-blockers are avoided because of their effects on left ventricular end-diastolic volume and cardiac output. Because severe left ventricular hypertrophy results in decreased ventricular compliance, the contribution of atrial systole to left ventricular preload becomes more crucial. Thus, loss of sinus rhythm may be quite detrimental, and efforts should be made to re-establish this rhythm. Echocardiography is very useful in assessing the degree of aortic stenosis and left ventricular function and hypertrophy. Cardiac catheterization provides a direct measurement of the transvalvular gradient and information regarding the aortic root and left ventricular function. Coronary angiography is recommended in patients older than 40 years of age or those with risk factors for coronary artery disease.

In chronic aortic regurgitation, the increased left ventricular diastolic filling and the increased stroke volume that are necessary to maintain adequate cardiac output result in increased left ventricular diastolic pressure and volume, diastolic wall stress, and eventually cavity dilatation. Compromised subendocardial perfusion due to decreased systemic diastolic pressure and increased left ventricular diastolic pressure is improved with faster heart rates and resultant higher systemic diastolic pressure and lower left ventricular diastolic pressure. Because an elevated afterload increases stroke work and left ventricular end-diastolic pressure, pharmacological reduction of systemic vascular resistance increases cardiac output by decreasing transvalvular pressure gradient during diastole and by reducing the amount of regurgitation. Beta-adrenergic agonists may increase stroke volume by increasing contractility and peripheral dilatation. Maintaining normal sinus rhythm in patients with aortic regurgitation is not as important as in aortic stenosis. Pulmonary vascular resistance is usually normal until severe end-stage left ventricular dysfunction develops. Echocardiography is important to follow the progression of aortic regurgitation as well as to identify any associated pathology. Cardiac catheterization permits assessment of the degree of aortic regurgitation, left ventricular dilatation, and left ventricular function. Again, coronary angiography should be performed in patients who are older than 40 years of age and those with risk factors for coronary artery disease.

ANESTHESIA

In patients with aortic stenosis, attempts should be made to avoid tachycardia with the choice of premedication and induction of anesthesia. Preload and afterload are closely monitored and maintained in the early stages of the operation. During induction and maintenance of anesthesia, an alpha-adrenergic agent, such as phenylephrine, may be necessary to sustain adequate systemic pressures. A narcotic-based anesthetic agent avoids myocardial depression, hypotension, and arrhythmias. Atrial flutter or fibrillation is treated with synchronized cardioversion to avoid reduction in cardiac output. If the patient's cardiac status deteriorates on induction, emergency institution of cardiopulmonary bypass may be required. Intraoperative transesophageal echocardiography is often helpful in assessing cardiac performance perioperatively.

In contrast to those with aortic stenosis, moderate tachycardia is not detrimental in patients with aortic regurgitation. Anesthetic management in these individuals is thus directed at maintaining myocardial contractility and heart rate. The anesthetic agent may be inhalational isoflurane or a narcotic with a muscle relaxant; anesthetic goals are to lower systemic vascular resistance and to maintain preload, contractility, and a moderate heart rate. Intraoperative transesophageal echocardiography is useful to monitor cardiac function.

OPERATION

Conventional aortic valve replacement

1 Full median sternotomy is the usual incision for aortic valve replacement, although a hemisternotomy can be used. After heparinization, the aorta is cannulated in the usual fashion, and the right atrium is cannulated with a two-stage venous cannula. In selected cases of reoperation, the femoral artery can be accessed for arterial return. Anterograde cardioplegia and aortic root vent catheter are placed in the ascending aorta just distal to the proposed aortotomy site. A pursestring suture is placed on the lateral aspect of the right atrium, followed by a stab incision and the placement of a retrograde cardioplegia cannula into the coronary sinus. Cardiopulmonary bypass is instituted, and the patient is systemically cooled to 32°C. A pulmonary artery vent is placed in the main pulmonary artery through a longitudinal stab incision. The aorta is cross-clamped. For patients with aortic stenosis without regurgitation, cardioplegic arrest can be adequately achieved in an anterograde fashion followed by retrograde cardioplegia.

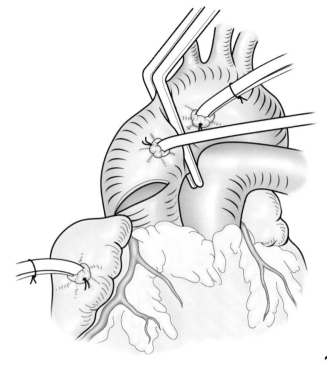

1

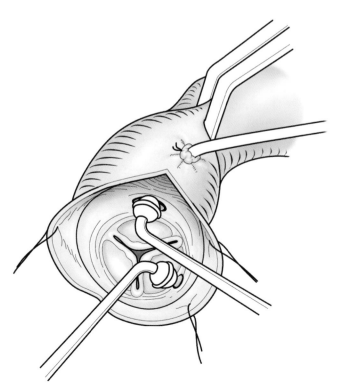

2

2 In those with aortic regurgitation, depending on the severity, the first dose of cardioplegia can be given into the coronary ostia via hand-held cannulae after an oblique aortotomy. Alternatively induction cardioplegia is given in a retrograde fashion concurrent with the aortotomy. During the operation, cardioplegic arrest is maintained with intermittent instillation of retrograde cardioplegia. Topical hypothermia is also used. An oblique aortotomy is made with the initial incision 2–4 mm above the sinotubular junction and 4–6 mm above the origin of the right coronary artery. The incision extends toward the noncoronary sinus, staying just above the level of the valve commissures. Sutures of 3/0 polyester are placed in the aortic wall for retraction and exposure.

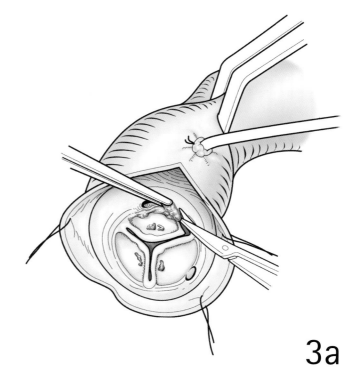

3a

3a, b
The anatomy of the aortic valve, sinuses, sinotubular junction, and anterior leaflet of the mitral valve is assessed. The diseased valve is sharply excised without damage to the aortoventricular junction and the annulus carefully debrided of calcific deposits using small rongeurs. Vigorous decalcification may result in aortic wall injury, injury to the anterior mitral valve leaflet, annular disruption, or left ventricular wall injury. Small calcific debris is evacuated by using high vacuum suction and cold saline irrigation of the left ventricle.

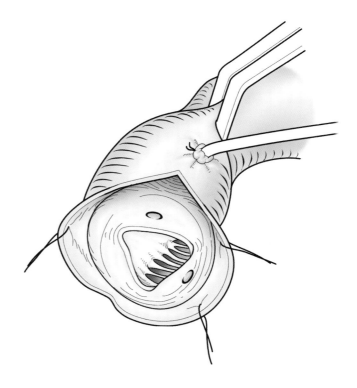

3b

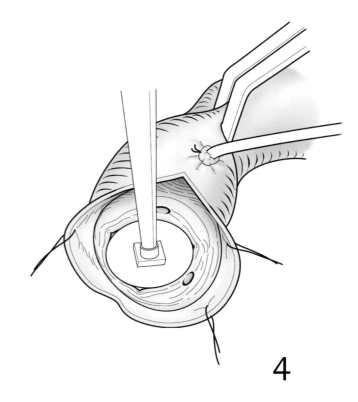

4

4, 5 The annulus is sized with a valve sizer, taking into consideration whether supra-annular or intra-annular placement is planned (Figure 4). Interrupted horizontal mattress sutures of 3/0 polyester are placed in the annulus (Figure 5). Sutures are positioned in a ventricle-to-aorta fashion for supravalvular valve placement or from the aorta-to-ventricle direction in cases of intra-annular valve placement. Care is taken in the region of the membranous septum, located inferior to the cupola formed by the commissure of the noncoronary and right coronary leaflets, so as to avoid injury to the bundle of His.

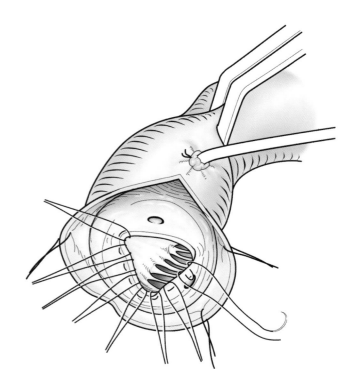

5

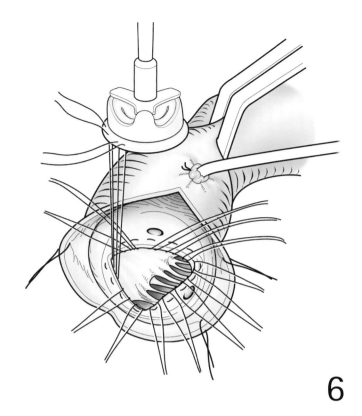

6

6, 7 The sutures are passed through the sewing ring of the valve prosthesis (Figure 6). For bileaflet mechanical prostheses, the prosthesis should be placed with the central axis parallel to the septum. Monoleaflet prostheses are positioned so the greater orifice opens toward the aortic arch. The valve holder is removed and the valve gently pushed into position. The sutures are tied and cut, and the competency of the valve is tested (Figure 7). The patient is gradually rewarmed.

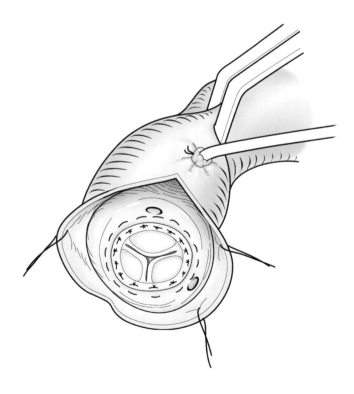

7

8 The aortotomy is closed using a 4/0 polypropylene continuous suture placed in an overlapping fashion beginning from the level of the sinus extending upward. After aortotomy closure, the aortic root vent is connected to suction, volume is added to the heart, the pulmonary vent is temporarily discontinued, the lungs are gently ventilated, and the left ventricle is gently massaged. The patient is placed in a steep Trendelenburg's position; the aortic cross-clamp is removed and the pulmonary vent resumed. The retrograde cardioplegia cannula is then removed and the site closed with 4/0 polypropylene suture. With the heart ejecting, the aortotomy is inspected for hemostasis. Additional deairing maneuvers are performed, including digitally inverting the left atrial appendage and permitting the heart to eject with the ascending aortic vent on suction. The pulmonary artery vent catheter is removed and the site repaired with a 4/0 polypropylene continuous suture. Assessment of intracavitary air can be facilitated with transesophageal echocardiography. The aortic root vent is removed. After adequate rewarming, the patient is weaned from cardiopulmonary bypass and the aortic and venous cannulae removed.

In cases of combined aortic valve replacement and coronary artery bypass grafting, the distal coronary anastomoses using vein or free arterial grafts are constructed first before the valve procedure. The distal internal mammary artery graft anastomosis is performed after the valve procedure and closure of the aortotomy. During a combined valve-coronary procedure, cardioplegia can be instilled anterograde via the vein (or free arterial) grafts and retrograde through the coronary sinus.

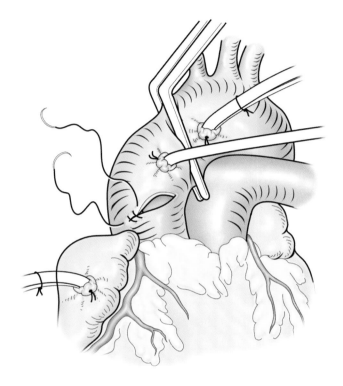

8

Aortic root enlargement

Smaller-sized stented bioprostheses and mechanical pros-theses can result with residual transvalvular gradients. For this reason, porcine bioprostheses smaller than 21 mm gener-ally are not used. In some patients, a 19-mm mechanical prosthesis may be implanted. Ideally, however, a patient with a small aortic annulus should be identified preoperatively, so that alternative techniques, such as an aortic root-enlarging procedure or a stentless bioprosthesis, might be considered. Occasionally, the precise size of the aortic annulus cannot be determined until the time of surgery.

One approach to the slightly smaller aortic annulus is to cant the valve at a slight angle to the plane of the annulus. After the sutures are placed in the annulus for a supra-annular valve placement, they are passed through the sewing ring and lowered into place so that the sewing ring is below the left and right coronary arteries but angled upward at the noncoronary sinus. The left and right annu-lus sutures are tied first, thereby securing the sewing ring to the annulus below the left and right coronary ostia. The sutures that correspond to the noncoronary annulus are tied last, allowing the valve to ride slightly above the annu-lus in this region.

9 Annular enlargement procedures are alternatives for those occasional patients in whom a prosthesis of at least 19 or 21 mm cannot be implanted. In many cases, enlarging the annulus by 2–4 mm may be sufficient. One technique associated with minimal increase in morbidity is to create a posterior annular split, leaving the anterior mitral leaflet and the left atrium intact. The aortotomy is carried down to the top of the noncoronary and left coronary commissure, just above the confluence of the intervalvular trigone, left atrial wall, and mitral annulus.

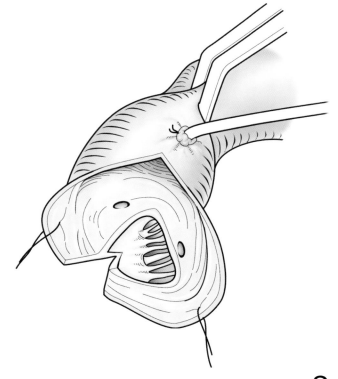

9

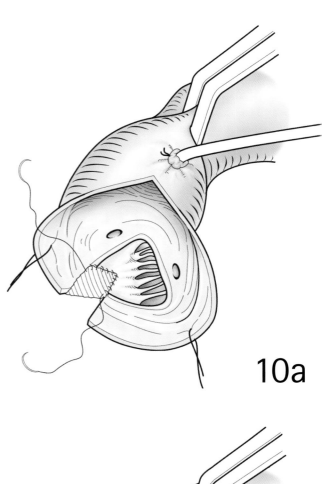

10a

10a, b An elliptical patch (pericardium or Dacron) is sutured to the incised fibrous trigone and aortic wall using continuous 4/0 polypropylene to enlarge the aortic annulus (Figure 10a). Interrupted horizontal mattress 3/0 polyester sutures are placed in the annulus (ventricle-to-aorta fashion for supra-annular valve placement), followed by the placement of similar sutures from outside in on the patch (Figure 10b). The valve prosthesis is then situated in a supra-annular fashion, and the sutures are tied and cut. The remainder of the patch is incorporated in the aortotomy closure.

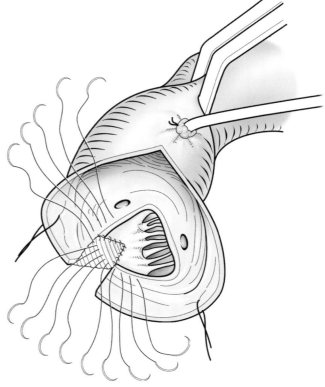

10b

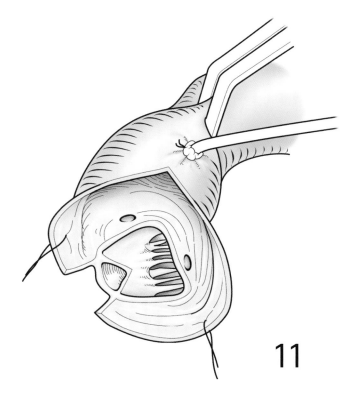

11

11, 12 When greater annular enlargement is desired, a posterior incision, as described by Manoughian, is made at the commissure between the left and noncoronary cusp and extended through the annulus and the intervalvular trigone into the center of the anterior mitral leaflet (Figure 11). The free edge and body of the anterior leaflet remain intact. The left atrium, which is entered at its attachment with the aortic root, can be opened further to facilitate exposure. An elliptical patch is used to close the defect in the anterior mitral leaflet (Figure 12).

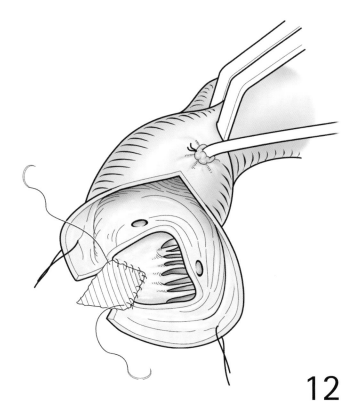

12

13a–e Interrupted horizontal mattress sutures are placed in the annulus and also through the patch (Figure 13a). The prosthesis is thus seated, using the patch as part of the annulus (Figure 13b). The incision in the left atrial wall is closed by continuous sutures by incorporating the atrial edges as the patch is sutured to the defect in the anterior mitral valve leaflet (Figures 13c and d). The superior portion of the patch is incorporated into the aortotomy closure (Figure 13e). Mitral regurgitation due to distortion of the anterior mitral leaflet rarely occurs.

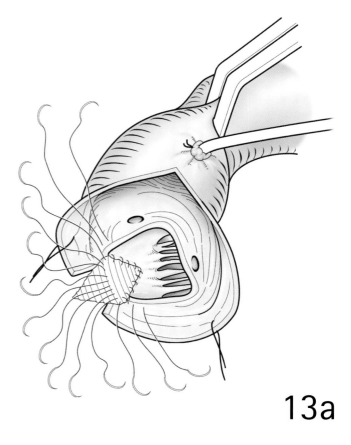

13a

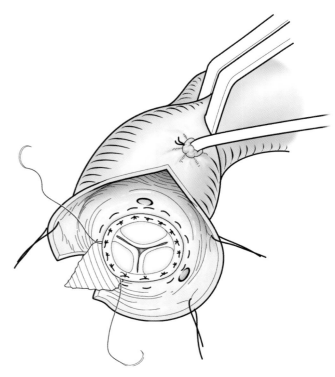

13b

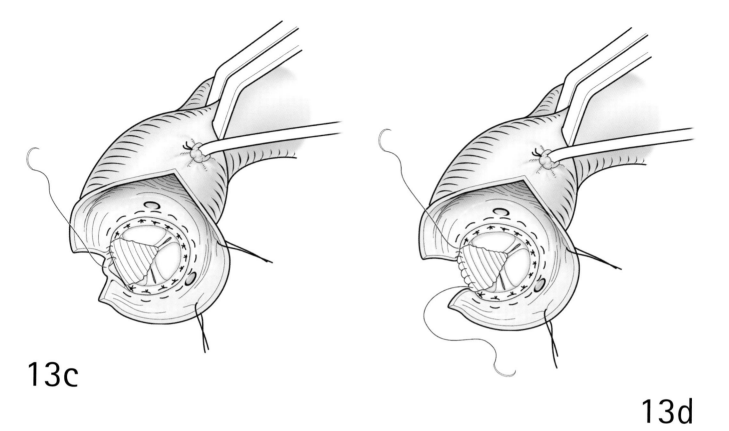

13c

13d

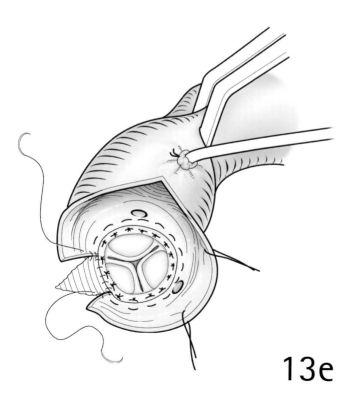

13e

Stentless bioprosthesis

14 The stentless porcine bioprosthesis has become increasingly popular, because it is associated with minimal residual transvalvular gradient and perhaps results in greater regression of left ventricular hypertrophy compared to the stented bioprosthesis. Stentless valves can be implanted in the subcoronary position, as an aortic root replacement, or as a root inclusion. Subcoronary implantation, aortic root replacement, and root inclusion are similar to techniques described for homograft replacement (see Chapter 19). The subcoronary technique for stentless valve implantation is presented here. A transverse aortotomy is made 1 cm above the level of the commissures and extended approximately three fourths of the aortic circumference. The aortic valve is exposed and excised as for conventional valve replacement. The annulus is sized by placing the sizer just inside the commissures. Care is taken to match the prosthetic valve with respect to the patient's aortic sinuses as well as annulus, because oversizing can cause distortion and incompetence of the prosthesis. If the indicated annular size is between consecutive implantation diameters, the slightly larger-sized prosthesis should be used, because the proximal end of the prosthesis may not stretch.

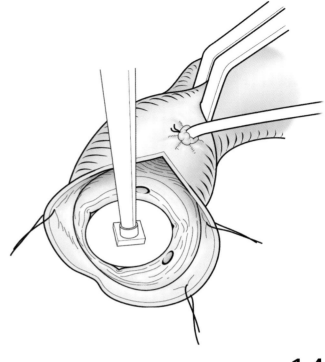

14

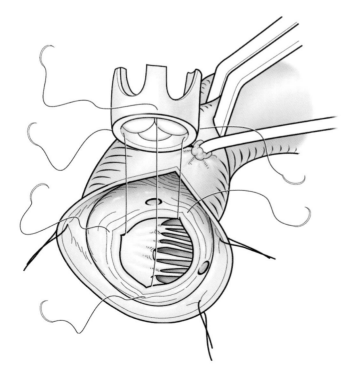

15 The stentless prosthesis is fashioned to permit subcoronary implantation. The muscle shelf portion of the prosthesis is oriented with the noncoronary annulus. Three 4/0 polypropylene sutures are placed in the annulus corresponding to the commissures. The sutures are brought through the fabric-reinforced region of the prosthesis, taking care not to injure the leaflets.

15

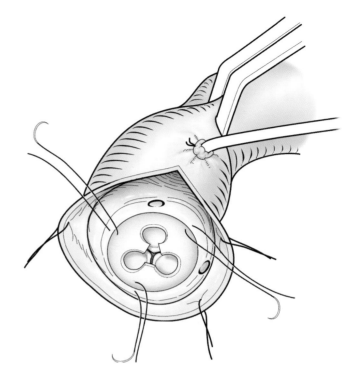

16a

16a, b The valve is lowered to the annulus and the sutures continued, approximating the prosthesis to the annulus from one commissure to the next. These sutures should follow a horizontal plane and not the scalloped shape of the native annulus. Alternatively, multiple interrupted 3/0 polyester sutures can be placed in the annulus. The sutures are oriented and evenly distributed so that placement into the fabric portion does not distort the prosthesis. The sutures are tied.

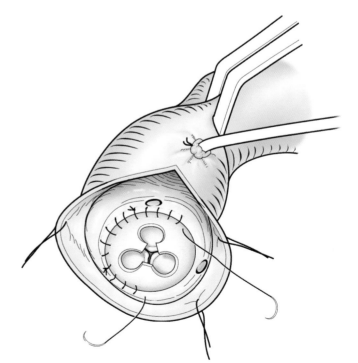

16b

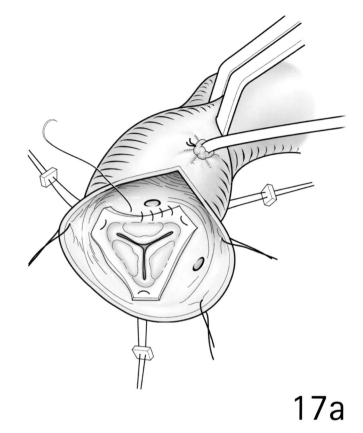

17a

17a, b The commissures of the prosthesis are secured to the patient's corresponding commissures using three double-armed 4/0 polypropylene sutures placed from inside out and tied outside the aorta. These sutures are used to approximate the prosthesis with the corresponding sinuses of the patient's aorta (Figure 17a). The sutures are begun from the commissures, brought through the aorta, and continued beneath each coronary ostium to the commissures; they are secured at the commissures (Figure 17b). The aortotomy is closed with 4/0 continuous polypropylene suture.

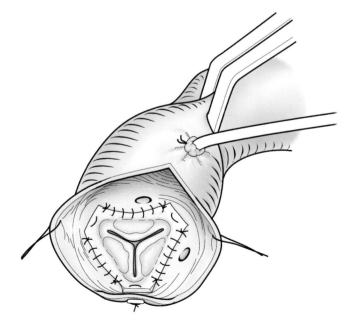

17b

POSTOPERATIVE CARE

Patients are closely monitored in the intensive care unit post-operatively; a pulmonary artery catheter may be helpful in assessing cardiac performance. Because they experience reduced left ventricular afterload, the majority of patients with aortic stenosis and left ventricular dysfunction have dramatic improvement after aortic valve replacement. Ejection fraction is improved, and the left ventricular end-diastolic volume and capillary wedge pressure are decreased. In those with low transvalvular gradients preoperatively, left ventricular performance may not improve significantly after aortic valve replacement, and intra-aortic balloon pump support may be required in the early postoperative period. Although myocardial function generally improves relatively rapidly, the hypertrophied ventricle requires an elevated preload to function normally. If the residual transvalvular gradient is low, left ventricular hypertrophy regresses over the ensuing months.

In patients who are recovering from aortic valve replacement for aortic regurgitation, left ventricular end-diastolic pressure and volume decrease immediately along with a decrease in wall stress; however, regression of left ventricular hypertrophy and dilatation is gradual. Postoperatively, adequate preload is important to fill the dilated left ventricle. Inotropic or intra-aortic balloon pump support may be required early postoperatively until left ventricular function improves. Patients with persistent left ventricular dilatation on follow-up are at increased risk for death.

OUTCOME

In our experience at Stanford, the operative mortality for isolated aortic valve replacement using porcine bioprostheses is 7 per cent. Others have reported operative mortality for aortic valve replacement with mechanical prostheses and bioprostheses in the general population to be 3–12 per cent. The operative mortality for aortic valve replacement using stentless prostheses is similar at 5 per cent. The strongest predictor of operative mortality is advanced age; this factor is associated with an operative mortality of upwards of 11 per cent for those older than 70 years of age. Other important risk factors include higher preoperative functional class, emergency operation, compromised renal function, associated coronary revascularization, and preoperative atrial fibrillation. Early morbidity includes myocardial infarction (2 per cent), stroke (1.7 per cent), wound complications (1.1 per cent), respiratory failure (2.9 per cent), tracheostomy (1 per cent), renal dysfunction requiring dialysis (0.7 per cent), reoperation for bleeding (11.5 per cent), and ventricular tachycardia or fibrillation (7.2 per cent).

Long-term survival rates in the Stanford experience for aortic valve replacement using a bioprosthesis have been observed to be 77 per cent, 54 per cent, and 32 per cent at 5, 10, and 15 years, respectively. For patients with aortic stenosis who underwent aortic valve replacement, the late survival rates were 85 per cent and 66 per cent at 5 and 10 years, respectively. Predictors of late mortality are advanced age, moderate to severe left ventricular dysfunction, coronary artery disease, peripheral vascular disease, atrial fibrillation, and renal dysfunction. In general, patients with aortic stenosis have a better long-term prognosis than those with aortic insufficiency after aortic valve replacement. The presence of left ventricular dysfunction has a significant impact on late survival. In patients with aortic insufficiency, the mean 5-year survival was 63 per cent for patients with depressed ejection fraction compared to 96 per cent for those with normal ejection fraction, emphasizing the importance of operation before the development of left ventricular dysfunction. The rate of reoperation is approximately 5–25 per cent at 10 years depending on the type of valve prosthesis, with an increased risk at reoperation approaching twice that of the first operation. It has been suggested that stentless aortic valve replacement confers a survival advantage compared to stented bioprosthesis. This survival advantage appears to be most prominent in younger patients (younger than 60 years of age), in whom the probability of death is fivefold greater with a stented bioprosthesis compared to a stentless valve. With advancing age, the benefits of stentless valves are diminished.

FURTHER READING

Bonow, R.O. 1994. Asymptomatic aortic regurgitation: indications for operation. *Journal of Cardiac Surgery* **9**, Suppl. 2: 170–3.

Cartier, P.C., Matra, J., Dumesnil, J.G., Pibarot, P., Lemieux, M. 1999. Midterm follow-up of unstented biological valves. *Seminars in Thoracic and Cardiovascular Surgery* **11**, 22–7.

Del Rizzo, D.F., Abdoh, A., Cartier, P., Doty, D., Westaby, S. 1999. The effect of prosthetic valve type on survival after aortic valve surgery. *Seminars in Thoracic and Cardiovascular Surgery* **11**, 1–8.

Fann, J.I., Miller, D.C., Moore, K.A., *et al.* 1996. Twenty-year clinical experience with porcine bioprostheses. *Annals of Thoracic Surgery* **62**, 1301–12.

Jones, E.L., Weintraub, W.S., Craver, J.M., *et al.* 1990. Ten-year experience with the porcine bioprosthetic valve: interrelationship of valve survival and patient survival in 1050 valve replacements. *Annals of Thoracic Surgery* **49**, 370–84.

Logeais, Y., Langanay, T., Leguerrier, A., *et al.* 1999. Aortic Carpentier-Edwards supraannular porcine bioprosthesis: a 12-year experience. *Annals of Thoracic Surgery* **68**, 421–5.

Lytle, B.W., Cosgrove, D.M., Taylor, P.C., *et al.* 1989. Primary isolated aortic valve replacement. *Journal of Thoracic and Cardiovascular Surgery* **97**, 675–94.

19

Aortic root replacement

CLIFFORD FREDERICK HUGHES AO, MBBS, FRACS, FACC, FACS
Clinical Associate Professor, Division of Surgery, University of Sydney Faculty of Medicine; Head, Cardiothoracic Surgical Unit, Royal Prince Alfred Hospital, and The Baird Institute for Applied Heart and Lung Surgical Research, Sydney, New South Wales, Australia

HISTORY, PRINCIPLES AND JUSTIFICATION

In 1968, Bentall and DeBono first described a procedure to replace the aortic valve and the ascending aorta and to re-implant the coronary arteries. Since then, the technique has been applied to diseases such as Marfan's syndrome, Ehlers–Danlos syndrome, annuloaortic ectasia, and even acute aortic dissection. Aortic stenosis with severe post stenotic dilatation and aortic regurgitation associated with a bicuspid aortic valve and dilated ascending aorta are both amenable to treatment with this technique. Elderly patients with atherosclerosis or syphilitic aneurysms and calcific aortic valve disease may also benefit. Advances in anticoagulant monitoring, education, and control have reduced the incidence of thromboembolic and hemorrhagic complications. Improved valve designs have resulted in better hemodynamics and left ventricular mass reduction. The long-term durability of mechanical valves ensures that a well-planned procedure is a definitive solution to a life-threatening problem.

This chapter therefore describes the use of a mechanical valve conduit to replace the root of the ascending aorta and aortic valve with reimplantation of the coronary arteries. Other modifications to the procedures, such as arch replacement or concomitant coronary artery bypass grafting, mitral valve replacement, and so forth, can be readily performed in association with these techniques.

PREOPERATIVE PLANNING AND PREPARATION

Aortic root replacement procedures are often prolonged and carried out in patients with other serious complicating conditions, such as aortic dissection. Meticulous attention to preoperative details is critical, particularly those factors that influence the choice of prosthesis. When possible, dental hygiene should be assured before any valve replacement. Coagulation mechanisms, including platelet count and function, should be normalized and antiplatelet agents such as aspirin, dipyridamole, nonsteroidal anti-inflammatory agents, and IIb/IIIa inhibitors discontinued well before the planned surgery. Many of these agents will continue to alter platelet function for as long as 10 days after they are ceased. Patients who are receiving warfarin (Coumadin) should have it ceased 5 days before surgery and, if necessary, should commence heparin until the morning of surgery. All patients older than 40 years should have coronary angiography. Appropriate radiology, plain x-ray, computed tomography scans, magnetic resonance imaging scans, or angiography may be necessary to plan the most appropriate procedure and cannulation sites. The patient is prepared and draped in such a way as to allow prompt management of all contingencies (i.e., saphenous vein harvest, arch replacement, or groin cannulation).

Since 1994, we have routinely used plateletpheresis to preserve platelet count and function. Platelet-rich plasma is harvested through a large-bore internal jugular venous cannula after the induction of anesthesia and as the patient is prepared and draped. Using a commercially available cell saver with a variable speed centrifuge (Electromedics AT 1000 – Electromedica, Boulder, Colorado or, more recently, Haemonetics Cell Saver 5, Haemonetics Coroporation, Baintree, Massachusetts), harvesting continues as the surgery begins but must be completed before the patient is heparinized. Approximately 25 per cent of circulating platelets can be collected and therefore protected from the effects of cardiopulmonary bypass. The technique provides fresh autologous platelets when the heparin is reversed and a platelet-based biological glue for topical hemostasis. The cell separator can be used after heparin is reversed as a cell saver or to wash cells if catastrophic postbypass hemorrhage occurs.

OPERATION

Incision and cannulation

1a, b For routine cases, a median sternotomy is performed, the thymus divided between ligatures, and the pericardium opened in the midline. Heparin is given and confirmed by the activated clotting time. The anatomy of the ascending aorta is then examined and an aortic cannulation site determined. In reoperations or if the entire ascending aorta or arch, or both, are aneurysmal, a transsternal 'clamshell' incision provides relatively quick and safe exposure. For localized aortic root pathology, it is usually possible to cannulate the extrapericardial ascending aorta. It is our aim to replace the entire aneurysmal intrapericardial aorta, and therefore, femoral arterial cannulation is often performed in the right groin. If severe atherosclerosis is present, this cannula can be introduced over a guide wire or the external iliac artery can be cannulated via the retroperitoneum.

We routinely use a two-stage atriocaval cannula inserted through a pursestring suture on the right atrial appendage. If the patient's condition is desperately urgent, he or she has had previous cardiac surgery, or the heart is displaced inferiorly and atrial cannulation is difficult, a long, retrograde transfemoral venous cannula (28 Fr) can be inserted over a guide wire introduced through the right saphenofemoral venous junction. An atrial cannula can be inserted later and connected to this venous line via a Y-connector if drainage is inadequate. Cardiopulmonary bypass is commenced but cooling delayed until the left ventricle is vented.

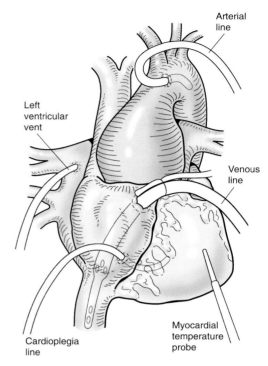

1a

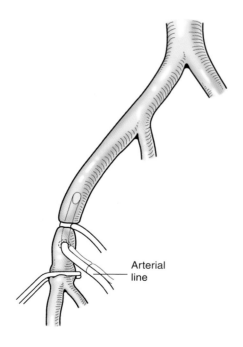

1b

A left ventricular vent is inserted through a pursestring suture on the anterior surface of the right superior pulmonary vein. A right-angled multi-fenestrated (20 Fr) catheter is inserted into the left atrium and manipulated through the mitral valve into the ventricle, if possible. It is carefully positioned so that it does not protrude into the ventricular myocardium at the apex. This type of vent is simple, safe, and very effective. It is easily positioned so that it is out of the surgical field.

For myocardial protection, a retrograde coronary sinus catheter is positioned in the coronary sinus through a pursestring suture on the free wall of the right atrium. Transesophageal echocardiography can provide assistance when cannulation of the coronary sinus is difficult. In the rare event that cannulation is not possible, we use direct coronary artery catheterization. After an initial dose of 750–1000 mL, blood-based cardioplegic solution is instilled every 20 minutes or on return of electrical or mechanical activity. Coronary sinus pressure is monitored during infusion.

Myocardial temperature is monitored to ensure effective myocardial cooling. The temperature probe is placed to the right of the interventricular septum, as this is the portion of the myocardium that is most susceptible to rewarming. At this stage, the anatomy can be reviewed and the necessary technique to treat the cephalad aorta selected. If the arch vessels are not involved and a closed technique is planned, we cool to a nasopharyngeal temperature of 25°C. If total circulatory arrest and 'open' techniques for the distal aorta are necessary, cooling is continued to 20°C. The techniques and planning for arch and distal resection as well as methods of cerebral protection are discussed elsewhere.

Mobilization of the aorta

2 While cooling continues, the aorta is gently mobilized and a heavy tape sling passed around the vessel (above the aneurysm if possible). After the pericardial reflection is incised, it is usually possible to develop a plane between the aorta and the right pulmonary artery. The safest way to do this is to use blunt dissection with the left finger and thumb surrounding the aorta until it is possible to lift it forward, and to carefully pass a large, blunt, curved vascular clamp behind it. The clamp is usually passed from right to left, guided by the left hand. When the tip of the instrument is seen between the pulmonary artery and the aorta, the remaining adventitia can be divided and the tape grasped and pulled gently around the aorta.

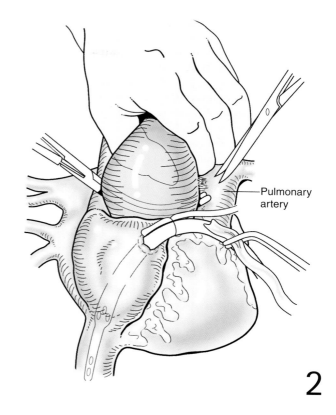

Pulmonary artery

2

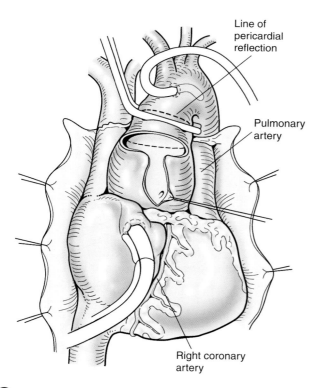

Line of pericardial reflection

Pulmonary artery

Right coronary artery

3

Excision of the aneurysm

3 When the heart fibrillates (usually 28°C), the aorta is cross-clamped immediately below the aortic cannulation site (or innominate artery if the femoral artery was cannulated), and blood-based cardioplegic solution is given. A longitudinal incision is made in the anterior surface of the aorta and continued superiorly until the neck of the aneurysm is reached. The aorta is then divided transversely, leaving sufficient cuff tissue below the cross-clamp to perform the distal anastomosis later. The transverse incision is continued carefully posteriorly around the aorta with care taken not to damage the pulmonary artery, particularly if the patient has adhesions from previous surgery or an aortic dissection. The original aortic incision is then carried inferiorly to a point just to the right of the commissure between the right and non-coronary cusps of the aortic valve, taking great care to avoid the right coronary ostium. A 4/0 monofilament traction suture is then placed on the left side of this incision, 1 cm from its inferior end.

4 The right side of the aneurysmal aortic root is then mobilized off the right atrium and divided immediately above the aortic annulus. This incision is continued posteriorly across the posterior commissure and on to the base of the left aortic sinus. Care is taken to avoid damage to the left atrium posteriorly and to avoid damage to the left main coronary artery. This dissection should stop halfway along the left aortic sinus. This part of the aneurysm is removed by carrying the line of incision superiorly, keeping to the right of the left main coronary artery to meet the distal line of transection.

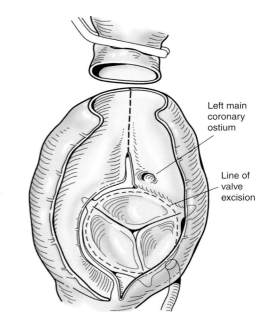

Left main coronary ostium

Line of valve excision

4

5 The left half of the aortic aneurysm wall is excised, commencing at the base of the original incision on the front of the aorta. The incision is carried carefully underneath the origin of the right coronary artery. The aortic wall is particularly thin here, and it is important to avoid damage to the underlying right ventricular outflow tract. The incision is continued until the commissure is reached.

The aortic wall is then incised to the left of the right coronary artery, and a large 'button' of aortic tissue containing the right coronary artery is mobilized. The superior portion of this button is left intact at this stage, but the coronary artery is mobilized for subsequent reimplantation.

Finally, the remainder of the aortic wall is excised, commencing at the left commissure and passing down the remainder of the left aortic sinus. At this point, the pulmonary artery is again at risk, as is the left main coronary artery, and care must be taken to visualize these structures before completing the excision. The excess aorta is then trimmed, leaving a large cuff of tissue around the left main coronary orifice. A generous portion provides a 'handle' to retract this coronary artery while the valve is being implanted.

The aortic valve is then excised from within the annulus, and the annulus is accurately sized. Any calcium or debris around the annulus is removed, particularly on the anterior leaflet of the mitral valve. The vent is clamped and the operative field irrigated, protecting the left coronary ostium with a small 'peanut' gauze on a hemostat. The vent is released.

If dense adhesions are present, the aneurysm wall can be left *in situ*, but we have found that our method enables much more precise graft and coronary placement. If it is decided to leave the wall in place, we would still transect the aorta immediately above the annulus as described, excising the two coronary artery buttons to reduce tension on these anastomoses.

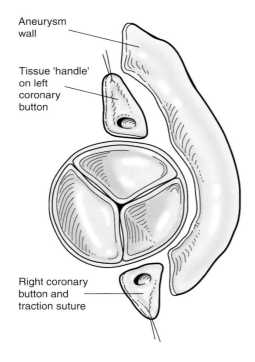

Aneurysm wall

Tissue 'handle' on left coronary button

Right coronary button and traction suture

5

Insertion of the valved conduit

6 The author uses an everting, interrupted mattress suture with Teflon pledgets for the lower anastomosis. 2/0 Ticron braided polyester sutures (Tyco Healthcare Group, Canada Inc., Quebec, Canada) (in a multi-pack of 20 sutures with alternating colored threads) are preferred. We have used several valved conduits, but our current preference is for the Medtronic-Hall device (Medtronic, Minneapolis, MN), which has a rotatable sewing cuff.

The first pledgeted mattress suture is placed at the posterior commissure. Both needles pass from the external aspect of the annulus into the left ventricular outflow tract. A second suture is placed immediately to its left, with the first needle passing through the pledget of the first suture and then through the annulus. Thereafter, the first pass of each suture is through the Teflon pledget of the previous one so that when the valve is finally seated, there is an interlocking layer of pledgets on the external aspect of the everted aortic annulus. Sutures are placed until the next commissure is reached, and all the sutures are secured with a single hemostat. Sutures are placed in the annulus of the right aortic sinus in a similar fashion, continuing in a clockwise direction. Finally, the sutures are placed in the noncoronary annulus. The second needle of the last suture must pass through the Teflon pledget of the first suture positioned, completing the Teflon reinforcement of the entire suture line.

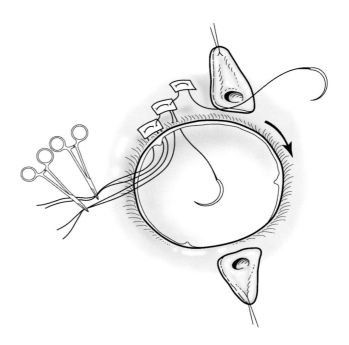

6

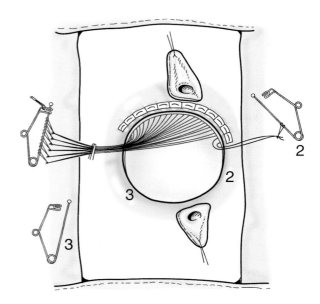

7a

SUTURE CONTROL

7 It is important to be certain that the sutures are not crossed or tangled, as this may lead to dangerous loops below the valve, incorrect seating of the valve, or paravalvular leak and hemorrhage. Many techniques are available to ensure that the multiple valve sutures remain organized, some of which use expensive disposable equipment. We use a very accessible and effective 'valve organizer': four instrument clips, found on most instrument trays.

One such clip is secured to each of four corners of the drapes around the wound. As each needle is passed through the annulus, the thread is clipped individually with a hemostat, the handle of which is then threaded over the valve organizer. When all the sutures on one aortic sinus are complete, the organizer is locked and all the threads secured with another hemostat.

The left aortic sinus sutures are initially placed on the upper right organizer. The sutures on the right aortic sinus are then placed on the upper left organizer. The remaining sutures are placed on the third, lower left valve organizer.

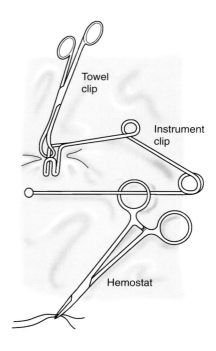

7b

SUTURE PLACEMENT ON THE VALVE

8 It is critically important to orient the valve correctly, particularly if it cannot be rotated within the sewing ring. It may help to mark the ring with three lines, corresponding to the commissures of the native valve. The three plications in the Dacron graft of the Medtronic–Hall valve serve this purpose well.

Now working in the reverse direction, and starting with the last needle on the noncoronary annulus, each suture is removed from the organizer, and the needle is passed through the valve annulus from below upward. As each pair of needles (i.e., one mattress suture) is passed through the sewing ring, their threads are clipped together and placed on the fourth (lower right) organizer. Placement of the sutures continues around the sewing ring of the valve until the next commissure is reached, whereupon the organizer is locked and the now empty third organizer is used to receive the next group of paired sutures.

When all the sutures have been placed, they are moistened, and the valve is lowered into position, taking care to avoid any redundant loops that occur underneath the valve. The valve handle is then removed, and all sutures are tied. To facilitate this step, the graft is retracted to the appropriate side, and the sutures are tied in the reverse order to which they were just placed on their organizer (i.e., clockwise). It is important to make sure that each pledget is seated correctly. If there is any difficulty in seating the valve, it may be helpful to tie the commissural sutures first.

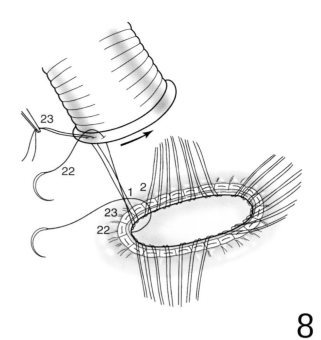

8

Once the valve is seated and before the sutures are cut, the valve disc motion is carefully assessed, and, if necessary, the valve is rotated. Ideally, when using a Medtronic–Hall valve, the greater orifice of the valve should face toward the non-coronary sinus, but the valve motion must not be impeded in any way. The everting technique ensures that the valve disk moves freely.

Reanastomosis of the coronary arteries

9 The Dacron graft is then cut to its appropriate length to facilitate the next step. A hemostat is placed on the anterior aspect of the superior end of the graft, and it is retracted inferiorly. With a pair of forceps holding the posterior wall of the graft, the site for the left coronary anastomosis is carefully determined. The author prefers to lay the graft onto the left coronary rather than to lift the coronary upward, possibly distorting it. When the appropriate site is determined, a hole, slightly larger than the ostium of the coronary artery, is cut in the Dacron graft using a high-temperature ophthalmic cautery unit.

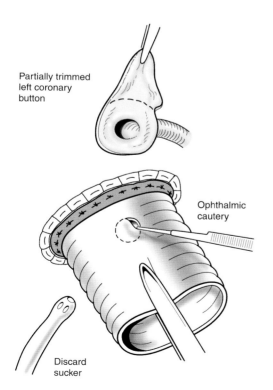

Partially trimmed left coronary button

Ophthalmic cautery

Discard sucker

9

10 The left coronary artery button is then trimmed to a size that is approximately 2–3 mm larger than the hole in the Dacron graft. The superior 'handle' on this button is left intact until the last minute, as it provides a good point of traction that does not damage the coronary ostium. The coronary ostium is then anastomosed to the Dacron graft with a continuous 5/0 monofilament polypropylene suture. The author uses a very small Teflon pledget and commences with a mattress suture inferiorly, beginning outside the coronary artery button and passing inside the graft. The first limb of the suture continues as a loose continuous suture along one half of the posterior wall of the anastomosis. As the suture line begins to turn upward along the graft, this suture is maintained on tension with a covered hemostat. The other half of the posterior wall of the anastomosis is then completed.

At this stage, general traction is applied to both sutures, and the graft is lowered onto the left coronary button. A fine nerve hook is used to ensure that each loop has pulled up securely and that the artery sits squarely on the graft. The sides of the anastomosis are then completed, the excess aortic tissue is trimmed, and the top suture line is completed.

When the anastomosis is completed, the final two sutures are passed through another small Teflon pledget. A nerve hook is used to pull up any loose loops, and the suture is secured. The anastomosis is then inspected from inside the Dacron graft. Any obvious defects can be corrected with a simple 5/0 polypropylene suture that is placed from within the Dacron graft and the coronary artery and tied externally.

The right coronary artery anastomosis is completed in the same way. It is particularly important to fill the heart before making the hole in the Dacron graft for this anastomosis. If the site is too low, the right ventricular outflow may 'roll over' the graft, kinking the artery as the heart distends.

Rewarming is commenced.

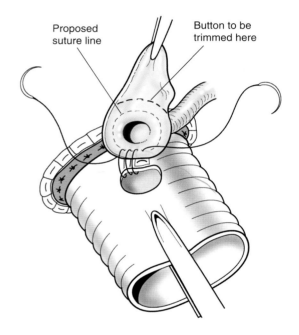

Proposed suture line

Button to be trimmed here

10

Preparation of the distal aorta

11a, b
The author uses a 'Teflon sandwich technique' for all distal ascending aortic anastomoses. This method provides great security and minimizes bleeding and the risk of dissection from the suture line. This technique is essential for the dissected aorta. We have tried various biological and glutaraldehyde resorcinol formalin glues in dissections but have discontinued their use. After the aorta is trimmed to length, a 1-cm Teflon strip is placed on the external aspect of the distal aorta, and a 0.7-cm Teflon strip is placed inside the lumen. Beginning posteriorly, these Teflon strips are secured with a running 4/0 polypropylene mattress suture.

The Dacron graft is then carefully measured and cut to length. The disparity in the size between the distal aorta and the Dacron graft must be carefully noted in planning the distal suture line. The incision in the graft is usually oblique and can be fashioned to minimize disparity. If the graft is too long, it may kink and may, in fact, obstruct the left coronary artery. If it is too short, it may distort or put too much tension on the left main coronary artery. The author prefers to leave the anterior aspect of the graft a bit longer and trim this as the suture line is completed.

The Dacron graft is then sewn into this Teflon sandwich with 3/0 polypropylene sutures. The first suture is a mattress suture that passes from outside the graft to inside. The suture is then passed inside to outside the Teflon sandwich and is tied firmly. Next, one limb of the suture is carefully passed behind the anastomosis, with particular care taken not to catch the left main coronary artery. The left side of the aortic anastomosis is then completed, with the sutures passing from outside the graft to inside and then from inside the distal aorta to outside. If there is significant disparity in size, the Dacron should be folded carefully into the graft, with each suture thus avoiding major 'teapot spouts.'

When the left side of this anastomosis is three fourths complete, the suture is held on traction while the right side is finished. Before the anastomosis is completed, the front of the graft is measured and trimmed. The suture line is completed while the left ventricular vent is turned off and blood is gradually returned to the patient.

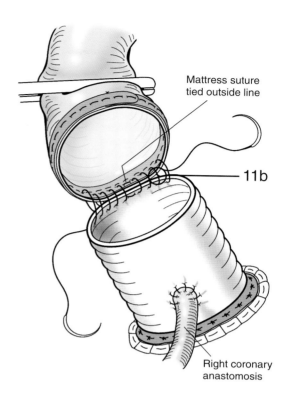

Mattress suture tied outside line

11b

Right coronary anastomosis

11a

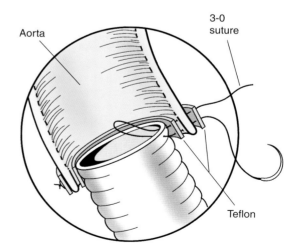

Aorta

3-0 suture

Teflon

11b

Deairing

Before the suture is finally tied, the heart, aorta, and graft are carefully deaired. This technique requires some attention and may take a few minutes. With the left ventricular vent turned off but still in position, blood is returned to the patient from the reservoir. At the same time, the lungs are inflated and sustained positive pressure applied. With the surgeon's left hand behind the heart, the fourth and fifth fingers can then invert the left atrial appendage while the remainder of the hand gently massages the left ventricle. At the same time, warm blood is infused through the retrograde cardioplegia line to flush any air out of the right coronary artery.

When the surgeon is satisfied that no air is present in the aortic root, the pump is turned off, the aortic cross-clamp slowly released, the surgeon's hand withdrawn, and the aortic suture tied and divided. The retrograde coronary sinus blood infusion is stopped, ventilation discontinued, the vent turned back on, and cardiopulmonary bypass reinstituted.

Hemostasis

At this stage, the suture line can be inspected carefully and completely. The small Teflon pledgets on the coronary anastomosis enable the surgeon to be certain that he or she has inspected the entire suture line. Any major bleeding can be secured with a 5/0 or 4/0 polypropylene suture. The roof of the left atrium is carefully inspected to ensure that no small venous bleeding points are present. The valve suture line is also inspected and, if necessary, reinforced with a 2/0 Ti-cron suture and pledgets. Teflon pledgets on the external annulus make it relatively easy to inspect this suture line. Finally, the distal suture line is inspected and any bleeding points secured with a 4/0 polypropylene suture, ensuring that each suture passes through the graft and through both layers of the Teflon sandwich.

Considerable 'ooze' may come from the suture lines and the graft at this stage. It should be borne in mind that the patient is fully heparinized and, if plateletpheresis has been used, he or she is relatively thrombocytopenic. The suture lines are then packed with oxidized cellulose gauze or Gelfoam, and preparations are made for decannulation.

Decannulation

The retrograde coronary sinus catheter is removed and the right atriotomy secured. The left atrial vent is removed. The vent is turned off, filling the heart and leaving some blood in the pericardium so that the cannula is withdrawn and the suture tied 'underwater' to prevent any air from entering the left atrium. Esophageal echocardiography is very useful in detecting air in the left ventricle at this stage. If significant air is detected, it should be removed via a large-bore needle passed through the highest aspect of the aorta while the ventricle is massed gently.

When the patient is fully rewarmed and hemostasis is secured, bypass is discontinued, the perfusion lines are removed, and protamine sulfate is given. Each cannulation site is then secured in the appropriate fashion. When the heparin has been completely reversed, the patient's platelets are reinfused slowly. The effect on blood loss is usually dramatic. If bleeding continues, the plateletpheresis console is used as a cell saver, and the coagulation mechanism is checked and corrected.

The oxidized cellulose 'gauze' is then removed and all suture lines inspected. It is important to be gentle when retracting the graft so that the coronary anastomoses are not excessively distracted. However, they can all be visualized, with the Teflon pledgets helping to identify the top and bottom of each anastomosis. Appropriate pacing wires (usually two ventricular and two atrial) are positioned and pericardial and mediastinal drains placed.

PLATELET GLUE

12 The plateletpheresis technique provides the surgeon with the opportunity to manufacture a biological glue using the patient's own platelets, topical thrombin, and calcium. This glue can be sprayed over each of the suture lines and a small piece of oxidized cellulose gauze reapplied. It is also useful to stop petechial bleeding from the surface of the heart, particularly in a reoperation. Some surgeons have suggested that this technique may improve wound healing. For this reason, the authors spray any remaining platelet glue along the edges of the sternum and in the subcutaneous wound. It is usually possible to cover the graft with pericardium or the mediastinal fat pad. The wound is then closed in layers in the routine fashion.

POSTOPERATIVE MANAGEMENT

The postoperative management protocols are the same as those for routine aortic valve replacement. Careful management of blood pressure, cardiac output, and rhythm are important. Protocols for hemostasis, transfusion, and reoperation should be standardized. Autotransfusion of shed mediastinal blood is another way to reduce exposure to homologous blood products. Since we began using plateletpheresis and the techniques just described, we have dramatically reduced the need for homologous blood or blood products and exposure to the associated risks. A significant proportion of our patients (41.5 per cent) were not given any homologous blood products. Furthermore, of those who did need homologous blood products, 46 per cent required three units or less.

In many of these patients, pericardial effusions develop early after operation. For this reason, a transthoracic echocardiogram is routinely performed the day before discharge (usually day 5). Patients are commenced on warfarin after the drains have been removed on the first postoperative day. Patients are given extensive education on the management of their anticoagulation and on antibiotic prophylaxis. They are reviewed at 6 weeks, after which they are returned to the care of their cardiologist or general practitioner, or both.

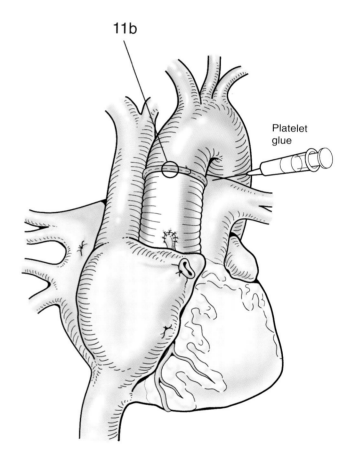

11b

Platelet glue

12

OUTCOME

Long-term follow-up should include transthoracic echo-cardiography at least every 12 months. Patients should be reviewed regularly by the surgeon (or cardiologist with current expertise in valve replacement) for the remainder of their life. They should wear a medallion or bracelet indicating that they have a valve *in situ* and that they are receiving anticoagulation. The valve make, model, and complete unique device identifier should also be recorded in the hospital note, the operation report, and the file of the attending medical practitioners.

In our experience, the long-term follow-up of these patients is excellent. Those who survive emergencies (aortic dissection, ruptured aneurysm, etc.) do remarkably well. Nevertheless, close cardiac, vascular, and hematological surveillance is mandatory for the life of the patient. With experience, the mortality of this procedure approaches that for isolated aortic valve replacement. On the other hand, patients who have had 'incomplete' procedures previously (for instance, aortic valve replacement in the presence of a dilated ascending aorta) frequently require reoperation, sometimes urgently. Reoperation in this setting may be hazardous in the extreme. The technique described here allows a safe and definitive aortic root replacement that should not require revision.

FURTHER READING

Bentall, H., DeBono, A. 1968. A technique for complete replacement of the ascending aorta. *Thorax* **23**, 338–9.

Dougenis, D., Daily, D.D., Kouchoukos, N.T. 1997. Reoperations on the aortic root and ascending aorta. *Annals of Thoracic Surgery* **64**, 986–92.

Gibson, J.L., Wajon, P.W., Hughes, C.F., Thrift, B. 1997. Intraoperative plateletpheresis for replacement of the ascending aorta and aortic valve with a composite graft. *Asia Pacific Heart Journal* **6**, 92–7.

Vallely, M.P., Hughes, C.F., Bannon, P.G., *et al.* 2000. Composite graft replacement of the aortic root after previous cardiac surgery: a 20 year experience. *Annals of Thoracic Surgery* **70**, 851–5.

20

Homograft aortic root replacement

MARK F. O'BRIEN FRACS, FRCS
Cardiac Surgeon and Director of Cardiac Surgical Research, The Prince Charles Hospital, Brisbane, Queensland, Australia

SUSAN HARROCKS RN, BN
Clinical Nurse Manager, Cardiac Surgical Research Unit, The Prince Charles Hospital, Brisbane, Queensland, Australia

HISTORY

Variations of implant techniques: justification for aortic root replacement

Since the first human implants of a homograft aortic valve for aortic valve replacement, varying methods of collection, sterilization, and storage preservation have confounded the interpretation of analyses of long-term homograft valve performance. The negligible risks of endocarditis and thromboembolism and the avoidance of the need for lifelong anticoagulation therapy became attributes of stentless tissue valves such as the homograft. Short donor death to retrieval times, early cryopreservation, and, in particular, host-donor age differences and the techniques of surgical implantation have remained the most powerful determinants of durability over the last 30 years of clinical analyses.

Three distinct technical methods of homograft valve implantation have evolved over the last three decades. Initially, the *subcoronary technique (two-suture line)* was used. This method had the added optional variations of inversion/eversion of the graft, with or without interrupted/continuous suture lines and with or without retention of the noncoronary homograft aortic sinus wall. Some inferior results due to leaflet distortion in some patient groups led to the introduction of the *cylinder (inclusion root) technique*. This homograft as a tube necessitated, in addition to the proximal and distal circumferential suture lines, the side-to-side homograft-host coronary artery ostial anastomoses. The host aorta was closed over the cylinder for hemostasis, representing a classic Bentall–De-Bono procedure. The third alternative technical implant procedure is the full *root replacement* with coronary artery button implantation. The unpredictable outcomes of the first two techniques (the subcoronary and the inclusion cylinder) can be due to the variations in asymmetry of the diseased host aortic root, leading to homograft leaflet distortion with subsequent varying degrees of postoperative incompetence. However, the full root replacement is virtually a 'stand alone' tube with minimal risk of distortion during implantation. The rationale for root replacement and its five advantages are:

1 The geometry of the homograft is maintained with less risk of distortion.

2 The homograft root virtually ignores the geometric variations in the host pathological anatomy.

3 Matching of graft-host sizes is far less critical compared to the more exact requirements with the two former techniques. The commissural posts of the homograft aortic wall are freestanding and not deformed as they may be with the intra-aortic nonroot techniques of implantation.

4 Root replacement is a simple, well-tried, well-performed technique as used with other devices such as mechanical valve conduits. Consequently, cardiac surgeons can readily accept and perform the procedure. The only difference is that the homograft root replacement requires gentleness in handling stentless tissue to avoid laceration and possible subsequent serious hemorrhage.

5 Clinical appraisal and echocardiography after root replacement confirm the superb hemodynamics.

The major and probable only disadvantage of the root replacement technique compared with other methods is the complete 'dismantling' of the native root, which may increase the complexity of subsequent redo replacement of the aortic valve or root. Nevertheless, of the total of 16 rereplacements of a cohort of 372 homograft root replacements that the authors' institution has performed from 1985 to 1999, nine reoperations have been possible with the insertion of a mechanical valve inside the homograft ascending aorta, and seven have had a second root replacement. In some the reoperation has not been an easy one, but all 16 operations have been successful.

Early after operation, root replacement homografts are competent or at the most demonstrate only a trivial incidence of valve regurgitation on echocardiography. They have a markedly reduced incidence of reoperation for technically caused early progressive regurgitation and a reduced incidence of hospital mortality and morbidity. These inferences and experiences have resulted from an analysis of 1022 homograft AVR implants from 1969 to 1998 at The Prince Charles Hospital and St. Andrew's War Memorial Hospital (29 years with a 99.3 per cent follow-up, failing to track seven patients only).

Over the past decades, many 'wet lab' workshops in several countries have addressed the issues of implantation techniques. Protagonists and antagonists for any one technique have published their opinions and results. Overall, the authors consider that the variations and complexities have unfortunately been deterrents to many 'trainee' surgeons (senior as well as junior). Consequently, stentless 'tissue valve' experience has not flourished, and the end result has been to impede the more frequent use of the homograft valve. Nevertheless, the inadequate supply of valves has restricted their preferential use for patients with active endocarditis and those (nonelderly) individuals who are unsuitable for lifelong anticoagulation.

The current technical recommendation by the authors is to use the homograft as a root replacement only, a policy carried out almost universally over the last 8 years. As of mid-1999, the *total* consecutive cohort of 372 patients received a homograft root replacement, with a 1.1 per cent hospital/30-day mortality, minimal return for early postoperative bleeding (1.4 per cent), and complete eradication of preoperative acute endocarditis in all 28 patients.

PREOPERATIVE PREPARATION

The patient has to have sufficient knowledge and informed consent as to why a homograft is the chosen device or the first choice, with other valves as second or third choices. Before operation it is helpful and instructive to assess the patient's valve pathology and root dimensions carefully. If a large supply of homografts is readily available, selection of the ideal size of valve can be made at the operating table. This situation, however, is unusual because of supply problems. In any case, the surgeon's experience, is achieved by prebypass knowledge of the aortic valve and root symmetry and of the valve annulus and sinotubular diameters (VAD and STD). Any obvious asymmetry can be determined with the preoperative or intraoperative echocardiogram. In addition, with active or healed endocarditis and in the case of some reoperations and perivalvular leaks, the presence, position, and size of abscess cavities are determined, and the subsequent operative procedure is planned. The presence of an acute or chronic dissection may necessitate a homograft with a long ascending aorta if the dissection is irreparable and valve suspension not possible.

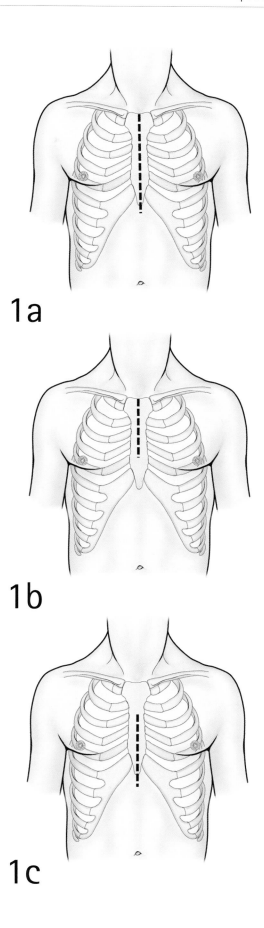

1a

1b

1c

OPERATION

Incision

1a–c The choices for operation are full median sternotomy (Figure 1a) or minimal access by upper (Figure 1b) or lower (Figure 1c) limited median sternotomy with or without lateral extension of the sternum in the fourth or second intercostal space, respectively. The authors consider that the results of homograft root replacement over the last 15 years have become predictable and extremely safe (1 per cent or less than 1 per cent for hospital/30-day mortality) with the use of the full median sternotomy. Nevertheless, the limited access approach is done successfully by some surgeons. However, critical appraisal of the margins for error, of the ability to be 'on top of' the operation, and of the avoidance of possible complications (including deairing procedures, absolute adequacy of cardioplegic delivery) is paramount for patient safety. Experience has now shown that bleeding is a rare complication with the forthcoming detailed technique. Limited access approaches must not increase the potential for morbidity.

General management

Important bypass procedures include the following:

1 Cannulation of the aorta high up near the innominate artery base to give good exposure of the aortic root. Groin vascular cannulation (usually iliac vessels) is used only if an aortic aneurysm, dissection, or reoperation with significant cardiac sternal adherence (rare) is present.
2 The authors prefer transatrial bicaval cannulation to maximize venous drainage and to minimize left heart blood suction. Carbon dioxide is insufflated into the pericardial cavity to minimize air embolism.
3 Left heart blood suction and cardiac decompression (if required) are carried out by right superior pulmonary venous cannulation. Suction is kept to a minimum.
4 Crystalloid or blood cardioplegia is delivered antegrade and retrograde, with all subsequent infusions given retrograde.
5 Antibleeding measures are considered very important, as the potential for postbypass bleeding is considerable. Therefore, aspirin and similar products are discontinued 7–10 days preoperatively where possible. Epsilon–aminocaproic acid (4–7 g total dose) or, more recently, aprotinin (especially for reoperation) is given in the moderate to high dose of 4–6 million units.

Homograft selection and preparation

To obtain the best long-term durability, the selected homograft should be one with the donor and recipient ages within 5 years of one another. The specific descriptive report on the homograft from the tissue bank is noted. A long length of ascending aorta may be desired, and the attached mitral valve leaflet is left *in situ* if required for closure of endocarditis abscess pockets. Ideally, providing the host VAD is known, the homograft can be thawed and trimmed before bypass. This step shortens cardiopulmonary bypass considerably and gives the opportunity for final careful inspection of the homograft, excluding, for example, thawing transverse tears of the aorta and any missed anomalies, such as an excessive number of leaflet fenestrations. The freezing and washing fluids and the final trimmings of the homograft are always sent for bacteriologic examination.

2 In trimming the graft, a 5-mm proximal cuff with its strong endocardium is left and, if required, much of the mitral anterior leaflet retained. The thickness of this proximal muscle cuff is 3–4 mm. The coronary arteries are cut flush with the aorta to be either oversewn later (with double-layer, continuous, over-and-over 6/0 polypropylene suture) or enlarged if this coronary ostium opposes the host coronary button satisfactorily. The long length of ascending aorta is left when needed to replace an aneurysmal or dilated aorta or more often to distend it with cardioplegic fluid to determine the exact site for the right coronary artery button implantation. The markings on the homograft are described later.

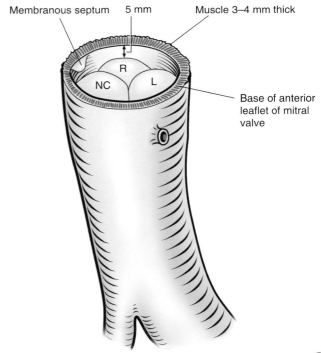

Membranous septum   5 mm   Muscle 3–4 mm thick

R
NC   L

Base of anterior leaflet of mitral valve

2

Intraoperative evaluation of the host aortic root

Before the insertion of a stentless valve, the surgeon is required to assess intraoperatively the pathological anatomy of the aortic root more carefully than would be done with a stented device. A more precise visualization of the geometry of the valve, the annulus, and the spatial relationships of the commissures to one another and to the coronary arteries is essential. Similarly, estimation of the way the pathological anatomy departs from that of the normal aortic root is important.

3 The homograft represents a normal aortic valve and root. This three-dimensional structure is a cylinder with length and breadth, the leaflets being at the base and the commissural posts and sinuses being part of its side wall. The transverse (annulus and sinotubular) and longitudinal axes are descriptive parts of this cylinder. All of these points, planes, or axes may be quite asymmetric in the diseased valve and root (see later). This situation should be identified so that appropriate mathematical readjustments can be made when the homograft is inserted as a root replacement. For instance, the distance between the coronary ostia and the VAD is important to calculate so that the coronary buttons are appropriately sited without overstretching, twisting, or angulation as they are sutured to the homograft sinuses. Any distortion of the homograft lessens leaflet coaptation, which in the normal young individual is as much as 40 per cent of each leaflet coapting with adjacent leaflet tissue. In addition to the need to assess the host aortic root, the important principle and objective is still to preserve the symmetry of the homograft. *The homograft should not be made to fit the host.* Consequently, distortion is minimized or abolished, and graft-host measurements become less critical when root replacement technique is used. The major judgment comes with the siting of coronary arteries for reimplantation. Here the 'freestanding' root is tethered, and without care improper siting can lead not only to coronary artery problems but also to some leaflet distortion. Lastly, the diameter of the aortic wall at its distal end requires measurement to match it approximately to the homograft distal aorta. A host reduction aortoplasty or distal Dacron graft may be necessary if ascending aortic dilatation or aneurysm is present or if the homograft aorta is of insufficient length.

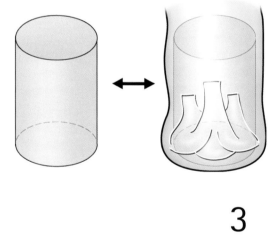

3

4 A brief outline of variations of an asymmetric diseased host root are summarized. This knowledge is perhaps most important for subcoronary and cylinder homograft valve techniques (and for stentless xenograft valve implantations as well). Younger and middle-aged patients are more likely to have either a severe, congenital, bicuspid calcific stenotic valve or an incompetent valve secondary to a congenital bicuspid aortic valve or to the varying etiologies of primary aortic wall pathology (medionecrosis, Marfan-like fibrillin abnormalities including idiopathic aortic root dilatation, etc.). Consequently, VAD and STD dimensions and their interrelationships may vary. The noncoronary sinus may be deeper than other sinuses. The horizontal plane of the annulus from sinus to sinus may be at a different angle, that is, not horizontal to the sinotubular junction.

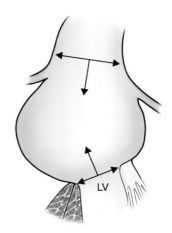

4

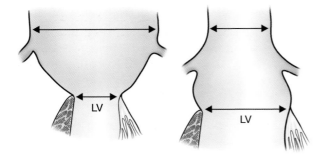

5a   **5b**

5a, b Unequal measurements of the VAD and STD may exist. Normally, the latter is 10 per cent smaller than the former. For example, a small VAD is less than STD (Figure 5a), and a larger VAD is greater than a large STD (Figure 5b).

Generally, only in the subcoronary and inclusion cylinder may it be necessary to perform reduction or enlargement of the VAD or STD diameters. These procedures are almost nonexistent with homograft root replacement, except in the following situations:

1. Severe tunnel aortic stenosis is present, necessitating a Konno or modified Konno procedure.
2. The large valve annulus, 30–35 mm, requires a reduction annuloplasty (see later).
3. The enlarged ascending aorta requires either replacement or a vertical aortoplasty to match, in size, the distal homograft wall diameter.

6a–c

In visualizing the aortic valve and annulus and comparing the intercommissural distances, the surgeon may see a variety of situations. In some bicuspid valves, after the leaflets and calcium around the rudimentary commissure are removed, the commissures may be almost at three equidistant points (Figure 6a). More frequently, with the bicuspid valve and particularly when the orifice is in an anteroposterior configuration, the noncoronary annulus is large and almost equal to or equal to the other two 'intercommissural' distances (Figure 6b). This situation becomes more important for subcoronary implantation to achieve correct intercommissural relationships. The coronary ostia are generally 120 degrees from one another, and this configuration presents no problem for a root replacement. However, less frequently the bicuspid valve has a transverse orifice, and the rudimentary commissure is anterior. With this scenario, invariably the right coronary artery (RCA) and left coronary artery (LCA) are directly 180 degrees opposite to one another (Figure 6c). This anatomy presents problems for subcoronary and inclusion cylinder implantation techniques and to a lesser extent for root replacements. At least one coronary button anastomosis will be close to a leaflet at the commissural post.

In essence, the position of the homograft commissure requires careful planning to ensure that no encroachment, deformation, or injury to the coronary ostia or leaflets occurs. This problem is greater with the subcoronary and cylinder techniques. With root replacement, the coronary button can be mobilized more, but gently and carefully, to allow an undistorted or nonoverstretched anastomosis to the homograft root. Some tricks assist in this maneuver and are outlined later. In summary, the stentless tissue valve autograft, homograft, and xenograft surgeon acquires all of this knowledge during his or her learning curve. This curve is shortened if maximum pre- and intraoperative assessment of all the previously mentioned factors is sought.

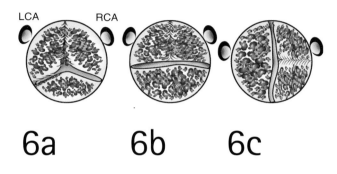

6a   6b   6c

Preparation of the host aortic root

7 If the homograft can be selected, thawed, trimmed, and checked as acceptable before bypass, the host aortic root can be fully prepared without interruption. The aorta is completely transected approximately 1 cm above both coronary ostia, and a T-shaped extension is made down into the noncoronary sinus. The exposure is generally excellent. The leaflets are excised, and the annular calcification is removed virtually completely, leaving sufficient strong tissue to prevent sutures from pulling out and to avoid polypropylene sutures fraying against residual calcific deposits. This maneuver restores annular extensibility, which can be maintained at least for some time after homograft implantation, as seen on our three-dimensional echocardiographic studies. Preparation of the rest of the root continues after the aortic valve orifice is measured. The importance of restoring such extensibility, a normal event during the cardiac cycle, is unknown in relationship to prolonging the durability of a stentless valve.

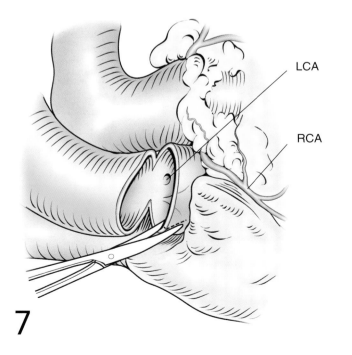

7

Preparation of the coronary buttons

8 The prevention of damage, twisting, and torsion while cutting out and suturing the buttons is the key to successful implantation. Damage to the button is minimized by dissecting close to the aortic wall, still leaving some adventitia, which serves well to close needle suture holes. If sharp dissection is carried out further away from the aortic wall, a greater risk of severing coronary branches exists, especially those of the right coronary artery. Twisting is prevented by not creating a circle to the button initially. Following the transverse aortotomy, a straight top or distal edge to the button exists once the rest of the circular aortic margins of the button are made. For example, the button is 'U'-shaped. The straight edge can always be kept distally, preventing rotation during suturing. Toward the finish of the suturing, the angled points at each end of the straight edge are cut to make the final circular button. In a similar way, the right coronary button has the same distal straight edge. Torsion kinking or overstretching of the coronary button is prevented by knowing the distance that the host coronary ostium was from its own aortic annulus and reproducing this distance from the homograft annulus. In addition, as outlined previously, distending the homograft aortic root with cardioplegic fluid assists in accurate siting of the right coronary button obviating problems with torsion.

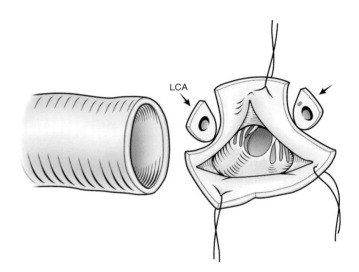

8

Implantation: alignment and specific markings on the homograft and host annulus

9 Correct implantation is facilitated and assured by appropriate markings on the homograft and host annulus. Matching without deformation is simplified. The homograft commissures are marked externally with a surgical pencil so that if new appropriate holes for the coronary anastomoses are necessary they will not be made too close to these external commissural markings. The homograft is implanted in the anatomical position. To ensure correct alignment of the graft and host at the annular level, 5/0 black silk marker sutures are placed in the host annulus, first under the left coronary ostium and then equidistantly at 120 degrees on either side (in the right coronary and noncoronary annuli). These points correspond to the nadir of each cusp of the allograft, which is marked with a surgical pencil on the graft's proximal cuff. In some situations with a bicuspid valve and a transverse orifice, the coronary ostia are 180 degrees opposite one another. This situation makes the implantation of a trileaflet valve more difficult. The coronary buttons cannot be anastomosed to the center of the homograft's coronary sinus, but with these markings and silk sutures the coronary buttons can be anastomosed to the aortic sinuses without impinging on or deforming a leaflet near its commissure. Fortunately, with the transverse bicuspid valve this scenario of coronary ostia 180 degrees opposite one another is not common. This occurrence should not preclude the selection and use of a homograft, but it does require the surgeon to take more time in planning, with the aid of the surgical pencil, where the coronary buttons can safely be anastomosed to the graft aortic sinuses. In summary, just as the artist or the architect may draw with perimeter markings to ensure correct proportion and alignment, the use of these markings simplifies and facilitates implantation with far less propensity to distortion of leaflets. The markings serve as an excellent guide for the young surgeon who is beginning his or her experience with stentless valves.

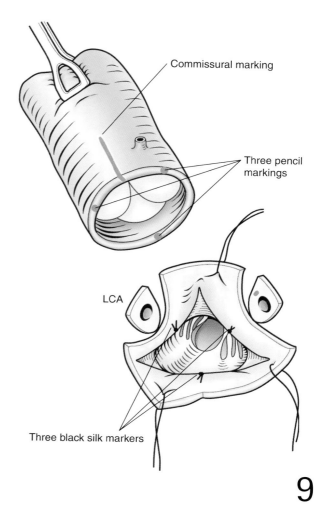

Commissural marking

Three pencil markings

LCA

Three black silk markers

9

Annular reduction, enlargement, and fixation

10 If the annulus is 30 mm or larger, some specific additional surgical procedure may be necessary to perform a reduction annuloplasty. Although this can be done with commissural plication or a pursestring suture method as described by Elkins, the authors prefer a reduction-fixation method, using Elkins' double 2/0 polypropylene pursestring suture first, followed by the incorporation of a Duran flexible ring within the continuous proximal suture line of the homograft. The host annulus, sized 30–35 mm, can be reduced accordingly to 27 mm or less with such a ring. The pure aortic valve incompetence due to the bicuspid aortic valve is the commonest reason for using this reduction annuloplasty. Annular fixation is also achieved.

The exceedingly small annulus, that is, 19 mm, generally requires no enlargement when a homograft is used. Occasionally, left ventricular hypertrophy is excessive, and a vertical left ventricular outflow tract myomectomy is required to remove subvalvular obstruction. Rarely is a posterior incision in the annulus (modified Nicks or Manouguian procedure) or even a Konno operation necessary. Charts that table the normal aortic annulus sizes according to body surface areas show surprisingly smaller root dimensions in adults than expected; that is, the annular diameter of a 2-sq m man averages 22.8 ± 1.7 mm, and the diameter of a 1.6-sq m woman is 20.3 ± 1.8 mm.

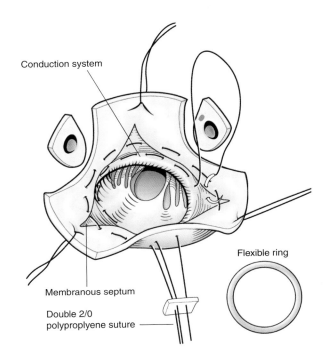

Conduction system

Membranous septum

Double 2/0 polyproplyene suture

Flexible ring

10

Proximal suture line

11 A continuous 3/0 polypropylene suture is used. Suturing begins at the left lateral side by passing the needle from outside to inside through the homograft at the base of its commissure between the right and left leaflets. The needle is then passed through the corresponding point of the host annulus. The first few sutures counterclockwise around the posterior annulus are backhand, whereas the rest are forehand. Good bites of host annulus and homograft tissue are taken approximately 2–3 mm apart. This posterior suture is continued toward the anterior portion of the noncoronary annulus, with the markers serving at appropriate matching points. The suture is tagged. The other arm of the continuous suture is then used to secure the homograft anteriorly from left to right. Sutures through the host annulus follow an imaginary horizontal line passing across the base of each commissure, rising anteriorly to avoid the conducting bundle. Most of the latter half of this anterior suturing through the muscular homograft cuff is done blindly, not visualizing the base of the valve leaflet. Occasionally, the one polypropylene suture is not long enough, and a second suture is necessary. The small half-circle needle is not only ideal but essential to negotiate any slightly difficult access points. A constant tension on the suture by the assistant ensures hemostasis. The tension is gauged by seeing the tissue being 'pulled up or elevated.'

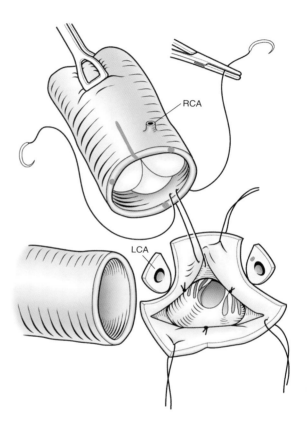

11

Coronary pedicle anastomoses

12a–d
Sometimes the host coronary buttons do not align ideally with the allograft coronary ostia. If such is the case, a new 7- to 8-mm hole is made by an aortic punch at the appropriate site. The homograft coronary ostium is then closed separately with a 6/0 double-layer, continuous polypropylene suture. The coronary anastomoses are carried out with continuous 5/0 polypropylene. This suture is more hemostatic than a 4/0 suture. A simple forehand technique again is used for the left and right anastomoses (Figure 12a, b). For the left anastomosis, the suture runs counterclockwise for the lower half and clockwise for the upper half. Suture spacing of 2–3 mm is critical. Before the right coronary anastomosis is commenced, the correct position should be verified. If a satisfactory length of homograft ascending aorta is available, a cardioplegic infusion line is inserted into the distal end of the homograft aorta after snugging around the line with infusion distending the aorta. In addition, if the right ventricle is distended by temporary clamping of the venous drainage line, a more precise position for the right coronary anastomosis can be determined. This cardioplegic infusion achieves left coronary artery flow, and the patency of the left anastomosis is checked at the same time. The right coronary anastomosis is then commenced after either a new punch hole is made or the homograft right coronary ostium is used. On most occasions a new punch hole is required (Figure 12b). The 5/0 suture is passed through the medial side of the homograft coronary ostium from outside to inside and then through the right coronary button from inside to outside. The suturing continues along the proximal or inferior half, tagging it on the right side. The anterior arm of the suture continues anteriorly over the remaining half to be tied on the right side with the other arm of the suture.

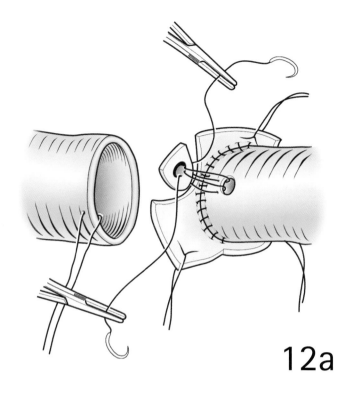

12a

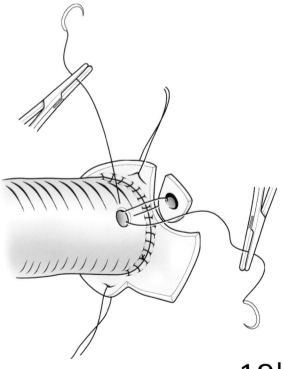

12b

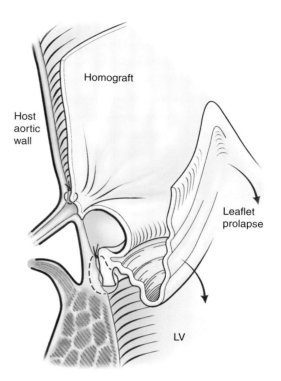

12c

On occasion, by using the homograft coronary ostium for the anastomosis instead of making a new hole in the homograft sinus, this inappropriate siting may lead to leaflet prolapse and distortion (Figure 12c, d). This situation is avoided by ensuring two steps. First, before the coronary buttons are fashioned, the distance from the center of the host coronary ostium to the host valve annulus should be noted. This distance has to be observed when siting the position in the homograft aortic sinus for the anastomosis. Second, distending the ascending aorta with cardioplegia infusion, as described, helps site the right coronary correctly. If the homograft ascending aorta is of insufficient length to distend it, an alternative is to complete the distal aortic anastomosis and then distend the aorta with cardioplegic fluid. Not opening the aortic cross-clamp may be wiser, as intracardiac air has not been removed at this stage.

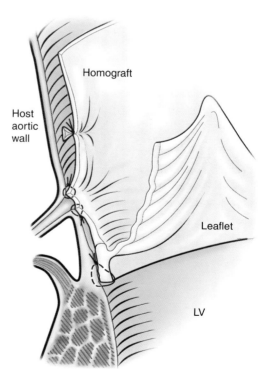

12d

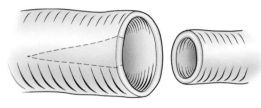

13a

Distal aortic anastomoses: vertical aortoplasty, ascending aortic replacement

13a–c The allograft is cut to length and tailored to the diameter of the host aorta. Some redundancy of the aorta is essential to avoid tension and stitch-hole bleeding, even though the homograft aorta is quite elastic and can comfortably adapt to size discrepancies with the host aorta. With 5/0 polypropylene, a forehand technique is again used, beginning on the left and proceeding posteriorly, stopping and tagging the suture on the right side anteriorly. The other arm of the suture from the left side is continued forehand anteriorly. If the host ascending aorta is dilated but not aneurysmal, a vertical aortotomy with a V-shaped excision produces more appropriate size matching of the two aortic ends for an anastomosis. If the aorta is aneurysmal, excision and replacement are necessary. Reconstitution is then made either by an interposition Dacron graft or by preserving the long segment of the homograft aorta if this is available.

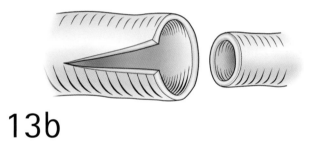

13b

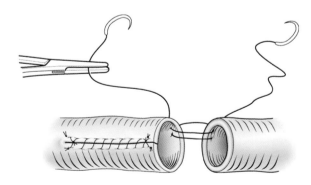

13c

OUTCOME

This technique of root replacement is an open appositional one without aortic wrapping. Excluding cases of external fixation and annular reduction, no Teflon/Dacron pledgeted sutures or glue are used. Hemostasis from these anastomotic suture lines has rarely been a problem (1.4 per cent). In addition, homograft aortic root replacement has been achieved with low mortality (four deaths in 375 aortic root replacements). The potential problem is that of reoperation and reroot replacement. This situation has been necessary for 16 patients for a variety of reasons (technical, $n = 3$; structural deterioration, $n = 8$; and endocarditis, $n = 5$). Extensive calcification of the homograft graft has been a problem only in young patients, mostly younger than 20 years of age.

The use of the homograft as a root replacement has increased the applicability of this valve for the treatment of virtually all pathological processes of the aortic valve and root. Strikingly obvious have been the excellent hemodynamics, the low incidence of reoperation for technical causes, and the more satisfactory outcome for patients with acute active endocarditis. Because of these advantages the root replacement technique has superiority over the subcoronary or intraluminal cylinder techniques. However, the long-term homograft valve durability of the three techniques, that is, the actuarial freedom from structural degeneration, has failed at this stage to show superiority of any one technique over the others.

Training of a 'tissue valve surgeon'

In addition to meeting the usual guidelines for the training of a cardiac surgeon, the trainee tissue valve surgeon who wishes to become adept in the use of stentless heart valves will succeed if the following steps are considered:

- A strong interest in stentless tissue valves is mandatory if patients are to receive optimal surgical standards under his/her care.
- The trainee surgeon should anticipate performing a reasonable volume of such operations to encompass the learning curve with the least mortality and morbidity.
- Implantation techniques should be practiced on animal hearts. Such 'wet lab' experience is invaluable. The trainee surgeon becomes familiar with the possible problems; and when the first human implant is being performed, the surgeon realizes that he/she has done this before (on animal hearts on a laboratory bench top!). We believe that no

surgeon should insert a stentless valve in a human without such laboratory practice.
- Repeated practice teaches the trainee surgeon some of the important techniques of gentleness in handling tissues. The minimization of bleeding from suture holes and of excess surgical manipulative 'trauma' can be achieved by the surgical technique of always withdrawing the suture needle in the line of its curve with the wrist action using a needle holder. The error is dragging the needle through the tissue, not in its curve, by using dissecting forceps and not the wrist rotating needle holder. This point is considered to be very important in the gentle handling of tissue.
- Ideally, the trainee should assist 'his/her senior' with these human operations and subsequently be assisted by 'an expert' when the trainee comes to do his/her first and possibly subsequent procedures.

This implantation of stentless tissue valves does require of the surgeon the act of spatial judgment, which is essential for valve repair work and especially congenital heart surgery. By obtaining the maximum information and gaining experience from each operation or laboratory practice, the surgeon's learning curve can and should be short.

FURTHER READING

Elkins, R.C., Knott-Craig, C.J., Howell, C.E. 1996. Pulmonary autografts in patients with aortic annulus dysplasia. *Annals of Thoracic Surgery* 61, 1141–5.

Lund O., Chandrasekaran V., Grocott-Mason R., *et al.* 1999. Primary aortic valve replacement with allografts over twenty-five years: valve-related and procedure-related determinants of outcome. *Journal of Thoracic and Cardiovascular Surgery* 117(1), 77–91.

Northrup, W.F., Kshetty, V.R. 1998. Implantation technique of the free-standing homograft or autograft root: emphasis on matching the host root to the graft. *Annals of Thoracic Surgery* 66, 280–4.

O'Brien, M.F. 1995. Allograft aortic root replacement: standardisation and simplification of technique. *Annals of Thoracic Surgery* 60, S92–4.

O'Brien, M.F., Finney, S., Stafford, E.G., *et al.* 1995. Root replacement for all allograft aortic valves: preferred technique or too radical? *Annals of Thoracic Surgery* 60, S87–9.

O'Brien, M.F., Harrocks, S., Stafford, E.G., *et al.* 2001. The homograft aortic valve: a 29-year, 99.3% follow-up of 1022 valve replacements. *Journal of Heart Valve Disease* 10(3), 334–45.

O'Brien, M.F., Harrocks, S., Stafford, E.G., *et al.* 2001. Allograft root replacement in 418 patients over a span of 15 years: 1985–2000. *Seminars in Thoracic and Cardiovascular Surgery* 13(54), 180–85.

21

Limited–access aortic valve surgery

DELOS M. COSGROVE MD
Chairman, Department of Thoracic and Cardiovascular Surgery, The Cleveland Clinic Foundation, Cleveland, Ohio, USA

JOHN H. ARNOLD MD, FACS
Staff Physician, Department of Thoracic and Cardiovascular Surgery, The Cleveland Clinic Foundation, Cleveland, Ohio, USA

HISTORY

Aortic valve surgery has traditionally been carried out through a 10–15-in. skin incision and a full midline sternotomy. This approach provides excellent exposure of the heart for cardiopulmonary bypass cannulation and exposure and replacement of the aortic valve. Results with this exposure have been excellent, and most centers report mortality rates well under 10 per cent, even in extreme cases. 'Routine' aortic valve procedures have much lower mortality rates.

During isolated aortic valve replacement, however, full exposure of the heart is generally unnecessary. Cannulation for cardiopulmonary bypass and work on the valve is concentrated in a very small area. Techniques, equipment, and procedures have been developed and modified to address aortic valve procedures through smaller incisions. The 'less invasive' moniker has been applied widely to procedures of which the overall goal is the development of techniques to do heart surgery less traumatically. We herein describe the development and application of our minimally invasive aortic valve surgical technique.

PRINCIPLES AND JUSTIFICATION

Many advantages exist for aortic valve replacement through smaller access incisions. Patient anticipation of the operation is improved. The overall procedure is less traumatic, with less bleeding, and there is theoretically less potential for wound infection. Application of the procedure results in shorter hospital stays with less pain and cosmetically more attractive incisions. Hospital costs are reduced, and this exposure has the added benefit of providing for safer reoperation, as we typically do not disturb the pericardium over the right ventricular outflow tract.

Determination to use the incision currently used by us involved development and/or evaluation of multiple exposures of the heart, including anterior thoracotomy, transecting sternotomy, and finally the implementation of an upper partial sternotomy. We herein discuss the progression of techniques up to our current technique. The push throughout this development has been to create and evaluate alternatives that allow delivery of the same quality of technical care to the patient while preserving the benefits of a procedure that costs less, is more acceptable to the patient, and potentially returns the patient to work sooner.

Successful application of minimally invasive procedures is a team approach combining the talents of cardiologists, cardiac surgeons, anesthesiologists, and the nursing support staff. Our current contraindications for this operation include pectus excavatum to the degree that the heart is displaced. Reoperation is a relative contraindication to the procedure, although some reoperations have been done at our institution. Similarly, a history of pericarditis is an indication that reduced mobility may preclude satisfactory operative exposure. Given the limited visualization of the epicardium provided by this incision, associated procedures, especially revascularization of the left side of the heart, remain contraindications.

Small incision aortic valve surgery was first applied at The Cleveland Clinic in January, 1996, using an anterior thoracotomy approach developed from our studies in the anatomy lab. A 10-cm vertical right parasternal incision with displacement or resection of the third and fourth costal cartilages provided excellent exposure of the ascending aorta and aortic root. However, we found it necessary in this exposure to cannulate our patients from the groin, and occasional patients had anterior chest wall instability after the procedure. Additionally, inadequate exposure of the aortic valve occasionally occurs, necessitating conversion to a full sternotomy. This situation requires a second parallel vertical incision, which sometimes sacrifices the intervening skin bridge leading to an unacceptable cosmetic result. Therefore, better approaches were sought.

We next evaluated the use of a horizontal incision, again approximately 10 cm in length, with a transecting sternotomy through the second or third interspace. Although this method provided excellent exposure, it frequently required direct or indirect sacrifice of one or both internal mammary arteries. In addition, occasional postoperative sternal instability was evident.

Since January 1997, our practice has been to expose the aortic valve using a partial upper sternotomy through an 8- to 10-cm skin incision. The breastbone is divided from the sternal notch through the third or fourth interspace on the right side. We have found this partial sternotomy to be widely applicable to both our minimally invasive aortic valve and mitral valve procedures, providing a single standard and widely applicable approach for both. Through this partial upper sternotomy, we are able to establish central cannulation and excellent exposure. The internal mammary arteries remain intact. Sternal stability using our standard sternotomy closure technique with monofilament stainless steel wire remains very reliable.

PREOPERATIVE ASSESSMENT AND PREPARATION

The patient is taken to the operating suite and placed on the operating table with the arms tucked. The anesthesiologist establishes appropriate monitoring lines and induces anesthesia, followed by intubation of the patient with a standard single-lumen endotracheal tube. To facilitate exposure during the procedure, a rolled towel is placed between the patient's shoulders. In deference to the reduced exposure, defibrillator patches are placed on the patient's back and anterior left chest wall.

A transesophageal echo probe is then positioned, and the heart is evaluated with specific attention given to the ascending aorta, aortic root, aortic valve, left ventricular outflow tract, and overall cardiac function. The use of transesophageal echocardiography is essential to the application of minimally invasive exposure. Echocardiography provides for the evaluation of the valve lesion and is used to determine whether the valvular lesion is mechanical, regurgitant, or a combination of these problems. Echocardiographic evaluation before the operation includes precise definition of the mechanism of the valve lesion, as well as the evaluation of cannulation sites in the ascending and/or descending aorta.

The assessment of the surgical results is highly reliant on the transesophageal echocardiography secondary to the reduced exposure. After surgery, traditional views may not be as readily reached by the echocardiographer, and special views, especially transgastric, may be required. Post procedure, transesophageal echocardiography is invaluable for evaluation of the valve repair or replacement; most importantly, it is used to determine the completeness of evacuation of air from the heart.

In addition to evolution of the surgical incisions and exposures, cannulation of the patient has evolved as we have refined our procedure. With our initial exposures, cannulation was carried out through the groin, via the femoral vessels. We found this approach added complexity and time to the operative procedures. We therefore moved to cannulate through our exposure at the chest, but found that the larger cannulas obstructed the rather limited view available. It was then determined that adding negative pressure to a hard-shell, closed-system cardiotomy venous reservoir would allow us to use much smaller cannulas, resulting in improved exposure. Vacuum-assisted venous drainage has the additional benefit of reducing our priming volume and hemodilution. This modification has resulted in a reduced rate of transfusion. In addition, no difficulty exists with airlock with this system. Exposure has been improved further with development and refinement of specialized venous cannulas designed to take advantage of the vacuum-assisted venous drainage system.

ANESTHESIA

The management of the anesthesia administered to patients undergoing less invasive aortic surgery is consistent with that used in standard full sternotomy procedures.

OPERATION

1 An 8- to 10-cm incision is made sharply beginning halfway between the sternal notch and the angle of Louis, and this incision is extended to the sternum with electrocautery. A sternal saw is used to divide the sternum in the midline and then brought out into the third or fourth interspace on the right, taking care not to injure the right internal mammary artery.

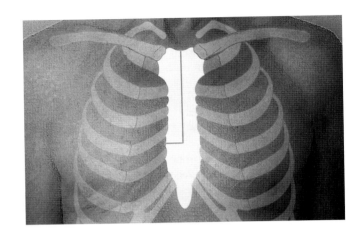

1

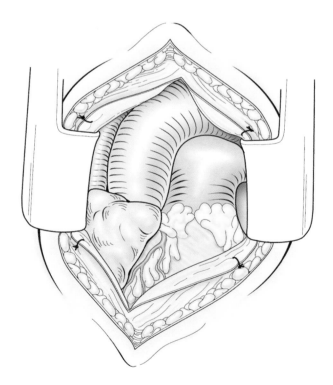

2 A Finochietto retractor is used to open the sternum and establish exposure. The thymus and mediastinal fat are divided between clamps and ligated. The pericardium is opened slightly to the right and suspended from the wound edges using silk sutures. The patient is heparinized. Arterial return is established with a 22-Fr Sarns soft-flow cannula at the pericardial reflection through a 2/0 silk pursestring secured with a Rumel tourniquet. Venous drainage is accomplished through the right atrial appendage with a 28-Fr cannula using vacuum-assisted venous drainage. We are routinely able to cannulate the coronary sinus from this exposure through an additional atrial pursestring. A needle vent is placed in the ascending aorta for delivery of antegrade cardioplegia as well as to facilitate deairing at the end of the case.

2

3 After heparinization and complete cannulation, the patient is placed on bypass. The ascending aorta is cross-clamped using a noncrushing occlusive clamp with a malleable handle (Cosgrove Flex Clamp), allowing the handle to be positioned out of the way during the case. Bolus cold blood cardioplegia is delivered antegrade, followed by delivery retrograde, to arrest the heart. If the aortic valve lesion is incompetent, the antegrade cardioplegia can be delivered via direct ostial cannulation after retrograde cardioplegia has been administered. Cardioplegia is repeated at appropriated intervals during the cross-clamp period. Exposure of the valve is accomplished through a transverse aortotomy that can be extended down towards the noncoronary sinus.

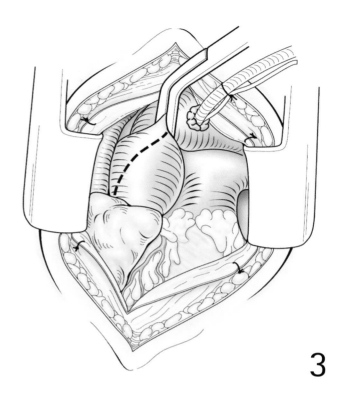

3

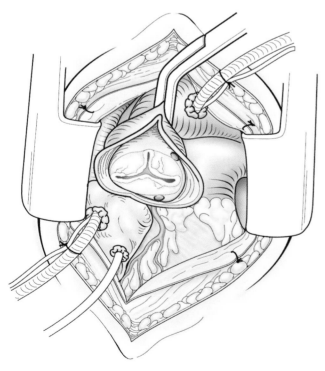

4 A single 2/0 silk suture is used to draw back the superior edge of the aortotomy. In addition, the patient is put in a slight degree of reverse Trendelenburg to facilitate exposure. A headlight provides reliable illumination within the surgical field.

4

5 If the valve cannot be repaired, it is resected sharply. The annulus is cleared of any remaining calcium. Once this maneuver is accomplished, pledgeted 2/0 horizontal mattress sutures are placed from the ventricular side at the commissures or commissural remnants. These sutures are tacked to the surrounding drapes with tonsil clamps under moderate tension to elevate the aortic root up into the surgical field. This maneuver serves to retract the aorta and maintain orientation of the aortic root, and it generally provides excellent exposure for placement of the remaining horizontal mattress sutures to secure an appropriately sized valve in the supra-annular position. The mattress sutures are of alternating colors to facilitate the progress of the case.

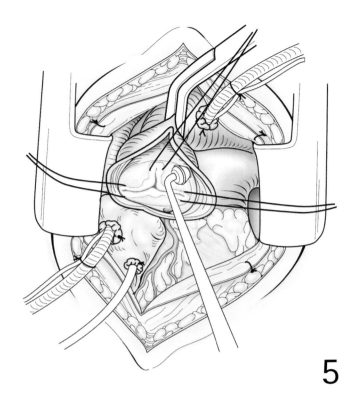

5

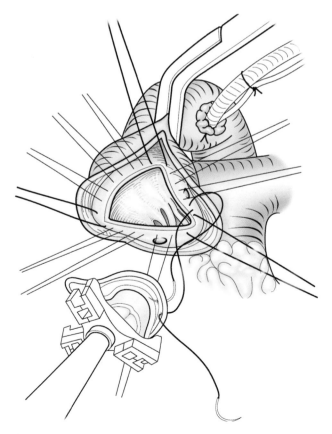

6

6 The left ventricle is not routinely vented other than to place a weighted basket sucker through the aortic root into the left ventricle to improve exposure. We have found that, with the vacuum-assisted venous drainage, this method of left ventricular clearance is satisfactory and also reduces the amount of intracardiac air. During the part of the operation when the heart is open, the surgical field is flooded with surgical grade carbon dioxide at 5–6 L/minute delivered through a thin plastic cannula sutured to the superior aspect of the wound. Carbon dioxide is used to reduce the amount of intracardiac air at the terminal portion of the case. Carbon dioxide is more dense than oxygen and nitrogen in the field. Any trapped carbon dioxide is highly absorbable into blood and plasma and therefore rapidly dissolves into solution once the aortotomy is closed.

Valve sutures are passed through the prosthesis annulus, and the valve is seated and tied into place. Before dividing the sutures, closure of the aortotomy can be facilitated by using the valve sutures for traction to expose the right aspect of the aortotomy. Once the corner stitch is placed, the valve sutures are cut and closure of the aortotomy is continued with running 4/0 Prolene.

7 Before completing the closure, the heart is filled and the lungs are inflated to force any remaining intracardiac air up and out of the heart. The aortotomy closure is then secured.

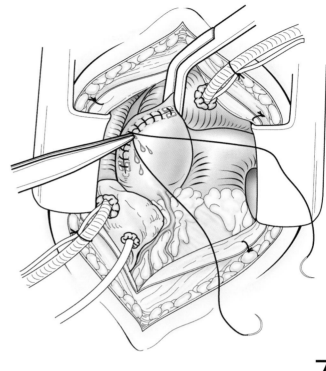

7

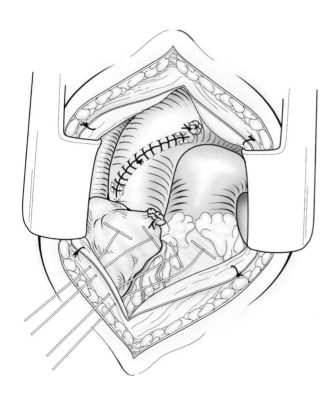

8

8 The patient is leveled on the table, and the cross-clamp is removed. Ventricular pacing wires are placed at the right ventricular outflow tract, and atrial wires are secured to the right atrium at this time on bypass to use the optimal exposure. The cross-clamp is partially applied along the most superior aspect of the aorta just distal to the aortic vent to trap and remove any remaining intracardiac air. Completeness of the evacuation of the air is evaluated by transesophageal echocardiography. Additionally, the function of the prosthesis (or repair) is closely evaluated. Once deairing is complete and the function of the heart and the aortic valve is judged to be satisfactory, the patient is weaned from bypass. Protamine is given to reverse the heparin, and the patient is decannulated. Once hemostasis is judged to be complete, a right angle chest tube is placed and directed so as to drain the diaphragmatic surface of the right pleura. An additional straight chest tube is placed so as to lie within the pericardial sac. The sternotomy is closed with monofilament stainless steel, and the soft tissues are closed with absorbable suture.

POSTOPERATIVE CARE

Patients are transported (intubated and sedated) to the surgical intensive care unit. Postoperative care proceeds in a routine manner. The patients are stabilized, and, if appropriate, weaned from the ventilator and extubated in the first 4–6 hours. Patients in stable condition are discharged from the intensive care unit the morning after their operation, after chest tubes and monitoring catheters are removed. Pacing wires are removed on the third postoperative day if the patient remains in sinus rhythm. Telemetry monitoring is continued until discharge, usually the fourth or fifth postoperative day. Patients begin a program of progressive ambulation and activity on the day after their procedure. We obtain a baseline postoperative transthoracic echocardiogram before discharge.

We do not routinely use warfarin (Coumadin) for our patients in sinus rhythm who have undergone valve repair or replacement with a tissue valve. These patients do receive one adult aspirin (325 mg) daily. Patients with mechanical valves are started on low-dose warfarin the day after operation, and the dosage is adjusted to maintain the international normalized ratio within the recommended range. Patients with atrial fibrillation unresponsive to therapy are also placed on anticoagulant therapy.

OUTCOME

The applicability of the exposure established through the upper partial sternotomy is not limited to aortic valve replacement alone. Additional procedures on the left ventricular outflow tract and ascending aorta can be accomplished with this exposure. These procedures include aortic valve repair and aortic root replacement with prosthetic material and/or autologous material, including homografts. In addition, lesions of the ascending aorta, such as aneurysms of the ascending aorta and arch, can be addressed using femoral cannulation.

From January 1996 through December 1999, 1400 patients have undergone valve surgery via a minimally invasive approach at our institution by one surgeon. Of these, 433 patients had aortic valve procedures. Patients undergoing aortic procedures using less invasive incisions had a mean age of 55.3 years (range, 18 to 87 years). Females comprised 31 per cent of our population. In this patient population, 85 per cent had normal or mildly depressed left ventricular function, and 15 per cent were classified as moderate or severe. Procedures performed included 95 (22 per cent) aortic valve repairs and 338 (68 per cent) replacements (179 tissue, 125 homograft, and 34 mechanical). Fifty-six multiple valve procedures were performed, including nine aortic valve plus revascularization procedures and 43 procedures involving repair or replacement of part or all of the ascending aorta or arch. Seven patients undergoing aortic valve procedures required conversion to full sternotomy, but these were early in our experience. Central cannulation is now uniformly successful, except where calcification of the ascending aorta requires that alternative cannulation sites be used. Pump and cross-clamp times were not lengthened relative to full access procedures. Only 45 patients (10 per cent) received blood products. Patients were discharged within 5 postoperative days 58 per cent of the time. Operative mortality in this group of patients was 0.9 per cent. Costs and charges were relatively less in the minimally invasive procedures group.

Thus, less invasive aortic valve surgery can be applied to a wide range of procedures in a safe and effective manner. Outcomes meet or exceed full sternotomy results for patient morbidity and mortality, rates of transfusion, intensive care unit and hospital lengths of stay, procedural costs, and patient acceptance.

FURTHER READING

Cohn, L.H., Adams, D.H., Couper, G.S., *et al.* 1997. Minimally invasive cardiac valve surgery improves patient satisfaction while reducing costs of cardiac valve replacement and repair *Annals of Surgery* **226(4)**, 421–6.

Cosgrove, D.M., Sabik, J.F. 1996. Minimally invasive approach for aortic valve operation. *Annals of Thoracic Surgery* **62**, 596–7.

Cosgrove, D.M., Sabik, J.F., Navia, J.L. 1998. Minimally invasive valve operations. *Annals of Thoracic Surgery* **65**, 1535–9.

Gillinov, A.M., Casselman, F., Cosgrove, D.M. 2000. Minimally invasive heart valve surgery: operative technique and results. In Yim, A.P.C. (ed.), *Minimal access cardiothoracic surgery*. Philadelphia, PA: W. B. Saunders, 555–62.

Minale, C., Reifschneider, H.J., Schmitz, E., *et al.* 1997. Single access for minimally invasive aortic valve replacement. *Annals of Thoracic Surgery* **64**, 120–3.

Svensson, L.G., D'Agostino, R.S. 1998. Minimal-access aortic and valvular operations, including the "J/j" incision. *Annals of Thoracic Surgery* **66**, 431–5.

22

Limited-access mitral valve surgery

WALTER RANDOLPH CHITWOOD, JR. MD
Chairman of Surgery, East Carolina University Brody School of Medicine; Cardiothoracic Surgeon, Department of Surgery, University Health Systems of Eastern North Carolina, Greenville, North Carolina, USA

L. WILEY NIFONG MD
Assistant Professor and Director of Surgical Research and Robotics, Department of Surgery, Division of Cardiothoracic Surgery, The Brody School of Medicine at East Carolina University, Greenville, North Carolina, USA

HISTORY

Minimally invasive, or limited-access, cardiac surgery has become popular over the past 5 years. Surgeons and patients alike expect excellent results, and early data suggest that these new operations are safe and effective and provide results comparable to those achieved with conventional operations. Elements constituting the ideal mitral valve operation are listed in Table 22.1. To attain these goals, surgeons have adopted an evolutionary implementation pattern. First, conventional approaches were modified and, in some hands, arrived quickly at micro and near port incisions. Then, video-assisted techniques were attempted. At East Carolina University (ECU), we have moved step-wise from using direct vision with smaller incisions (level I), to video assistance (level II), to video-directed, voice-activated robotic techniques (level III), and recently, to complete robotic mitral valve repairs (level IV). This classification was proposed by Loulmet and describes this ascension accurately (Table 22.2). A series of 'camps,' or comfort levels, has been established premonitory to advancing toward a completely endoscopic mitral valve operation. Although some currently are achieving near endoscopic valve repair/replacements, surgeons should rely on results of longitudinal patient studies before setting a new standard.

Microincisions are considered as being 4–6 cm, and *port incisions* connote those 3–4 cm or less in length. *Video assistance* indicates that 50–70 per cent of the valve repair or replacement is done while viewing the operative field through a monitor, and *video direction* implies that nearly all of the operation is done videoscopically. Lastly, *robotic assistance* really means *computer-enhanced surgery*, where electro-mechanical devices intervene between the surgeon's hands and patient. At our institution, we have safely performed over 100 mitral valve operations using limited-access methods described in this chapter.

Table 22.1 *Ideal mitral valve operation*

Tiny chest incisions – ports only	Excellent intra-atrial exposure
Tactile feedback	Same or better quality operation
Eye–brain-like visualization	Valve repairs 60–80%
Facile, secure valve attachment	Reoperation 1–2%
Minimal cardiopulmonary bypass	Mortality 1–2%
Central antegrade perfusion	Surgical pathway memory to teach learners
Minimal blood product usage	Radiographical instrument positioning and tracking
Minimal ventilatory and inte. ve care unit times	
Dexterous intracardiac access	
Subvalvular facility	
Complete valve topography	
No instrument conflicts	

Table 22.2 *Minimally invasive cardiac surgery Carpentier/Loulmet classification*

Level I
 Mini-incision (10–12 cm)
 Direct vision
Level II
 Micro-incisions (4–6 cm)
 Video-assisted
Level III
 Micro (4–6 cm) or port (3–7 cm) incision
 Video-directed
Level IV
 Port incision—robotic instruments
 Video-directed

PRINCIPLES AND JUSTIFICATIONS

The most popular limited-access incisions and techniques for mitral surgery are the upper hemisternotomy with standard aortic clamping and direct vision, and a right minithoracotomy with aortic occlusion using an endoaortic balloon and direct visualization. Right parasternal incisions seem to have faded away because of chest wall complications. For minimal access mitral surgery, Carpentier prefers a **C**-shaped midsternotomy, and Doty now uses lower hemisternotomy. In an effort to decrease postoperative discomfort and hospitalization and return patients to normality quickly, we use videoscopic techniques and 4–6 cm incisions for nearly all cases of isolated mitral valve disease. We have bypass grafted two patients simultaneously through a small left chest incision. However, at present, we do not suggest combined surgery. Obesity and age have not been contraindications for this type of surgery.

Both rheumatic and myxomatous valve replacement and repairs are amenable to these techniques. The operation is particularly applicable to younger women, who desire a very cosmetic operation. Incisions can be placed so that even scanty clothing will not reveal them. We have been impressed with videoscopy for repairing and replacing mitral valves in patients who have had previous coronary operations. Hypothermic fibrillation provides a quiet, safe mode for approaching the valve without aortic clamping. Our series includes over 60 reoperative mitral valve cases, and the method seems particularly applicable. Early in the series, we were reluctant to attempt videoscopic repairs for anterior leaflet pathology. Now, we advocate anterior leaflet chordal transfers, replacements, and segmental patching using videoscopic means.

Despite our liberal use of these techniques, relative contraindications include previous pleural scaring, previous right thoracotomy, severe pulmonary hypertension (pulmonary artery systolic [PAS] greater than 70 torr), severe posterior annular calcification, a calcified or highly atherosclerotic ascending aorta. Patients should be selected on an individual basis; however, each of these contraindications has occasionally been ignored with a good outcome. We remain concerned when pulmonary hypertension is severe and a small right coronary artery exists. In this instance, suboptimal myocardial protection may result more easily in right ventricular dysfunction, especially if any air is embolized.

Preoperatively, patients are counseled regarding the most common potential risks, which include stroke, myocardial infarction, bleeding, heart failure, and death. Thus far, our ECU operative mortality has been less than 2 per cent, and we have had 2 strokes, no infarctions, and residual heart failure. Postoperative bleeding is much less common (0.9 per cent) than in sternotomy patients. Currently, when the articulated daVinci robotic device (Intuitive Surgical, Mountain View, CA) is used for mitral valve surgery, patients and family are informed additionally. Early operations were done on a U.S. Food and Drug Administration Institutional Review Board-approved study. Now that da Vinci has been FDA approved we use it routinely.

VIDEO-ASSISTED AND VIDEO-DIRECTED MITRAL VALVE SURGERY

The ECU 'micro-mitral' operation (MMO) embraces the combined benefits of a 5–6 cm minithoracotomy, direct percutaneous transthoracic aortic clamp occlusion, telescopic video assistance, centrifugal pump-assisted venous return, and instrument development. Peripheral arterial perfusion was selected initially because of convenience and wide exposure. Nevertheless, with femoral vessel cannulation and retrograde flow, higher potential for arterial injury, aortic dissection, and deep venous thrombosis exists. Central arterial cannulation is becoming more feasible, even in closed chests. Recently, voice-activated robotic camera operation also has been added to provide direct 'surgeon-cerebral' camera manipulation. The combination of these and other modalities has brought us close to our videoscopic goal in a relatively short time.

ANESTHESIA AND PRESURGICAL PREPARATION

Generally, single left-lung ventilation has been used to obtain intrathoracic exposure. In some centers, bronchial blockers are used to deflate the right lung. A left internal jugular vein Swan-Ganz catheter is inserted and floated to a near wedge position. For superior vena caval (SVC) drainage, a right internal jugular 17-Fr Biomedicus cannula (Medtronic Inc., Minneapolis, MN) can be inserted over a guidewire using coaxial dilators and positioned with the tip located near the right atriocaval junction. This procedure is best done by the anesthesiologist before surgical draping. Independent SVC drainage is especially important when using robotic devices. Here, the transthoracic aortic clamp must be placed posteriorly (dorsal) and can cause SVC kinking with ventral atrial retraction. After heparin reversal, when withdrawing this catheter after surgery, hemostasis is obtained easily with pressure alone.

1 A transesophageal echocardiographic (TEE) probe is then positioned and a study done. All air removal strategies are inadequate without close TEE monitoring. External defibrillator patches should be placed on the right posterior scapula and on the left anterior chest, subtending the greatest cardiac mass. The patient should then be positioned with the right chest elevated 40 degrees and the shoulders tilted back slightly. The right arm is suspended across the chest. The patient is then prepared and draped in a sterile manner. Generally, we topographically mark the midsternal line and right second to fifth intercostal spaces. At this time, the Aesop 3000 (Intuitive Surgical Inc, Sunnyvale, Calif., Santa Barbara, CA) robotic arm is positioned as shown.

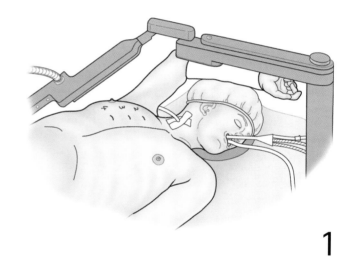

1

PREOPERATIVE MITRAL VALVE FUNCTIONAL ASSESSMENT

Accurate valve function assessment is necessary both preoperatively by TEE and intraoperatively either by videoscopy or direct vision. As micro incision operations provide less opportunity for direct assessment, a detailed preoperative TEE study is essential and should include four-chamber, short-axis, and transgastric views. The transgastric view has been particularly helpful in localizing pathology in prolapsing valves, as specific leaflet segment leakage can be masked in other views. Modern repair surgeons must have expertise in echocardiography, as individual anatomical valve repairs become predicated on personal ability to plan the reconstruction. After the atrium is opened, a pressurized saline test should be done and compared to echo assessment. Just as in our sternotomy-based repairs, we have applied Carpentier's functional categories to our endoscopic repair philosophy.

Type I – normal leaflets

In this situation, the posterior mitral annulus has become dilated along the muscular portion, changing the normal D-shaped geometry to a more spherical configuration. Thus, the posterior leaflet edges become distracted radially away from the normal coaptation points along the anterior leaflet, resulting in a central leak. Anterior annular deformation is unusual because of the fibrous complement. Type I insufficiency most commonly occurs with global ischemia and/or cardiomyopathy. However, type II and III insufficiency also may affect secondary annular dilation, eventuating in additive type I leakage. The simplest endoscopic repairs have been in patients with type I pathology. Annuloplasty ring implantation generally promotes sufficient leaflet coaptation and valvular competence.

Type II – leaflet prolapse

Type II regurgitation occurs most commonly with ruptured or elongated chords. However, acute and chronic ischemia may result in either papillary muscle elongation or rupture and leaflet prolapse. Repairs for type II insufficiency, either by resection, chordal transfer, or polytetrafluoroethylene neochord insertion, must re-establish natural chordal geometry and length. Except in children, an annuloplasty always should be added to the repair. Edge-to-edge (Alfieri) leaflet approximation is an option for repairing isolated segmental prolapse in a large annulus. The latter method promises to be a good way to repair severe bileaflet or Barlow's valves using videoscopy. Severe Barlow's disease is the most difficult type to repair videoscopically, as variable chordal elongation exists among valve regions. Individual chordal shortening is difficult with two-dimensional videoscopic means. However, segmental resections, polytetrafluoroethylene chord implantations, and Alfieri techniques are amenable to videoscopic repairs of anterior leaflet problems. We still prefer a full sternal approach to repair ischemia-related papillary muscle ruptures. Also, for multi-segment Barlow's pathology, either full or modified sternotomy and direct vision approaches or robotic methods are preferred, especially when commisural involvement exists.

Type III – restrictive leaflets

Rheumatic fever still is the most common cause of restrictive insufficiency. Ventricular dilatation, from either acute or chronic ischemia, also can cause restriction by lateral displacement of papillary muscles, which distract chords toward the cardiac apex during systole. Resultant tethering of leaflet edges causes an asymmetric leak jet. Most frequently, remodeling by a standard complete ring implantation corrects ischemic insufficiency. In type III rheumatic insufficiency, deformed subvalvular structures cause retraction of leaflet edges. In type III situations, either anteriorly or posteriorly directed echo jets suggest either rheumatic chordal shortening or transient dyskinesia with regional chordal tethering. In the latter circumstance, the saline test may appear normal and an asymmetric annuloplasty ring may work. In insufficient rheumatic valves, the plane of leaflet coaptation must be re-established either by papillary fenestration, cusp extension, chordal resection (perhaps with polytetrafluoroethylene replacement), or chordal plasty. Repairs of complex rheumatic valves are best approached conventionally; however, valve replacements are quite amenable to videoscopic surgery.

OPERATIVE TECHNIQUE

2a–d

For peripheral cardiopulmonary perfusion, a 2-cm infrainguinal ligament transverse incision is made over the femoral vessels. Both the femoral artery and vein are identified, with little dissection around the vessels. A 4/0 Prolene (Ethicon, Inc., Cincinnati, OH) longitudinal-oval, purse-string suture is placed on the surface of each vessel for cannula introduction. Using the Seldinger technique with guide wire and dilators, either a 17- or 19-Fr Biomedicus femoral arterial cannula is inserted and passed as far as the iliac-aortic junction. Similarly, a long 23-Fr DLP (Medtronic, Inc., Minneapolis, MN) femoral venous cannula is passed to the right atrium under echo control. Care should be taken to follow the guide wire–directed dilators, and no force should be exerted. To date, we have had no retrograde aortic dissections; however, these can be disastrous. For small or atherosclerotic femoral arteries, central cannulation of the ascending aortic arch can be done safely. A Biomedicus catheter can be introduced either through the incision or a second interspace port. Newer ascending aortic arch Endodirect cannulas (Cardisvations, Somerville, NJ) have been shown to be effective for central antegrade perfusion. For this technique, a double pursestring suture is placed in the lateral aorta, just below the innominate artery, and the catheter is inserted over progressive dilators. It is best to have the thoracoscopic camera in place before doing this less-controlled maneuver. The combination of percutaneous femoral and internal jugular venous drainage has been ideal. The anesthesiologist inserts this cannula before patient positioning.

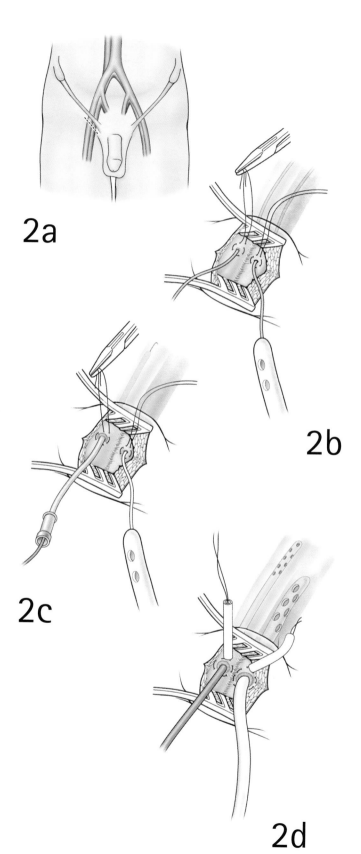

2a

2b

2c

2d

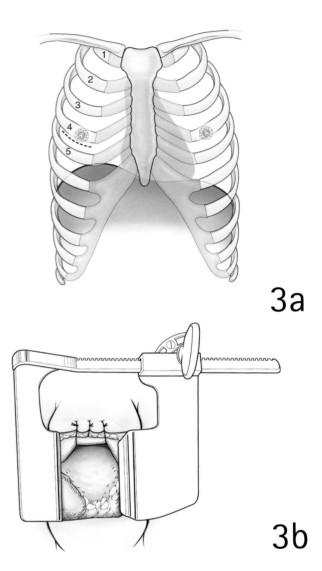

3a

3b

3a, b A 4–6 cm submammary incision is performed. A pectoral flap is elevated cephalically to the level of the fourth rib anteriorly, and after the right lung is deflated, the fourth intercostal space is entered into the free pleural space. A short thoracic retractor (ESTECH Danville, California) is used to spread soft tissues and elevate the upper chest wall with almost no rib spreading. A longer lift retractor and some rib retraction will become necessary for large patients. Carbon dioxide is continuously flushed into the chest cavity to minimize post operative intracardiac air.

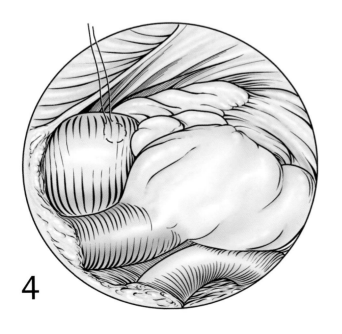

4

4 The pericardium is opened longitudinally, 2 cm anterior (ventral) to the phrenic nerve, under direct vision. The incision is carried anterior to the SVC and on to the aortopericardial reflection. Several 2/0 silk retention sutures are placed between the anterior pericardial edge and the skin edge. These are tied very tight, rotating the heart and aorta toward the incision. After cardiopulmonary bypass is established using assisted (suction) venous return, a transthoracic skewer or suture puller is passed through the chest wall. 2/0 Silk sutures are placed on the most cephalic and inferior portions of the posterior pericardial edge and pulled through the chest wall for lateral retraction of the pericardial edge. After bypass is established, these sutures are tied around small rubber tubes, distracting the dorsal pericardial edge even more toward the incision, which pulls the aorta even more toward the incision. In many cases, the ascending aorta is quite visible by direct vision.

5a, b The Aesop 3000 should have been placed on the left side of the table near the head with the arm positioned across the chest, before prepping the patient. The surgeon should be positioned near the right shoulder with a good view of the monitor. The monitor should be oriented parallel to the surgeon's plane of vision. Voice activation of Aesop 3000 by the surgeon allows 'in/out,' 'right/left,' and 'up/down' types of movements of the 5-mm camera-telescope tip placed posterior to the incision via a trocar in the fourth interspace. This robot can also memorize three separate camera positions with instant electromechanical position recall. Other types of manual camera holders also work well.

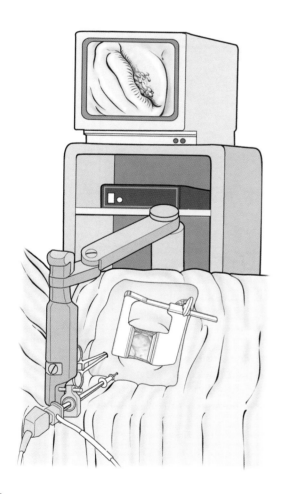

5a

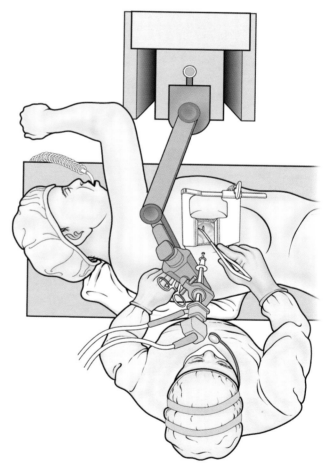

5b

6 The surgeon's position is shown.
Cardiopulmonary bypass is established with the systemic temperature lowered to 26°–28°C. An antegrade cardioplegia cannula is placed along the anterior ascending aorta, under either direct or assisted vision. Retrograde cardioplegia is used occasionally by cannulating the right atrial wall through the incision.

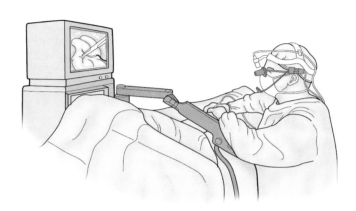

6

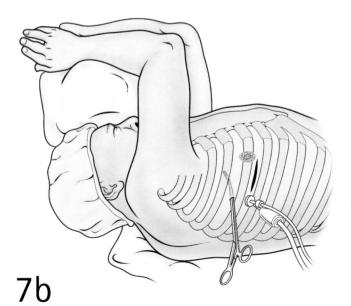

7a

7b

7a, b For introduction of the Chitwood transthoracic aortic clamp (Scanlan International, Inc., Saint Paul, MN), a 4-mm incision is made in the third intercostal space, just cephalad to the fifth intercostal space videoport, and along the midaxillary line. Under video-assisted guidance, the clamp is positioned with the immobile 'prong' passed behind the ascending aorta and through the transverse sinus. Care should be taken to prevent injury to either the right pulmonary artery, left atrial appendage, left main coronary, or aorta. The entire transverse sinus can be viewed with the camera during clamp deployment.

8 After cross-clamping, administration of cold antegrade blood cardioplegia, and asystole, a small (3–4 cm) left atriotomy is made just medial to the right superior pulmonary vein entrance.

8

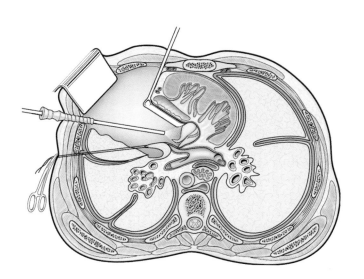

9

9 A transthoracic retractor (ESTECH, Danville, Calif). is introduced to provide atrial septal displacement and valve exposure. When the interatrial septum is retracted ventrally, the anterior mitral leaflet hangs free, much like a curtain. In large left atria, the lateral walls tend to 'fall in,' and early placement of commissure sutures helps establish anatomical topography and orientation. The surgeon is then ready to operate through the incision and 'voice-drive' the camera simultaneously. A small intra-atrial sucker will keep the operative field completely dry.

10 The valve being approached is shown through the incision. The camera is supplying all visual input to the surgeon. Early placement of either 2/0 Ticron (Davis & Geck, Hamilton, Bermuda) or 2/0 Cardioflon (Peters Inc. Paris, France) annuloplasty sutures facilitates visualization during more complex repairs.

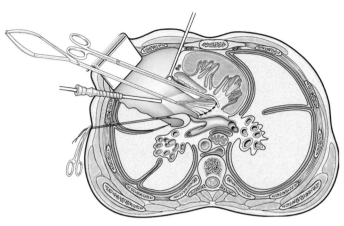

10

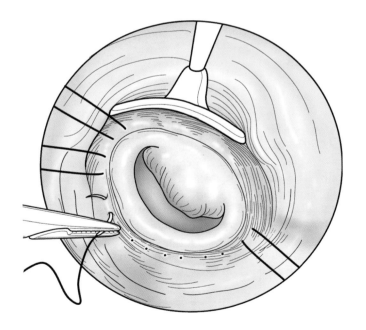

11

11 Moving along the anterior annulus, much like a 'technical climber,' new sutures are placed before releasing the preceding position. Exposure for each subsequent suture becomes predicated on retraction of the previous one. Generally, we begin at the left commissure or fibrous trigone and proceed counterclockwise. After placement, sutures should be arranged serially and suspended tightly from external Gabbay-Frater suture guides (Genzyme Surgical, Inc., Boston, MA). We measure the annulus and intercommisural distance after these sutures are placed. Often, the atrial incision is small, and sizers must be detached from the handle and passed with a clamp. Leaflet resections, papillary reconstructions, and chord insertions or transpositions should be done after annular sutures are completed.

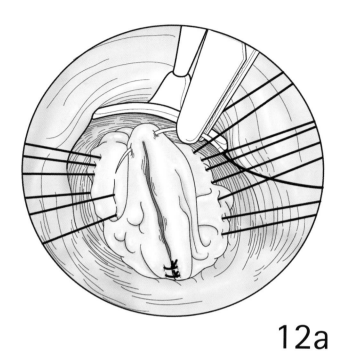

12a

12a, b Closure of a posterior leaflet defect with 4/0 Cardionyl (Peters, Inc., Paris, France) is demonstrated after a P$_2$ prolapse quadrangular resection. Using a specialized device, knots are made extracorporeally and tightened with the 'tail-hook' end. To prevent 'air' knots, while snugging sutures and securing annuloplasty rings, care must be taken to make the first knot a 'two half-hitches' slip-knot.

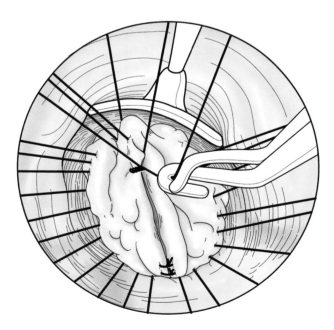

12b

13 For both repairs and replacements, anterior sutures usually require video assistance; however, posterior sutures sometimes can be placed by direct vision. When passing suture needles through the mitral annulus, a thin-bodied, short-jawed holder is best for providing needle stability. Varied needle positions and angles are required for optimal flexibility during suturing. Tissue torque tends to dislodge or rotate needles, and specialized shafted holders are a must.

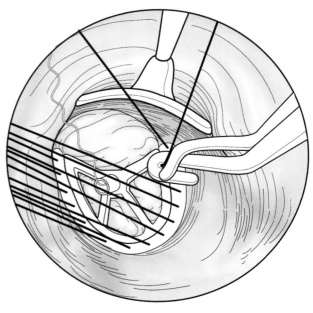

13

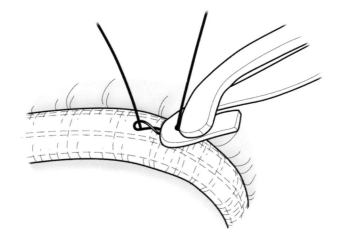

14

14 After completion of annular sutures, they are passed through the annuloplasty ring or band, and the extrathoracic prosthesis is lowered into position through the small atriotomy. We use specialized instruments to seat the prosthetic valve/rings and tie all knots, as well as to cut sutures to uniform lengths.

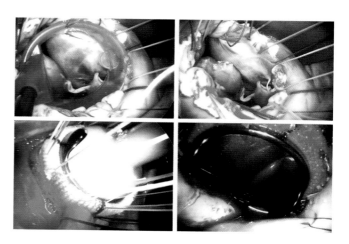

15 A videoscopic mitral valve replacement with a St. Jude mechanical prosthesis (St. Jude Medical, Inc., Minneapolis, MN) is shown.

15

16 A completed repair using a Cosgrove-Edwards annuloplasty band (Edwards Lifesciences, Irvine, CA) and a Carpentier-Baxter Physio ring (Baxter-Edwards, Inc., Irvine, CA) are demonstrated.

Finally, the left atriotomy is closed under direct vision. Before aortic clamp release, carbon dioxide is insufflated into the left atrium, while venous return is decreased and both lungs are ventilated. This maneuver helps to purge pulmonary veins of residual air. Multiple partial aortic occlusions during cardiac ejection are done to ensure cardiac air expulsion through the aortic vent. Complete air removal from the heart and aorta is confirmed by TEE. Usually, a single ventricular pacing wire is placed on the right ventricular anterior wall. After clamp removal, the posterior aorta should be inspected for injury using the camera, and then the patient is weaned from cardiopulmonary bypass using standard methods. A 30-Fr silastic chest tube is placed through the camera portsite, and the incision closed. In the event of right coronary air trapping, low-dose dopamine is of help for weaning.

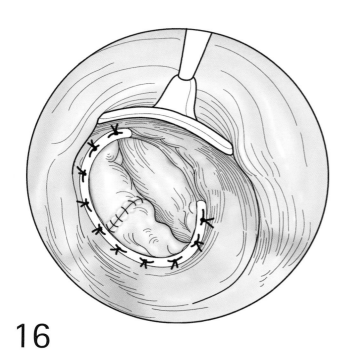

16

POSTOPERATIVE CARE AND OVERALL RESULTS

After final echocardiographic assessment of the valve and ventricular function, the double-lumen endotracheal tube should be changed to a single lumen tube. Most patients can be extubated within 3–6 hours after surgery. Generally, chest tube drainage is minimal; but if it becomes excessive, chest wall bleeding should be considered. In the above group, only one re-exploration for bleeding was needed. Prophylactically, we maintain patients on 3 µg/kg per minute of dopamine for 12 hours after surgery for complete right ventricular recovery. Pacing wires usually are removed on the first postoperative day, followed by the chest tube. An immediate postoperative chest x-ray is always obtained to ensure full right lung expansion and correct endotracheal tube placement. Cardiac function is monitored until extubation with either a simple central venous pressure or flow-directed pulmonary artery catheter. Most patients are ambulating on the first postoperative day with a discharge target of two or three more days.

OUTCOME

Since 1996, our group at ECU has performed over 300 videoscopic MMOs, with total series mortality of 1 per cent. One patient died 27 days postoperatively of an arrhythmia. For the entire series, one stroke occurred. One patient required re-exploration for bleeding. Three MMO patients had conversions to a sternotomy because of central cannulation site, left atrial and aortic bleeding. Two dialysis patients required late reoperation for endocarditis, and one was reoperated on immediately for a failed repair. Total operative, perfusion, and cross-clamp times have fallen markedly with experience, as have ventilatory and intensive care unit times. Perfusion times remain at 158 minutes with arrest times averaging 110 minutes. These have fallen from 183 and 136 minutes, respectively, as noted in our first 31 patients. For the entire series, the average length of stay is 4.5 days, compared with 5.1 days in our first cases. Both experience and robotic camera assistance have been added to improving every time-based parameter. With the addition of the Aesop 3000 robot, perfusion and cross-clamp times have decreased additionally to a mean of 144 and 94 minutes, respectively. We have seen no additional major complications or mortality in the complete series of over 300 patients and now maintain an 80 per cent repair rate. As mentioned earlier, most types of pathologies are now amenable to videoscopic minimal access mitral surgery.

Endoscopic robotic mitral valve surgery – the final answer?

17a-d

Computer-assisted cardiac surgery has taken on a new importance, although still in its infancy. One of the newest additions to limited-access mitral valve surgery is a true surgical robot – daVinci – that conceptually works by telepresence and remote instrument activation. Long instruments placed through small incisions lack the finest instrument and needle-positioning control. To regain as good or better finger control than sternotomy-based operations, surgeons no longer manipulate valve tissue directly, but through tiny electronically activated robotic instruments. Operators sit at the master control unit at a distance from the patient-side slave unit. A high-power, three-dimensional camera transmits the operative topography accurately, while two 1-cm transthoracic robotic arms emulate precise finger motions at the intracardiac instrument tips. Superhuman hand control is possible, through computer-assisted motion scaling, wrist-position clutching, and tremor filtration. Seven degrees of freedom are possible compared with three to four degrees with a human hand, impeded by long instruments and a limited-access incision.

Recently, our center obtained the first U.S. Food and Drug Administration Investigational Device Exemption to perform mitral valve surgery using daVinci. We also have finished a location FDA trial. The surgical preparation, perfusion tech-

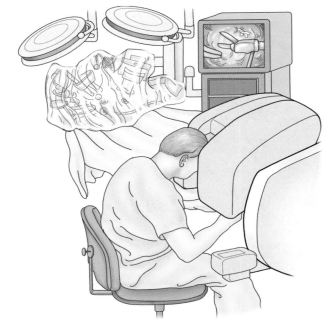

17a

niques, and limited-access incisions were exactly as described for the MMO. However, all intracardiac portions of each operation were done robotically from the master console, located 10 ft. from the operative site. Previously, approximately 20 mitral operations were done in Europe using similar methodology. By December 2003, we had performed 115 complete mitral valve repairs with daVinci. In most patients, trapezoidal P_2 resections were followed by interrupted annular and leaflet closures. Subsequently, Cosgrove annuloplasty bands were sutured intra-atrially using the daVinci robot and individual sutures. We had done sliding plastics and chord replacements transfer as well. All patients have done well despite longer perfusion and cross-clamp times that approached those of our first series of video-assisted operations. We have had no operative mortality. Operative times are following the same decrement as the MMO. Although robotic methods offer promise, surgeons must remain circumspect and pursue a defined evolutionary path toward the ideal mitral operation. There are many prudent, safe ways to improve patient care. Because of experience with open procedures, cardiac surgeons are in a unique position to innovate and develop 'cardiac microsurgery.' Technology developments and patient requirements will drive these needed changes.

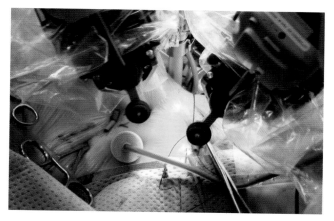

17b

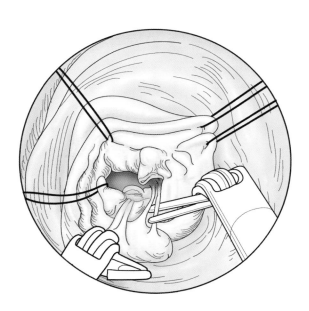

17c

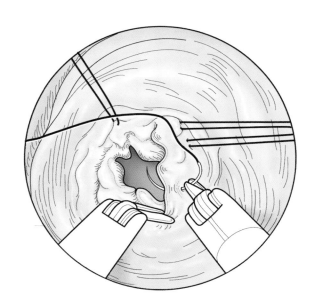

17d

FURTHER READING

Chitwood, W.R., Jr. 1999. Video-assisted and robotic mitral valve surgery: toward an endoscopic surgery. *Seminars in Thoracic and Cardiovascular Surgery* **11(3)**, 194–205.

Chitwood, W.R., Jr, Nifong, L.W., Elbeery, J.E., *et al.* 2000. Robotic mitral valve repair: trapezoidal resection and prosthetic annuloplasty with the daVinci surgical system. *Journal of Thoracic and Cardiovascular Surgery* **120(6)**, 1171–2.

Chitwood, W.R., Jr, Wixon, C.L., Elbeery, J.R., Moran, J.F., Chapman, W.H., Lust, R.M. 1997. Video-assisted minimally invasive mitral valve surgery. *Journal of Thoracic and Cardiovascular Surgery* **14**, 773–80.

Cohn, L.H., Adams, D.H., Couper, G.S., *et al.* 1997. Minimally invasive cardiac valve surgery improves patient satisfaction while reducing costs of cardiac valve replacement and repair. *Annals of Thoracic Surgery* **226**, 421–6.

Cosgrove, D.M., Sabik, J.F., Navia, J.L. 1998. Minimally invasive valve surgery. *Annals of Thoracic Surgery* **65**, 1535–8.

Falk, V., Autschbach, R., Krakor, R., *et al.* 1999. Computer-enhanced mitral valve surgery: toward a total endoscopic procedure. *Seminars in Thoracic and Cardiovascular Surgery* **11(3)**, 244–9.

Kypson, A.P., Nifong, L.W., Chitwood, W.R., 2003. Robotic mitral valve surgery. *Surg Clin North Am* **83**, 1387–403.

Nifong, L.W., Chu, V.F., Bailey, B.M., Maziarz, D.M., Sorrell, V.L., Holbert, D., Chitwood, W.R., 2003. Robotic mitral valve repair: experience with the da Vinci system. *Annals of Thoracic Surgery* **75**, 438–42.

Mitral valve repair and reconstruction

FRANCIS C. WELLS FRCS
Associate Lecturer of Surgery, University of Cambridge School of Clinical Medicine; Consultant Surgeon, Cardiothoracic Surgical Unit, Papworth Hospital National Health Service Trust, Cambridge, UK

HISTORY

The essential contribution of the intact mitral valve to normal left ventricular (LV) function is now widely appreciated. This complex anatomical interdependence has brought about increased efforts to conserve the valve and its subvalvar apparatus whenever possible. An exhaustive review of the physiology of this relationship is not within the scope of this chapter, but this is the cornerstone for the understanding of the surgical techniques described herein.

Current surgical techniques are based on the functional classification of valve dysfunction as described by Professor Carpentier. Before this important contribution, abnormalities of the valve were described in the context of the underlying pathological process. Although an appreciation of the pathology is important, it does not lend itself to a coherent method of valve reconstruction.

Using his functional classification, Carpentier devised a series of surgical techniques that have been robust enough to allow widespread dissemination to surgeons of average ability and that have stood the test of time. The proper use of these surgical techniques requires accurate intraoperative evaluation of the valve anatomy. Herein lies the key to a successful outcome for the patient. Although preoperative and intraoperative echocardiography are valuable in assessing the likelihood of achieving a repair, the technology is not sophisticated enough to be able to predict the precise surgical procedure that will be necessary. This level of information is only available on direct examination of the valve itself.

The main advantages of conservation and repair of the valve are better hemodynamic performance and the minimization of thromboembolic problems while obviating the need for long-term anticoagulation in patients who retain sinus rhythm.

FUNCTIONAL CLASSIFICATION OF VALVE DYSFUNCTION

Three categories of valve dysfunction, either independently or in combination, describe the full range of abnormalities that may be encountered in all patients. They are as follows:

Type 1: Normal leaflet motion
Type 2: Excessive leaflet motion
Type 3: Restricted leaflet motion

1a Type 1 dysfunction consists of annular dilatation, leaflet perforation, or a combination of the two. The leaflet perforation may be congenital as part of a spectrum of congenital cleft anterior leaflet (with or without partial atrioventricular canal defect), or it may follow an episode of endocarditis.

1b Type 2 lesions (excessive leaflet motion) are a result of elongation or rupture of cords or papillary muscles. Pathology relating to the papillary muscles may result from degeneration or ischemia. The most commonly affected leaflet is the posterior, but lesions of either leaflet or both leaflets are common. The easiest and most stable repairs are associated with degenerative posterior leaflet problems.

1c Type 3 lesions also affect both anterior and posterior leaflets and principally are a result of rheumatic heart disease. The number of valves that can be repaired in this group is understandably much lower than that of the type 2 category. Percutaneous balloon valvotomy has become an accepted alternative treatment for many of these patients. Open valvotomy continues to have a role, but valve replacement with preservation of the subvalvar apparatus is an excellent operation with sound long-term results.

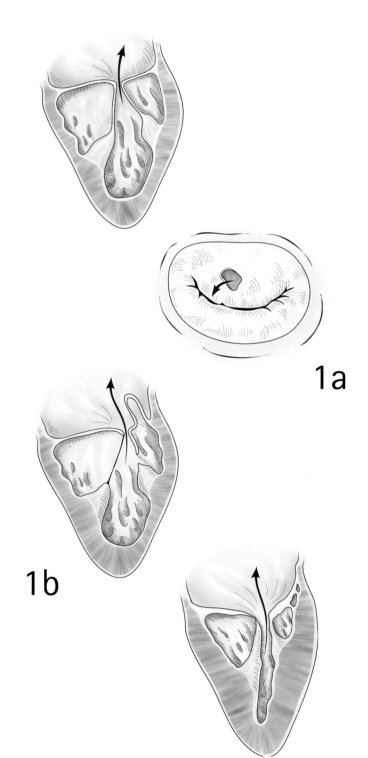

1a

1b

1c

INDICATIONS FOR MITRAL VALVE REPAIR

The indications for, and the timing of, surgical intervention in mitral valve disease has changed in the recent past. The decline in functional capacity of a patient with mitral valve disease is often slow. For many patients, precipitous change only occurs with the development of atrial fibrillation or the rupture of a cord. This natural history has led to the significant delay of referral of a patient for surgery until the change in ventricular function is very advanced. At this time, complete recovery of ventricular function is unlikely. This delay was as a result of the complications seen in association with valve replacement, especially if the subvalvar apparatus was resected. With the validation of safe, reproducible, and durable valve repair techniques, the situation has changed. Much earlier referral is now encouraged. It is particularly advantageous to the patient if repair can be done before the onset of atrial fibrillation and significant dilatation of the LV. The association between these two morbid factors has been established. Not only does timely repair obviate the need for anticoagulation, but it significantly improves mid- and long-term survival. An increase in LV diastolic dimensions of greater than 20 per cent should bring about a referral for surgery.

Early intervention on types 1 and 2 prolapse is most likely to result in repair in the hands of an experienced surgeon. The chance of a repair in type 3 prolapse is probably no more than 30 per cent, and some deferment is still acceptable. Surgery should not be long delayed after the onset of atrial fibrillation.

OPERATION

Safe and reproducible surgery on the mitral valve requires cardiopulmonary bypass. For most surgeons, this requirement means a midline sternotomy and aortic and bicaval cannulation with the use of caval snares. The heart is arrested using cold cardioplegia, and the patient is systemically cooled to 28°–30°C. Some form of cardiac venting via the aortic root, LV apex, or pulmonary artery is used.

Exposure is the critical factor in achieving a sound result. The main routes of access to the valve are as follows:

2a, b *A vertical incision in the left atrium just posterior to the interatrial groove.* This groove can be developed for quite a distance with sharp dissection carrying the incision closer to the mitral valve. The incision extends beneath the superior vena cava cephalad and the inferior vena cava caudad. Elevation of the posterior margin of the left atrial incision with a suture attaching it to the pericardium helps to rotate the atrium toward the operator and, hence, deliver the valve into view.

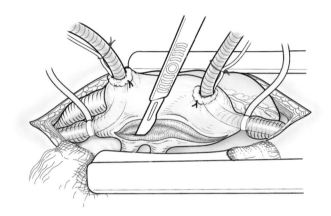

2a

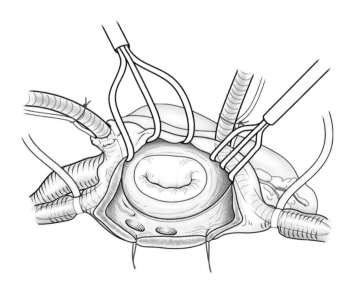

2b

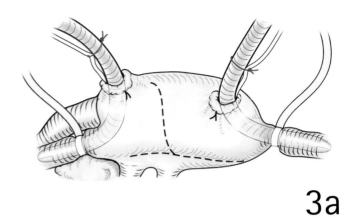

3a

3a, b *A transatrial incision as described by Dubost.* An incision is made in the wall of the right atrium directed posteriorly towards the interatrial groove. This incision is then carried through the septum up to the edge of the mitral valve annulus. This manouvre brings the mitral valve into excellent view in even the smallest of atria.

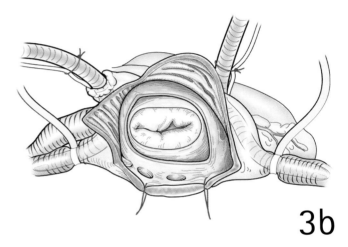

3b

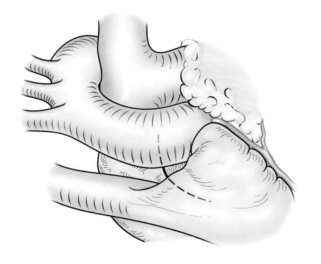

4

4 *The roof of the left atrium.* The incision is placed between the aorta and the superior vena cava directed transversely. This incision also gives good exposure, but it runs the risk of damaging the sinus node artery in some patients and cuts through the weakest part of the atrial wall, increasing the risk of hemorrhage post-repair.

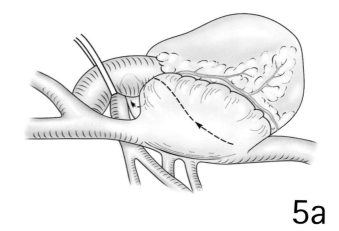

5a

5a–c A combination of the incisions depicted in Figures 3 and 4 is described as the Supracristal approach. Although this approach offers excellent exposure, it involves a great deal of repair work and, in my experience, is rarely necessary.

Should coronary bypass surgery be needed, it is generally better to complete the distal anastomoses to the native coronary arteries before carrying out the valve surgery. If aortic valve surgery is also required, my preferred order of proceedings is to excise the aortic valve and size the aortic annulus to select the appropriate valve, then carry out the coronary anastomoses before repairing the mitral valve. The left atrium can then be closed and the prosthetic aortic valve sewn into place. Deairing can then be carried out before removal of the cross-clamp and completion of the aortic anastomoses of the arterial or venous grafts. The judicial use of additional aliquots of cardioplegia may be used at suitable intervals during the operation.

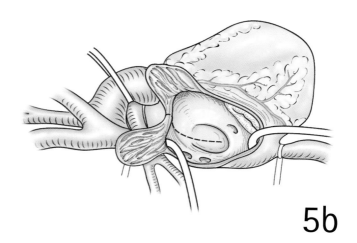

5b

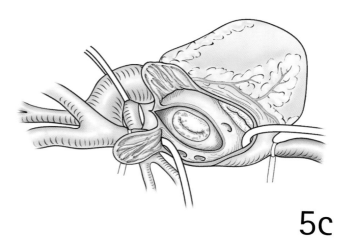

5c

Assessment of valve anatomy

A sound knowledge of mitral valve anatomy is essential. Assessment of the valve anatomy can be carried out as follows:

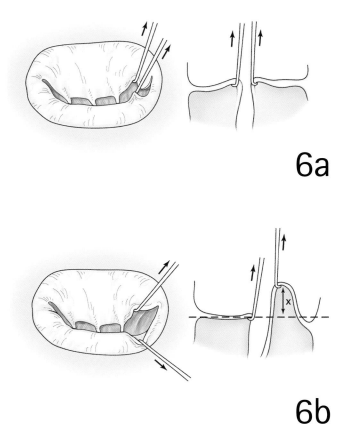

6a **6b**

6a, b Begin at the portion of the posterior leaflet next to the anterolateral commissure. Draw it out with a nerve hook, and do the same with the opposing portion of the anterior leaflet. Good apposition of the leaflet edges should exist with a coaptation length of 5–10 mm. The operator should then move along the leaflets, assessing coaptation of the anterior and posterior leaflets for the whole commissure. Sites of prolapse or restriction of one leaflet or the other are noted.

Most surgeons operate on the mitral valve with cardioplegic arrest. This situation gives rise to nonphysiological prolapse of both leaflets as a result of relaxation of the LV muscle and the associated papillary muscles. Thus, some experts have suggested that, to derive the most accurate assessment of the valve pathology, this leaflet assessment should be carried out with the heart fibrillating. Although the presence of tone in the heart may be a more realistic situation, the degree of prolapse of both leaflets after the administration of cardioplegia is likely to be the same for both leaflets. For practical purposes, examination of the valve after cardioplegic arrest is acceptable, provided that this difference is appreciated.

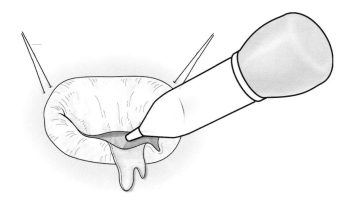

7

7 Another technique that is worth using as part of the assessment process is the forceful injection of saline through the valve with a bulb syringe. Provided that the aortic root remains closed, this maneuver will demonstrate prolapse of any portion of the valve that is present. Traction on sutures that have been placed at each of the commissures will elevate the annulus and allow a better appreciation of the valve.

8 In addition to leaflet and subvalvar lesions, attention needs to be paid to the shape and size of the annulus. Any significant annular dilatation will usually be obvious. Annular dilatation usually occurs in the region of the LV free wall (corresponding to P2/P3).

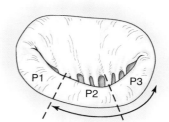

8

9

9 A common and important anatomical finding is the presence of scallops in the posterior leaflet. These scallops are important because a deep one on either side of the prolapsing segment can cause distortion of the repair, leaving significant residual regurgitation. Closure of such a defect may be necessary. If sufficient apposing anterior leaflet exists to fill the gap, however, it may be left safely.

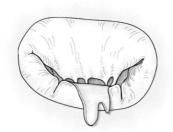

Surgical management of annular dilatation

Annular dilatation invariably accompanies mitral valve leaflet prolapse and, indeed, may be the primary pathological process. Uneven loading of the subvalvar apparatus may lead to stretching and rupture of cords and papillary muscles. In the absence of any leaflet prolapse, the dilatation may be corrected by the implantation of a remodeling annuloplasty ring. A great deal of discussion has taken place about what sort of ring should be used.

The normal mitral annulus reduces its orifice by approximately 40 per cent in systole. Normal basal motion of the LV is an important accompaniment of normal LV function. Evidence exists that has been derived from animal experimentation to show that this function is significantly impaired by the insertion of a rigid ring. Theoretically, the implantation of a flexible ring should allow better preservation of LV systolic function. However, very little evidence has been derived from the human subject who has suffered mitral regurgitation for many years. Whether such a diseased annulus can ever function normally again is not known. If that is the case, then it is unlikely that the choice of a flexible ring (which may lose its flexibility over time) will make a measurable difference to outcome in the long term.

An inadequate repair will give rise to problems. Implantation of a standard rigid Carpentier-Edwards annuloplasty ring will achieve a demonstrably good result, because the whole of the annulus is brought up into the same plane and the anterior leaflet is fully developed. This ring allows the best assessment of leaflet coaptation. Semiflexible and flexible rings exist, as do complete and partial varieties of each. A full discussion of the merits of each is beyond the scope of this text.

10 Other techniques exist for annular remodeling, including suture plication of the Paneth and Wooler varieties. Although not frequently used now, circumstances exist in which the knowledge of these simple methods is a useful adjunct to the procedure at hand.

Reduction of the annular circumference using the technique of quadrangular resection is also very acceptable; this technique will be described later. The most common technique remains the insertion of an annuloplasty ring. The insertion techniques are broadly similar for all. The method for the insertion of the standard rigid type is therefore described.

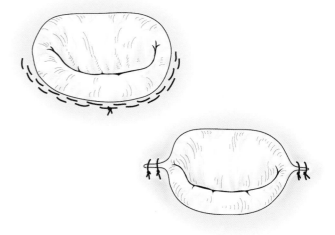

10

11 First, place a suture through the annulus at each commissure. The distance between these two points is measured, and the appropriate sized ring is selected. Account should be taken of the surface area of the anterior leaflet, as the end result must bring about good coaptation between anterior and posterior leaflets for the entire length of the line of coaptation.

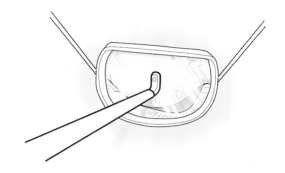

11

12 Sutures are then placed around the whole circumference of the annulus. Usually two sutures will be needed on either side of the center of the septal annulus. Care must be taken to avoid the atrioventricular node, which lies close to the anterolateral end of the commissure. When placing the sutures around the mural portion of the annulus, the other anatomical structures that lie in close proximity must be avoided. These structures are the circumflex coronary artery and the coronary sinus.

Spacing of the sutures in the annuloplasty ring must take account of the annular remodeling that is necessary.

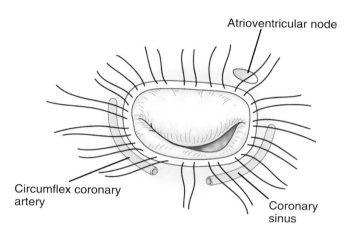

Atrioventricular node

Circumflex coronary artery

Coronary sinus

12

13 The ring is then slid into place and the sutures tied.

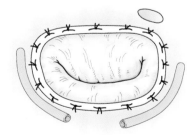

13

Repair of leaflet perforation

14 The most common etiology of leaflet perforation is endocarditis. Any residual granulation tissue or excrescences should be excised, leaving edges that are normal. The hole may then be patched using glutaraldehyde-fixed pericardium. A point to note is that the patch should be significantly larger than the hole to be patched (approximately 10–20 per cent larger), so that the suturing does not place undue tension on the leaflet and cause retraction.

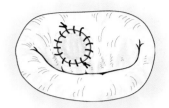

14

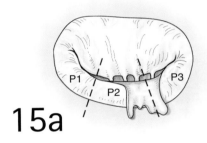

15a

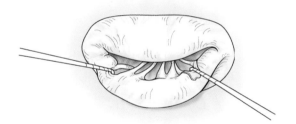

15b

Repair of posterior leaflet prolapse

15a, b This lesion is the most common affecting the mitral valve, and the one that is most amenable to a good long-term result. The prolapse can occur anywhere along the length of the leaflet but is most commonly found in the region of P2/P3. Often, more than one cord is ruptured or elongated.

16 The precise anatomical location of the prolapse and its full extent must be appreciated before the prolapsing segment is excised. This assessment is done by drawing up the leaflet with a nerve hook and comparing it with the opposing portion of anterior leaflet. Passing a fine suture around the first normal cord on each side of the prolapse will mark out the extent of the resection that is required.

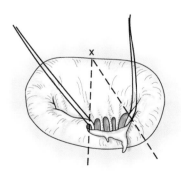

16

17a Imaginary lines are drawn, radiating from the top dead center of the septal annulus. These mark out the lines of resection of the leaflet. Resection of a little less than that which is necessary is wise, as the redundant portion can be incorporated in the sutures, adding strength to the repair.

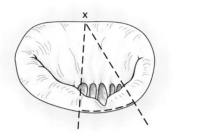

17b The mobilized portion of the leaflet is then resected from the annulus, leaving a rim of leaflet measuring approximately 1 mm in height. This resection ensures the integrity of the annulus.

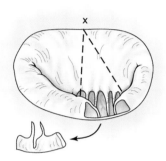

18a If the resected portion is not large (less than 20 per cent of the mural annular length), reconstruction can be by direct plication with 1–3 nonabsorbable sutures. Having these sutures pass through the annulus itself and not the atrium or the ventricle is essential, as the strength of these tissues is in the annulus.

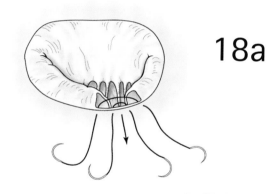

18b The center of the portion to be plicated is then drawn backwards, and each suture is firmly tied. No small holes should be left, as they can result in high-pressure jets, which in turn can give rise to hemolysis.

This procedure draws the resected edges of the posterior leaflet back together again without tension. The fact that the resection has been along radial lines from the center of the septal annulus also ensures that the leading edge of the posterior leaflet is under no tension at all.

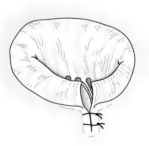

19 Sutures are then placed through the leading edge of the valve to line the leaflets up appropriately. The edges are then sewn together with interrupted fine monofilament sutures with the knots buried on the underside.

When the repair is complete, an annuloplasty ring may be inserted to ensure long-term stability of the repair.

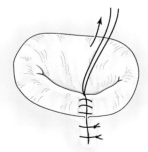

Sliding annuloplasty

20 In situations in which more than 20–30 per cent of the annulus must be resected, a sliding annuloplasty may be used. In addition, if the posterior leaflet is excessively high, a significant chance exists that the anterior leaflet will be forced into the LV outflow tract during systole (systolic anterior motion). This situation can be prevented by reducing the height of the posterior leaflet with triangular resection of the mobilized portions of the posterior leaflet. These resections do not have to be very extensive, as some of the redundant tissue may be taken up with the sutures giving more strength to the repair.

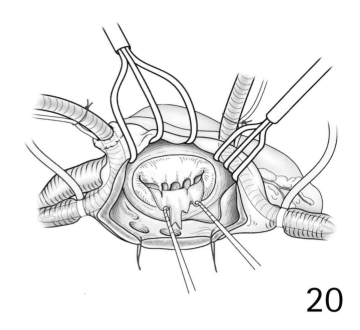

20

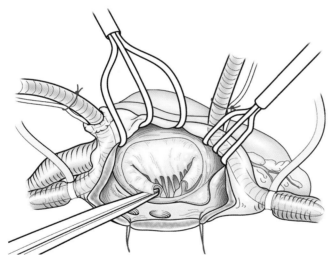

21 The first steps are as previously described for the simple leaflet resection.

21

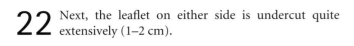

22 Next, the leaflet on either side is undercut quite extensively (1–2 cm).

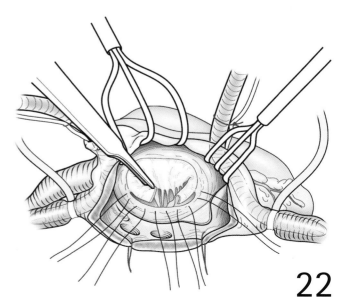

22

23 Each of these sutures is then plicated and tied individually. This maneuver will bring the leaflets back into alignment.

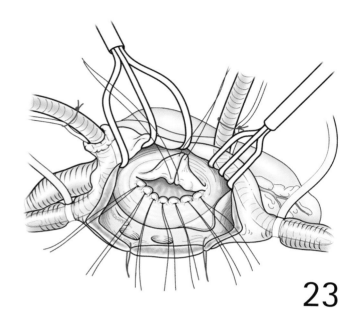

23

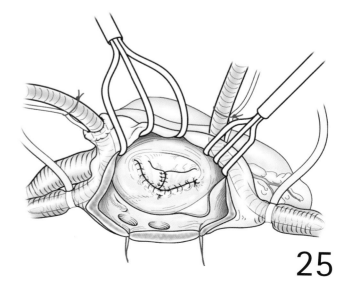

24

24 A suture is then placed through the leading and trailing edges of the leaflet. The suture through the trailing edge is then passed through the annulus at the point where the leaflets are equally placed over the posterior annulus. This suture is then tied.

Each end of the stitch is then used to resuture the leaflet back to the annulus. A separate suture is used at the opposite end of the suture line. The leaflet edges are then reapproximated with interrupted sutures, as described previously.

25 This method has the advantage of stabilizing a significant length of the mural annulus and may obviate the need for an annuloplasty ring. This theory remains unproven.

These two procedures cover the vast majority of posterior leaflet problems and also give rise to the most stable long-term results. Mastery of these two surgical techniques will allow repair of 70 per cent or more of mitral valve lesions.

25

Annular decalcification

26a Occasionally, the surgeon will encounter an annulus that is heavily calcified. The calcification may extend from one commissure to the other. Not only might this situation prevent satisfactory valve repair, but replacement may be very difficult. Techniques to deal with heavy calcification are therefore useful and important.

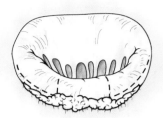

26a

26b The first step is to cut the posterior leaflet away from the calcified annulus with a knife for the full extent of the lesion. Then, with a scalpel, carefully pare the calcified tissue away. This step will often leave the fat of the interatrial groove exposed.

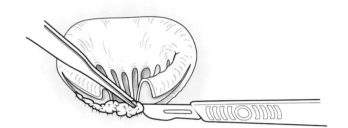

26b

26c

26c When complete, take a glutaraldehyde-fixed patch and sew it to the edges of the defect.

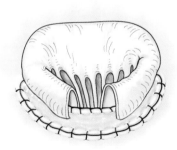

26d The leaflets can then be reattached to the annulus, completing the repair.
The long-term durability of such a repair has been reported by David and others.

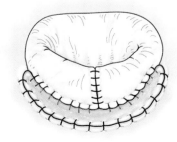

26d

Anterior leaflet prolapse

Extensive prolapse of the anterior mitral valve leaflet does not lend itself easily to satisfactory durable reconstruction. Initial encouraging reports of anterior leaflet triangular resection that extended back to the annulus have subsequently been called into question and have been shown not to be durable.

Chordal shortening has also been shown not to be durable in many patients and has been replaced by chordal reconstruction using Gore-Tex sutures as replacement chords.

27 A pledgeted 4/0 Gore-Tex suture is placed through the fibrous portion of the papillary muscle and then through the annulus, each end of the suture being passed through twice. The suture is then tied under gentle tension so as not to retract the ventricular wall beyond its normal position. This step may be repeated as often as needed to achieve satisfactory resuspension of the ventricle.

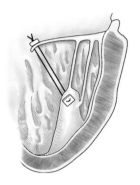

27

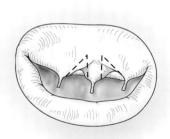

28a

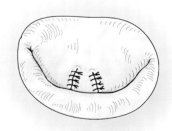

28b

28a, b Smaller areas of anterior leaflet prolapse between supportive chords may be resected with limited triangular resections. These areas can then be resutured to restore a normal leaflet surface.

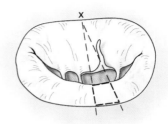

29a

29a–c For very discrete anterior leaflet lesions, a normal apposing section of posterior leaflet can be resected and flipped over. When sutured to the surface of the anterior leaflet, this patch will overcome the anterior leaflet prolapse.

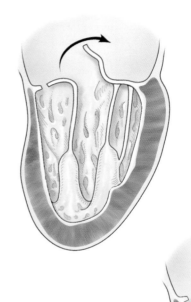

29b

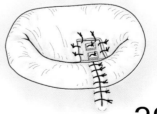

29c

Commissural lesions

30a, b Lesions involving the commissures can be so complex and extensive as to be irreparable. However, many local lesions can be repaired with resection of the prolapsing portion and plication of the annulus at that point. The leaflet can then be reconstructed using interrupted nonabsorbable sutures.

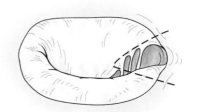

30a

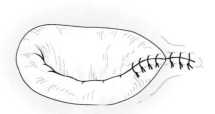

30b

Restricted leaflet motion

Type 3 lesions are most commonly a result of rheumatic disease. Several lesions are also associated with ischemia and a few other rare conditions. The amount that can be achieved with these lesions is limited, but attention to the detail of the lesion can result in a worthwhile result.

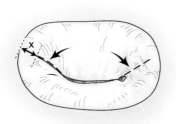

31a

31a Commissurotomy in the presence of flexible leaflets, although an excellent procedure, is rarely presented to the surgeon because of the effectiveness of percutaneous balloon valvotomy. The incision in the commissure should not extend closer to the annulus than 3–5 mm.

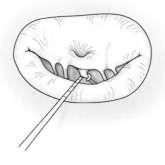

31b

31b Tethering of the leaflet by retracted secondary chords can be relieved by resection of those chords. They are sought out using a nerve hook and cut away. Fused and thickened principle chords can be fenestrated and 'freed up' to allow better motion and improved flow across the valve.

Testing the result of the repair

32 At the end of the procedure, assessment of valve function is important before closing the atrium and separation from bypass. This process may be achieved by the injection of saline across the valve under pressure. An alternative method is to perfuse the LV via an LV vent until the ventricle is distended and the valve pressurized.

Any remaining areas of significant prolapse should be attended to before closure of the atrium. Once deairing has been completed and bypass discontinued, the result can further be assessed using transesophageal ultrasound.

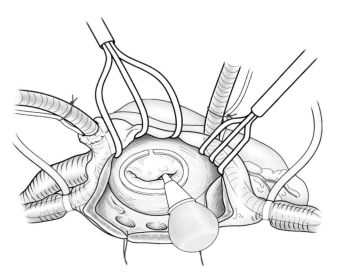

32

POSTOPERATIVE CARE

The patient is allowed to wake slowly while being observed in a high-dependency unit. Uncomplicated cases can be returned to the ward within 24 hours, and many within 6 hours. Patients with pulmonary hypertension may need to be taken slower to remove the risk of a hypoxic pulmonary hypertensive crisis.

Anticoagulation is begun as soon as bleeding has stopped and continued for 6 weeks unless the patient is in atrial fibrillation, an independent need for life-long anticoagulation.

OUTCOMES

Operative and early hospital deaths after mitral valve repair procedures are consistently less common in reported series than are early post-operative deaths following mitral valve replacement. To what extent these improved survival statistics reflect a clustering of poorer pre-operative status in those patients who are not suitable for mitral repair and require valve replacement versus a better tolerated operative experience in repair versus replacement patients cannot be determined. Whatever the explanation, the improved operative survival in patients having mitral repair versus mitral valve replacement mandates an attempt at repair whenever possible.

Other factors affecting early and late outcome after mitral valve repair surgery include pre-operative left ventricular function, the presence and degree of pulmonary artery hypertension, and perhaps most influential is the status of pre-operative right ventricular function. When there is substantial pulmonary hypertension and right ventricular dilation and dysfunction associated with chronic mitral valve regurgita-

tion, concurrent tricuspid valve annuloplasty may be required to ameliorate early post-operative right heart failure.

For the vast majority of patients requiring mitral valve repair for even severe mitral regurgitation, however, valve repair is very safe and effective. The concurrent application of an annuloplasty ring is especially important for a patient with a dilated left ventricle. Valve repair alone in such a patient may fail early after surgery because of progressive left ventricular dilation. Valve repair patients should be followed regularly with echocardiograms to look for evidence of recurrent regurgitation. In the rare patient with a regurgitant jet associated with incomplete closure of the posterior leaflet at the line of leaflet excision, the patient may develop hemolytic anemia from mechanical red cell damage at the point of regurgitation.

FURTHER READING

Carabello, B.A. 1993. The mitral valve apparatus: is there still room to doubt the importance of its preservation? *Journal of Heart Valve Disease* 2(Editorial), 250–2.

Carpentier, A. 1983. Cardiac valve surgery—the "French correction." *Journal of Thoracic and Cardiovascular Surgery* 86, 323–37.

David, T., Feindel, M., Armstrong, S., Sun, Z. 1995. Reconstruction of the mitral annulus: a ten year experience. *Journal of Thoracic and Cardiovascular Surgery* 110, 1323–32.

Deloche, A., Jebara, V., Relland, J., et al. 1990. *Journal of Thoracic and Cardiovascular Surgery.* 99, 990–1002.

Lee, E.M., Shapiro, L.M., Wells, F.C. 1995. Mortality and morbidity after mitral valve repair. *Journal of Heart Valve Disease* 4(5), 460–70.

van Rijk-Zwikker, G., Delemarre, B., Huysmans, H. 1994. Mitral valve anatomy and morphology: relevance to mitral valve replacement and valve reconstruction. *Journal of Cardiac Surgery* 9(2 Suppl.), 255–61.

Surgery for valvular endocarditis

J. R. PEPPER MA, MCHIR, FRCS
Professor of Cardiothoracic Surgery, Department of Surgery, Imperial College of Science, Technology and Medicine;
Consultant Cardiothoracic Surgeon, Department of Surgery, Royal Brompton Hospital, London, UK

PRINCIPLES AND JUSTIFICATION

Infective endocarditis is an uncommon condition with a prevalence of 0.3–3.0 per 1 000 hospital admissions worldwide or approximately 16 patients per million of the population per year. This entity is commonly classified into native valve endocarditis (NVE) and prosthetic valve endocarditis (PVE). Between 55 and 75 per cent of patients with NVE have a definite predisposing condition: rheumatic heart disease, congenital heart disease, mitral valve prolapse, degenerative heart disease, or intravenous drug abuse. Despite advances in antibiotic treatment and improved surgical intervention, the mortality of NVE remains high at 20–30 per cent. Early diagnosis is crucial so that appropriate treatment can be started. Delay in diagnosis may lead to increased mortality.

PVE accounts for between 7 per cent and 25 per cent of cases of infective endocarditis and has a high mortality of 23–70 per cent. These cases are usually divided into early and late infections, with early PVE occurring within 60 days of surgery. With increasing experience the dividing line between early and late is more sensibly set at 12 months. The incidence of PVE peaks at approximately 5 weeks after operation and levels off to a stable rate by 12 months. Early PVE is rare, caused by skin organisms, usually staphylococci, and carries a very high mortality. Analysis of the microbiology indicates that PVE that occurs within the first year after operation is commonly due to coagulase-negative staphylococci (Staphylococcus epidermidis), gram-negative bacilli, and fungi, organisms indicative of hospital-acquired infection. Late PVE is caused by the same organisms as NVE and carries an intermediate mortality, which is organism dependent, between that of early PVE and NVE.

In order of frequency, the aortic, mitral, tricuspid, and, rarely, pulmonary heart valves are infected, although any heart valve can be infected in NVE. Because of the fibrous continuity between aortic and mitral valves, infection on one may spread to the other, commonly from the aortic onto the anterior leaflet of the mitral valve. Infection tends to run a more virulent course on the aortic valve. Indications for operation in NVE are essentially the failure of medical treatment. Indications include (1) persistent fever despite appropriate antibiotics with adequate drug trough levels; (2) vegetations found by echocardiography on a valve, especially if the vegetations are enlarging; (3) evidence of peripheral embolism; (4) conduction disturbances or renal failure; (5) the presence of annular or myocardial abscesses; and, most important, (6) a deterioration in the hemodynamic status of the patient.

When a portal of entry can be identified, the most common sites are wound infections and the next commonest are intravascular catheters. Patients with early PVE usually have infection that involves the junction of the prosthetic sewing ring and the native valve annulus. Paraprosthetic leak is common in this situation, and further extension of the infection may cause tissue destruction, abscess cavity formation, and fistulas into adjacent cardiac chambers such as the right atrium or right ventricle. The presence of vegetations on the prosthesis creates the danger of embolization, and approximately 25 per cent of patients have evidence of peripheral embolism before operation.

The poor prognosis for PVE arises from the fact that the valve sewing ring is a foreign body, and foreign body infections are extremely difficult to treat. Relatively few microorganisms are required to establish these infections. Organisms adherent to the foreign body are less accessible to leukocytes and macrophages. Poor penetration of antibiotics into the foreign material is another factor.

PREOPERATIVE ASSESSMENT AND PREPARATION

The diagnosis of PVE should be as secure as possible. Multiple blood cultures should be taken at a time when the patient is not receiving antibiotics. Evidence of peripheral embolism and echocardiographic imaging abnormalities should be present. The decision to start antibiotics in a patient who has a prosthetic heart valve is a major one and should not be undertaken without first obtaining blood cultures.

The definition of active PVE depends upon confirmation of at least two of the following criteria:

1   A clinical picture of sepsis with features of congestive heart failure, peripheral embolization, and constitutional symptoms of malaise and weakness,
2   Blood cultures that are positive for micro-organisms,
3   Anatomical features of active endocarditis, specifically annular or myocardial abscess, vegetations, or paraprosthetic leak.

Transesophageal echocardiography (TEE) has revolutionized the management of PVE. In most cases the echocardiographic findings are obvious, but, especially in early cases of PVE, TEE features may be subtle. If the patient has had a routine echocardiogram after a primary valve replacement, those subtle changes may be easier to identify. TEE is essential for scanning the aortic valve and ascending aorta, as these are the commonest sites of abscess.

Because of the risk of dislodging vegetations from an infected prosthetic aortic valve, coronary angiography is usually avoided. In today's population of patients who undergo valve surgery, however, many also have coronary artery disease and may have had previous coronary artery bypass grafts.

Medical treatment of prosthetic valve endocarditis

All patients with suspected or proven PVE should be placed on intravenous antibiotics that are appropriate for the organism involved. If the valve remains without evidence of any anatomical abnormality on echocardiography, the diagnosis is uncertain, and antibiotics are continued. If the patient's fever does not resolve, a search is undertaken for an extracardiac source of infection. The chances for a successful combined medical–surgical cure are better if the operation is undertaken before extensive tissue destruction has occurred. Antibiotics should be continued preoperatively as long as clinical improvement is occurring, but we proceed to operation in almost all instances. We are particularly aggressive in the presence of *Staphylococcus aureus* because of its well-known propensity for local tissue destruction.

A patient with evidence of systemic infection who does not have evidence of sewing ring infection but has vegetations on the prosthetic valve is treated surgically in our institution. However, false-positive diagnoses of prosthetic valve vegetations do occur. Continued signs of infection such as fever or peripheral embolization are an indication for operation. Echocardiography is repeated weekly; and if the vegetations increase in size, operation is advised.

Aortic root abscess

Infective endocarditis that affects the aortic valve may be complicated by an abscess cavity in the aortic root, and this complication is more frequent and serious in prosthetic than in native valve infections. The terminology of aortic root abscess is misleading. Strictly speaking, uncontrolled infection causes a mycotic aneurysm of one of the sinuses of Valsalva, which is in free communication with the aortic root above the valve leaflets. This situation often results in paravalvular regurgitation directly into the left ventricular (LV) outflow tract. A true enclosed abscess cavity very rarely, if ever, develops. Several clinical features suggest abscess formation in infective endocarditis. These signs include new onset or worsening of congestive cardiac failure, involvement of the aortic valve, staphylococcal infection, poor clinical response to antibiotics, appearance of new high-degree atrioventricular block, and pericarditis.

TEE is now the imaging method of choice for most cases of infective endocarditis and is mandatory in suspected PVE. TEE offers particular advantages in the diagnosis of complications of endocarditis in the aortic root and the area of the aortic-mitral intervalvular fibrosa. Transthoracic echocardiography can give useful information about vegetations, the hemodynamic consequences of valvular regurgitation, and aortic root abscess. TEE can provide a useful anatomical definition of annular involvement and whether the cavity extends to involve the subaortic curtain or upper interventricular septum.

Principles of operation

1   The timing of surgery should be based on clinical considerations, not the length of antibiotic treatment.
2   Radical excision of all infected material including all suture material.
3   Restoration of valve function by repair or replacement, using simple sutures without pledgets placed into normal healthy tissue.
4   Use of biological material whenever possible .

The use of biological material has clear advantages. Aortic valve homografts are particularly useful in aortic root abscesses. They enable the abscess cavity to be completely excluded from the circulation, they are more resistant to infection than any other valve substitute, and their use allows a flexible approach to the operation.

The indications for surgery in PVE are uncontrolled sepsis, progressive congestive heart failure, peripheral emboli, and vegetations on echocardiography. These patients are often seriously ill, with hemodynamic instability and multi-system organ dysfunction.

OPERATION

Approach

All procedures are carried out through a midline sternotomy. Cardiopulmonary bypass is established with two caval cannulae and an aortic cannula. Caval cannulae are preferred to a single atrial cannula because this approach is more flexible if, for example, a fistula is found communicating with the right atrium. Separate snared caval cannulae also provide better myocardial protection for the septum, an important consideration in difficult redo procedures.

Myocardial protection

We use cold blood cardioplegia for these procedures. The details of our technique are described elsewhere, but two thirds of the initial dose (150 mL/m^2) is given anterogradely into the coronary ostia and one third retrogradely via the coronary sinus. Additional maintenance doses of cardioplegia are given by the retrograde route approximately every 20 minutes. Shortly before the aortic cross-clamp is removed, warm reperfusion (hot shot) is given retrogradely. Over the

last 10 years, the operative treatment has improved due to better myocardial protection, increased surgical experience, aggressive débridement of tissue, better management of the circulation with alpha agonists and pitressin, the use of homografts, and better management of blood loss. Nevertheless, the early mortality for PVE remains 10–20 per cent.

Homograft insertion

Two approaches can be used to implant a homograft valve. The first is to use the homograft as a freestanding root with reimplantation of the coronaries. This approach effectively excludes the root abscess from the circulation. If the tissue destruction has spread to involve the mitral valve, the anterior leaflet of the mitral valve belonging to the homograft can be used to replace the infected area in continuity with the aortic valve.

An alternative approach that is suitable for situations in which less tissue destruction has occurred is to use the original two-layer, subcoronary implantation technique. The proximal suture line is placed well below the abscess cavity, using interrupted fine sutures without tension and without pledgets. Inclusion techniques such as the 'mini-root' are not recommended, as they commonly give rise to distortion of the leaflets and thus compromise the long-term result. Intraoperative TEE is an important adjunct to this type of surgery, for it can help to ensure the integrity of the coronary anastomoses and the absence of turbulence, which, if present, may suggest distortion.

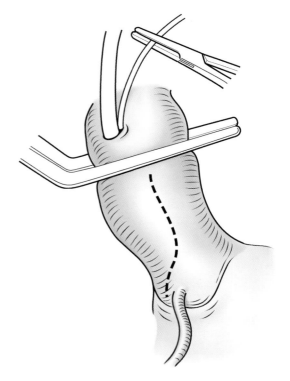

1a

1a, b The aorta is opened by a longitudinal incision to allow maximum exposure, which is particularly helpful in small aortic roots. If the aortic root is enlarged, a transverse incision 2 cm distal to the origin of the right coronary artery is very effective, especially if the incision is continued posteriorly and the aorta is transected.

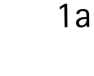

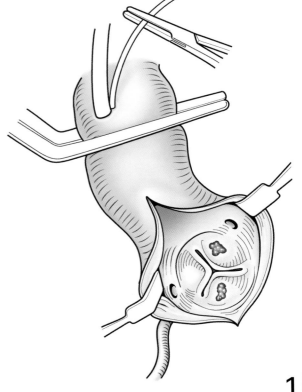

1b

2a All infected material is removed, including, in the case of PVE, all suture material, pledgets, and remnants of the valve sewing ring. Specimens are sent for microscopy and culture.

2b Endocarditis is limited to the leaflets of the valve with destruction of the margins and perforation. A two-layer subcoronary technique is appropriate in this setting.

2c Aortic root abscess is present at and above the level of the annulus. One or more coronary sinuses are destroyed, and partial (occasionally total) ventriculoaortic discontinuity exists. This situation is best handled by a freestanding homograft aortic root.

2d More extensive destruction involving the anterior leaflet of the mitral valve but with preservation of the chordae is shown in Figure 2c. This degree of destruction is more commonly seen in PVE. A freestanding aortic homograft root with the anterior leaflet of the mitral valve still attached can be used to repair the entire defect. This approach avoids the use of prosthetic material.

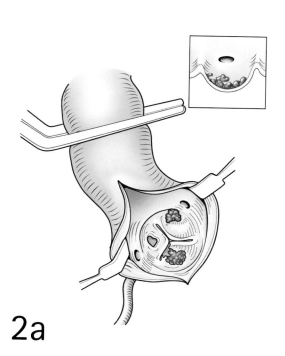

2a

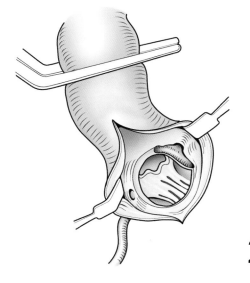

2c

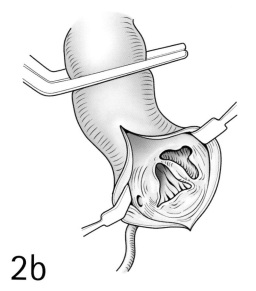

2b

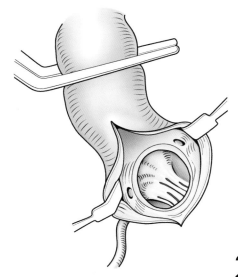

2d

3a
A subcoronary, two-layer homograft implantation is shown in Figure 3a. The proximal anastomosis is secured with interrupted sutures of 4-0 Ethibond. The use of fine suture material and small knots is desirable. The sutures are placed into the LV outflow tract into healthy tissue proximal to the infected area. Sutures placed deep into the muscle may be required. The knots should be tied firmly but carefully as apposition sutures. Pledgets are avoided because they are unnecessary and a potential site for recurrent infection.

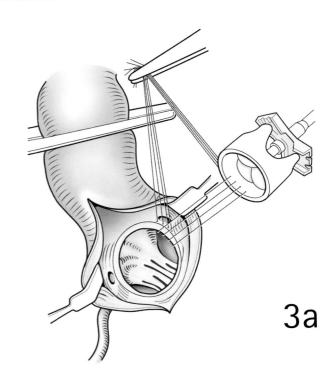

3a

3b, c
The posts of the homograft are secured approximately 1 cm 'above' the top of the original native commissure. This technique is most appropriate when three evenly spaced (120 degrees apart) commissures are present. The commissural sutures should not be tied down until the distal running suture is complete, as this maneuver aids exposure. The homograft has been inserted in the subcoronary position with the abscess cavities lying outside the circulation between the proximal and distal suture lines.

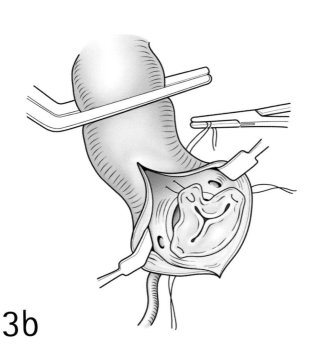

3b

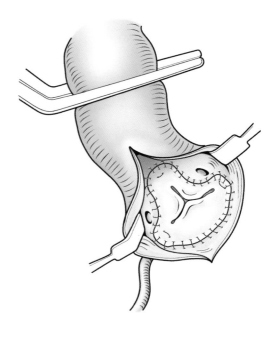

3c

4a Aortic root abscess is present above and below the level of the annulus.

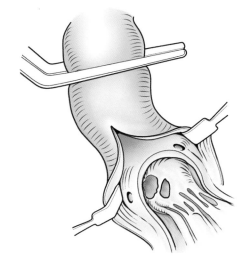

4a

4b The proximal suture line of the homograft is placed in healthy tissue within the LV outflow tract proximal to the abscess cavities. The attached mitral leaflet can be used not only to replace part of the mitral valve but also to patch abscess cavities on the septum by rotating the homograft through 120 degrees.

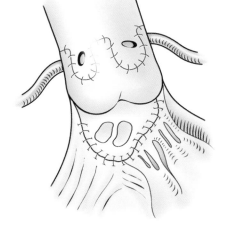

4b

4c Freestanding aortic homograft replacement with the proximal suture line placed proximal to or 'below' the abscess cavities is shown in Figure 4c.

Some authors have advised the use of a pulmonary autograft to provide a 'living graft,' but this approach is controversial, as the risks and benefits are finely balanced. Living valve tissue is more likely to be resistant to infection, but a less viable valve must still be placed in the right ventricular outflow tract. We have used this approach in patients with acute endocarditis, native and prosthetic, but have avoided it in elderly individuals with comorbidity.

If an aortic homograft is not available, a pulmonary homograft or a freestanding glutaraldehyde-preserved stentless valve can be used. The long-term fate of both of these valves is unknown, and they should be used cautiously. These valve substitutes may become aneurysmal; therefore, close observation with regular echocardiographic examination under the supervision of a cardiac surgeon is mandatory.

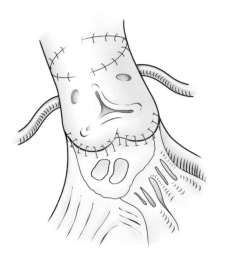

4c

Mitral valve surgery

Our approach is to attempt a repair if feasible. The use of the aortic homograft to replace the anterior leaflet of the mitral valve has been mentioned. The so-called drop lesions of the anterior leaflet that are seen in association with aortic endocarditis can be simply repaired with autologous pericardium. More extensive repairs of a commissure are frequently possible. Extensive destruction of the posterior annulus requires removal of all infected and devitalized tissue and replacement with either autologous pericardium or, if not available, bovine pericardium. A running 4/0 Prolene suture is used on the atrial and the ventricular aspects of the patch. A mechanical or bioprosthetic valve is then inserted using multiple simple sutures of 2/0 polyester material.

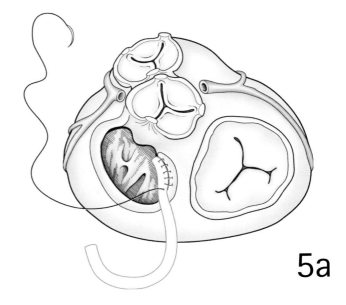

5a Circumferential reconstruction of the mitral valve (MV) annulus with autologous pericardium is shown in Figure 5a.

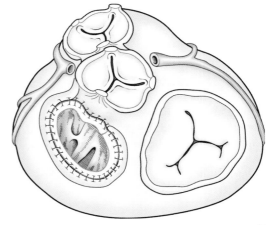

5b The pericardial strip has been placed and is made slightly redundant to facilitate the placement of sutures for the prosthetic valve (PV) insertion.

Tricuspid valve surgery

Infection of the tricuspid valve usually responds to medical treatment. Failure to do so implies the presence of resistant organisms, multiple organisms, or neglected disease. Fungal infection invariably requires surgical intervention. Similarly, if the patient has an indwelling transvenous pacing lead, operation is required. As with the mitral valve, we set out to repair the valve, if possible. If the valve is totally destroyed, the use of a mitral homograft in the tricuspid position is an effective solution. We do not favor total excision of the valve in line with other authors in view of the poor long-term results.

OUTCOME

The presence of an annular abscess is a significant predictor of future endocarditis and strongly associated with early recurrence. Patients with streptococcal infections do significantly better than those with nonstreptococcal infections in terms of recurrence of infection. Reinfection is common in drug abusers. Several case series of operations for PVE have been published. Larbelestier *et al.* reported a 5-year survival rate for 47 patients with PVE of 50 per cent, and a further 14 per cent required reoperation during the study period. Lytle had an overall survival rate of 82 per cent at 5 years, and freedom from reoperation was 75 per cent. Nineteen survivors (15 per cent) underwent another operation after their procedure for PVE.

Despite the decreasing in-hospital mortality for reoperation, the occurrence of PVE is still a major adverse event. The documented low incidence of endocarditis for patients who undergo a mitral valve repair or aortic valve replacement with a homograft is a strong argument for the use of these procedures as primary operations.

FURTHER READING

David, T.E., Komeda, M. 1989. Surgical treatment of aortic root abscess. *Circulation* 80, Suppl. 1: I-269–74.

Larbelestier, R.I., Kinchla, N.M., Aranki, S.F., Cohn, L.H. 1992. Acute bacterial endocarditis: optimizing surgical results. *Circulation* 86, 68–74.

Lytle, B.W. 1995. Surgical treatment of prosthetic valve endocarditis. *Seminars in Thoracic and Cardiovascular Surgery* 7, 13–19.

O'Brien, M.F., McGiffin, D.C., Stafford, E.G. 1989. Allograft aortic valve implantation. Techniques for all types of aortic valve and root pathology. *Annals of Thoracic Surgery* 48, 600–9.

Perreas, K., Rayner, A., Pepper, J. 1999. A simple and flexible blood cardioplegia delivery system. *European Journal of Cardiothoracic Surgery* 16, 482–4.

Petrou, M., Wong, K., Albertucci, M., Brecker, S.J., Yacoub, M.H. 1994. Evaluation of unstented aortic homografts for treatment of prosthetic valve endocarditis. *Circulation* 90, Suppl. II: II-198–204.

25

Use of pulmonary autograft for aortic valve replacement

THOMAS L. SPRAY MD

Alice Langdon Warner Professor of Surgery, Department of Cardiothoracic Surgery, University of Pennsylvania School of Medicine; Division Chief of Cardiothoracic Surgery, The Children's Hospital of Philadelphia, Philadelphia, Pennsylvania, USA

HISTORY

Replacement of the aortic valve by transfer of the patient's native pulmonary valve was first accomplished by Ross in 1967. Advantages of the pulmonary autograft include the fact that the valve is viable, has growth potential, can repair itself, has ideal hemodynamic characteristics, does not require anticoagulation, and has a very low risk of thromboembolism. Early results with the Ross operation were complicated by technical problems with harvesting the autograft and early failures related to technical problems with implantation. With the wide availability of multiple types of aortic valve substitutes for adults, the Ross operation has been used relatively infrequently in adults. Nevertheless, the optimal hemodynamics of the Ross procedure and modifications of technical features of implantation have eliminated most of the late concerns, and the Ross operation is now being met with renewed enthusiasm, especially on younger patients and possibly older patients who require valve replacement and have contraindications to anticoagulation.

PRINCIPLES AND JUSTIFICATION

Multiple valve replacement options are available for adults. However, no perfect valve substitute exists, and any choice of valve is associated with late complications, valve deterioration, infection, or potential for reoperation. Therefore, selection of a valve choice for any young or old adult patient demands a selection among potential late complications and the implications of these complications for each individual patient.

Advantages of the Ross pulmonary autograft operation for aortic valve replacement in adults include the fact that the valve is autologous tissue and has long-term viability, which may make it especially suitable in patients with endocarditis. The valve has optimal hemodynamic performance with an extremely low valve gradient after implantation and may even improve ventricular remodeling in long-standing aortic stenosis or insufficiency. The lack of valve noise and the low valve failure and reintervention rate on the autograft are favorable, along with the freedom from anticoagulation and anticoagulation-related hemorrhage. An extremely low incidence of thromboembolism has been reported with the pulmonary autograft valve.

Indications for consideration of the Ross operation for valve replacement in adults include single aortic valve pathology, mechanical or bioprosthetic valve failure, endocarditis of the aortic root, valve replacement in athletes or young adults in whom anticoagulation is contraindicated, patient age up to 50 years, and possibly older patients, if not debilitated. The indication of single aortic valve pathology is relative, because associated mitral valve repair can be performed with the Ross operation, and the Ross autograft replacement may be optimal in patients with a very small aortic root, even in the face of the requirement for other valve replacement or tricuspid valve repair. In patients without aortic root dilation but with valvar, subvalvar, and supravalvar aortic disease, the Ross operation with root replacement is the optimal treatment.

Indications for the Ross operation for previous prosthetic valve failure include inability to adequately anticoagulate a patient, recurrent thromboembolism despite anticoagulation, valve thrombosis on anticoagulant therapy, recurrent gastrointestinal bleeding or significant interference with the patient's lifestyle due to anticoagulation or valve noise, infection of the prosthetic valve, and early bioprosthetic failure. Certainly, patients who have early failure of a homograft valve should be considered for other types of valve reconstruction.

Endocarditis of the aortic root is a situation in which the viability of the autograft is desirable and use of the root replacement technique can exclude abscesses. The only true contraindication in the face of endocarditis to the Ross operation is infection of the pulmonary valve.

Use of the Ross operation in athletes or young adults with a contraindication to anticoagulation is desirable, because optimal hemodynamics are achieved. The major hemodynamic burden after the Ross operation is on the right ventricle (RV) due to gradients across the RV outflow tract reconstruction with homografts. RV hypertension is well-tolerated but may limit the functional result. Women of childbearing age are also good candidates for the Ross operation, as are patients with lifestyle contraindications to anticoagulation.

Contraindications to the Ross operation include connective tissue diseases, such as Marfan's syndrome, which affect the pulmonary artery and aortic annulus. Patients with significant immune complex disease, such as rheumatoid arthritis, lupus erythematosus, and active rheumatic heart disease, have potential for inflammatory change of the autograft with early failure. Nevertheless, large series of Ross operations for patients with rheumatic heart disease have been reported if the disease is not active with ongoing inflammation at the time of the procedure. Other potential contraindications to the Ross operation have been suggested, including advanced three-vessel disease, other severe valve pathology requiring valve replacement, severely depressed left ventricular (LV) function, and multi-system organ failure along with older age (greater than 60 years) and severe calcification of the aortic root. Most of these potential contraindications are only relative, because the optimal hemodynamics of the autograft valve may actually improve overall LV function postoperatively and other valve replacement does not preclude the Ross procedure. Significant calcification of the aortic root compli-cates any type of valve replacement and does not, in and of itself, contraindicate the Ross procedure. Older patients may actually benefit from the Ross operation by optimal hemodynamics if they are not generally debilitated and if coronary artery disease can be addressed at the time of the operation, as in other valve replacement.

The major absolute contraindication to the Ross operation is abnormal pulmonary valve anatomy. Patients with quadricuspid valves or distortion of the commissural attachments of the pulmonary valve should not have the autograft used as an aortic valve replacement, because leakage will almost inevitably recur.

PREOPERATIVE CARE

Patients considered for the Ross operation should undergo hemodynamic evaluation as necessary, and the indications for aortic valve replacement are similar to those for the use of other types of aortic valve prostheses. If the patient has had a previous operation, including ventricular septal defect closure or other operations that may have required suturing near the pulmonary valve annulus and could distort the pulmonary valve anatomy and function, additional information should be sought; preoperative echocardiography showing a normal-size pulmonary valve annulus with normal anatomy and without significant leakage is required before considering the pulmonary autograft operation. Mild leakage of the pulmonary valve may be well-tolerated or improved when placed under the higher hemodynamic load in the aortic position and does not contraindicate use of the pulmonary valve if it is otherwise structurally normal.

ANESTHESIA

Anesthetic techniques for the Ross operation are similar to those used for any major open heart operation for valve replacement.

OPERATION

A standard median sternotomy incision is used. After suspension of the heart in a pericardial cradle, aortic cannulation is done as distally in the aorta as near the innominate origin as possible to allow clamping of the aorta distally and improve access to the aortic root. Bicaval cannulation with venting of the LV through the right superior pulmonary vein is generally used. Retrograde cardioplegia can be administered through the coronary sinus or antegrade cardioplegia given directly into the coronary ostia as desired. Myocardial protection is provided with moderate systemic hypothermia to 28°C and cardioplegic administration.

1 Before arresting the heart, mobilization of the fat pad at the proximal aorta to identify the origin of the right coronary artery is advisable, and dissection of the pulmonary artery away from the ascending aorta with mobilization of the pulmonary artery branches is useful to facilitate reconstruction of the RV outflow tract after the autograft has been harvested.

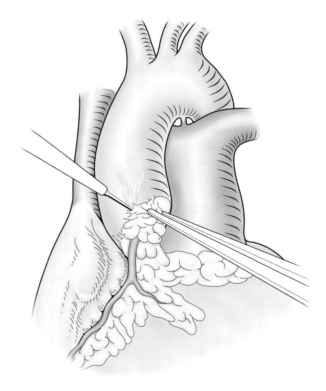

1

2a, b With the aorta cross-clamped and after cardioplegia administration, a transverse aortotomy is made approximately 1.5 cm distal to the origin of the right coronary artery, and the aortic valve is examined. If the aortic valve is not repairable, the valve is excised, and additional cardioplegia is injected antegrade into the coronary ostia as necessary. The pulmonary artery is incised at the origin of the right pulmonary artery, and the incision is carried obliquely to the origin of the left pulmonary artery anteriorly, allowing adequate exposure to examine the pulmonary valve. Careful examination is performed to ensure that the pulmonary valve is anatomically normal and, therefore, useable as an autograft valve replacement. If the pulmonary valve is anatomically suitable, the transection of the pulmonary artery is completed. If the pulmonary valve is bicuspid but otherwise anatomically suitable, and if the Ross operation is clearly the most preferable procedure, then use of the bicuspid pulmonary valve can be considered, although the late results of the use of these valves are not known. More significant valvular abnormalities, such as abnormal commissural attachments or extra or diminutive cusps, have been associated with early failure, and the valve should not be used in this circumstance. If the pulmonary valve is abnormal, the pulmonary artery can be closed, and valve replacement of the aortic valve is performed with any of the numerous other potential prosthetic valve options.

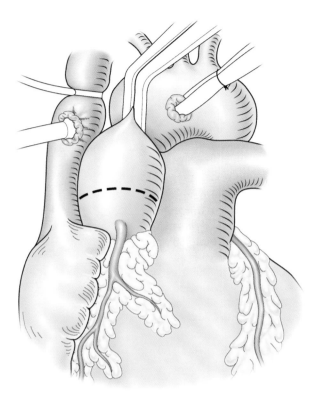

2a

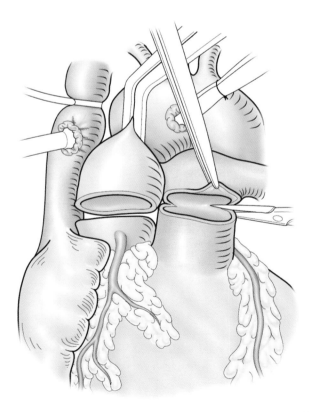

2b

2c If the autograft is useable, the pulmonary valve is retracted anteriorly, and initial dissection is begun on the posterior aspect of the proximal pulmonary artery adjacent to the pulmonary artery until septal myocardium is encountered. Staying close to the posterior aspect of the pulmonary valve will avoid the left coronary artery. Use of electrocautery dissection in this area is advantageous to cauterize any small epicardial vessels that may cause troublesome postoperative bleeding.

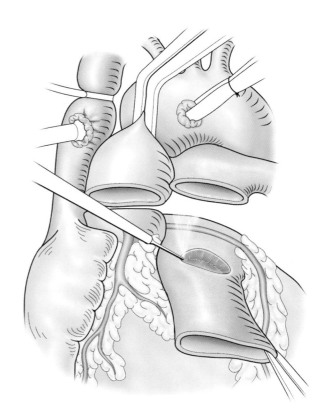

2c

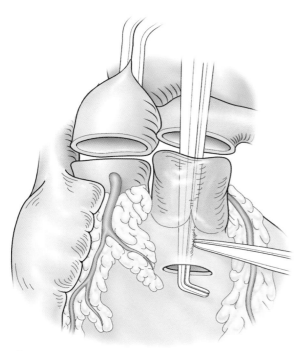

2d

2d After mobilization of the posterior aspect of the pulmonary valve, a right angle clamp is placed through the pulmonary valve approximately 4–5 mm below the pulmonary valve annulus where the anterior aspect of the RV outflow tract can be identified, and a small transverse incision is made below the pulmonary valve annulus in the outflow tract. It is important to make this incision lower than one would normally expect to avoid damaging the pulmonary valve, which sits lower than one expects in the outflow tract. Once the incision is made in the RV and the pulmonary valve leaflets are readily visible, it is possible to extend the incision in the outflow tract anteriorly and posteriorly, staying approximately 4 mm from the pulmonary valve annulus and avoiding major epicardial coronary branches.

2e Completion of the enucleation of the pulmonary autograft from the RV outflow tract is performed by partially incising the posterior ventricular muscle of the septum. A fat pad and plane of dissection is usually present in the plane of penetration of the first septal perforator off the anterior descending coronary artery, which traverses the septal musculature toward the conal papillary muscle of the tricuspid valve. Care is taken to avoid interference with this vessel; if care is taken to keep the dissection in the plane adjacent to the anterior muscle of the septum, it can be readily avoided. Often a fibrous tissue connection (i.e. the conus tendon) is present between the pulmonary artery and the aortic annulus, which may require sharp division to complete the enucleation of the autograft.

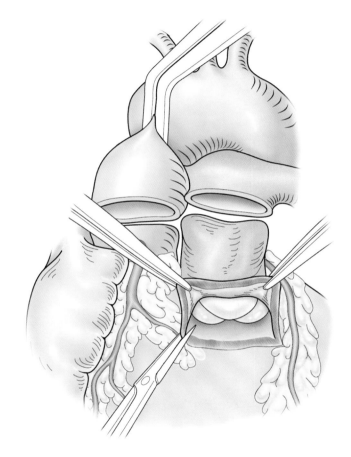

3 After enucleation of the pulmonary valve and pulmonary artery, the muscle beneath the pulmonary valve should be trimmed 2–3 mm below the valve annulus. It is often advantageous to bevel the muscle to thin the muscular annulus, which will then be placed in the LV outflow tract to avoid potential subaortic narrowing.

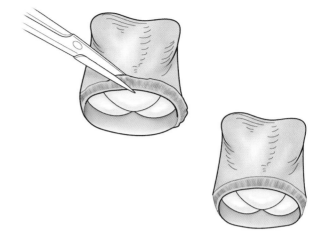

3

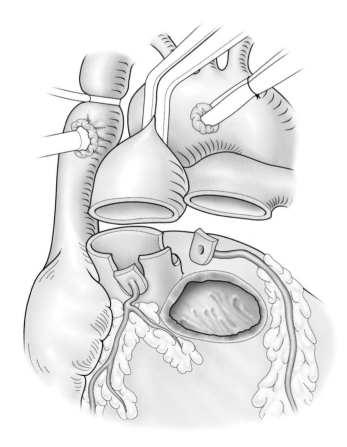

4 The left and right coronary ostia are then mobilized with a button of aortic wall for reimplantation into the autograft, and the remaining proximal aorta is trimmed down to within 3–5 mm of the aortic annulus to allow reinforcement of the proximal aortic suture line.

A major consideration for the pulmonary autograft implantation is size-matching between the autograft valve and the aortic annulus. In patients who have dilation of the aortic root such that the aortic root is larger than the pulmonary autograft, annular reduction may be necessary. The annular reduction procedure can be performed in several ways, including simple reinforcement of the annulus with a Dacron or Teflon strip at implantation of the autograft, downsizing the aortic root circumferentially as these sutures are tied. Direct annular narrowing can be performed either with plication sutures at the areas of the commissures of the aortic valve annulus with pledgeted sutures, or a with continuous annuloplasty suture as described by Elkins.

4

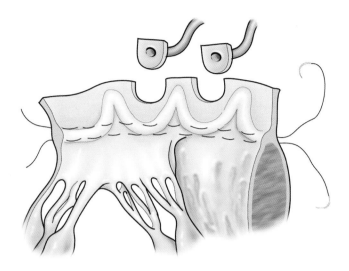

5a

5a, b In the annuloplasty technique described by Elkins, a double layer of continuous Prolene 2/0 or 3/0 polypropylene sutures are placed at the level of the aortic valve annulus in a transverse fashion and brought exteriorly, where they are placed through a pledget that is then tied over a Hegar dilator or valve sizer of the appropriate size for the patient's body surface area.

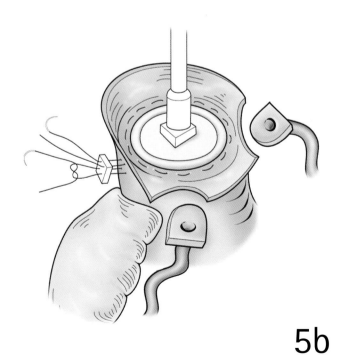

5b

6 Direct suture narrowing of the annulus can be performed beneath the level of the commissures at the aortic annulus with pledgeted sutures as an alternative. If the pulmonary autograft is larger than the aortic annulus, the excision of the aortic valve usually allows the annulus to dilate to match the pulmonary autograft, although incision into the LV outflow tract 5–6 mm to the left of the right coronary ostium will allow enlargement of the annulus to create an adequate size match in most cases. More extensive enlargement of the annulus requires the Ross Konno modification, which is described in Chapter 51.

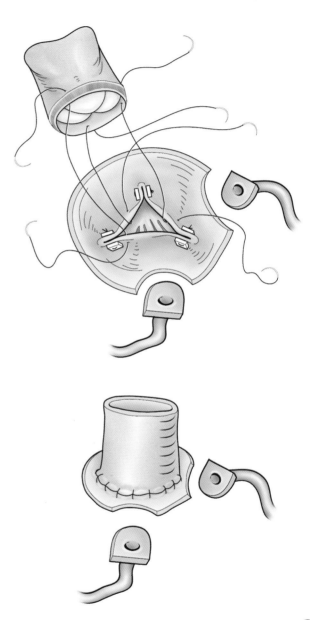

6

7 Implantation of the autograft is performed by orienting the autograft such that the pulmonary valve sinuses line up with the reimplantation sites for the coronary ostia. A suture is placed at the base of each commissure of the pulmonary autograft and positioned in the aortic annulus such that the aortic annulus is trifurcated by the three sutures. Because the pulmonary valve sinuses are equal in size and the aortic valve sinuses are rarely equal in aortic valve pathology, adjustment of these sutures is necessary to align the autograft in the aortic valve annulus.

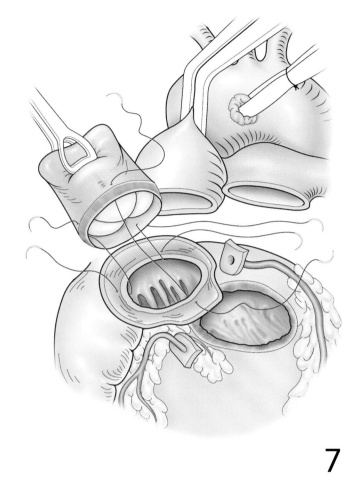

7

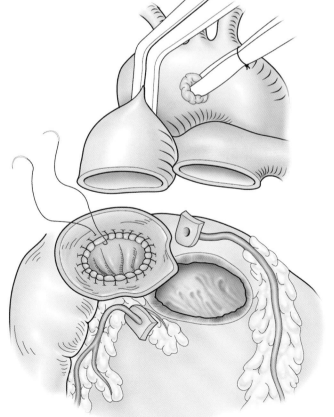

8

8 The autograft valve can then be inverted into the LV outflow tract, and additional interrupted sutures are placed at equally spaced intervals along the annulus; alternatively, the previously placed sutures can be tied and a running suture used to complete the proximal anastomosis.

9 If the annulus is to be fixed, as is recommended in virtually all adult patients with the Ross operation, the sutures should be placed through a continuous strip of Dacron or Teflon felt; alternatively, with the interrupted technique, the sutures can be tied over a strip of Dacron graft material to fix the aortic annulus at a set size. The aortic valve is then everted, and care is taken to inspect the valve leaflets to ensure that no injury has occurred.

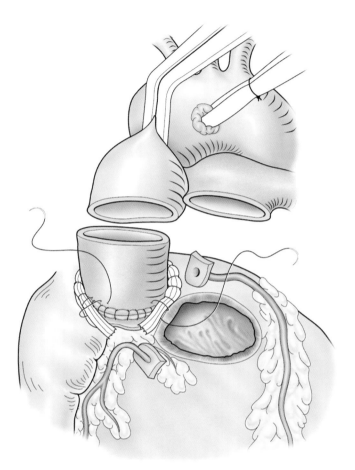

9

10 The proximal aortic wall is oversewn in a continuous fashion over the suture line, taking partial-thickness sutures into the autograft epicardial wall to reinforce the suture line to prevent hemorrhage posteriorly, where it can be difficult to control. When the autograft is implanted either with continuous or interrupted sutures in the proximal suture line, the sutures are taken in the area of the aortic annulus near the membranous septum to avoid interference with the conduction tissue. After reinforcement of the proximal aortic suture line at suitable sites on the wall of the autograft, buttons of pulmonary artery are excised, and the buttons of aorta with coronary ostia are reimplanted into the autograft using running 5/0 or 6/0 polypropylene suture.

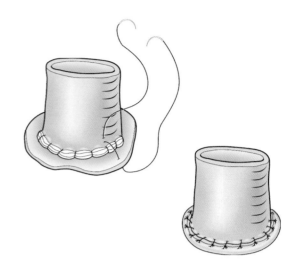

10

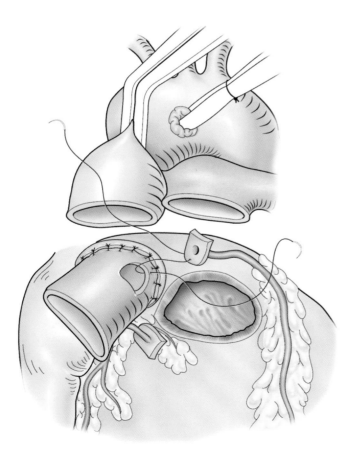

11

11 Both the right and left coronary arteries can be implanted at this time, or the left coronary can be initially implanted and the distal suture line created to allow the pulmonary autograft to distend to better judge the location for reimplantation of the right coronary, which can be higher than normal on the autograft wall.

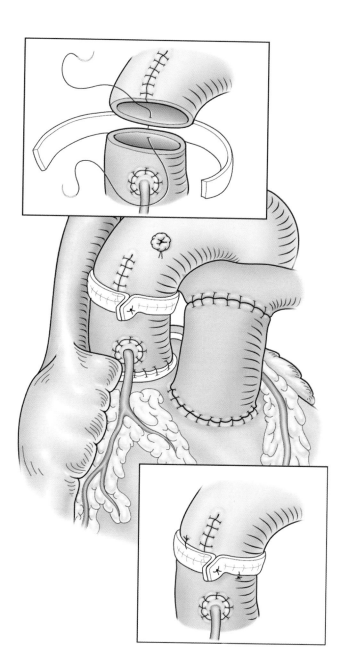

12 After completion of the coronary implantation, the distal suture line to the ascending aorta is created. It is often advisable to trim the aorta to shorten it by approximately 1.0–1.5 cm to account for the length of the pulmonary autograft. In addition, it may be necessary to tailor the distal aortic size to be equal to the autograft diameter by excision of a wedge of tissue anteriorly. It is also preferable to reinforce the aortic suture line if there is any potential size discrepancy using a strip of Teflon felt or Dacron graft material. After completion of the reconstruction, cardioplegia can be injected through the aortic suture line just before tying to ensure dilation of the aortic root without autograft insufficiency and to check for any potential bleeding sites.

At this time, the aortic clamp can be released, if desired, to test the integrity of the suture lines and to ensure the absence of aortic insufficiency. It may be necessary to manipulate the perfusion pressure if additional sutures are necessary in the autograft suture lines at this time. However, meticulous hemostasis should be secured before the RV outflow tract reconstruction is begun.

12

13 The RV outflow tract is reconstructed with use of a pulmonary homograft. Recent modifications of cryopreservation have improved the lack of antigenicity of homografts, which may improve late results. A pulmonary homograft of a suitable adult size is selected, thawed, and then trimmed to match in length and in width of the subpulmonary muscle tissue, the excised pulmonary autograft. After the aortic clamp is released, the distention of the autograft may actually make exposure to the pulmonary bifurcation more difficult for suturing of the pulmonary homograft; therefore, in some centers, the entire procedure is done with the aorta cross-clamped. The distal anastomosis of the homograft is then created, and the proximal anastomosis of the homograft to the RV outflow tract is created with a running polypropylene suture with care being taken to place the posterior suture line superficially in the septal muscle to avoid interference with the septal perforators of the anterior descending coronary artery.

After completion of the pulmonary homograft insertion, the patient is rewarmed to normothermia, the vent is removed, and the patient is weaned off cardiopulmonary bypass. Transesophageal echocardiography is routinely performed in the operating room to assess the pulmonary autograft function; only trace insufficiency is generally seen. Moderate or greater insufficiency of the autograft is an indication for either revision or replacement with a different prosthesis.

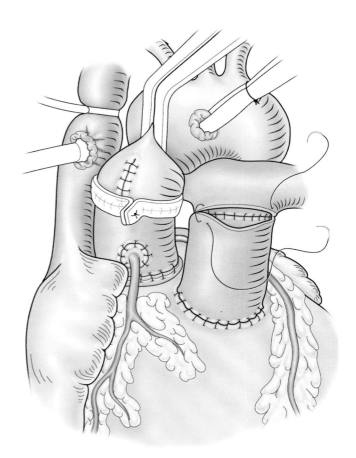

13

POSTOPERATIVE CARE

Meticulous hemostasis is necessary in the operating room, because extensive suture lines are present with the autograft valve replacement operation. Use of aprotinin or other antifibrinolytic agents can aid in achieving intraoperative hemostasis. Postoperative management is similar to that of other valve replacement procedures and includes avoidance of hypertension, which can exacerbate bleeding. In the absence of significant chest tube drainage, early extubation is desirable. Early postoperative arrhythmias are common, but they are generally minor and usually do not require more than short-term medical therapy.

OUTCOME

The Ross operation can be performed with an operative risk that is no higher than, and possibly less than, other types of aortic valve replacement. The overall operative risk reported in the large registry of Ross procedures has been approximately 2.5 per cent, and postoperative complications are not different from those seen in a similar patient population undergoing other types of prosthetic aortic valve replacement.

Patients with the Ross operation are not anticoagulated, and thromboembolism has been virtually nonexistent on late follow-up in these patients. Because anticoagulation is not used, gastrointestinal hemorrhage is not a consideration. Frequent echocardiographic follow-up is necessary, however, because two valves are replaced in this operation, and echocardiographic assessment every 3–6 months early after the operation, and yearly thereafter, is desirable.

A major concern for the use of the Ross operation is the development of late autograft insufficiency and valve failure requiring reoperation. In a large series from Dr. Ron Elkins of over 200 Ross operations, freedom from reoperation on the autograft valve was 92 ± 3 per cent at 5 years. In a larger experience with the Ross registry reported in 1999, the freedom from autograft explantation was 80 per cent at 25 years and approximately 90 per cent at 9 years. Thus, the late valve failure rate is superior to that of most bioprosthetic valves currently available.

In spite of the excellent results with the autograft valve, reports have been published of dilation of the autograft aortic root requiring reintervention. Dilation of the root is common early after the procedure, but appears to stabilize. Valve failure can occasionally be repaired; approximately 50 per cent of reoperations on the autograft require replacement of the autograft with a different prosthetic valve.

The major weakness of the Ross operation is the fate of the pulmonary outflow tract. Progressive narrowing of the RV outflow tract at the homograft conduit has been reported in every major series of the Ross operation, and balloon dilation has generally been unsuccessful in relieving this obstruction. Conduit replacement or patching of the narrowing has generally been required and has been accomplished with very minimal morbidity. Whether these processes are related to an immune response to the homograft valve is not known; however, currently processed cryopreserved homografts may have improved overall characteristics and limit the development of this complication. In the large series by Dr. Elkins, freedom from homograft reoperation was 93 ± 3 percent at 8 years; in the Ross registry data, freedom from RV outflow tract replacement or repair was approximately 83 per cent at 25 years.

Patient satisfaction with the pulmonary autograft valve replacement has been excellent. Patients are able to resume a normal lifestyle with minimal restrictions. Exercise tolerance in athletes after the operation has been excellent, with essentially normal exercise tolerance and only mild RV outflow tract gradients on exercise.

Although the Ross operation has generally been reserved for younger patients requiring aortic valve replacement, recent reports of Ross operations in patients older than 60 years of age have shown similarly low mortality with excellent hemodynamics and possibly less RV outflow tract obstruction than that occurring in similar patients done at younger ages. Thus, expansion of the use of the Ross operation into elderly populations may be considered.

FURTHER READING

Elkins, R.C., Knott-Craig, C.J., Howell, C.E. 1996. Pulmonary autografts in patients with aortic annulus dysplasia. *Annals of Thoracic Surgery* 61, 1141–5.

Elkins, R.C., Lane, M.M., McCue, C. 1996. Pulmonary autograft reoperation: incidence and management. *Annals of Thoracic Surgery* 62, 450–5.

Kouchoukos, N.T., Davila-Roman, V.G., Spray, T.L., Murphy, S.F., Perrillo, J.B. 1994. Replacement of the aortic root with a pulmonary autograft for aortic valve disease in children and young adults. *New England Journal of Medicine* 330(1), 1–6.

Oury, J.H., Hiro, S.P., Maxwell, J.M., Lamberti, J.J., Duran, C.M. 1998. The Ross procedure: current registry results. *Annals of Thoracic Surgery* 66(6 Suppl), S162–5.

Ross, D., Jackson, M., Davies, J. 1992. The pulmonary autograft – a permanent aortic valve. *European Journal of Cardio-thoracic Surgery* 6, 113–16.

Schmidtke, C., Bechtel, J.F., Noetzold, A., Sievers, H.H. 2000. Up to seven years of experience with the Ross procedure in patients >60 years of age. *Journal of the American College of Cardiology* 36, 1173–7.

SECTION IV

Surgery for Heart Failure

26

Heart transplantation

MICHAEL A. ACKER MD
Section of Cardiac Surgery, Division of Cardiothoracic Surgery, Department of Surgery, University of Pennsylvania School of Medicine, Philadelphia, Pennsylvania, USA

DAVID ZELTSMAN MD
Assistant Professor of Surgery, Division of Thoracic Surgery, Thomas Jefferson University, Jefferson Medical College, Philadelphia, Pennsylvania, USA

HISTORY

The technique of the orthotopic cardiac transplantation was developed and popularized by Richard Lower and Norman Shumway. The authors used moderate hypothermia, cardiopulmonary bypass, and an atrial 'cuff' anastomosis, a technique that became the standard for cardiac transplant. The world's first successful human-to-human heart transplant was performed on 3 December 1967 in South Africa by Christian Barnard. However, over the next several years, poor early clinical results led to few heart transplantation attempts, and only the most dedicated centers continued experimental and clinical work in the field. The introduction of cyclosporine for the management of immune reactions and rejection episodes greatly facilitated heart transplantation. The number of transplants dramatically increased from only 106 in 1980 to over 4000 cases in 2002 worldwide.

Cardiac failure, however, remains the leading cause of death in the United States, affecting more than 5 million people with greater then 700 000 deaths annually. Approximately one third of heart failure patients are in New York Heart Association class III/IV. The cost of caring for these patients is growing and approaches $50 billion per year. Cardiac transplantation remains the gold standard of surgical therapies for advanced end-stage heart failure and is a valuable tool in the armamentarium for the treatment of end-stage heart disease. Transplantation is reserved for patients with New York Heart Association class IV symptoms when other modes of medical and surgical treatment fail. The 1-year survival rate after heart transplant is 85 per cent and 68.5 per cent at 5 years. This procedure is now offered at 142 cardiac transplant centers in United States alone, with more than 2000 heart transplants performed annually. Many more transplants are being done elsewhere, primarily in countries with sophisticated cardiac surgery programs.

PRINCIPLES AND JUSTIFICATION

Selection criteria for recipients

In general, patients with irreversible end-stage heart disease who failed maximum medical therapy, exhausted other surgical options, and have an estimated 1-year survival of less than 25 per cent are considered appropriate candidates for heart transplantation. It is assumed that a transplant candidate will be able to resume a relatively normal active life and be compliant with the rigorous medical regimen postoperatively. In most transplant centers, a fully integrated, multidisciplinary committee of surgeons, heart failure cardiologists, nurses, and social workers select potential recipients and ensure that there is an equitable allocation of available donor organs to patients with the greatest chance of postoperative survival and rehabilitation. Optimal donor organ allocation is achieved through improved risk stratification of potential recipients and prediction of successful outcomes for cardiac transplantation. Severe pulmonary hypertension (greater than 6 Wood units), concurrent malignancy, positive human immunodeficiency virus status, active systemic infection, end-stage kidney or liver disease, and advanced age constitute some of the factors precluding successful transplantation. Transplantation in patients up to the age of 65 is routine, with some centers considering patients up to the age of 70 years. Selected recipients are prioritized for transplant based on several factors, including medical urgency, proximity of the potential donor to the patient, and duration on the transplant list. Given the persistent and worsening shortage of donors, waiting times continue to increase and are often greater than several months for even the sickest of patients (i.e. status I).

Criteria for selection of organ donor

Although 3573 patients were on the UNOS national patient waiting list as of October 2003, fewer than half can be expected to proceed to heart transplantation. The persistent donor organ shortage has led several European countries to adopt Presumed Consent legislation, whereby organ donation will occur in individuals shown to be brain dead, unless the individual had specifically requested otherwise. In the United States, however, organ donation may be confirmed by the donor's immediate family, even when a documented pre-consent has been given by the donor. Criteria used to establish brain death includes loss of cortical function, apnea, absence of brain stem reflexes, and irreversibility over a 24–48 hour period. Metabolic disturbances, pharmacological agents, and hypothermia must be ruled out as a possible reversible cause for the patient's impaired neurological status. Donor evaluation includes age, height and weight, gender, ABO blood type, hospital course, cause of death, hemodynamic support necessary to sustain the donor, and routine laboratory data including tests for cytomegalovirus, human immunodeficiency virus, and hepatitis B and C viruses; chest x-ray; arterial blood gas; and echocardiogram. Right heart catheterization is helpful, whenever possible. Coronary angiography in the donor is indicated for male donors older than 45 years and female donors older than 50, in those others with significant risk factors for atherosclerotic coronary artery disease. Intraoperative assessment of the heart with direct visualization and palpation is a final step in the evaluation for suitability of the donor heart.

Basic matching criteria of a potential recipient with a possible donor are based primarily on ABO blood group compatibility and body size. Traditionally, donor weight should be within 30 per cent of recipient weight except in pediatric patients, for whom closer size matching is attempted. To avoid early post-transplant right ventricular (RV) failure in recipient patients with elevated pulmonary vasculature, a larger donor may be preferred. Currently, prospective human lymphocyte antigen matching is not a requirement for successful recipient-donor match because of limits on ischemic time of the cardiac allograft and current allocation criteria.

OPERATION

Donor heart procurement

A key component of successful transplantation is effective communication between the procurement team at the remote site of organ harvest and the surgical team at the parent institution, to minimize the ischemic time and to ensure the proper timing of the recipient's preparation for the transplantation. This condition is especially important because multi-organ procurement by different organ harvest teams is common, time consuming, and occasionally unpredictable.

A skin incision is performed from the sternal notch to the pubis, and median sternotomy is done in a standard fashion. Incising the pericardium longitudinally and tacking up the cut edges to the skin with stay sutures creates the pericardial well. The heart is inspected visually and palpated for any evidence of atherosclerosis, wall motion abnormalities, thrills, or degrees of acute injury. When this final cardiac assessment is completed, the surgical team at the recipient's hospital is notified and given an approximate time for expected donor cardiectomy and return to the parent institution.

The superior vena cava (SVC) and inferior vena cava (IVC) are mobilized circumferentially. The SVC is encircled with heavy silk ties, left untied at this time, distal to its junction with the azygos vein. The IVC is freed from its loose attachments to the diaphragm and mobilized to its full supra-diaphragmatic length. The ascending aorta is then mobilized to the innominate artery distally, dissected free from the pulmonary artery (PA), and encircled with umbilical tape. Ideally, once the mediastinal IVC is clamped, the abdominal IVC is vented to a bag, decompressing the abdominal organs. If the liver surgeon prefers the venous drainage to be into the chest, then the right pleural cavity from the pericardium is widely opened to divert warm venous blood away from the heart once the cardiectomy has begun. Up to and including this stage of the operation, it is important to maintain the donor normothermic to prevent arrhythmias.

1 Once preparation for explantation of abdominal organs is completed, the patient is administered 30 000 U of heparin intravenously. A cold University of Wisconsin cardioplegic solution is placed in the pressure bag and hung, ready for infusion. Any central venous or Swan-Ganz catheters are withdrawn from the SVC. The SVC is then ligated or stapled distal to the azygos vein and divided. The heart is then retracted superiorly and the IVC is divided. Placing a clamp on the IVC is advisable and preferred, if venous drainage is obtained via infradiaphragmatic IVC by the liver harvest team, to divert warm blood away from the chest and facilitate exposure for the cardiectomy. When venous drainage is directed into the chest, the suction catheters are placed in the IVC, pericardium, and pleural cavity to aspirate the blood and clear the operative field. The distal IVC is left open for cardiac venting. The heart is allowed to eject several times and the aortic cross-clamp is applied at the takeoff of the innominate artery. A single flush cardioplegia (1000 mL) is infused with a 14-gauge needle placed in the distal ascending aorta. It is important to keep the heart decompressed, and additional venting can be obtained rapidly by amputating the tip of the left atrial (LA) appendage (if lungs are being procured), or by incising the right superior pulmonary vein. Topical ice saline is applied to achieve rapid cardiac cooling. Once cardiac arrest is achieved and the cardioplegic solution has been given, the heart is retracted cephalad, and pulmonary veins are divided individually or the LA is opened between pulmonary vein orifices and the coronary sinus (if the lungs are being harvested). With the LA mobilized, the main PA is divided proximal to the bifurcation. The aorta is divided just proximal to the cross-clamp, making most of the ascending aorta available for the implant procedure. One may mark longitudinally the anterior surface of the SVC and IVC with the marking pen to prevent malalignment during the bicaval implantation.

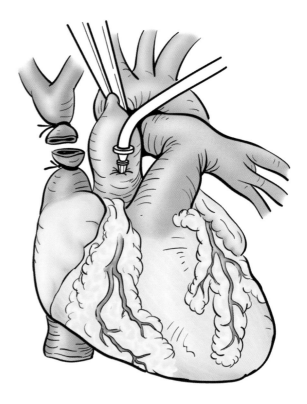

1

2 The heart is removed from the donor's chest and taken to the back table, where it is placed in the cold saline for inspection. The aorta is separated completely from the PA, the confluence of the right and left PAs is opened, the cardiac valves are inspected, and the atrium is examined for the presence of a patent foramen ovale, which, if present, is closed with 4/0 polypropylene suture. The orifices of the pulmonary veins are incised widely to create the LA cuff.

The heart then is placed in the bowel bag filled with ice-cold saline. Three sterile bowel bags are used, and each is filled with cold saline and securely closed. The bags are tied separately and placed on ice in a cooler for transport. The estimated time of arrival should be confirmed with the recipient team. A total ischemic time for harvest and transport of the donor heart should be less than 4 hours. Early graft dysfunction is increasingly likely as the procurement ischemic interval exceeds 4 hours.

Recipient cardiectomy

We prefer placement of a Swan-Ganz catheter in all patients, as knowledge of PA pressures, pulmonary vascular resistance, and central venous pressure may be required for optimal postoperative care. Once adequate general anesthesia is achieved, a midline incision is performed, and a median sternotomy is carried out. In the case of a redo sternotomy, the oscillating saw is used with care to preserve patent grafts and anterior cardiac structures. Systemic heparin is given to maintain the activated clotting time at greater than 400 seconds. After a pericardial well is created, the aorta is cannulated high at the level of the innominate artery. Bicaval cannulation is used. We prefer an angled metallic-tip SVC cannula and a straight, single-stage IVC cannula. The SVC cannula is placed directly into the SVC, and the IVC cannula is placed as low as possible near the IVC/right atrial (RA) junction. Umbilical tapes are passed around the SVC and IVC. The right PA must be carefully protected during SVC mobilization. We generally await arrival of the donor heart before initiating cardiopulmonary bypass. Systemic hypothermia to 32°C is achieved, and the aortic cross-clamp is applied just proximal to the aortic cannula.

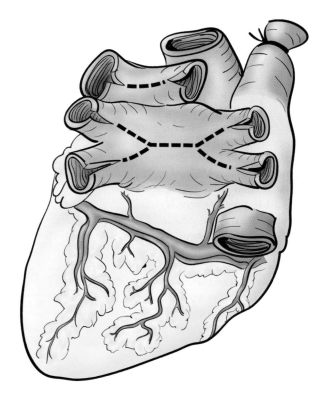

2

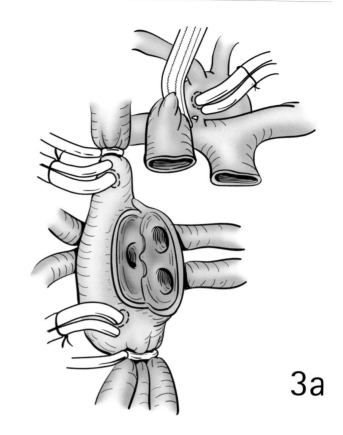

3a, b After the heart fibrillates, the caval snares are tightened and the aorta is transected at the sino-tubular junction (in non-redos). The main PA is divided just above the pulmonary valve and can be trimmed back, depending on the length of the donor PA. The RA is opened at the appendage, and the incision is carried down along the atrioventricular groove to the coronary sinus orifice, with care taken to preserve an adequate cuff at the IVC orifice for the anastomosis. The coronary sinus and appendages are excised. The incision is continued into the LA via the septum and is extended to the area of the LA appendage, which is removed. The LA walls are divided along the atrioventricular groove. As much of the native atrium as possible is removed. We find it useful to use electrocautery on the cut surfaces of the atrial cuffs for hemostasis. By removing the atrial appendage, coronary sinus, and extra atrial tissue, relatively small atrial cuffs are left. If bicaval anastomoses are to be used, the IVC and SVC cuffs are fashioned after a standard cardiectomy.

3a

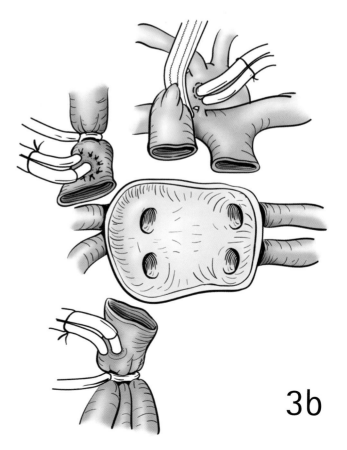

3b

4 Redo sternotomy in patients who have undergone previous placement of an implantable left ventricular assist device (LVAD) may be especially challenging and often requires up to 2 hours to allow safe dissection and cannulation for cardiopulmonary bypass. In this situation, communication with the procurement team may be especially important to avoid increasing donor organ ischemia because of prolonged cardiectomy maneuvers. The previous sternotomy incision is reopened. If the LVAD is intra-abdominal, we do not enter the abdomen to remove the LVAD until after the cardiac transplant is completed. Care should be taken at the time of VAD implantation to ensure that the outflow graft is to the right of the midline so that reopening the median sternotomy with the oscillating saw does not injure the graft. Usually, the outflow valved conduit can be palpated to the right of the level of the xiphoid, which can facilitate safe dissection of the sternum off the heart and outflow graft conduit. A well-developed fibrous capsule usually surrounds the outflow graft, which can be opened to allow easy access to the graft at its junction with the aorta. With the graft and aorta exposed, the RA and SVC are dissected out and cannulated in the standard manner. The inflow cannula–apical connection is not dissected out until the aorta is cross-clamped. The outflow graft is cut, and the device is aspirated of blood. The inflow cannula is then removed from the heart and transected at the lead of the diaphragm. The LVAD itself is left in place in the abdomen until after completion of the transplant, when protamine has been given and the patient is hemodynamically stable. It is essential that the diaphragm be reconstructed after removal of the LVAD.

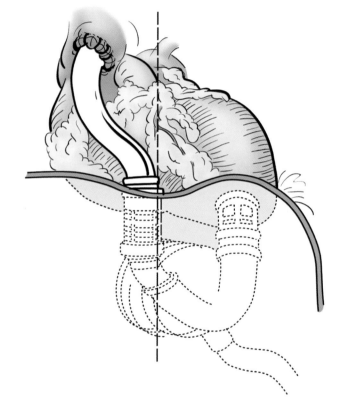

Cardiac implantation

The donor heart is removed from the sterile transport bags, carefully inspected, and prepared for implantation. The SVC is oversewn with 4/0 polypropylene if biatrial implantation is to be performed. Implantation is begun with LA anastomosis using a long (48″) 3/0 double-armed polypropylene suture. The donor heart is lowered into the chest in the anatomical position and then rotated 180 degrees toward the left to expose the LA cuff. The running suture starts at the base of the LA appendage and is carried out to the IVC orifice.

4

5a, b We use an everting technique to assure endocardium-to-endocardium opposition. The anterior portion of the LA anastomosis is completed using the second arm of the polypropylene suture, connecting the interatrial septum and sewing anteriorly toward IVC, thus completing the LA anastomosis. We intermittently apply cold saline on the RV to maintain the local hypothermia.

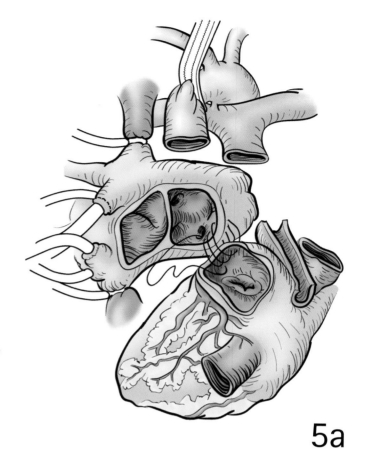

5a

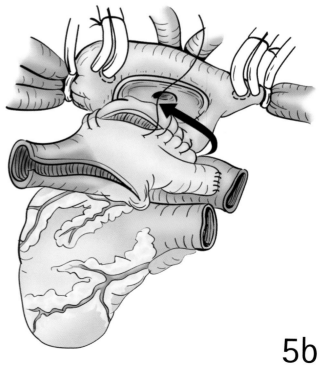

5b

6 In the case of a standard biatrial implantation, the right atrial anastomosis is performed next. The RA is tailored with an incision made on the donor RA from the IVC orifice up toward the right atrial appendage, taking care to avoid the sinoatrial node area near the junction of SVC and RA. Alternatively, the RA incision can be made from the IVC orifice up and through the cut end of the SVC. The length of that incision approximates the recipient's right atrial opening. Again, we use 3/0 (48″) double-armed polypropylene and perform the septal (posterior) suture line first. We start the running suture at the superior portion of the septum and continue it to the IVC area, taking care to avoid encroaching on the orifice of the coronary sinus. The anterior suture line is completed in a similar fashion with a second suture arm in a running manner.

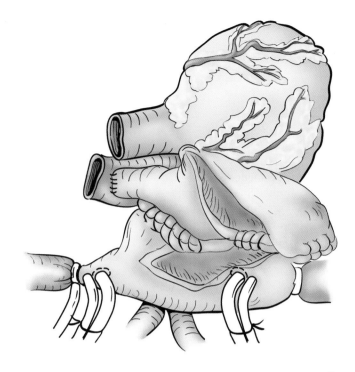

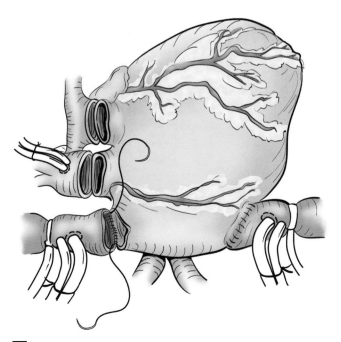

7 If bicaval anastomoses are being performed, on completion of the LA connection, we proceed with IVC anastomosis. It is crucial to preserve an adequate cuff during the recipient cardiectomy and assure that no twisting has occurred. We use two 4/0 double-armed polypropylene sutures at the 3 and 9 o'clock positions and begin the posterior suture line first, where the sutures are tied. This prevents a possible pursestring effect when tying the sutures on completion of the anastomosis. The SVC anastomosis is performed similarly. Again, the 3 and 9 o'clock stabilizing sutures are placed to prevent the pursestringing. Although use of the bicaval implantation technique is being performed increasingly often, clear evidence of benefit is lacking. Purported benefits include decreased tricuspid regurgitation, improved atrial contractility, and decreased incidence of heart block.

The PA anastomosis is performed next. The donor PA is trimmed back to approximately 5 mm above the attachments of the pulmonic valve. The aorta and PA are completely separated both in the donor heart and in the recipient heart. It is important to avoid any redundancy of the PA, as it is prone to kink or twist when there is excessive length, resulting in a pressure gradient between the RV and PA.

8 We use a single 48″ 4/0 polypropylene suture. The posterior suture line is performed first, followed by the completion of the anterior row, making up any difference in the size between the donor and recipient PAs. We do not tie the sutures at this time, but place a temporary PA vent and secure the suture line once the RV is contracting well after release of the cross-clamp.

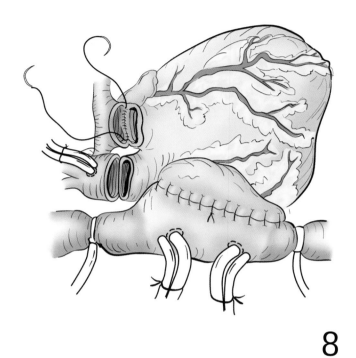

8

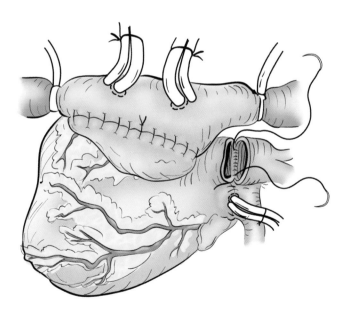

9

9 At this point, we anastomose the aortas, and systemic rewarming is begun. The donor aorta is trimmed, but some redundancy is acceptable, because this will facilitate access to the posterior aortic suture line for additional suturing if needed for hemostasis later. Our preference is to use 4/0 long double-armed polypropylene suture. Again, any circumference discrepancy is made up during closure of the anterior aspect of the anastomosis. After the aortic sutures are tied, an aortic root vent is placed, secured, and put to suction.

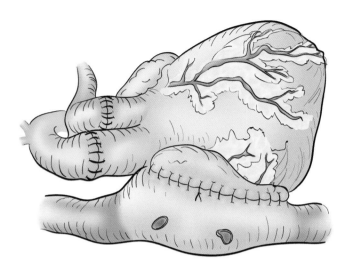

10a

10a, b 500 mg of Solu-Medrol is given, and the cross-clamp is removed with the patient in the Trendelenburg position. Completed biatrial (Figure 10a) and bicaval (Figure 10b) orthotopic cardiac transplant is demonstrated.

All anastomotic sites are carefully examined for bleeding, especially the LA and the posterior PA, as it may be difficult to evaluate these areas once the patient is weaned off cardiopulmonary bypass. We place two ventricular and two atrial temporary pacing wires (on the donor atrium), making sure that the threshold is low, as it may be necessary to maintain the wires for prolonged periods of time. Isoproterenol infusion is initiated at a dose of 0.02 µg/kg per minute. If needed, the heart is atrially paced between 100 and 120 beats/minute. Effectiveness of deairing is evaluated with transesophageal echocardiography, which is routinely used in all cases. Additionally, inotropic support is instituted, as necessary. We prefer low-dose epinephrine (0.02–0.05 µg/kg per minute) and milrinone (0.25–0.5 µg/kg per minute). If RV failure is still present associated with pulmonary hypertension, high central venous pressure, and low or borderline cardiac output, inhaled nitric oxide can be added. Once the cardiac function is adequate, metabolic derangements have been corrected, oxygenation is sufficient, and deairing is complete, the aortic root vent is removed and patient is weaned off cardiopulmonary support.

It is not uncommon to detect some degree of RV dysfunction at this time. A Swan-Ganz catheter is advanced into the PA to assess the PA pressure. It is also possible to detect a gradient across the pulmonary anastomosis at this time. The chest is irrigated with antibiotic solution (vancomycin 1 g/L), mediastinal and pleural chest tubes are placed, and the sternotomy is closed in the usual fashion. The patient is transferred to the surgical intensive care unit for further management.

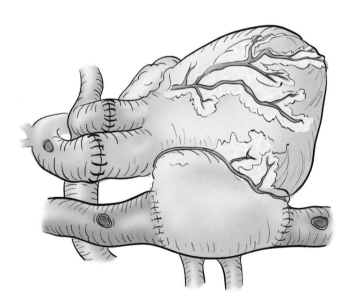

10b

INTENSIVE CARE UNIT AND PERIOPERATIVE CARE

Inotropic support is continued until the patient is hemodynamically stable. If pulmonary hypertension persists, inotropic support and pacing, if needed, is weaned over 2–3 days to allow the RV to slowly adapt to high afterload. Echocardiography (two-dimensional and transesophageal) is used extensively to guide the therapy. Special consideration is given to facilitate early extubation and removal of intravenous lines, tubes, and catheters. Isoproterenol is weaned off over the course of 24–48 hours, starting on postoperative day 2, while maintaining a heart rate of greater than 100 beats/minute. Further management continues in a telemetry ward, where aggressive physical therapy and ambulation is instituted. If the patient has an uncomplicated postoperative course, he or she is routinely discharged home within 14 days.

Immunosuppression

We routinely use a triple drug immunosuppression protocol for heart transplant patients, with a gradual wean from steroids, whenever possible. Solu-Medrol, 500–1 000 mg i.v., is given intraoperatively just before removal of the aortic cross-clamp. Postoperatively, Solu-Medrol, 125 mg i.v. every 8 hours, is administered for the next 24 hours and then replaced with prednisone by mouth, which is tapered over the next 2 weeks until 30 mg/day is reached. The patient is weaned off steroids by post-transplant week 40, if no major rejection episodes have occurred.

Cyclosporine therapy usually is initiated postoperatively within 24 hours. The oral form is given, 5 mg/kg per 24 hours, and divided in two doses. If the patient cannot resume oral intake, an intravenous cyclosporin is used at 0.25–1.00 mg/kg per 24 hours. The dose is adjusted to maintain the serum levels at 200–300 µg/L for the first 6 months postoperatively, with a gradual decrease to 100–200 µg/L subsequently. Mycophenolate mofetil, 1 g i.v., is started on call to the operating room and continued at 1 g i.v. twice a day postoperatively.

Lymphocytolytic induction is not part of our routine post-transplant immunosuppression protocol. It can be initiated, however, if pretransplant serum creatinine is greater than 2.0 mg/dL, postoperative serum creatinine is greater than 2.5 mg/dL, or oliguria persists for longer then 24 hours. Patients with serum creatinine of 1.5–2.5 mg/dL should be maintained on low-dose cyclosporine. Efficacy of immunosuppression is assessed by routine RV endomyocardial biopsies. The first postoperative biopsy is performed within 7–10 days.

OUTCOME

The mortality rates for patients undergoing heart transplant remain low. Perioperative (30 days) mortality for heart transplant patients is approximately 7 per cent. Eighty-three per cent of patients survive at 1 year, greater than 70 per cent survive at 5 years, and 22 per cent of cardiac transplant patients survive 18 years.

FURTHER READING

2000 Annual Report of the U.S. Scientific Registry of Transplant Recipients and the Organ Procurement and Transplantation Network. Transplant Data 1989–2000. Rockville, MD and Richmond, VA: HHS/HSRA/OSP/DOT and UNOS. Retrieved May 28, 2001 from the World Wide Web: http://www.unos.org/Data/anrpt_main.htm.

Barnard, C.N. 1967. A human cardiac transplant: an interim report of a successful operation performed at Groote Schuur Hospital, Capetown. *South African Medical Journal* **41**,1271.

Keck, B.M., Bennet, L.E., Rosendale, J., Daily, O.P., Novick, R.J., Hosenpud, J.D. 2000. Worldwide Thoracic Organ Transplantation: A report from the UNOS/ISHLT International Registry for Thoracic Organ Transplantation. *Clin Transpl*, 35–49.

Miller, L.W. 1998. Listing criteria for cardiac transplantation: Results of an American Society of Transplant Physicians–National Institutes of Health conference. *Transplantation* **66(7)**, 947–51.

Transplant Patient Data Source (2001, May 11). Richmond, VA: United Network for Organ Sharing. Retrieved May 28, 2001 from the World Wide Web: http://www.patients.unos.org/data.htm

Yacoub, M., Mankad, P., Ledingham, S. 1990. Donor procurement and surgical techniques for cardiac transplantation. *Seminars in Thoracic and Cardiovascular Surgery* **2(2)**, 153–61.

27

Heart–lung transplantation

JOHN WALLWORK FRCS(ED), MB CHB, FRCS, FRCP, MA
Consultant Cardiothoracic Surgeon and Director of Transplantation, Department of Cardiac Administration, Papworth Hospital National Health Service Trust, Cambridge, UK

STEVEN S. L. TSUI BA, MB BCH, MA, MD, FRCS(Eng), FRCS(C-Th)
Consultant Cardiothoracic Surgeon, Papworth Hospital National Health Trust, Cambridge, UK

HISTORY

Animal experimentation in heart-lung transplantation began in 1907, with sporadic attempts in humans from 1968. However, clinical success with heart-lung transplantation remained elusive. Dehiscence of the tracheal anastomosis and infection of the pulmonary allograft invariably led to the death of all early recipients. With the discovery of cyclosporin A and improved surgical techniques, Reitz and colleagues demonstrated that it was possible to achieve long-term survival in a primate model after heart-lung transplantation by the late 1970s. The use of cyclosporin made it possible to reduce the doses of steroids in the early post-transplant period. This advance allowed proper healing of the tracheal anastomosis and virtually eliminated the problem of airway dehiscence. Reitz and colleagues subsequently achieved the first successful human heart-lung transplant at Stanford University in 1981. Once satisfactory survival of heart-lung recipients had been demonstrated, many other established transplant centers with experience in cardiac transplantation also embarked on their own program of heart-lung transplantation.

PRINCIPLES AND JUSTIFICATION

Before the successful application of heart-lung transplantation, no effective treatment existed for patients suffering from advanced pulmonary parenchymal, and pulmonary vascular disorders. The development of heart-lung transplantation, and subsequently lung transplantation, provided new therapeutic options for patients with end-stage lung diseases. The earliest patients treated by heart-lung transplantation were limited to those suffering from severe pulmonary hypertension (e.g. primary pulmonary hypertension and Eisenmenger's syndrome). This procedure has since been successfully performed in patients suffering from most other forms of lung failure. A certain overlap exists between the indications for heart-lung, single-lung, and bilateral-lung transplantation. Each major transplant center has its own evolving strategy based on its experience and preferences.

We would consider all patients with severe, combined end-stage heart and lung failure for heart-lung transplantation. The commonest indications for heart-lung transplantation at Papworth Hospital are Eisenmenger's syndrome, primary pulmonary hypertension, and other pulmonary vaso-occlusive diseases with concomitant right ventricular failure. We also consider patients with bilateral lung failure without heart failure for heart-lung transplantation, particularly those younger than 40 years of age. This strategy includes most patients with cystic fibrosis and young patients with other septic lung conditions. In addition, we sometime offer heart-lung transplantation to selected patients who are on the lung transplant waiting list if suitable heart-lung blocks become available. This approach has included patients with fibrosing alveolitis, pulmonary lymphangioleiomyomatosis, emphysema, and alpha$_1$-antitrypsin deficiency.

Some transplant centers have raised concerns regarding the use of heart-lung transplantation for patients with isolated lung failure. Because of the severe shortage of donor organs exists, this approach might not make maximal use of the available donor organs. Another concern is that it is unnecessary, and indeed may be disadvantageous, to transplant the heart as well as the lungs in patients who are suffering from isolated lung failure.

In Papworth Hospital, we feel that our approach is entirely justified. Patients with isolated lung failure who are fortunate enough to be offered a heart-lung transplant routinely donate their excised heart for domino heart transplantation. Therefore, the fact that these patients receive the complete heart-lung block does not compromise the actual number of donor hearts available for heart transplantation. Furthermore, implantation of a heart-lung block is technically simpler than that of bilateral single-lung transplant. As a result, earlier reperfusion of the donor organs is feasible, thereby reducing organ ischemic times. In the current era, survival following heart-lung transplantation is as good as, and in our experience better than, that of bilateral single-lung transplant.

In addition, the results of heart transplantation from live domino donors are superior to those from cadaveric heart donors. Therefore, major centers with extensive experience in heart-lung transplantation continue to adopt this approach. We believe that heart-lung transplantation in these patients, coupled with domino heart donation, provides the maximal patient benefit from a single heart-lung block.

PREOPERATIVE ASSESSMENT AND PREPARATION

All patients who are experiencing significant functional restrictions due to severe cardiopulmonary failure can be referred for the consideration of heart-lung transplantation. In general, most suitable candidates should have end-stage, irreversible disease on maximal medical therapy and have a life expectancy limited to 1 or 2 years. The list of investigations provided in Table 27.1 is useful in assessing potential candidates for heart-lung transplantation.

Table 27.1 *Diagnostic and prognostic investigations for potential heart-lung transplant candidates*

Full pulmonary function tests
Exercise tolerance as measured by a 6-min walk
Electrocardiogram
Echocardiogram
High-resolution computed tomography of the thorax in patients with parenchymal disease, pleural disease, previous thoracic surgical procedures, and complex congenital anomalies
Coronary angiogram in patients >45 yr old with risk factors for coronary artery disease who may be domino donors

Prognostic data are available for many conditions that can be treated by transplantation. Such data help to determine the optimal timing of transplantation. For example, in patients with cystic fibrosis, an FEV$_1$ less than 30 per cent predicted, PaO$_2$ less than 7.3 kPa (55 mm Hg), or PaCO$_2$ greater than 6.7 kPa (50 mm Hg) correlates with a 2-year survival of less than 50 per cent. Furthermore, those patients who have developed life-threatening complications as a result of their underlying condition should also be listed early. These complications include massive hemoptysis, severe cor pulmonale, and multiple syncopal episodes; in cases of primary pulmonary hypertension, those who are refractory to treatment with prostacyclin should also be included. Current contraindications to heart-lung transplantation are listed in Table 27.2.

Table 27.2 *Contraindictions to heart–lung transplantation*

Absolute
  Infection with human immunodeficiency virus
  Hepatitis B antigen positivity
  Hepatitis C infection
  Recent malignancies
  Active extrapulmonary infections
  Requirement for invasive ventilation
  Overt psychiatric illness
Relative
  Age >55 years
  Extensive pleural adhesions
  Severe peripheral vascular disease
  Significant neurological impairment
  Progressive neuromuscular disorder
  Severe renal impairment
  Steroid dependence (daily dose of prednisolone >30 mg)
  History of substance abuse

Management of patients awaiting heart–lung transplantation

Patients awaiting heart-lung transplantation should be followed up closely to prevent further deterioration of their condition and to maximize their chances of survival until suitable donor organs become available. Cystic fibrosis patients with recurrent sinus infections may require sinus drainage procedures. Patients with severe primary pulmonary hypertension sometimes respond to treatment with prostacyclin infusions. Balloon atrial septostomy may also be considered for these patients as a bridge to transplantation. Steroid doses should be kept to a minimum. Adequate nutritional intake is ensured to avoid cachexia and is supplemented via an enteral feeding tube when indicated.

Donor–recipient matching

ABO blood group compatibility between donor and recipient is mandatory, as in all other solid organ transplantations. As part of the assessment process before patients are accepted for transplantation, they should be tested for the presence of pre-formed anti–human lymphocyte antigen (HLA) antibodies using a panel of lymphocytes of known HLA type. If cytotoxic activities occur against 20 per cent or more of the panel, pre-transplant direct cross-matching between donor lymphocytes and the serum of the potential recipient is required. Finally, the donor lungs have to be matched to a recipient with the appropriately sized chest cavity. No real consensus exists on how this size matching is best achieved. In Papworth Hospital, we compare the predicted total lung capacity of the donor with that of the recipient from normograms based on sex and height and accept a difference of up to 15 per cent. Other centers compare chest circumference together with vertical and transverse thoracic dimensions as measured on donor and recipient chest radiographs.

ANESTHESIA

Heart-lung transplantation is performed under general anesthesia. The patient is intubated with a single-lumen endotracheal tube. After induction of anesthesia, a small test dose of aprotinin (50 000 units or 5 mL) is administered by slow intravenous injection for the detection of allergy. A loading dose of 2 000 000 units (200 mL) is then given by intravenous injection over 20 minutes, and 2 000 000 units are added to the priming fluid of the extracorporeal circuit. The maintenance dose of aprotinin is 500 000 units/hour (50 mL/hour) until the end of the operation.

OPERATION

1a, b **Incision and pleural inspection** Heart-
lung transplantation is performed through a
median sternotomy incision. This approach allows excellent
exposure of all the mediastinal structures, as well as access to
the hilum of both lungs. This incision may be extended above
the sternal notch if the innominate vein is to be cannulated
for cardiopulmonary bypass.

Once the sternum has been divided, each pleural space is
entered to assess the amount of pleural adhesions. Sometimes
these adhesions can be highly vascular, division with electrocautery before systemic heparinization is advisable. When
hemostasis of the divided pleural adhesions has been secured,
the patient is given heparin intravenously for systemic anticoagulation (300 units/kg to achieve an activated clotting
time of greater than 700 seconds). The anterior pericardium
is opened with an inverted-**T** incision. Two strong stay-
sutures are placed on either side of the pericardial edge.
Traction on these sutures will facilitate subsequent exposure
of the hilar structures.

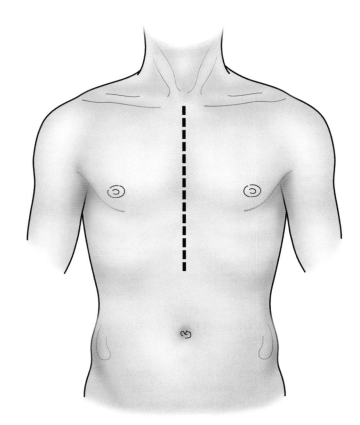

1a

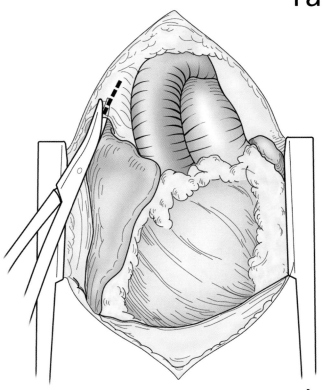

1b

2 **Cannulation for cardiopulmonary bypass** The ascending aorta is separated from the pulmonary trunk. The venae cavae are dissected free and encircled with nylon tapes. Standard high ascending aortic cannulation is performed with a 24-G aortic cannula for arterial return. If the heart of the recipient is diseased and is to be discarded, the venae cavae are separately cannulated with two 30-G venous cannulae. These cannulae should be placed as far laterally and posteriorly as possible to facilitate subsequent anastomosis of the right atrial cuff. An alternative method of cannulation for cardiopulmonary bypass is used if bicaval anastomosis is employed for implanting the donor heart-lung block (Figure 17). Cardiopulmonary bypass is commenced, the patient is cooled to 30°C and ventilation is discontinued.

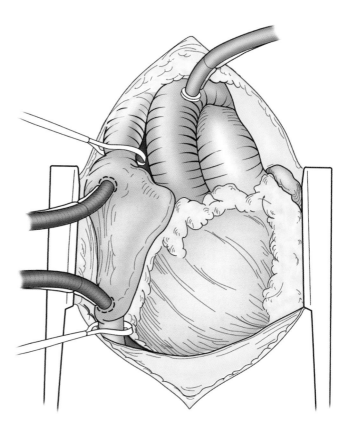

2

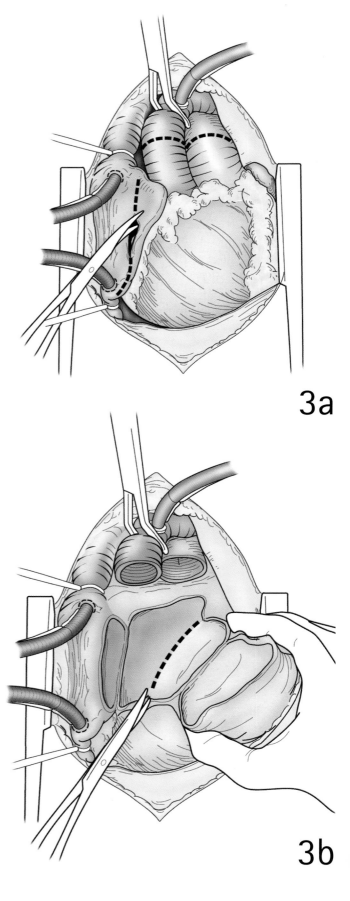

3a

3b

3a, b

Recipient cardiectomy One of the most important aspects of heart-lung transplantation is to avoid injury to the phrenic nerves, the vagus nerves, and the left recurrent laryngeal nerve of the recipient. This goal can be achieved by careful dissection and excision of the recipient heart and lungs with the following steps. The aorta is cross-clamped, and the nylon tape is tightened around each caval cannula with a snare. The recipient cardiectomy is essentially the same as the standard cardiectomy performed for heart transplantation. The right atrium is incised along the right atrioventricular groove. This incision is carried cranially between the superior vena cava (SVC) and the ascending aorta, excising the right atrial appendage, and caudally towards the coronary sinus. This incision should be at least 1 cm away from the caval cannulation sites to leave an adequate cuff of tissue for subsequent right atrial anastomosis. The ascending aorta and the main pulmonary trunk are now transected at a level 2 cm below the aortic cross-clamp. The heart is lifted forward and removed by cutting along the left atrioventricular groove.

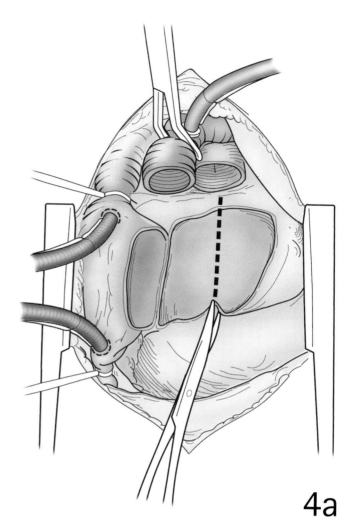

4a–c **Posterior pericardial dissection** Once the heart has been excised, the remaining posterior left atrial wall is divided in the midline. This maneuver has the effect of separating the right and left pulmonary veins. Each side of the bisected left atrial cuff is retracted forward in turn to divide the posterior pericardial reflections behind the left atrium. The plane of dissection should be kept close to the atrial surface to avoid injury to the branches of the vagus nerves on the surface of the esophagus.

4a

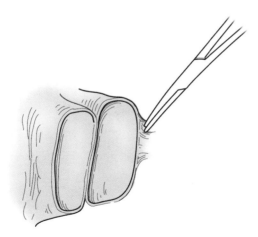

4b

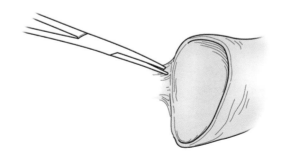

4c

5a-c Preparation of the pulmonary artery patch

The next step is to bisect the pulmonary trunk at its bifurcation into the right and left pulmonary arteries. Because the left recurrent laryngeal nerve passes under the aortic arch adjacent to the ligamentum arteriosum, special care has to be taken in this area to avoid its injury. A dimple on the inner surface of the left pulmonary artery marks the site of the ligamentum arteriosum. A 1-cm disc of pulmonary artery is left intact around this dimple to preserve the left recurrent laryngeal nerve. The use of electrocautery is avoided, and bleeding points should be controlled with Ligaclips (Ethicon, Somerville, NJ 08876, USA). The rest of the left and right pulmonary arteries are dissected free laterally.

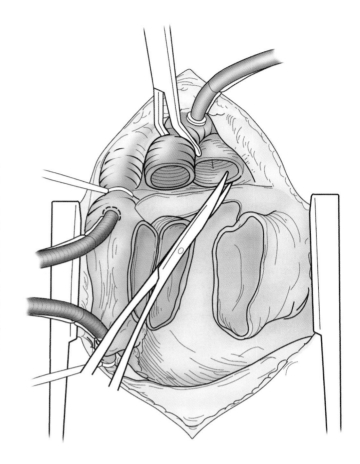

5a

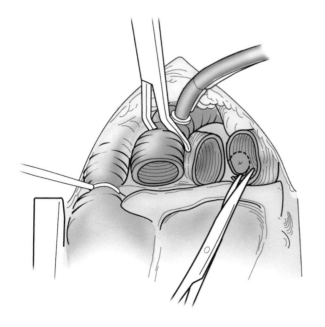

5b

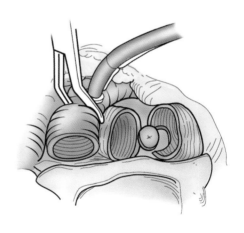

5c

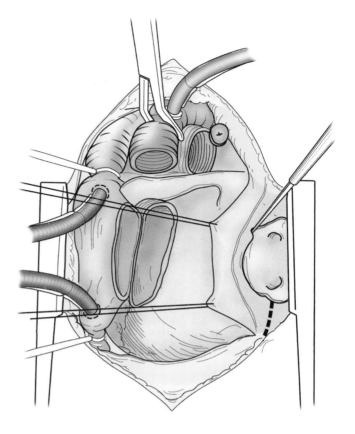

6a

6a, b Dissection of the anterior hilum of the left lung   The anterior pleural is widely opened, and the left-sided pericardial stay sutures are retracted over to the right to expose the hilum of the left lung. The lung is initially mobilized by dividing the pulmonary ligament with electrocautery. The pleural reflection overlying the left pulmonary artery and veins is incised next. The left phrenic nerve is clearly seen on the pleural surface of the pericardium coursing towards the diaphragm, and it is usually a good distance anterior of the lung hilum. As the pericardial sac is cut open adjacent to the hilar vessels, the left atrial cuff, together with the stump of the left pulmonary artery, can be delivered into the pleural cavity. Traction on these structures will allow the incision in the pericardium to encircle these vessels. This maneuver creates a small window in the lateral aspect of the posterior pericardial sac. To facilitate subsequent passage of the left donor lung through this pericardial window, it is widened by extending an incision inferiorly toward the diaphragm.

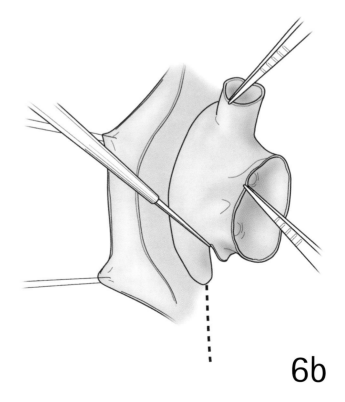

6b

7 **Dissection of the posterior lung hilum** The whole left lung is now brought out of the wound and retracted to the right of the midline to expose the posterior aspect of the left hilum. The vagus nerve courses inferiorly in the posterior mediastinum behind the bronchus. Even though it may not be easily identifiable at this stage, the vagus nerve is often stretched across the surface of the bronchus by this maneuver. To avoid injury to this nerve, the pleural reflections overlying the left main bronchus are incised close to the lung substance. The pleura is then swept away from the surface of the bronchus toward the mediastinum using a dental swab. Branches of the bronchial artery are controlled with Ligaclips. Once this step has been completed, the intact left vagus nerve is often seen lying close to the cut edge of the pleural reflection on the surface of the esophagus.

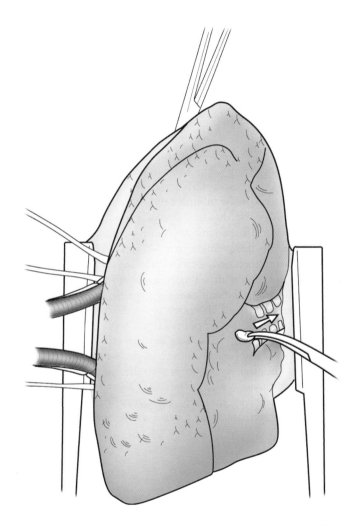

7

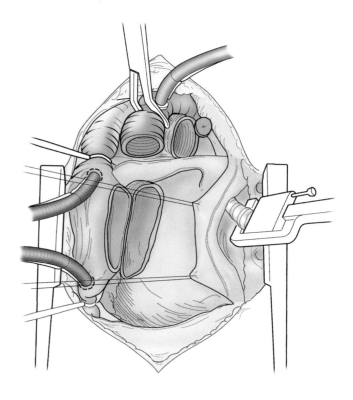

8a

8a, b Division of the bronchus and removal of the lung After the left lung has been returned to the pleural cavity, the left main bronchus is skeletonized by dividing the remaining soft tissue and lymph nodes on its anterior surface with electrocautery. The bronchus is closed with a TA-30 stapling device. Cutting the bronchus distal to the staples allows removal of the lung without contamination of the operative field by the bronchial stump.

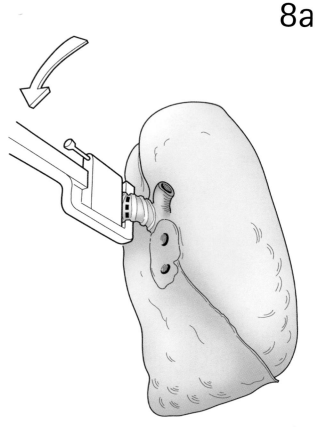

8b

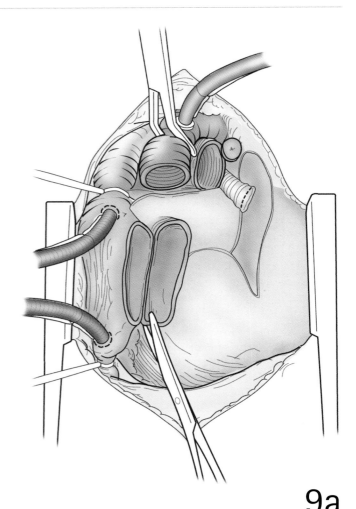

9a

9a, b Dissection of the right pulmonary venous cuff from the right atrium

The right pulmonary venous cuff is separated from the right atrium by cutting the remaining left atrium away from the back of the interatrial septum. The right lung is excised in the same way as the left lung by repeating the steps outlined in Figures 6–8. The phrenic nerve on the right tends to lie much closer to the lung hilum than the nerve on the left, and special care has to be taken to avoid its injury.

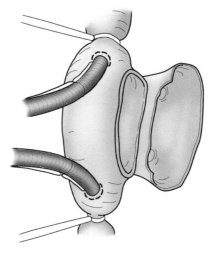

9b

10 **Carinal dissection** At this stage, the two stapled bronchial stumps are just visible through the defect in the posterior pericardium. The anesthetist clears the trachea of secretions with a suction catheter, and 30 mL of 10 per cent aqueous Betadine solution is used to wash out the lumen of the tracheal stump. The tracheal carina can be brought into the operating field by downward traction on tissue clamps applied to the two bronchial stumps. Access to the tracheal carina can be enhanced by rotating the aortic cross-clamp 90 degrees counterclockwise to widen the space between the SVC and the ascending aorta.

Electrocautery is used to make a transverse opening in the envelope of soft tissue on the tracheal carina. This incision should be made as low as possible to leave the blood supply of the distal trachea undisturbed. The distal carina and the bronchial stumps are skeletonized by blunt dissection using a dental swab. To expose the posterior surface of the carina, the tissue clamps on the two bronchial stumps are retracted upward. At this point, both vagus nerves are at risk of injury as they become displaced with the bronchus on each side. Keeping the plane of dissection right on the surface of the airways and avoiding the use of the electrocautery are imperative.

At this stage, dissection of the mediastinum is almost complete. Before proceeding any further, meticulous hemostasis of all the posterior mediastinal structure has to be carried out, because these areas will become inaccessible once the donor organs have been inserted.

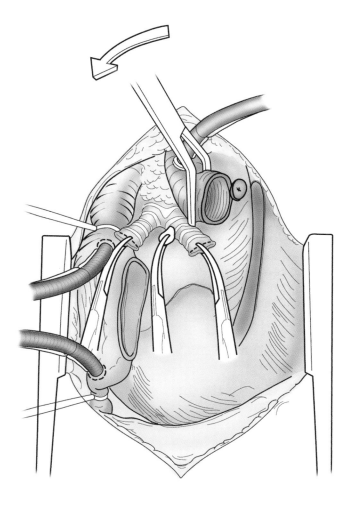

10

11 **Preparation of the donor trachea for implantation**
The donor trachea is transected 2 cm above the carina. Secretions are aspirated from the donor airways for culture and microbiological examination. Each bronchus is gently washed out with 20 mL of normal saline to remove retained secretions. The trachea is trimmed to its final length, which is just one cartilage ring above the carina.

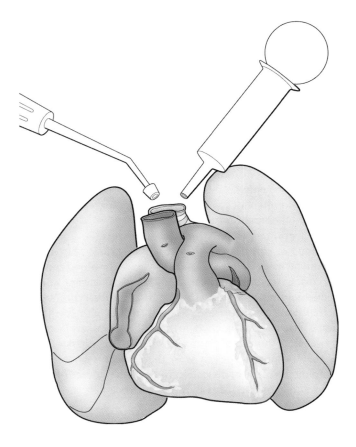

11

12a–c Preparation of the recipient trachea for implantation

Once the donor organs are ready for implantation, the recipient trachea is opened just above the carina. Use of electrocautery in this area must be avoided, and the peritracheal soft tissue is left undisturbed to preserve the blood supply to the trachea anastomosis. The incision is carried around the anterior two thirds of the trachea with scissors. At this stage, traction on the tracheal stump is maintained through the membranous part of the trachea to prevent it from retracting back into the superior mediastinum. Once a 3/0 polypropylene suture has been passed into the recipient trachea, division of the membranous part of the trachea can be completed and the carina excised.

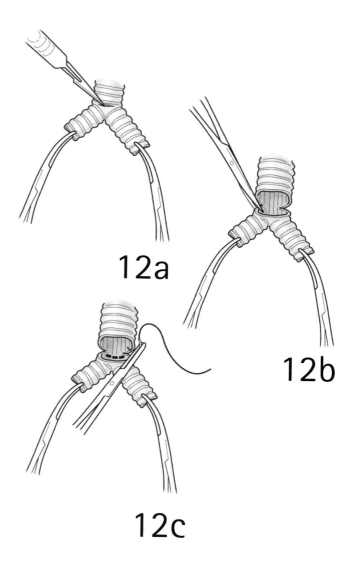

12a

12b

12c

13a, b   Delivery of the heart-lung block into the recipient for tracheal anastomosis

The donor heart-lung block is partially wrapped in cold, wet swabs. The tracheal anastomosis is performed with the 3/0 polypropylene suture that has already been placed in the recipient trachea. The first two or three passes of the running suture are made with the donor block still on the abdominal surface of the recipient. The donor block is then lowered into the recipient chest cavity. The surgeon supports the weight of the donor organs by placing the right hand behind the donor heart. The left hand is used to maneuver the right donor lung beneath the right atrial cuff of the recipient and through the pericardial window, into the right pleural cavity. At the same time, the assistant gently pulls up on the two ends of the 3/0 polypropylene suture to approximate the donor and recipient trachea. The left lung is then maneuvered through the corresponding pericardial window into the left pleural cavity. Finally, the donor heart is lowered into the pericardial cavity. At this stage, the orientation of each lobe of the lungs must be checked to ensure that they have not been twisted around their axis during passage through the respective pericardial windows.

Traction of the donor aorta forward and downward provides exposure for the completion of the tracheal anastomosis. The row of running suture for the membranous part of the trachea is placed from inside the trachea, moving from left to right. The same suture is continued onto the cartilaginous part of the trachea, and the anterior row of suture is placed from outside the trachea. Once the tracheal anastomosis is complete, the donor and recipient peritracheal soft tissue is approximated with a running 4/0 polypropylene suture to cover the anastomosis. The anesthetist aspirates any blood that has been spilt into the airways during the performance of the tracheal anastomosis. The lungs are gently reinflated and ventilated with a tidal volume of 5 mL/kg from this point onward. This maneuver does not usually interfere with the rest of the implant operation.

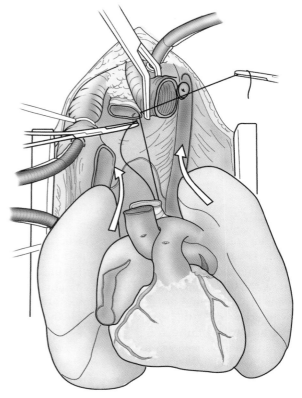

13a

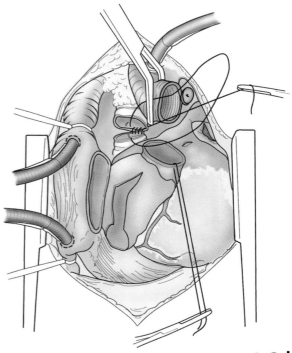

13b

14 **Right atrial anastomosis** The donor SVC is closed with a 4/0 polypropylene suture. The donor right atrium is opened by making an incision from the lateral aspect of the inferior vena cava (IVC) toward the right atrial appendage to match the size of the recipient right atrial cuff. Patent foramen ovale or defects in either the donor or recipient atrial septum should be closed. The right atrial anastomosis is performed with an extra long 3/0 polypropylene running suture (120 cm), which is left untied for later deairing of the heart.

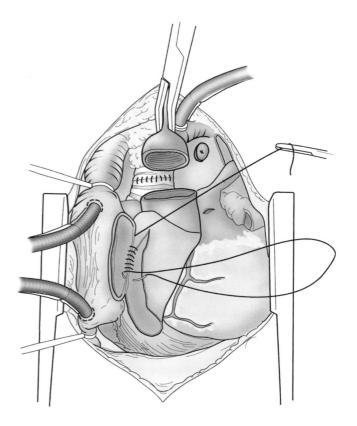

14

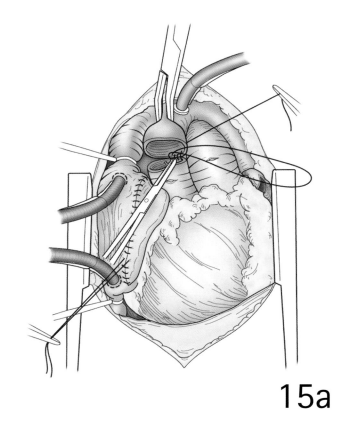

15a

15a, b
Aortic anastomosis and deairing of the heart Gradual rewarming of the patient to 37°C is commenced. The aortic anastomosis is performed with a 4/0 polypropylene running suture. The patient is placed steeply head down in preparation for deairing of the heart. The nylon tapes around the venae cavae are removed, and the venous line of the extra-corporeal circuit is partially occluded to allow filling of the heart. The right atrium is thoroughly deaired before the suture line is tied. Next, the right ventricle is deaired through the pneumoplegia site in the pulmonary trunk. The tidal volume of the ventilator is increased to 10 mL/kg. As more blood is allowed to flow across the pulmonary vasculature, deairing of the left heart can be accomplished through the tip of the left atrial appendage and the cardioplegia site of the aortic root. The aortic cross-clamp is then removed, and reperfusion of the implanted organ is commenced.

At this stage, we routinely start an isoprenaline infusion (0.02 μg/kg per minute) and a dopamine infusion (5 μg/kg per minute) to decrease pulmonary vascular resistance and increase cardiac contractility. Further deairing of the heart is undertaken before the deairing sites in the pulmonary trunk, the left atrial appendage, and the aortic root are closed with 4/0 polypropylene sutures.

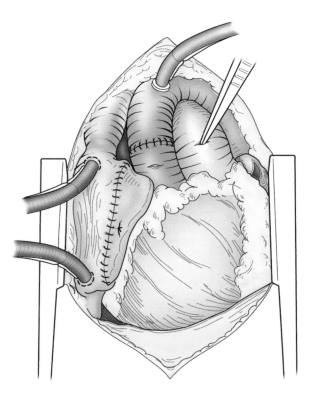

15b

15c Temporary pacing wires are secured to the donor right atrium and right ventricle and brought out through the skin below the incision. Chest drains are inserted (Figure 16). When normothermia is achieved, the patient can be weaned off cardiopulmonary bypass. Overdistention of the heart must be avoided at this stage. When the venous cannulae have been removed, residual heparin is reversed with protamine sulphate (3 mg/kg). Clotting factors and platelets are routinely administered, as postoperative hemorrhage is a frequently encountered complication of heart-lung transplant. Finally, the aortic cannula is removed, and hemostasis is secured before the sternotomy is closed.

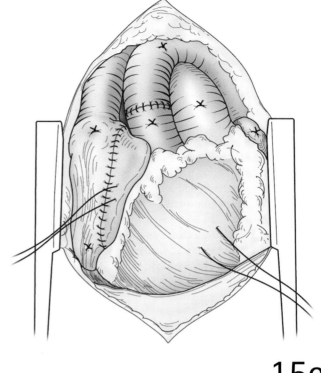

15c

16 **Positioning of chest drains**   Careful positioning of chest drains is crucial after heart-lung transplantation to enable early detection of postoperative hemorrhage and to prevent collections from accumulating inside the chest cavity. A pleural drain is inserted in the mid-axillary line on each side. Each drain is directed toward the posterior costophrenic angle and then along the paravertebral gutter to the apex of the pleural cavity. Additional side holes are cut into the drains at the level of the costophrenic angle. Two mediastinal drains are positioned anteriorly, one to lie in the back of the pericardial cavity and the other one retrosternally. These drains are connected to bottles with underwater seals and placed on a suction of 7 kPa.

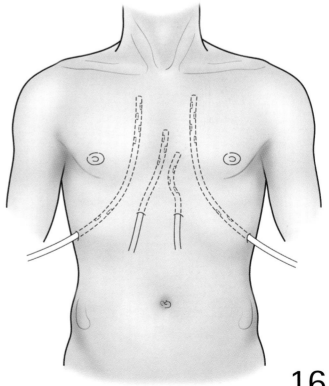

16

17 Direct cannulation of innominate vein for cardiopulmonary bypass As an alternative to cannulating the SVC via the body of the right atrium for cardiopulmonary bypass, direct cannulatation of the innominate vein or high SVC is possible to provide venous drainage. This modification is necessary when a heart-lung transplant recipient donates a domino heart for transplantation. In fact, this is our preferred method of cannulation for cardiopulmonary bypass in all heart-lung transplants.

A 5/0 polypropylene pursestring suture is placed in the innominate vein. The pursestring is approximately 8 mm wide and 15 mm long. A forceps is used to grasp the vein on each side of the pursestring, and a 12-mm longitudinal incision is made with a No. 11 knife blade. A 22-G venous cannula is inserted into the vein to a depth of 1 cm, and the pursestring suture is tightened with a snare. Securing this venous cannula against the wound edge is advisable to prevent its displacement during the rest of the procedure.

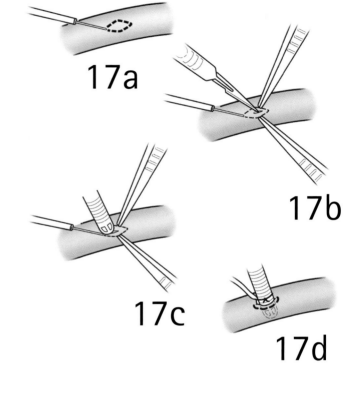

17a

17b

17c

17d

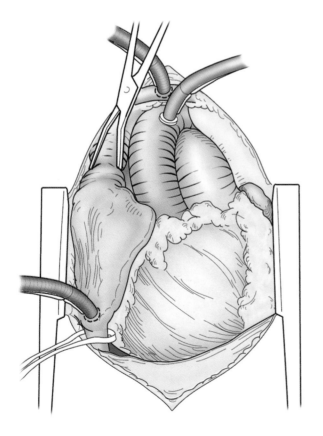

18 Control of the superior vena cava The aorta and IVC are cannulated as before, and cardiopulmonary bypass is instituted. Instead of using a nylon tape and a keeper to control the SVC, an angled pediatric vascular clamp is used. This clamp acts to maintain the correct orientation of the SVC once it has been divided. Furthermore, the clamp does not compress the SVC into a small 'rose-bud' and thereby facilitates its subsequent anastomosis.

18

19 **Division of superior and inferior venae cavae**
A cross-clamp is applied to the distal ascending aorta. If the heart of the recipient is used for domino donation, cardioplegia is delivered into the aortic root for myocardial preservation, and cold saline is added to the pericardium for topical cooling. Once the heart is arrested, the IVC can be controlled with a nylon tape, and the heart of the recipient can be excised. The SVC is divided 1 cm above the right atrium to preserve the sinoatrial node. The IVC is divided so as to leave a 1-cm cuff of atrial tissue around the IVC cannula. The rest of the cardiectomy is similar to that of a cadaveric donor heart, with division of the individual pulmonary veins, distal pulmonary trunk, and ascending aorta. Excision of the lungs and preparation of the distal trachea are carried out as described in Figures 5–13.

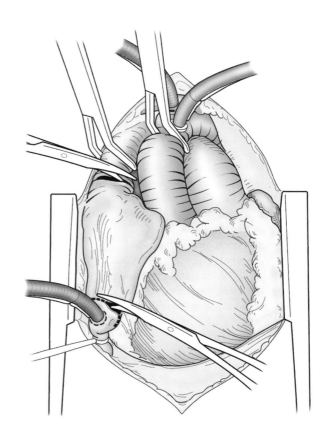

19

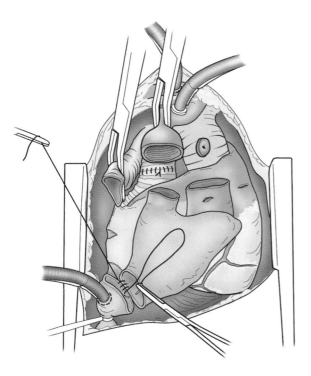

20 **Caval anastomosis**   Once the tracheal anastomosis has been completed, attention is turned to the IVC. As this structure lies deep within the pericardial cavity, access can be difficult. Exposure for this anastomosis is enhanced by displacing the heart through the left pericardial window into the left pleural cavity. The IVC anastomosis is performed with an extra-long 3/0 polypropylene running suture. The heart is then returned to the pericardial cavity, and the SVC anastomosis is completed using a 4/0 polypropylene running suture, taking care to avoid twisting of the donor or recipient SVC. The rest of the procedure is carried out as described in Figures 15 and 16.

20

POSTOPERATIVE CARE

Early postoperative care is directed toward the prevention of ischemic/reperfusion pulmonary edema, infection, and rejection. Chest drains are left *in situ* for at least 48 hours or until the cessation of any air leak.

Immediate postoperative care

No special isolation facility is necessary. Patients are kept sedated and ventilated with close monitoring of all hemodynamic parameters, arterial blood gases, urine output, and chest tube drainage. The ventilator is set to provide a tidal volume of 10 mL/kg, peak inflation pressures of less than 25 mm Hg, PEEP of 5–10 cm H_2O, and the lowest inspired oxygen concentration to provide PaO_2 of greater than 12 kPa. Once hemodynamic stability is achieved and excessive hemorrhage is excluded, patients are weaned from the ventilator. Most patients are extubated within 6–12 hours of transplant and are ready for discharge from the intensive care unit after 24–48 hours. Crystalloid infusion is restricted to 30 mL/m² per hour for the first 24 hours, and a loop diuretic is given six times per hour to 'run the patients dry.' Low-dose infusions of dopamine and isoprenaline are continued for 48 hours to maintain urine output and minimize pulmonary vascular resistance. Aggressive physiotherapy and early mobilization are essential in the prevention of pulmonary infection.

Immunosuppression regimens

In Papworth Hospital, immunosuppression for heart-lung transplant recipients is initiated on induction of anesthesia with intravenous azathioprine and methylprednisolone. Rabbit antithymocyte globulin (RATG) is commenced as soon as patients are on cardiopulmonary bypass, and further doses are given on day 1 and day 2 post-transplant. A second dose of methylprednisolone is given intravenously on reperfusion of the organs. Cyclosporin is only commenced on day 3 or thereafter to minimize the risk of renal dysfunction in the early post-transplant period. Maintenance immunosuppression is currently achieved with a triple-drug regime consisting of methylprednisolone, azathioprine, and cyclosporin. Details of our current immunosuppressive regime are shown in Table 27.3.

Infection prophylaxis

All recipients receive intravenous prophylactic antibiotics to cover gram-positive and gram-negative organisms at the time of transplantation. We currently use cefotaxime (2 g every 12 hours) and vancomycin (1 g every 12 hours) for the initial 48 hours. For cystic fibrosis patients who are known to be colonized by Pseudomonas species, cefotaxime is substituted with ceftazidime and tobramycin, or other agents as guided by sensitivities. Subsequent use of antibiotics depends on information obtained from bacteriological studies on the donor and the recipient.

Prophylaxis for cytomegalovirus (CMV) is necessary if either the donor or the recipient has been tested positive for CMV. Ganciclovir is administered intravenously for the first week and then orally for 3 months. As prophylaxis against *Pneumocystis carinii* pneumonia, a single oral dose (480 mg) of Septrin (a mixture of trimethoprim and sulfamethoxazole in a proportion of 1 part to 5 parts, respectively) is commenced when patients are able to take oral fluids. This drug is continued for a minimum of 6 months or until the dose of prednisolone is reduced to 0.1 mg/kg per day.

Table 27.3 *Immunosuppression regime for heart-lung transplant recipients*

Drug	Timing	Route	Dosage instructions
Azathioprine	On induction	i.v.	2 mg/kg
	Post-transplant	oral	2 mg/kg per d; decrease dose if leukocyte count $<5 \times 10^6$/dL
Methylprednisolone	On induction	i.v.	500 mg
	On reperfusion	i.v.	500 mg
	Postoperative	i.v.	125 mg at 8 h, 16 h, and 24 h
Corticosteroids maintenance (prednisolone)	Oral post-transplant	1 mg/kg per d	In 2 divided doses; reduce by 5 mg/d down to a dose of 0.2 mg/kg per d, maintained for 6 mo
RATG	On cardiopulmonary bypass	i.v.	1 mg/kg; to run over 10 h
	Days 1 and 2	i.v.	1 mg/kg; reduce to 0.5 mg/kg if T-cell level <5%
Cyclosporin	After cessation of RATG	oral	Commence with 100 mg daily in 2 divided doses, increasing by 100 mg/d to reach a total dose of 8–10 mg/kg per d; dose adjusted according to trough levels with target of 300–400 µg/L

RATG = rabbit antithymocyte globulin.

OUTCOME

Early complications and outcome

Since 1981, over 2500 patients have undergone heart-lung transplantation worldwide. Operative mortality has decreased significantly with accumulating experience. In our series of nearly 300 consecutive heart-lung transplants, operative mortality is 14 per cent. Donor organ dysfunction used to be an important cause of early death after heart-lung transplantation. With the introduction of an active donor management program, this problem has become much less common. We routinely employ Swan-Ganz catheters and hormone replacement therapy (triiodothyronine T3, vasopressin, and insulin) to resuscitate multi-organ donors before organ procurement. This strategy has the effect of optimizing donor organ function. Furthermore, this routine has enabled us to identify and discard organs that are likely to fail in the immediate post-transplant period. Occasionally, severe interstitial pulmonary edema still occurs as a result of the 'reimplantation response.' This complication can be difficult to manage, but sometimes it responds to inhaled nitric oxide at a dose of 20 parts per million.

Bleeding in excess of 750 mL in the first 24 hours post-transplant is found to be associated with a threefold increase in the risk of death after heart-lung transplantation. Patients who have undergone previous cardiac or thoracic surgery and those with extensive pleural adhesions are more likely to develop this problem. Careful surgical dissection, meticulous hemostasis, and the routine use of aprotinin have reduced the incidence of this difficulty. However, a significant number of patients still require surgical re-exploration to control the bleeding. The two most common bleeding sites are bronchial arteries in the mediastinum and pleural adhesions on the chest wall. Access to these areas through a median sternotomy incision is often unsatisfactory. Depending on which of the drains the bleeding appears to be coming from, a lateral thoracotomy may provide better access for re-exploration and securing hemostasis.

Another common problem seen after heart-lung transplantation is periodic pulmonary dysfunction with hypoxia and diffuse interstitial shadowing on the chest x-ray. This finding may be accompanied by pleural effusions. Such a clinical syndrome may either be due to acute allograft rejection or pulmonary infection. The only way to reliably distinguish between these two causes is to perform fiberoptic bronchoscopy and transbronchial biopsy to obtain tissue samples for histopathological evaluation and microbiological studies. In contrast with patients who have had heart transplantation alone, the incidence of isolated cardiac rejection after heart-lung transplantation is very low. As a result, our policy has been to avoid routine biopsy of the right ventricle after heart-lung transplantation.

Acute rejection episodes often respond to treatment with boluses of intravenous methylprednisolone (1 g on 3 consecutive days). For resistant rejection episodes, steroid boluses may be supplemented by a 3-day course of rabbit antithymocyte globulin. With the routine use of ganciclovir prophylaxis when either the donor or the recipient is CMV-seropositive, CMV pneumonitis has become rare post-transplant. Commonly encountered pathogens include multi-resistant *Staphylococcus aureus*, Pseudomonas, Candida, and Aspergillus. Despite careful surveillance and the aggressive use of antibiotics, infection remains a major cause of early and late mortality after heart-lung transplantation.

Late outcome

The Registry of the International Society for Heart and Lung Transplantation shows a 1-year actuarial survival of 61 per cent following heart-lung transplantation. Individual centers with extensive experience often obtain much better results. The Stanford group reports a 1-year survival rate of 73 per cent. In Papworth Hospital, the 1-, 5-, and 10-year survival rates are 75 per cent, 51 per cent, and 27 per cent, respectively. Our longest survivor received her heart-lung transplant in 1985.

Beyond the first year of heart-lung transplantation, bronchiolitis obliterans (OB) becomes a significant cause of morbidity and mortality. This problem can occur as early as 2–3 months after transplantation and may be present in 30 per cent of recipients by 6 months. Affected individuals first notice a fall in their FEV_1 on portable spirometry, which is later accompanied by a dry cough and progressive breathlessness on exertion. Histologically, OB is characterized by an acellular fibrous plugging of the lumina in the terminal bronchioles.

Current evidence suggests that OB represents chronic rejection of the pulmonary allograft. A strong correlation exists with early CMV infection, and OB appears to be more common with greater degrees of HLA mismatch between donor and recipient. At the earliest stages, OB may respond to augmentation of immunosuppression. Unfortunately, once the disease becomes established, no effective treatment is available and progressive deterioration is relentless. In some cases, reduction of immunosuppression may be preferred to decrease the frequency and severity of infective episodes. At present, OB remains the Achilles' heel in the long-term success of heart-lung transplantation.

In contrast with heart transplantation, cardiac allograft vasculopathy is an uncommon problem after heart-lung transplantation. Although it accounts for 2–4 per cent of late deaths, vasculopathy invariably occurs in patients who have already developed advanced OB. Because pravastatin has been shown to improve medium-term outcome after heart transplantation and may also reduce the incidence of cardiac allograft vasculopathy, we now routinely prescribe pravastatin after heart-lung transplantation as well.

In summary, heart-lung transplantation has become an established form of treatment for patients with end-stage cardiopulmonary failure. Currently, it represents the only therapeutic option in selected patients with otherwise untreatable conditions. Successful heart-lung transplantation provides symptomatic relief and increases life expectancy. However, the severe shortage of donor organs has limited its expansion and has restricted the number of patients who can benefit from this treatment. More effective means of using the diminishing donor pool, together with aggressive resuscitation of marginal donors, are essential to maintain a supply of organs for an increasing number of patients. Although a significant number of heart-lung recipients survive beyond 10 years, long-term success of heart-lung transplantation has been hampered by the development of OB. Advances in immunosuppressive strategies, together with an improved understanding of immunotolerance, hold the best hope for a brighter future for all transplant recipients.

FURTHER READING

Heart and Heart-Lung Transplantation. Baumgartner, Reitz and Achuff. 1990 W.B. Saunders Company.
Thoracic Transplantation. Shumway and Shumway. 1995 Blackwell.
Comprehensive Atlas of Organ Transplantation. Kuo, Dafoe, Bollinger and Davis. 2004 Lippincott Williams and Wilkins.

28

Mechanical ventricular assistance

ROHINTON J. MORRIS MD
Associate Professor of Surgery, Division of Cardiothoracic Surgery, University of Pennsylvania Health System – Presbyterian Medical Center, Philadelphia, Pennsylvania, USA

HISTORY

Mechanical assistance to the failing heart has taken numerous forms, from the partial support of the intra-aortic balloon pump to the full support of a centrifugal pump and cardiopulmonary bypass (CPB). Since the first successful use of the left ventricular assist devices (LVADs) in the 1960s, and their clinical success as a bridge to transplantation, patients in both acute and chronic heart failure have been supported for long periods of time until recovery or replacement. Ventricular assist devices (VADs) can be grouped into acute and chronic support, but strategies for placement and intraoperative management are similar. Morbidity and mortality of these operations are high, but better selection of patients, early intervention, and newer pharmacological support continues to decrease the daunting complications of this life-saving operation.

PRINCIPLES AND DEVICE SELECTION

Heart failure, with attendant organ malperfusion, secondary to acute myocardial infarction, or in the operative or perioperative period, requires urgent intervention with an acute device. The principles of an acute device should be simple and rapid deployment, decompression of the myocardium, and maintenance of end-organ perfusion.

Two current devices are in wide use for acute support: the Abiomed BVS 5000 (Abiomed Cardiovascular Inc., Danvers, MA) and the Thoratec VAD (Thoratec Laboratories Corporation, Pleasanton, CA). Cannulation of the atria or ventricle allows complete decompression of the strained myocardium, and the pneumatically driven pump delivers pulsatile flow back into the aorta or pulmonary artery via grafts. Both devices can be used for univentricular or biventricular support, and their pump housings are located extracorporeally, allowing for sternal closure. These devices also require anticoagulation to minimize thromboembolism. The BVS-5000 is simpler in principle, using gravity drainage and manipulation of vascular resistance to maintain end-organ perfusion, but it also has a shorter (i.e. days to weeks) duration of use. The Thoratec VAD uses vacuum-assisted drainage and manipulation of systolic time, rate, and drive pressure to achieve pulsatile flow. With proper care and attention, the Thoratec VAD can be maintained for months.

Chronic support of the left ventricle (LV) should entail long-term reliability, portability, and adequate cardiac flow for active patients. Two devices currently on the market are widely used: the TCI vented-electric HeartMate LVAD (Thermocardiosystems, Woburn, MA) and the Novacor LVAD (Baxter Healthcare Corporation, Oakland, CA). Both pumps have inflow cannulas, which are placed in the LV apex for drainage. These cannulas are connected to a pump body, which then is connected to an outflow cannula and graft that is subsequently sewn onto the ascending aorta. The conduits to and from the main pump housing contain bioprosthetic valves to obviate regurgitation. The pumps are placed either intraperitoneally (personal preference) or in a pocket in the abdominal wall, and an electrical driveline from the pump exits the patient via a subcutaneous tunnel in the right lower quadrant of the abdomen. Our preference for use is the TCI vented-electric HeartMate LVAD because of the avoidance of anticoagulation.

PREOPERATIVE ASSESSMENT AND PREPARATION

Earmarking of the patient with severe cardiac dysfunction can simplify the decision making when difficulty ensues. Signs of cardiogenic shock with decreased end-organ perfusion can herald the use of ventricular assistance. Intractable arrhythmias also constitute a major indication for VAD support. Transesophageal echocardiography is used on all cases and is essential, not only to assess ventricular and valvular function, but to detect air, thrombus, cannulae misplacement, and so forth.

OPERATION

Chronic devices

1a After median sternotomy, cannulation for CPB should be planned, with eventual placement of VAD grafts in mind. Aortic cannulation should be placed as high as possible, close to the arch; saphenous vein grafts (SVGs) should be placed on the lesser curvature, leaving enough room for a side-biting clamp and eventual VAD graft to the lateral wall of the ascending aorta. Any saphenous vein graft should also have enough length so as not to be impinged with a graft to the pulmonary artery in case of right ventricular (RV) support. Single two-stage venous cannulation will suffice in the majority of cases, but bicaval cannulation may afford better drainage, and in the case of an RV device, the appendage can be used for venous return with the VAD cannula.

The abdominal cavity is entered, and space created for the pump. Alternatively, a pump pocket can be created by dissecting the rectus abdominis from the posterior rectus fascia. We have found greater bleeding and incidence of infection by using a pump pocket in the abdominal wall, and we have found that most patients tolerate intra-abdominal placement without difficulty.

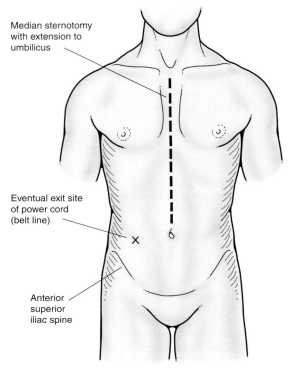

Median sternotomy with extension to umbilicus

Eventual exit site of power cord (belt line)

Anterior superior iliac spine

1a

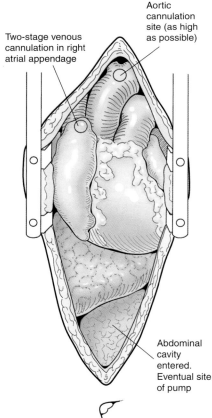

Aortic cannulation site (as high as possible)

Two-stage venous cannulation in right atrial appendage

Abdominal cavity entered. Eventual site of pump

1b

1b, c Preparation of the device is performed on a back table while the sternum is opened and the patient prepared for cannulation. The outflow grafts are immersed in albumin and autoclaved, or, alternatively, prepped with unheparinized blood from the patient and thrombin. The devices are flushed, taking care to keep the electrical cord dry and protected.

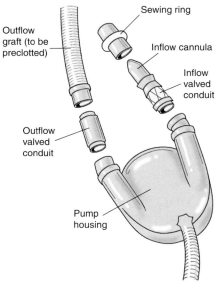

Outflow graft (to be preclotted)

Sewing ring

Inflow cannula

Inflow valved conduit

Outflow valved conduit

Pump housing

1c

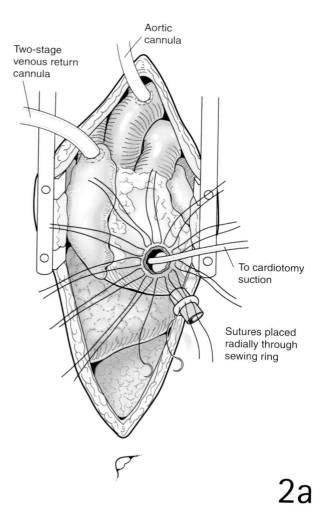

Two-stage
venous return
cannula

Aortic
cannula

To cardiotomy
suction

Sutures placed
radially through
sewing ring

2a

2a, b Placement of the VAD can be performed with the heart warm and beating, but cardioplegic arrest may be necessary to minimize blood in the field while cannulating the LV apex or left atrium through the pulmonary veins. Transesophageal echocardiography is used on all cases, and it must be used to assess for patent foramen ovale or aortic insufficiency. If either is present, it must be corrected before placement of the pump. Moderate to severe aortic insufficiency can either be repaired or the aortic valve can be completely closed with a pericardial patch.

The heart is elevated on lap pads, and a point is chosen for inflow cannulation approximately 2 cm to the left of the left anterior descending artery at the apex. Coring of the ventricle is performed with a 14-Fr coring device, taking care to direct the cut toward the LV cavity and not toward the septum. Multiple mattressed, pledgeted sutures of 0-Tevdek are placed circumferentially around the ventriculotomy. The LV cavity can be emptied with a flexible cardiotomy sucker, and any thrombus should be removed before placement of the inflow cannula. The sutures are brought through the sewing ring on the inflow cannula and tied down. After making an opening in the diaphragm, the inflow cannula can be connected to the pump in the abdominal pocket. Alternatively, the diaphragmatic attachment to the ribs may be detached with a 2-cm rim to allow ease of connection. The heart should be allowed to fill at this point, permitting passive filling of the pump. The pump should be agitated to evacuate as much air as possible.

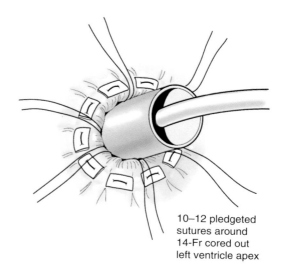

10–12 pledgeted
sutures around
14-Fr cored out
left ventricle apex

2b

3a, b

The outflow valved conduit and graft are then attached, and the graft is left clamped. The graft is stretched and measured to the ascending aorta. A side-biting partial occlusion clamp is placed on the greater curvature of the aorta, and the graft is sewn with a slight bevel using 4/0 Prolene. The aorta should have a small button excised to avoid any gradients, and thought should be given to leaving enough aorta for cardiac transplantation. A gentle curve to the graft should be used so that it does not remain in the midline for re-entry.

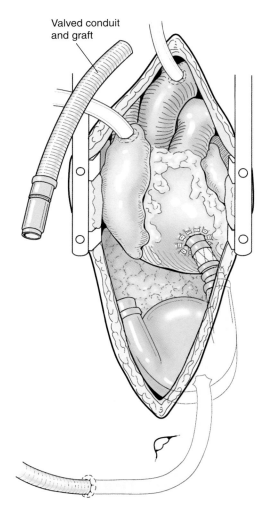

Valved conduit and graft

3a

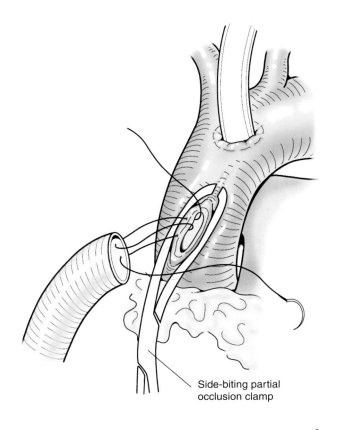

Side-biting partial occlusion clamp

3b

4 A deairing vent is placed in the ascending portion of the graft, and the graft is allowed to fill both retrograde from the aorta as well as antegrade from the pump. Transesophageal echocardiography should be used with gentle ventilation to assess any remaining air. The heart should also be filled, with decreases in CPB flows to fill the VAD. Gentle hand-pumping should effectively remove all remaining air. The device should be started with the patient on partial CPB and in the Trendelenburg position.

When weaned from CPB, the right heart should be assessed for a short period of time before reversing anticoagulation. Pulmonary hypertension by itself is not a clear indication for RV support. Heavy bleeding, with resultant massive transfusion, will often lead to RV failure and should be corrected before weaning from bypass.

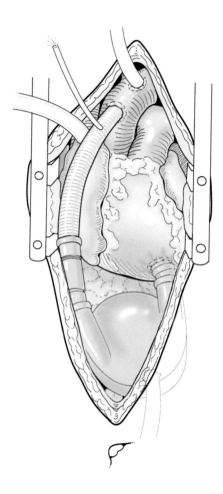

4

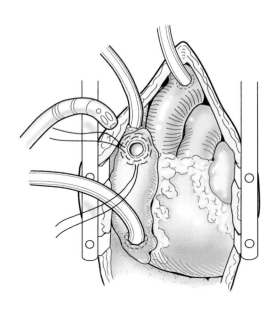

5a

Acute ventricular assist device placement

5a, b For acute VADs, it is imperative to plan cannula placement on the chest wall before cannulation. Arterial grafts should be stretched before sizing and can easily be manipulated once the other end is brought through the chest wall. A deairing needle should be placed at the highest point in these grafts through a purse-string suture. The venous return cannulae are generally placed before pulling through the chest wall, and they should be placed through a double pursestring suture that is reinforced with pledgets. Approximately 2–4 cm of the cannula should be inserted into the right or left atrium, taking care not to insert it through the mitral or tricuspid valves. The valve mechanism may get entangled in the cannula and thereby block venous return.

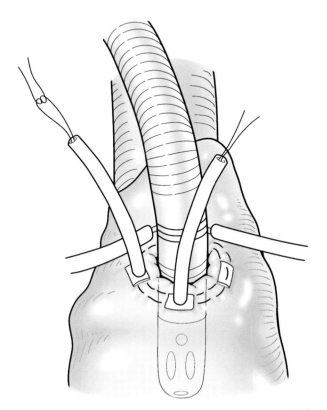

5b

5c Thoratec® Ventricular Assist Device (VAD) and three cannulation approaches for univentricular left heart support (Panel A), and biventricular support (Panels B and C). Ao = aorta. LA = left atrial appendage, pulmonary artery, RA = right atrium, Apex = left ventricular apex, IAG = cannula inserted via the interatrial groove and directed towards LA roof. Note that the VADs in Panel C are turned over on the sides of the chest that are opposite of those in Panel B. (Modified from Farrar DJ *et al. New England Journal of Medicine* 1988; 318: 333–340. Copyright 1988, Massachusetts Medical Society).

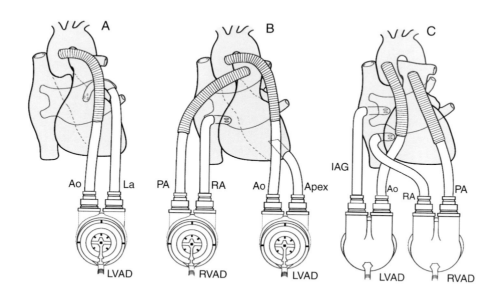

5c

POSTOPERATIVE CARE

Bleeding problems are paramount in these patients. Strict hemostasis is essential, and minimizing blood transfusion reduces the risk of right heart failure. Adjunctive agents, such as aprotinin, are extremely helpful in combating coagulopathy. Because both acute VADs and the Novacor device require anticoagulation, extra time is spent in the operating room until the field is as dry as possible. We fully reverse the heparin with protamine at the end of the procedure, and we generally start anticoagulation within the next 24 hours, before chest tubes are pulled. Significant bleeding and attendant transfusion are also implicated in right heart failure when placing an LVAD. RV failure that requires an acute VAD occurs in 5–10 per cent of cases having primarily left heart failure. Inotropes may have to be continued in the immediate postoperative period to assist the RV.

Driveline infections occur commonly (50–70 per cent) in various series, but truly life-threatening infection with pocket abscess formation or sepsis is only seen in 5–10 per cent of cases. Dressing changes and wound care must be carried out in a sterile fashion, and early institution of antibiotics for wound drainage is standard.

Device malfunction has occurred only rarely and is the basis for anecdotal reports.

OUTCOME

The mortality rate for VAD placement ranges from 25 to 40 per cent in various series. The outcome is obviously different for acute and chronic devices. Factors that play key roles in acute placement of VADs include timing of implant, duration of shock, presence or absence of cardiac arrest, underlying disease states, and age. The most common cause of death is multi-system organ failure. Life-threatening hemorrhage and late infection with sepsis also contribute to the mortality associated with these devices.

Over the last few years, most transplant programs, including ours, have allowed patients to go home with chronic VADs and resume a 'normal' life. Although reversal, both histologically and clinically, of heart failure has been reported, the majority of VADs is being used as bridge-to-transplants. A significant cohort of patients now exists that has used chronic VADs for years, which points to the eventual use of these devices as 'destination' therapy.

FURTHER READING

Argenziano, M., Oz, M.C., Rose, E.A. 1997. The continuing evolution of mechanical ventricular assistance. *Current Problems in Surgery* 34, 317–88.

Pennington, D.G. 1994. Mechanical circulatory support. *Seminars in Thoracic and Cardiovascular Surgery* 6(3), 129–94.

Goldstein, D.J., Oz, M.C., Rose, E.A. 1998. Implantable left ventricular assist devices. *New England Journal of Medicine* 339(21), 1522–33.

Fischer, S.A., Trenholme, G.M., Costanzo, M.R., Piccione, W. 1997. Infectious complications in left ventricular assist device recipients. *Clinical Infectious Diseases* 24, 18–23.

McCarthy, P.M., Nakatani, S., Vargo, R., *et al.* 1995. Structural and left ventricular histologic changes after implantable LVAD insertion. *Annals of Thoracic Surgery* 59, 609–13.

29

Use of conventional techniques: revascularization and valve repair

STEVEN F. BOLLING MD
Professor of Surgery and Attending Surgeon, Section of Cardiac Surgery, University of Michigan Medical School, Ann Arbor, Michigan, USA

VINAY BADHWAR MD
Chairman, Tampa Bay Heart Institute, St. Petersburg, Florida, USA

IVA A. SMOLENS MD
Section of Cardiac Surgery, University of Michigan, Ann Arbor, Michigan, USA

HISTORY

Along with the introduction of cardiopulmonary bypass nearly half a century ago, attempts were made to surgically manage patients with advanced heart failure. Early poor outcomes from these efforts discouraged surgeons from offering these patients any surgical alternatives other than transplantation. Consequently, patients with dilated cardiomyopathy of idiopathic, ischemic, or valvular origin were limited to medical therapy alone.

More recently, this practice has been re-examined with a renewed appreciation of the mechanics and pathophysiology of heart failure. With the ability to identify hibernating myocardium that is capable of resuming postoperative myocardial function has come the means to apply conventional surgical techniques to these unconventional patients. Proper preoperative medical management combined with refined conventional surgical techniques has now led to the successful application of coronary revascularization and mitral valve reconstruction to patients with advanced heart failure.

PRINCIPLES AND JUSTIFICATION

Congestive heart failure has become a major public health problem in the United States. An estimated 4.7 million Americans are living with heart failure, resulting in 900 000 hospitalizations, over 10 billion dollars in health costs, and approximately 250 000 deaths each year. Despite significant improvements in medical management, more than half of the patients who present with congestive heart failure die within 3 years. Furthermore, of the 500 000 patients who are newly diagnosed each year in the United States, fewer than 2900 heart transplantations are performed due to the limited number of donor hearts that are available and the inapplicability of transplantation in older patients or in those with comorbid medical conditions.

It is well recognized that coronary artery disease and mitral regurgitation (MR), when present in patients with cardiomyopathy, are each an independent predictor of poor survival. Moreover, recent evidence has revealed that early surgical intervention in these cohorts results in significant improvement in survival and quality of life that may equate with or even surpass that of transplantation. When feasible, surgical restoration of normal mechanics and physiology has clear benefits over the immunosuppression-related 'disease exchange' of transplantation.

Coronary artery bypass graft

We have known for nearly 20 years, via the Coronary Artery Surgery Study (CASS), European Coronary Surgery Trial (ECST), and Veterans Administration studies, that revascularizing patients with left ventricular dysfunction can result in a greater than 25 per cent improvement in long-term survival. Early enthusiasm was tempered by reports of high operative mortality in patients with a low ejection fraction (EF). Since then, as success with the medical and surgical management of heart failure and transplantation grew, so did the interest in applying this experience to patients with ischemic cardiomyopathy. Successful revascularization can now be performed on patients with an EF of less than 30 per cent, with hospital mortalities as low as 5 per cent.

The premise behind the improvements in EF, long-term survival, and quality of life of these patients is believed to be postoperative myocyte recruitment. Restoration of perfusion resuscitates dormant viable myocardium and serves to protect the previously functioning portions of the ventricle from further ischemic insults, arrhythmias, and infarction.

To minimize morbidity, a multidisciplinary approach to the preoperative management of heart failure is essential. Patients ideally suited for coronary artery bypass grafting (CABG) are those medically optimized, with or without angina, who have good distal coronary targets, functional hibernating myocardium identified preoperatively, and no evidence of right ventricular dysfunction. As experience in managing these patients increases, many surgeons have operated on patients with EFs of less than 10 per cent, including those who are undergoing reoperation and those with moderate elevations in pulmonary artery pressure. Nevertheless, patients with clear documentation of poor right ventricular EF, clinical right-sided congestive symptoms, or fixed pulmonary hypertension above 60 mm Hg systolic should be approached cautiously, as these individuals may be better suited for transplantation.

Mitral valve repair

Many patients with cardiomyopathy develop MR. Moreover, severe MR affects almost all heart failure patients as a preter-minal or terminal event. Mortality is not only related to the severity of ventricular systolic dysfunction but also to the presence of mitral insufficiency. The progressive dilation of the left ventricle (LV) gives rise to MR, which begets more MR and further ventricular dilation. This cycle of heart failure is often manifested as an escalation of congestive and low-output symptomatology. Therefore, the goal of surgical intervention is to interrupt this cycle of dilation through the restoration of normal cardiac physiology and ventricular mechanics.

Fundamental to the management of MR in heart failure is a firm understanding of the functional anatomy of the mitral valve. The mitral valve apparatus consists of the annulus, leaflets, chordae tendineae, and papillary muscles, as well as the entire LV.

Therefore, maintenance of chordal, annular, and subvalvular continuity is essential for the preservation of mitral geometrical relationships and overall ventricular function. Adherence to this principle is vital when dealing with patients who have compromised LV function. During the era when the only surgical treatment for MR was mitral valve replacement, the dependence of ventricular function on annulus–papillary muscle continuity was not fully appreciated. Consequently, patients with low EF who underwent mitral valve replacement with removal of the subvalvular apparatus had prohibitively high mortality. In an attempt to explain these outcomes, the concept of a beneficial 'pop-off' effect of MR was conceived. This idea erroneously proposes that mitral incompetence provides a low-pressure relief during systolic ejection from the failing ventricle and that removal of this effect through mitral replacement is responsible for deterioration of ventricular function. Consequently, mitral valve replacement in patients with heart failure was discouraged. More recent studies documenting the importance of maintaining the integrity of the subvalvular apparatus in preservation of postoperative LV function have led to surgical techniques that have been applicable to patients with end-stage heart failure. Accordingly, preservation of the mitral valve apparatus in mitral surgery has been demonstrated to enhance ventricular geometry, decrease wall stress, and improve systolic and diastolic function. This geometrical restoration is the premise behind the success of mitral reconstruction in heart failure.

1a, b Functional MR is a complication of end-stage cardiomyopathy, and its pathogenesis is multi-factorial. With normal ventricular geometry, the redundant mitral leaflets are responsible for a zone of coaptation that is more than twice the area of the mitral valve orifice. In the absence of organic mitral disease, as the failing ventricle dilates, MR develops as a result of the concomitant progressive dilation of the mitral annulus, which results in incomplete leaflet coaptation and a central regurgitant jet of so-called functional insufficiency. Therefore, in heart failure the most significant determinant of leaflet coaptation and MR is the diameter of the mitral valve annulus. The left ventricular dimension is of less importance in functional MR, as the lengths of the chordae and papillary muscles are similar in myopathic hearts regardless of whether MR is present. This situation may explain why mitral annular reduction and reconstruction can be applied to patients with diminished EFs.

With ischemic cardiomyopathy, the mechanisms that contribute to MR are more complex. Functional MR from annular dilation is compounded by ischemic changes to the subvalvular structures of the entire ventricle. 'Papillary muscle dysfunction' is not an isolated disorder of the papillary muscle; it is a disturbance in the coordination of the lateral ventricular walls and the mitral valve apparatus. Thus, the combination of annular dilation and ischemic changes in the subvalvular structures leads to an alteration in the functional geometry of the mitral valve.

The mechanisms behind the success of mitral valve repair in cardiomyopathy center on the restoration of ventricular mechanics and physiology. The preoperative adaptations to severe MR include increases in ventricular preload, wall tension, and stroke volume. With nearly half of the stroke volume being ejected into the left atrium during presystole, the contractile efficiency of the ventricle is limited. Furthermore, this reduction in effective cardiac output combined with increased left ventricular wall stress serve to restrict further coronary flow reserve. Thus, regardless of the preoperative EF, surgical elimination of the regurgitant flow results in an augmented effective cardiac output, reduced ventricular volume and wall stress, and improved coronary flow reserve.

A systematic approach should be used when considering a patient for mitral valve repair in the setting of congestive heart failure. Indications to undergo mitral valve repair in cardiomyopathy include symptomatic, medically optimized patients with 3+ to 4+ MR as confirmed by echocardiography. It is preferred that patients are free of cardiac ischemia. However, a combined approach to address the coronary pathogenesis as well as the MR may be necessary. Furthermore, those patients with a prior sternotomy or cardiac operation should not be denied mitral repair, as these patients can be approached through a right posterolateral thoracotomy. As with CABG for heart failure, con-

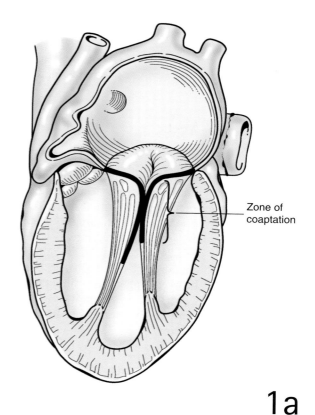

Zone of coaptation

1a

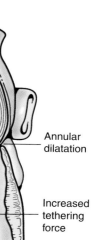

Annular dilatation

Increased tethering force

Weak closing force

Widening of interpapillary distance

1b

traindications to mitral repair include severe right ventricular dysfunction and irreversible primary pulmonary hypertension. As with all cardiac procedures, surgical morbidity and mortality can be effectively minimized in cardiomyopathy patients with a thorough preoperative evaluation.

PREOPERATIVE ASSESSMENT AND PREPARATION

Regardless of the underlying etiology, patients with advanced left ventricular dysfunction manifest clinical signs of heart failure. These signs may range from mild shortness of breath and fatigability to episodic and debilitating congestive symptoms that require active medical support. For any patient with heart failure who is being considered for either CABG or mitral surgery, the importance of a thorough preoperative evaluation cannot be overemphasized. Although somewhat controversial, many heart failure surgeons now believe that with proper preparation, no EF is too low to attain a satisfactory long-term surgical outcome.

Coronary artery bypass graft

The process of preoperative investigation should coincide with optimizing the patient's medical management. This treatment should entail an aggressive regimen of diuretic and vasodilator therapy to minimize ventricular afterload and normalize the patient's circulating blood volume. For patients with severe heart failure, a brief period of inotropic therapy for ventricular resuscitation may be necessary to optimize their medical management. Inability to be weaned from this support is often indicative of severe myocardial injury and poor overall prognosis with any surgical therapy other than mechanical ventricular assistance or transplantation.

Preoperative investigations should begin with transthoracic echocardiography to evaluate ventricular function and identify any underlying valvular pathology. Baseline screening physiological studies of oxygen consumption, pulmonary function, and cardiopulmonary endurance are recommended. Identification of reversible ischemia by means of a nuclear study can be helpful; however, for patients with angina, many centers proceed directly to coronary angiography.

Although angina may be indicative of living ventricular muscle, perhaps the most important correlate of a successful surgical recovery is the quantification of myocardial viability Therefore, before subjecting hearts with limited ventricular function to the temporary stunning of cardiopulmonary bypass, a determination of myocardial contractile reserve is essential. Not only is this useful to ensure that the patient can be safely separated from bypass, but this information is predictive of recovery of ventricular function and long-term survival after operation.

Although thallium 201 perfusion scans may distinguish myocytes with membrane integrity from scar, positron emission tomography (PET) scanning and dobutamine stress echocardiography have emerged as the most useful tests to identify preoperative myocardial viability and to predict postoperative function. With the use of systemically administered tracers, PET scanning has the ability to detect a mismatch between myocardial blood flow and myocyte function. Scanning for the metabolic substrate fluorodeoxyglucose (FDG) provides identification of aerobic cellular activity. When comparing this activity to the assessment of myocardial flow, hypoperfused areas of the myocardium that take up FDG are noted to be viable or hibernating. Despite the high specificity of PET scanning, its cost and relative lack of availability have limited its widespread use.

Dobutamine stress echocardiography involves the administration of incremental doses of dobutamine while observing for changes in segmental wall thickness and recruitment of segmental ventricular function. A biphasic response to the introduction and withdrawal of inotropy can be highly predictive of contractile reserve and an indicator of the patient's tolerance of cardiopulmonary bypass and functional recovery. Although this test is less expensive and more widely available than a PET scan, it requires the expertise of a trained cardiologist and may be observer dependent. Therefore, the optimal test for myocardial viability depends on the facilities that are available at one's institution. After severe systemic comorbidity, malignancy, and other contraindications to surgery are excluded, fully evaluated and medically optimized patients may safely proceed to surgery.

Patients with dilated cardiomyopathy and MR usually present with symptoms of severe congestive heart failure. Symptoms of decreased cardiac output and pulmonary congestion increase proportionally to the progression of MR. Before surgical intervention, these patients require careful investigation and preoperative management. Like those who are being considered for CABG, all patients with cardiomyopathy should be optimized with a medical regimen that includes aggressive diuresis, digoxin, and afterload reduction with agents such as angiotensin-converting enzyme inhibitors or vasodilators.

Mitral valve repair

Physical examination of MR in cardiomyopathy typically reveals a hyperdynamic cardiac impulse and a characteristic blowing holosystolic murmur that may radiate from the apex to the axilla, back, or neck. Radiographically, patients usually have an enlarged cardiac silhouette that is indicative of left ventricular or atrial enlargement. Typical electrocardiographic findings include left atrial enlargement and ventricular hypertrophy.

A preliminary transthoracic echocardiogram is helpful to assess ventricular function noninvasively and estimate the severity of MR. Left ventricular performance is best inferred from the diameter of the LV at end systole. Measurements of end-systolic dimension are less dependent on preload than EF and thus provide a more accurate assessment of contractile function.

Color Doppler analysis provides a semiquantitative analysis of MR. This method is often sensitive to load conditions, driving pressure, jet eccentricity, and left atrial size and, thus, may lead to incorrect estimations of the true degree of MR. Proximal flow convergence analysis, which calculates the regurgitant volume by measuring the flow proximal to the mitral valve orifice, may be a preferable method to quantify the extent of regurgitation accurately in patients with heart failure. Once MR is identified, it is essential to define clearly the mitral pathoanatomy by transesophageal echocardiography. A detailed understanding of leaflet and chordal excursion including the character of the regurgitant jet is helpful to plan the correct operative approach effectively. In the vast majority of these patients, ventricular geometrical distortion results in a symmetrical central jet of regurgitation from mitral annular dilation. In cases of anatomical distortion of the valve anatomy, the regurgitant jet may be eccentrically located. These patients may require a more complex repair to correct leaflet prolapse or chordal rupture.

Before mitral repair, coronary angiography should be performed to identify and to assess the extent of native coronary disease as well as the patency of any prior grafts in patients who have undergone previous revascularization. If occlusions are detected, a study to assess myocardial viability in the distribution of the occluded vessel is advocated to determine if a preoperative percutaneous or concomitant surgical revascularization procedure is warranted. Although cardiac catheterization is not necessary to establish the diagnosis of MR, it is useful to ascertain the etiology of heart failure when a discrepancy exists between clinical and noninvasive study findings. Occasionally, right heart catheterization is required if concerns of pulmonary hypertension cannot be adequately assessed by echocardiography.

ANESTHESIA

In patients with heart failure who have limited contractile reserve, the induction of anesthesia should be performed in such a manner as to avoid dramatic swings in arterial pressure and ventricular preload. For this reason, Swan-Ganz and arterial pressure catheters should be placed before anesthetic induction. With restricted coronary reserve, forward flow is often dependent on volume adaptation and a heightened catecholamine state; and therefore, volatile inhalational anesthetics and medications that can result in vasodilatation are avoided. Some surgeons have advocated the use of a preoperatively placed intra-aortic balloon to protect coronary perfusion against dramatic changes in pressure during induction of

anesthesia. However, as experience is gained managing the anesthetic of these patients, few continue this practice.

A safe and effective method of anesthesia for these patients is often comprised of a high-dose narcotic combined with a muscle relaxant. Pancuronium is preferred, as its slight sympathetic activity tends to counteract the bradycardia that is seen with high-dose narcotics. This combination allows for a smooth physiological induction with little heart rate variability.

After induction, transesophageal echo (TEE) probe placement for intraoperative echocardiography is performed. This maneuver permits the assessment of the integrity of the mitral valve as well as a real-time evaluation of contractile function. TEE monitoring has proven helpful in guiding postcardiopulmonary bypass hemodynamics.

OPERATION

Coronary artery bypass graft

Median sternotomy, conduit harvesting, and cannulation are performed in a routine atraumatic fashion. Whenever appropriate, a pedicled internal thoracic artery graft should be prepared and used. Any unnecessary manipulation of the arrhythmogenic ventricles should be avoided until cardiopulmonary bypass is instituted. Absolute attention to myocardial protection and the judicious use of anterograde and retrograde cold blood cardioplegia should be encouraged. Delivery of cardioplegia to all regions throughout the procedure minimizes ventricular dysfunction and helps to avoid difficulty in weaning from cardiopulmonary bypass. Some surgeons advocate temperature-directed grafting, where regions with higher myocardial temperature are grafted first, followed by cardioplegic delivery down completed grafts. Regardless of the technique used, a strategy for homogenous myocardial protection should be used.

The fundamental premise behind a successful operation is to attain an expeditiously performed and yet complete revascularization. As the failing myocardium is particularly intolerant to further episodes of ischemia, careful consideration should be given to the quality of the distal vessels and the ease with which good anastomoses can be achieved. Operative time expended grafting small or extensively diseased vessels, or performing additional techniques such as endarterectomy, may be counterproductive. Because the price to pay for incomplete revascularization or transient ischemia may be severe, off-pump techniques may not be ideally suited for these patients unless performed flawlessly.

Mitral valve repair

2 A median sternotomy is the incision most commonly used for approaching the mitral valve; however, a right anterior thoracotomy also affords good access to the mitral valve and is especially useful in the reoperative patient. As the key to successful mitral valve surgery is adequate exposure, bicaval cannulation with an approach via the interatrial groove is preferred for almost all patients undergoing mitral valve procedures. When cardiopulmonary bypass has been instituted, the aortic cross-clamp is applied, and diastolic arrest of the heart is achieved with the use of cold blood cardioplegia delivered either in an anterograde, retrograde, or combined approach. The left atrium is then opened with an incision just posterior to the interatrial groove, and it may be extended inferiorly to the back of the heart and superiorly behind the superior vena cava (SVC). The use of a specially designed self-retaining retractor greatly facilitates exposure of the mitral valve.

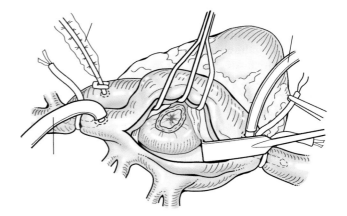

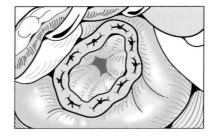

2

3 In cardiomyopathy patients the etiology of the mitral insufficiency is most often due to mitral annular dilation; and therefore, the goal of effective repair is to re-establish the zone of coaptation with mitral annular remodeling. Annular sutures should be securely placed through the fibrous annulus, rather than into the leaflet or the atrial wall. To achieve effective geometrical remodeling in these patients, the surgeon should 'undersize' the annuloplasty ring to 'overcorrect' the zone of leaflet coaptation with a complete circumferential ring. Once the valve repair is completed, the atrium is closed, appropriate deairing maneuvers are performed, and the patient is separated from cardiopulmonary bypass.

On completion of high-risk coronary revascularization and mitral valve repair in myopathic patients, separation from cardiopulmonary bypass may be challenging. Patients with chronic heart failure have increased circulating plasma catecholamine levels and depleted myocyte stores of norepinephrine. After long-term exposure to elevated catecholamines, myocyte beta-adrenoreceptors become down-regulated and desensitized. This situation results in a reduction of intrinsic cyclic adenosine monophosphate (cAMP) production and a reduced positive inotropic effect of exogenous beta-adrenoreceptor agonists. Therefore, in the face of reduced basal myocyte cAMP availability, one can use the increased inotropic effect of phosphodiesterase inhibitors that are not dependent on beta-adrenoreceptors. With the combination of these two agents, however, exogenously administered norepinephrine acts to replenish depleted myocyte stores and stimulate cAMP production, which in turn serves to augment the positive inotropic effects of phosphodiesterase inhibition. Therefore, for these reasons, a combination of norepinephrine and milrinone is used to successfully wean the patient with heart failure from cardiopulmonary bypass.

With greater experience in heart failure surgery, the requirement for postoperative mechanical support is becoming infrequent. Most centers report intra-aortic balloon use in fewer than 15 per cent of cases of CABG, and even less often following mitral repair. Moreover, with proper preoperative and operative preparation, ventricular assist devices are now rarely necessary.

POSTOPERATIVE CARE

In addition to the routine postcardiotomy management, the patient with advanced left ventricular dysfunction requires tight control of volume loading in the initial postoperative period, followed by reintroduction of the full complement of the preoperative antifailure medical therapy. This treatment should include a diuretic regimen in combination with afterload reduction therapy. The introduction of beta-blockade for arrhythmia prevention or the use of emerging multifunctional drugs such as carvedilol has proven to be helpful. Judicious follow-up of these patients is necessary to assure the

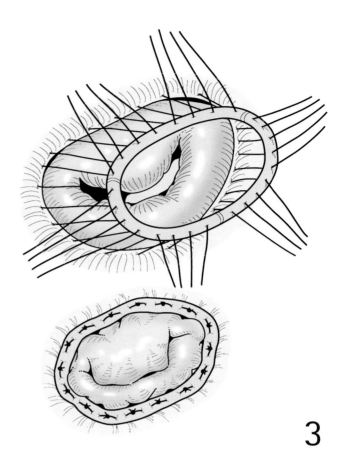

3

tight maintenance of the patient's circulating volume. A thorough rehabilitation regimen is essential to promote mobilization and to hasten postoperative recovery.

As operative intervention does not correct the underlying myocardial composition and myocyte structure, one must be observant for the existence of low-output or arrhythmia complications that may occur with cardiomyopathy patients. For the rare occurrence of ventricular arrhythmias that are unresponsive to pharmacological therapy, the use of implantable defibrillators may significantly enhance postoperative recovery as well as long-term survival.

OUTCOME

The 3-year survival of patients with cardiomyopathy is less than 50 per cent. When these patients have concomitant coronary artery disease or MR, the 1-year survival has been reported to be as low as 30 per cent. The surgical treatment of cardiomyopathy with coronary revascularization or mitral valve repair provides these patients with new alternatives to attain improvements in quality of life and long-term survival.

Coronary artery bypass graft

Multiple groups have been uniformly successful in demonstrating improvements in survival, ventricular function, and functional status with coronary revascularization in patients with ischemic cardiomyopathy. Series outlining long-term outcomes from CABG on patients with EFs less than 25 per cent have been reported by groups from Yale, New York's Mount Sinai, Toronto, Duke, and The University of Verona, among others.

The 5-year survival with transplantation ranges from 62 per cent to 82 per cent, whereas with medical therapy alone, it is less than 30 per cent. Most series report survival following CABG for ischemic cardiomyopathy ranging from 85 per cent to 88 per cent at 1 year, 75 per cent to 82 percent at 2 years, 68 per cent to 80 per cent at 3 years, and 60 per cent to 80 cent at 5 years. Operative mortality has been reported from 3 per cent to 12 per cent, with the main predictor of increased risk being urgency of operation. It is encouraging to note that the long-term survival of CABG patients is equivalent to that of transplantation in most series. The superior survival of CABG over transplant in the first 2 years postoperatively may be due to early attrition from rejection or infection in the latter group. Although little data have been reported on patients with EFs of less than 10 per cent, one can infer that these individuals would have a similarly better outcome than their nonrevascularized, medically treated counterparts. As experience with heart failure surgery expands, refinements in preoperative and operative management of CABG patients will be reflected in the uniformity of future long-term results.

Improvement of EF after revascularization can be correlated to the amount of viable ischemic myocardium noted preoperatively. In addition to improved EF, patients with viabilities of greater than 20 per cent of the ventricular mass noted by PET have documented increased survival and quality of life after revascularization. With dobutamine stress echocardiography, similar positive outcomes are recognized to be proportional to the number of preoperatively responsive ventricular segments.

When compared to medical therapy, revascularized patients have significant improvements in quality of life. Most series report considerable enhancements in patient mobility, peak oxygen consumption, and functional status. The average preoperative New York Heart Association (NYHA) class of 3.5 reportedly drops to 1.5 after revascularization. Postoperatively, the numbers of hospitalizations for heart failure substantially decrease, and many patients return to work.

With adequate preparation, coronary revascularization can now be performed on heart failure patients of any EF with minimal morbidity and mortality. The ensuing revival of hibernating viable myocardium restores ventricular function as well as the patient's functional status. Thus, with adequate documentation of preoperative viability, even patients with EFs of less than 10 per cent are capable of attaining a successful outcome.

Mitral valve repair

In an attempt to decrease the volume overload of heart failure and restore optimal ventricular geometry, the University of Michigan has instituted a program of mitral valve repair in patients with severe heart failure. Since the program's inception, more than 120 patients with refractory end-stage cardiomyopathy and severe MR have undergone mitral reconstruction. All of these patients had pure geometrical distortion of the LV with annular dilation and were repaired with an undersized flexible annuloplasty ring. No patients in the study required complex mitral valve repair. The group was evenly divided between ischemic and nonischemic cardiomyopathies, with a mean EF of 14 per cent. Although annular reconstruction alone seems intuitive for patients with the central regurgitation of dilated cardiomyopathy, this procedure may not be appropriate for management of the eccentric MR of ischemic cardiomyopathy. It is encouraging, however, that statistical analysis did not reveal any differences in outcome when these two etiologies were compared. The overall 30-day operative mortality was 5 per cent, with only one intraoperative death from right ventricular failure. With a mean duration of follow-up of 38 months, the 1- and 2-year actuarial survival has been 80 per cent and 70 per cent, respectively, with 26 late deaths. All patients have remained on medical therapy for their congestive heart failure. The NYHA class has improved an average of two functional classes, and all patients reported subjective improvements in quality of life. Reduction in sphericity index and improvements in left ventricular EF, cardiac output, and end-diastolic volumes have been observed in all patients.

Groups from the Cleveland Clinic, and Boston's Brigham and Women's Hospital have recently reproduced these results. At the Cleveland Clinic, 35 patients with severe left ventricular dysfunction underwent mitral repair. These patients all demonstrated improvements in NYHA functional class, with their 1- and 2-year actuarial survival rates being 89 per cent and 86 per cent, respectively. At the Brigham and Women's Hospital, 81 patients with an EF less than 30 per cent underwent mitral valve repair, and more than 60 of them underwent concomitant coronary revascularization. Similarly, these patients were noted to have significant improvements in EF and NYHA class, with 1- and 2-year actuarial survival rates of 73 per cent and 68 per cent.

Mitral reconstruction in cardiomyopathy safely restores mitral competency and left ventricular geometry. This procedure can now be performed with reproducible long-term results and minimal operative mortality. The physiological improvement in contractile efficiency and cardiac output affords patients improvements in functional status and quality of life.

The successful use of coronary revascularization and mitral reconstruction has transformed the management of cardiomyopathy. These options now provide patients who would normally have no other alternative with a reliable method of attaining long-term survival and a better quality of life. Together with transplantation and assist devices, the refined conventional techniques of coronary bypass and mitral repair should be included in the armamentarium of the heart failure surgeon.

FURTHER READING

Bolling, S.F., Pagani, F.D., Deeb, G.M., *et al.* 1998. Intermediate-term outcome of mitral reconstruction in cardiomyopathy. *Journal of Thoracic and Cardiovascular Surgery* **115**, 381–8.

Chen, F.Y., Adams, D.H., Aranki, S.F., *et al.* 1998. Mitral valve repair in cardiomyopathy. *Circulation* **98**, Suppl. II: 124–127.

Di Carli, M.F., Maddahi, J., Roshsar, S., *et al.* 1998. Long-term survival of patients with coronary artery disease and left ventricular dysfunction: implications for the role of myocardial viability assessment in management decisions. *Journal of Thoracic and Cardiovascular Surgery* **116**, 997–1004.

Marwick, T.H., Zuchowski, C., Lauer, M.S., *et al.* 1999. Functional status and quality of life in patients with heart failure undergoing coronary bypass surgery after assessment of myocardial viability. *Journal of the American College of Cardiology* **33**, 750–8.

Mickelborough, L.L., Carson, S., Tamariz, M., *et al.* 2000. Results of revascularization in patients with severe left ventricular dysfunction. *Journal of Thoracic and Cardiovascular Surgery* **119**, 550–7.

Senior, R., Kaul, S., Lahiri, A. 1999. Myocardial viability on echocardiography predicts long-term survival after revascularization in patients with ischemic congestive heart failure. *Journal of the American College of Cardiology* **33**, 1848–54.

30

Left ventricular reconstruction for ischemic cardiomyopathy

PATRICK M. McCARTHY MD
Surgical Director, Kaufman Center for Heart Failure, Department of Thoracic and Cardiovascular Surgery, The Cleveland Clinic Foundation, Cleveland, Ohio, USA

HISTORY

Left ventricular (LV) reconstruction for ischemic cardiomyopathy has been in the repertoire of cardiac surgeons since the earlier aneurysm repairs more than 40 years ago. The technique has evolved from simple linear repairs of the infarcted free wall of the LV to more complete repairs involving not just the free wall but also the infarcted LV septum. A tremendous variation exists in the extent of infarction, the distribution of scar between the septum and free wall, and the degree of subsequent ventricular dilatation. The effectiveness of linear repair versus more complete repair is related to this variation. The remodeled dilated ventricle increases wall stress in areas remote from the LV aneurysm. The fundamental mechanism behind improved LV function after repair of an aneurysm in the left anterior descending (LAD) distribution is improved function in the circumflex and right coronary artery territories due to reduction in wall stress in these areas remote from the aneurysm.

PRINCIPLES AND JUSTIFICATION

Most patients who undergo this surgery have additional indications for cardiac operations such as three-vessel or left main coronary artery disease. Many patients also have significant (3+ or greater) mitral regurgitation, usually due to ventricular dilatation with apical tethering of the papillary muscles causing restricted motion of the posterior leaflet and a central jet of mitral regurgitation. However, some patients undergo this operation because of a discreet LAD scar with a history of progressive LV dilatation and reduction in ejection fraction, typically associated with symptoms of congestive heart failure. The average ejection fraction in our series was 23 per cent. Most often in our experience, the operation is performed for patients who have a discreet infarcted area in the LAD territory, only rarely with additional infarctions in the circumflex and/or right coronary territories. In our experience, approximately 60 per cent of patients have had a true aneurysm (dyskinesia), and the other 40 per cent have had akinetic areas of infarction with a dilated ventricle. Patients are selected for surgery based on ventriculography (ideally biplane) and 3-D imaging studies such as 3-D echocardiogram or cardiac magnetic resonance imaging. The final decision on whether to proceed with LV reconstruction may be made in the operating room. Some patients who were thought to have scar preoperatively were found to have thick muscle at the time of surgery. Unless magnetic resonance imaging indicates extensive nonvisible subendocardial scar, then the LV reconstruction will be aborted, and only bypass and/or valve repair will be performed.

The majority of patients (over 85 per cent) have an isolated LAD infarction when chosen for this surgery. Occasionally, we have used the same techniques of reconstruction for patients with lateral wall or posterior wall infarctions. Also, similar techniques of reconstruction can be used for patients with postinfarction ventricular septal defect or contained free wall rupture. Also, occasionally, the techniques can be performed for patients with acute myocardial infarction (usually undergoing ventriculotomy to remove an underlying LV thrombus), although much greater care must be taken in placing sutures and tying the pursestring suture.

OPERATION

1 The operation is typically performed through a full median sternotomy incision. With a transmural LAD infarct, frequently extensive adhesions exist between the pericardium and the LV aneurysm. In our experience, approximately 40 per cent of the operations were performed for akinetic areas (not dyskinetic true aneurysms), and then adhesions to the pericardium may not be present. The operation is performed under normothermic full cardiopulmonary bypass. Separate caval cannulae are used for concomitant mitral valve surgery. Alternatively, a two-stage venous cannula can be used if mitral valve repair is not needed.

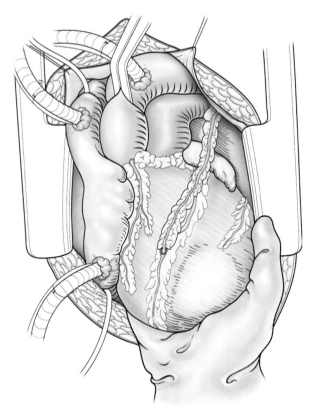

1

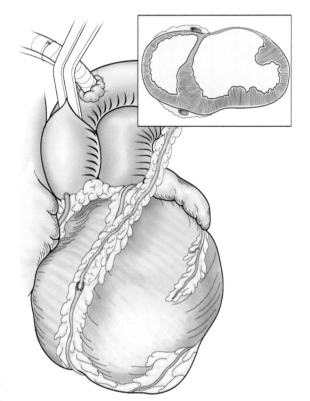

2

2 Coronary artery bypass is performed in approximately 90 per cent of patients. If a true LV aneurysm exists with no remaining areas of viable muscle and a cord-like LAD, then the LAD is not grafted. However, especially with akinetic areas, the LAD is grafted if areas of remaining viable myocardium are present and also to supply collaterals to the right coronary system. Coronary artery bypass surgery is usually performed first, after the aortic cross-clamp is applied and cardioplegia is administered antegrade and retrograde. Cardioplegia is also given down saphenous vein grafts when those are used.

3 Mitral valve repair has been used in 43 per cent of our patients. The mitral valve is exposed through a standard left atriotomy with annuloplasty using a small ring. The small ring coapts the leaflets, which are apically tethered in the enlarged ventricle. We have been evolving from a partial flexible band (illustrated) to a complete remodeling ring.

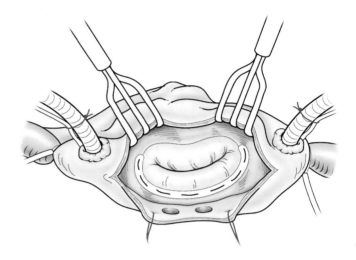

3

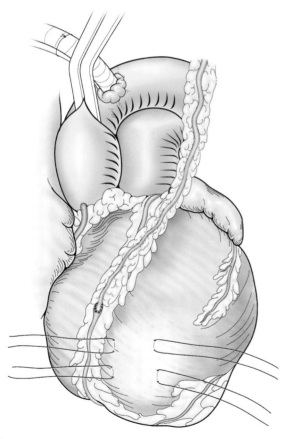

4 After the coronary artery bypass grafts, the mitral valve repair, and the proximal anastomoses are completed, the aortic cross-clamp is removed. Reconstruction of the infarcted ventricle is performed on the beating heart. The LV apex is exposed with traction sutures and sponges behind the heart.

4

5 The LV is opened through the thin-walled aneurysm approximately 12 cm to the left of the LAD. The incision of the ventricle is typically 4–6 cm long, extending from the apex along the proximal LAD. The table is rotated toward the surgeon to facilitate exposure of the septum and LV cavity. Stay sutures are placed to retract the wall of the aneurysm.

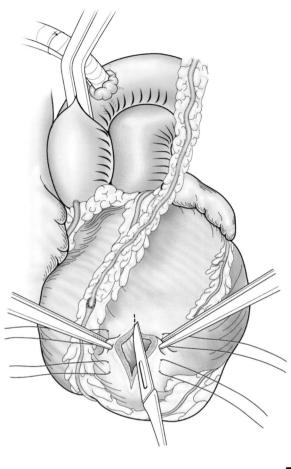

5

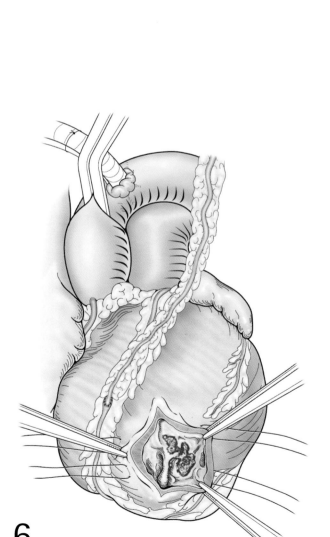

6

6 Approximately 30 per cent of patients have some LV thrombus. At this point, the LV thrombus is carefully removed, including the areas of thrombus that may be trapped within trabeculations. One must be careful in the beginning phases of the operation not to manipulate the heart until the aortic cross-clamp is placed, especially if adhesions to the pericardium or a recent myocardial infarction are present.

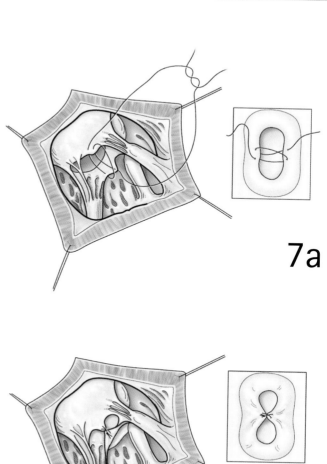

7a

7a, b, c Some patients with severe mitral regurgitation are also treated with an edge-to-edge approximation of the anterior and posterior leaflets of the mitral valve (i.e. Alfieri repair). This procedure can be performed through the left atrium; but when a LV reconstruction is planned, visualization of the areas to be approximated is easier through the LV. The free edge of the anterior and posterior leaflets are approximated in the mid-portion (where the cords from the anterior and posterior papillary muscles reach the edge of the valve leaflets) using two Ethibond 4-0 sutures (as illustrated). This manoever creates a figure eight appearance of the mitral valve when seen on short axis by echocardiography. The Alfieri repair is never performed for patients with thick valve leaflets (or a history of rheumatic fever), to avoid creating possible mitral stenosis. We have also used the edge-to-edge technique to close the posterior commissure (not illustrated) between A3 and P3.

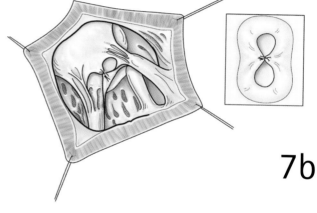

7b

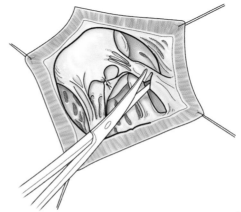

7c

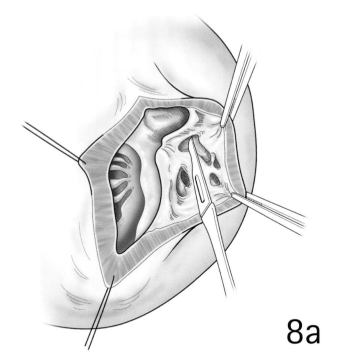

8a

8a, b For patients with a discreet endocardial scar, a sub-endocardial resection is performed. The scar is stripped away from the areas of the septum and free wall, until the border zone is reached between infarcted and normal myocardium. If a small opening is made through the ventricular septum, it can be easily identified by filling the heart on cardiopulmonary bypass, and then closing the small opening with a pledgeted suture.

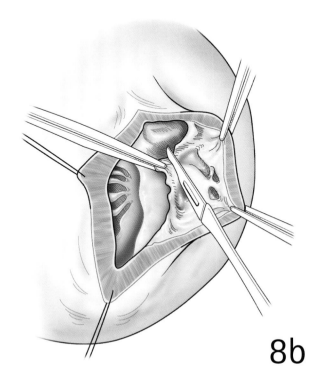

8b

9 For patients with a history of ventricular tachycardia, a cryoprobe is placed on the border zone between infarcted and normal muscle, the typical site of macro re-entry circuits causing ventricular tachycardia. Cryolesions are placed at –60°C for 2 minutes each. Their lesions placed sequentially until the entire border zone has been ablated. For a posterior aneurysm, the lesion should include the isthmus between the infarct and the mitral valve annulus.

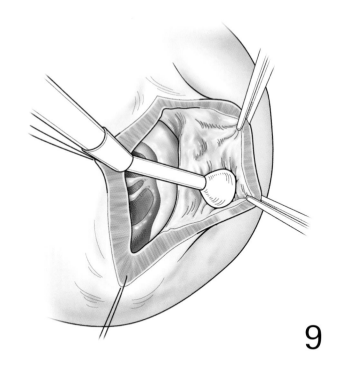

9

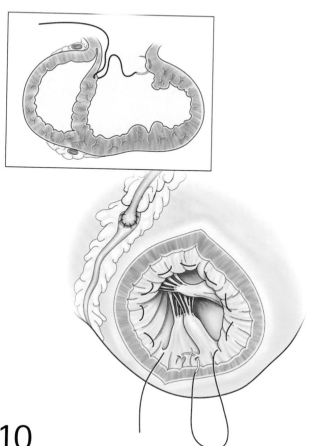

10 Reconstruction of the ventricle begins by determining the proper location to place the pursestring sutures that will exclude the infarcted LV wall from remaining normal muscle. In most patients with mature infarcts, the border zone between the scarred, infarcted myocardium and the normal myocardium in the distribution of the circumflex and right coronary arteries is clearly evident. In patients with a more recent infarct and patients with an akinetic area, palpation with the heart beating may be very useful to clearly delineate the areas of myocardium that will contract versus the akinetic areas. With transmural chronic LV aneurysms, the trabeculations have largely disappeared from the scarred area, so the border zone is clear. With more recent infarcts and in patients with akinetic areas, trabeculations may remain, and palpation may be the only way to determine the border zone.

10

11 A pursestring suture of #0 Prolene on an M0-6 needle is then placed through the border zone between infarcted and normal myocardium. This position also corresponds to the area of contracting versus akinetic myocardium. The goal of the pursestring suture is to reduce the opening and clearly separate the excluded scar tissue from the remaining myocardial chamber, which will then be surrounded by normal myocardium. In placing the pursestring suture, an important consideration is that the remaining myocardial chamber should be at least 100 cc. Some surgeons use a balloon to help judge the remaining myocardial cavity. The bites for the needle are typically placed 2–4 mm into the scarred portion of myocardium, and they are placed quite deep so that they hold tension well when the suture is tied.

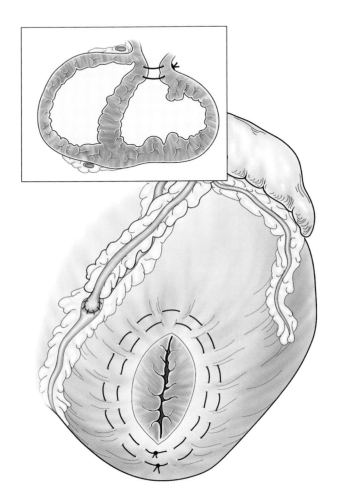

11

12 The first pursestring suture has been tied, reducing the orifice typically to 1–3 cm. At this point, we usually place a second pursestring suture 2–4 cm superficial to the first pursestring suture. When the second pursestring suture is tied, this double cerclage excludes the infarcted area from the myocardial chamber, and only a small opening remains.

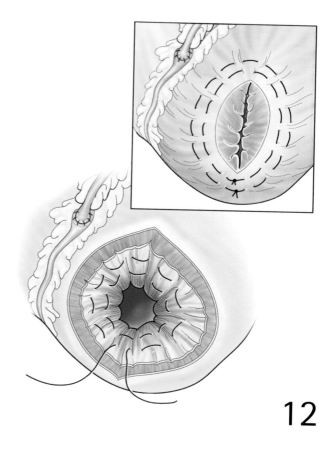

12

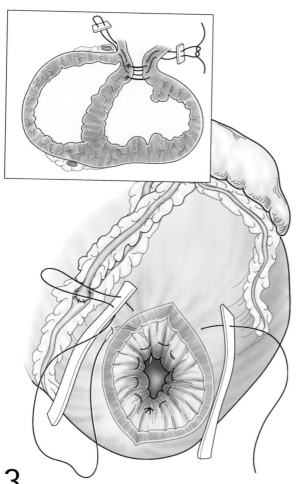

13

13 Two strips of felt are then placed lengthwise on the epicardial surface and are used to support the closure from outside the myocardium. 2-0 polypropylene sutures on an MH needle are used as horizontal mattress sutures and are passed through the level of the myocardium at the level of the first pursestring suture. Typically, we bring the sutures out on the left side of the LAD and are careful to avoid obstructing the LAD, in case doing so may precipitate arrhythmias.

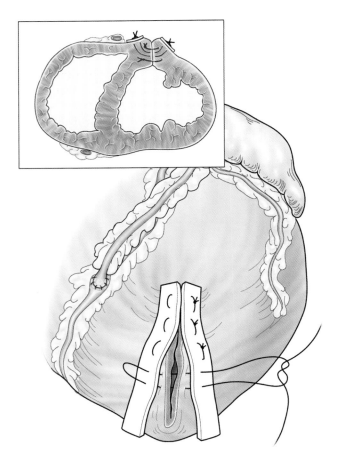

14 While the heart is still beating, the mattress sutures are tied. Typically, a small amount of blood is exiting through the opening in the ventriculotomy during this portion of the closure. An aortic vent is in place and on suction. Since the heart is elevated, any air is rising to the apex and is evacuated through the ventriculotomy.

14

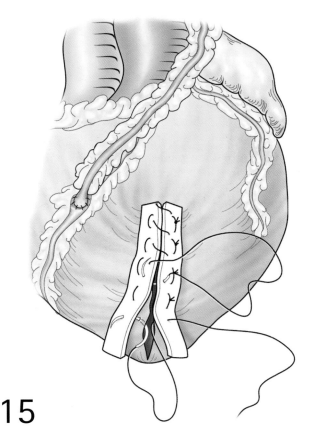

15 When the horizontal mattress sutures are tied, the ventriculotomy is further closed in two layers with running 2-0 polypropylene sutures on an MH needle. With this very secure closure, the risk of reoperation for bleeding has been very low (less than 2 per cent). Intraoperative transesophageal echocardiography is used to be certain that air has been evacuated from the heart. A needle can be passed through the LV apex suture line, although usually this step is not required.

15

16 The completed reconstruction is best demonstrated in cross section. The myocardial chamber is now largely surrounded by normal myocardium. However, the akinetic infarcted area that has been excluded from the LV chamber is still visible by 2-D echocardiography along the anterior wall. Because 2-D echocardiography focuses on wall motion, these estimates of cardiac function are less accurate (unless extensive scar has been resected and removed). More accurate measurements of ejection fraction are based on quantitative volumetric measurements, either with 3-D echocardiography or cardiac magnetic resonance imaging. These techniques calculate end-diastolic and end-systolic volumes, stroke volume and, therefore, quantitative ejection fraction. 2-D estimates based on observations of regional wall motion function are less precise.

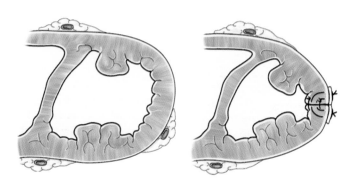

16

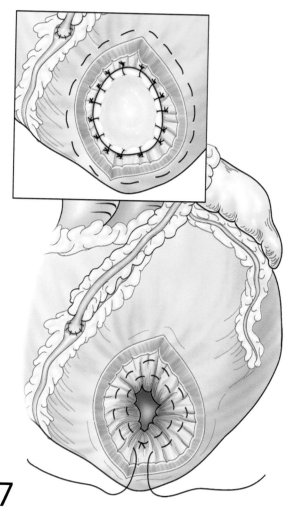

17 Using the technique as described, we rarely use a patch to reconstruct the ventricle, but in three circumstances it may be useful. Patients with a calcified LV aneurysm have little flexibility in the LV wall, and the pursestring sutures do not draw the ventricular wall together. The calcium is removed, similar to a subendocardial resection. These patients may be best served with a patch closure. The patient with a huge LV cavity requires a patch because the edges cannot be drawn together by the pursestring suture, but this situation is rare. Patients with a reconstructed, small LV cavity may have a low stroke volume and diastolic dysfunction. These patients may need patch reconstruction to maintain an LV end-diastolic volume of approximately 100 cc. Altogether, less than 5 per cent of patients in our recent experience have required a patch because of a calcified aneurysm or to maintain adequate ventricular volume. The patch is typically placed after the first pursestring suture has been tied. Usually, we use autologous pericardium for the patch; but also bovine pericardium, Hemashield, or even endocardial scar may be used for the patch. The patch can be secured to the scar tissue at the level of the pursestring suture using running 3-0 polypropylene suture or horizontal mattress sutures of pledgeted 3-0 polypropylene suture.

17

18 Once the patch has been secured, theoretically the ventriculotomy does not need to be closed further. However, because of bleeding from the edge of the ventricular muscle and epicardial surface, we usually close the remaining LV scar over the patch.

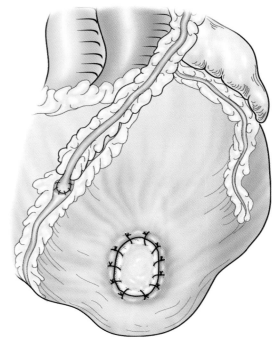

18

OUTCOME

Despite the poor cardiac function and history of congestive heart failure, operative mortality has been low (2 per cent in more than 250 patients), and long-term freedom from recurrent heart failure has been excellent.

FURTHER READING

Athanasuleas, C.L., Stanley, A.W.H., Buckberg, G.D. et al. 2001. Surgical anterior ventricular endocardial restoration (SAVER) for dilated ischemic cardiomyopathy. *Seminars Thoracic Cardiovascular Surgery* **13**: 448–57.

Calderia, C., McCarthy, P.M. 2001. A simple method of left ventricular reconstruction without patch ischemic cardiomyopathy. *Annals of Thoracic Surgery* **72**: 2148–9.

Di Donato, M., Sabatier, M. Dor, V., et al. 1997. A kinetic versus dyskinetic postinfarction scar: relation to surgical outcome in patients undergoing endoventricular circular patch plasty repair. *American College of Cardiology* **29**: 1569–75.

Dor, V. 1997. Reconstructive left ventricualr surgery for post-ischemic akinetic dialatation. *Seminars on Thoracic Cardiovascular Surgery* **9**: 139–45.

Mickleborough, L.L., Carson, S., Ivanov, J. 2001. Repair of dyskinetic or akinetic left ventricular aneurysm: results obtained with a modified linear closure. *Journal of Thoracic Cardiovascular Surgery* **121**: 675–82.

SECTION V

Thoracic Aortic Disease

31

Aortic arch aneurysms

JOSEPH E. BAVARIA, MD
Associate Professor of Cardiothoracic Surgery, University of Pennsylvania School of Medicine; Director, Thoracic Aortic Surgery Program, University of Pennsylvania Medical Center, Philadelphia, Pennsylvania, USA

HISTORY

Aortic arch surgery has always been limited by the critical necessity to protect the brain during arch anastomosis. In 1966, Borst *et al.* first reported the use of hypothermic circulatory arrest (HCA) for repair of the aortic arch. The next seminal report regarding successful surgery of the aortic arch was published by Griepp *et al.* in 1975, describing the successful use of HCA in a series of patients. Surgical reconstruction of the aortic arch was then advanced as HCA was used with increasing frequency. Diseases such as fusiform and saccular aneurysm of the aortic arch, acute type A dissection of the thoracic aorta, and chronic dissecting aneurysmal disease were all successfully treated during this period with improving results. A landmark publication by Svensson and Crawford in 1993 describing the results of 656 consecutive aortic arch procedures using HCA, as well as the large series by Drs. Ergin and Griepp in 1999, further advanced aortic arch reconstruction.

Surgical techniques to reduce perioperative mortality and stroke risk were proposed, such as the concept of 'open distal anastomosis' for treatment of type A aortic dissection. During much of the 1980s and early 1990s, continuing clinical research advanced our understanding of the effects of HCA on the cerebral cortex. In the early 1990s, led by the Japanese cardiac surgeons, the concept of retrograde cerebral perfusion (RCP) was advanced. Circulation management techniques were improved and modified over the next 5 years as the combination of HCA with RCP was used by aortic arch surgeons worldwide. However, the fact that circulatory arrest times longer than 50–60 minutes require improved antegrade cerebral perfusion (ACP) techniques to maintain low stroke and mortality rates became well recognized in recent years.

Surgical technique also improved and modifications of standard aortic arch procedures were developed. These advancements included the 'elephant trunk' procedure, which allowed simpler distal arch anastomosis as well as provided for an easier second stage descending thoracic aortic procedure if necessary. More experience with simultaneous brachiocephalic vessel repair as a separate adjunct to aortic arch reconstruction was also advanced. Cannulation techniques improved, including the use of routine Dacron graft side arms and more routine use of axillary/subclavian artery cannulation, therefore allowing easier ACP during aortic arch reconstruction.

PRINCIPLES AND JUSTIFICATION

Aortic arch aneurysms can present in many ways. Some will present asymptomatically after the patient has obtained a chest x-ray or computed tomography (CT) scan of the chest for another reason. Many patients present with chest pain and, more specifically, back pain referred to the intrascapular region. This symptom usually signifies an enlarging aneurysm and can be more pronounced during periods of hypertension. Aortic arch aneurysms can also present with mediastinal compressive symptomatology. Large fusiform aneurysms of the aortic arch as well as saccular aneurysms of the lesser curve of the aortic arch can present with hoarseness as the recurrent laryngeal nerve is stretched over the aneurysmal wall. Additionally, left phrenic nerve involvement with resultant left hemidiaphragmatic dysfunction has been reported. In many cases of aortic arch aneurysm, the trachea is deviated to the right with a significant curvature and, in some cases, the patient has simultaneous left mainstem stenosis. This problem can be quite critical during endotracheal tube placement perioperatively and especially during double-lumen endotracheal tube placement by anesthesia.

The etiology of aortic arch aneurysms is quite diverse. Most aneurysms are related to atherosclerotic disease, and this fact is especially true of saccular aneurysms of the aortic arch. Chronic aortic dissecting aneurysms are also quite frequent. This observation is especially true after completion of a previous acute type A aortic dissection repair and recurrence of a chronic dissecting aneurysm of the aortic arch years later. Marfan's Syndrome also predisposes to aortic arch aneurysm, again especially after aortic dissection. Syphilitic aneurysms are still noted, and pathological analysis of aortic arch aneurysms occasionally reveal very significant inflammatory cell processes. Proximal aortic arch aneurysms, usually in combination with ascending aortic aneurysm, are quite common with congenital bicuspid aortic valve disease. These aneurysms usually do not extend distal to the ligamentum arteriosum.

The indications for aortic arch aneurysm surgery have continued to evolve. Numerous reports have documented the dismal natural history of large thoracic aortic aneurysms. As in all cases of surgical repair of aneurysmal disease, the decision whether to surgically correct the lesion is dependent on the balance between the natural history of the disease and the present state of the art of the surgical reconstruction. As aortic arch aneurysmal repair was more morbid than many other aneurysm procedures (e.g. ascending aortic or infrarenal abdominal), the historical indication for repair was a larger diameter than in other segments of the human aorta. Generally accepted indications for surgery include (1) an absolute diameter of greater than 7.0 cm; (2) a documented growth rate, using serial imaging studies, of greater than 0.5 cm per year; or (3) the presence of pain and symptoms referred to the aortic arch aneurysm. This situation would include symptoms of chest and back pain, as well as occasional progressive aneurysmal compressive symptoms, such as hoarseness, pulmonary artery obstruction, tracheal or left mainstem bronchus obstruction, and any evidence of aortic leak or rupture.

PREOPERATIVE EVALUATION

Aortic arch anatomy can be well assessed through present radiological techniques. The magnetic resonance angiogram and the CT angiogram are the preferred aortic imaging techniques and can offer extensive insight into aortic arch and branch vessel anatomy. Additionally, in some cases, thoracic aortography is necessary. Additionally, duplex scanning of the carotid arteries and transesophageal echocardiography (TEE) can yield very important information. Preoperative evaluation of patients with aortic arch aneurysms consists of an assessment of the aneurysm rupture risk and a full evaluation of comorbidity to assess whether the patient is an operative candidate and exactly what operative morbidity and mortality can be expected.

An assessment of aortic anatomy as well as related arterial anatomy is critical in these cases. Knowledge of aneurysm diameter and aneurysmal extent (length) is critical in planning for these operations. The magnitude of the operative procedure depends on whether the aortic aneurysm is limited to the arch or has a significant descending or ascending aortic component. Additionally, aneurysmal extension into the brachiocephalic vessels, such as the innominate, left common carotid, or left subclavian arteries is important. Fundamentally, complex circulation management techniques (to be discussed in Aortic arch procedures (Classification)) are determined by how much time the aortic arch reconstruction must take. In general, aortic arch reconstructive times requiring an open aortic arch less than 30 minutes are well tolerated with simple HCA. HCA with RCP is also used extensively in these procedures. Aortic arch reconstruction with procedure times less than 50 minutes can usually be satisfactorily reconstructed using deep HCA with RCP as a circulatory adjunct. However, in most instances, any arch reconstructive technique requiring longer than 50 minutes should be performed with the addition of an ACP technique to preserve optimal brain function postoperatively. In addition, the use of intraoperative neurocerebral monitoring with electroencephalography (EEG) and sensory-evoked potentials may be beneficial in more complex aortic arch reconstructions.

A rigorous comorbid workup reviewing all major organ systems is essential in planning for aortic arch aneurysm surgery. Preoperative studies, other than imaging studies of the aorta itself, include cardiac catheterization, carotid artery Doppler studies, pulmonary function studies, assessment of myocardial and cardiac valvular function by echocardiography, studies of renal function, peripheral artery assessment, and studies of the coagulation system and platelet function. Additionally, a complete review of all medications is in order with special attention to cardiac, neurological, and hematological medications. In some cases, especially if there is a history of previous transient ischemic attacks or cerebral vascular accidents (CVA), a CT scan of the brain should be obtained. Cardiac catheterization is performed as many cases have concomitant coronary artery disease that can be treated and managed during the aortic arch procedure. Knowledge of cardiac valvular function is essential. This point is especially true in cases approached via the left chest as ventricular fibrillation is very poorly tolerated in the presence of aortic valve insufficiency. Knowledge of the status of the carotid arteries is essential. If high grade internal carotid artery stenoses exist, these may be best treated preoperatively because antegrade and RCP techniques could be hazardous or less dependable in the presence of secondary carotid artery lesions. Knowledge of the patient's pulmonary function is essential, as perioperative prognosis after complex aortic arch surgery can be substantially affected by significant obstructive or restrictive pulmonary disease. Femoral artery and femoral vein cannulation is occasionally necessary during these procedures that mandate peripheral artery studies to fully assess these structures.

After completion of all preoperative studies, a critical surgical decision regarding aortic arch aneurysms is the determination of which incision and approach must be used. Most true aortic arch aneurysms can be reached via median sternotomy, and this approach would usually be preferred.

However, many distal arch diseases, especially if combined with a concomitant descending aortic process, should be approached via a left thoracotomy. Other less used approaches can include hemisternotomy and left anterior thoracotomy. Only after a complete assessment of the aortic anatomy and the patient's comorbid status can these decisions be made correctly.

Aortic arch procedures (Classification)

1a–d
Aortic arch procedures for aneurysms can be generally defined into four different categories. The first is a 'total aortic arch' which is generally

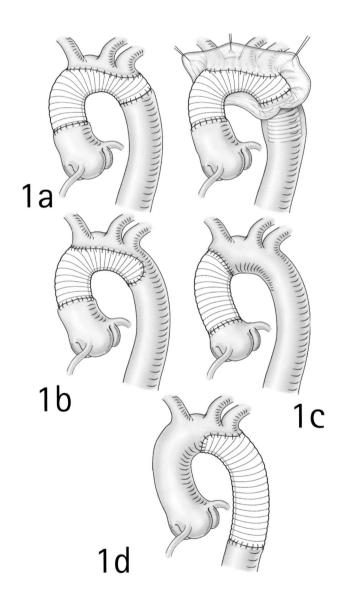

1a

1b

1c

1d

referred to as an *aortic arch reconstructive procedure* consisting of a distal anastomosis, distal to the subclavian artery orifice with a separate Carrel patch of brachiocephalic vessels and a proximal anastomosis in the ascending aorta or, if there is more reconstruction proximally, a graft-to-graft proximal aortic anastomosis. The distal anastomosis in a total aortic arch is often performed using an elephant trunk technique. Many surgeons prefer the elephant trunk technique even if they are not expecting a subsequent distal descending thoracic aortic procedure. This preference is because the elephant trunk technique allows for an easier technical distal anastomosis. The second type of aortic arch reconstruction is a 'hemi-arch' technique. This technique is used often as it can replace the great bulk of the aortic arch and only requires one continuous suture line. Additionally, many surgeons prefer to use an 'open proximal anastomosis' for a subsequent distal thoracic aortic procedure. This operation uses cardio-pulmonary bypass and HCA through a left thoracotomy; therefore, an elephant trunk technique is not necessary and a hemi-arch is very satisfactory. The third aortic arch technique is a simple 'open distal anastomosis' that is usually used for either repair of an acute type A aortic dissection or as an adjunct to an ascending aortic aneurysm repair. The fourth aortic arch technique is an 'open proximal anastomosis' that is an aortic arch repair via the left chest. This technique usually requires a beveled anastomosis into the aortic arch with complete replacement of the distal arch, including the isthmus, and is often accompanied by a descending aortic replacement.

PERIOPERATIVE MONITORING (ANESTHESIA)

Aortic arch procedures usually require standard cardiac anesthesia with the addition of measures to occasionally provide for double-lumen endotracheal intubation and single-lung ventilation. In addition, attention must be paid to the trachea as it often has an abnormal anatomy secondary to the compressive nature of the aneurysm itself. Many aortic arch aneurysm procedures are performed with EEG and sensory-evoked potential monitoring as well as other methods of cerebral cooling that require input from the anesthesiologist. Intraoperative TEE is extremely helpful. Use of anesthetic agents with neurodepressive effects is quite controversial and must be discussed with the anesthesiologists. This approach includes long-acting and short-acting barbiturates. Additionally, neuroprotective agents, such as steroids, lidocaine, magnesium, and mannitol, are often administered during aortic arch procedures. Control of bleeding is a very important part of successful aortic arch surgery; therefore, a discussion with anesthesia regarding aprotinin or aminocaproic acid (Amicar) use is beneficial.

Circulation management

2a, b Intraoperative circulation management during repair of aortic arch aneurysms is extremely important and is the key feature distinguishing these operations from all others. The surgeon has to evaluate the patient and the type of reconstructive procedure necessary in a very detailed manner before operation. Circulation management decisions include whether to proceed with HCA with or without RCP, or whether use of an ACP technique is more appropriate. This decision is dependent on the time needed to reconstruct an open aortic arch. Occasionally, the surgeon has to make a change in circulation management strategy before the initiation of cardiopulmonary bypass or even during the actual reconstructive procedure. Therefore, all circulation management options during an open arch should be available to the surgeon during the course of the procedure.

RCP is usually delivered via the superior vena cava (SVC) at a target central venous pressure (CVP) of approximately 20–25 mm Hg in a slight Trendelenburg position. The RCP has an inflow temperature of between 10° and 12°C. Usually, flow rates at these CVP pressures approximate 150–300 cc/minute. Dark black blood is seen emanating directly from the brachiocephalic orifices during the open aortic arch procedure. RCP delivered at these pressures is safe and offers the following advantages: (1) the ability to eliminate arterial debris, (2) provision of a brain 'epidural cooling jacket', and (3) an excellent deairing mechanism. Whether RCP delivers any cortical metabolic substrate is highly controversial.

ACP is usually delivered via the innominate artery or the innominate artery and left common carotid artery. Direct cannulation or balloon-equipped endovascular catheters are routinely used. General guidelines for ACP include a flow rate approximating 10 cc/kg/minute at 20°C or an ACP flow rate which can achieve a pressure of 40 mm Hg in the radial arterial line.

Generally, aortic arch procedures of less than 40–50 minutes can be accomplished with very acceptable morbidity and mortality using HCA with RCP. Most surgeons at this time believe that the addition of RCP to HCA decreases overall morbidity and mortality and is a very simple and easy

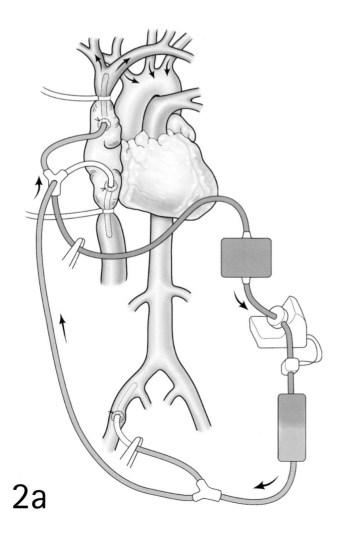

2a

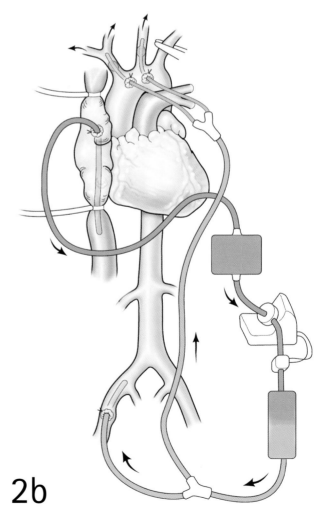

2b

circulatory adjunct to implement. Routine use of an ACP technique is also becoming more common. Initially, it was thought that ACP contributed to higher focal stroke rates, usually secondary to brachiocephalic vessel cannulation, but recent ACP techniques during arch reconstruction are safe with very low rates of global cerebral dysfunction.

Conduct of operation (Sequence)

The conduct of operation during aortic arch surgery is complex. Management of cardiopulmonary bypass, with the overall goal of minimizing total CBP time, is a very important concept during the performance of these operations. In general, if ascending aortic cross-clamping is tolerated, proceed with as much proximal aortic dissection and operation as possible until adequate cooling is achieved. Once target cooling has been achieved, proceed directly to the aortic arch component of the procedure as the remainder of the procedure usually can be completed during the rewarming phase. Using this sequence, the most efficient use of cardiopulmonary bypass time is achieved. Again, the overall goal is to try to minimize any 'standing-and-waiting-around time' during rewarming. The surgeon tries to avoid performing the

aortic arch procedure last, as this sequence increases total cardiopulmonary bypass time.

The role of neurocerebral monitoring is controversial. Many groups have shown that the optimum end point for cooling is not a particular temperature or cooling time, as these are extremely variable in human populations. A documented flat-line EEG is the most sensitive indicator of adequate cooling at this time. In addition, achieving a flat-line EEG can be important and quite useful information in optimizing the circulation management sequence during aortic arch reconstruction. Many patients achieve a flat-line EEG before 30 or 45 minutes of cooling, which then allows for earlier initiation of HCA and, therefore, less total cardiopulmonary bypass time and rewarming time. Conversely, potential cerebral ischemia in patients who cannot reach a flat-line in 30–45 minutes would be avoided if patients were monitored by EEG during the cooling phase.

OPERATION

Incision and exploration

3a, b The standard incision for aortic arch aneurysms is the median sternotomy. Approximately 80–90 per cent of all aortic arch aneurysms presenting in the aortic surgery clinic can be approached through a median sternotomy. A rare aneurysm, especially one involving the left subclavian artery, needs to be exposed through a hemisternotomy with anterior thoracotomy in the fourth interspace. For these incisions, we usually use an inframammary skin incision and then create a small pectoral flap to expose the fourth interspace laterally. The patient is usually 'bumped up' into a 30 degree position with the left side up. This position provides excellent exposure to the full anterior mediastinum, ascending aorta, aortic arch, and the distal aortic arch. For distal aortic arch aneurysms, especially those associated with a proximal descending thoracic aneurysm, the approach is usually a left thoracotomy. This is addressed in a subsequent section on distal aortic arch aneurysms (Chapter 33). The median sternotomy incision also allows for a left or right anterior sternocleidomastoid 'extension' if the innominate artery or left common carotid artery needs simultaneous reconstruction. For patients with poor pulmonary function and low forced expiratory volume in 1 second, the median sternotomy incision is well tolerated, especially compared to any exposure through the ribs.

Once the chest is open, a thorough examination of all cardioaortic structures is performed. An exact understanding of the extent of the aneurysm is undertaken. The relationship of the key intrathoracic nerves, including the vagus, phrenic, and recurrent laryngeal nerves, is identified. Additionally, the relationship of the major venous structures of the mediastinum to the aortic arch aneurysm is completed. This assessment is especially important for the innominate vein and SVC.

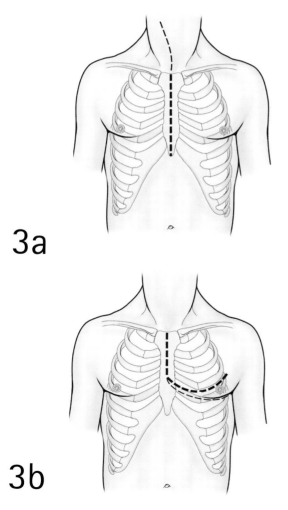

3a

3b

3c A standard posterolateral thoracotomy is used for exposure of the distal aortic arch. If the entire descending thoracic aorta is to be replaced, in addition to the distal aortic arch, then resection of the fifth rib greatly facilitates complete exposure of the aortic arch and the distal thoracic aorta. If the distal aortic arch alone is the main focus of the operation then a fourth interspace incision is best. The posterolateral thoracotomy is made in a standard fashion, and the ribs are spread. The retractor is placed, and a full exploration of the left chest and distal aortic arch is then performed. Great care is taken to identify the left vagus as well as the left phrenic and left recurrent laryngeal nerve. The left lung is deflated on single-lung ventilation. The remainder of the operative technique regarding distal aortic arch reconstruction via a left chest approach is contained in the following sections on complete arch repair and distal arch aneurysms (see Chapters 33 and 34).

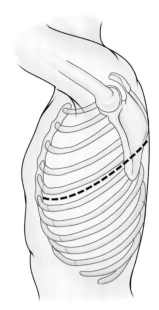

3c

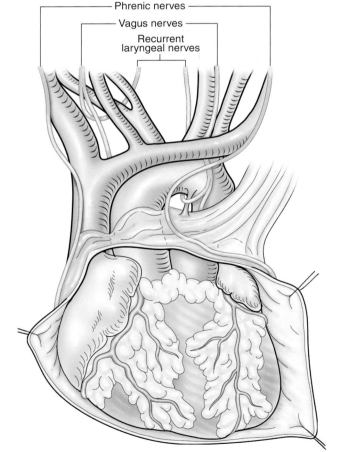

Phrenic nerves
Vagus nerves
Recurrent laryngeal nerves

Operative exposure of the aortic arch

4 A median sternotomy is made, the thymus is divided, and a pericardial cradle is constructed. The left pleural space is entered, as access to the proximal descending aorta may be needed during full arch reconstruction. Dissection of the distal ascending aorta and the aortic arch is then begun. The ascending aorta is encircled, and full exposure of the aortic arch is performed. The innominate vein is dissected free, allowing wide exposure of the superior aspect of the middle mediastinum. The orifice of the innominate artery is fully exposed as it emanates off the aortic arch. The right lateral aspect of the pericardial reflection onto the very distal ascending aorta is dissected off the aortic arch. Great care should be taken at this level to avoid the use of high energy electrocautery because the right recurrent laryngeal nerve and right phrenic nerve can be in this general vicinity. This concern is especially true if there is significant distortion of normal mediastinal anatomy from large aneurysmal disease. Next, the origin of the left common carotid artery is identified. The pericardial reflection off the aortic arch is dissected free. At the level of the ligamentum arteriosum, the left main pulmonary artery is released inferiorly off of the pericardial reflection and aorta. This maneuver frees the left pulmonary artery from the lesser curve of the aortic arch. Likewise, the greater curve of the aortic arch is mobilized off the superior aspect of the pericardial reflection. The left phrenic and recurrent laryngeal nerves are identified and carefully dissected off the left lateral aspect of the aortic arch. In performing a total arch repair, careful division of the ligamentum, without injury to the recurrent nerve, is performed. Aortic arch aneurysms commonly present with hoarseness and

4

recurrent laryngeal nerve (and even phrenic nerve) paralysis or paraparesis. However, postoperative complications can be minimized with retention of these nerves and good function of the left hemidiaphragm and left vocal cord. If these structures are not well visualized from within the pericardium medially, one should visualize the nerves via an opening of the left pleural space through the median sternotomy. Occasionally, passage of a Penrose drain around this large pedicle of left vagus and phrenic nerves is helpful, thereby having full exposure and identification of these two important nerves at all times during the aortic arch reconstruction. These nerves can usually be retracted laterally and out of the way of the distal anastomosis. As was performed with the innominate and left carotid arteries, the left subclavian artery is also identified at its origin off the aortic arch and exposed. Beware of the thoracic duct in this general vicinity, again especially if significant anatomical distortion exists owing to aneurysm size.

Once full exposure of the entire aortic arch has been achieved, with separation of the aortic arch from its pericardial attachments as well as separation of the left pulmonary artery from the ligamentum arteriosum, the patient is prepared for cannulation. Venous cannulation is performed using a standard double-stage angled venous cannula and a smaller cannula placed into the SVC. A caval tape is placed around the SVC at the cavoatrial junction distal (heart side) to the confluence of the azygos and SVC.

Arterial cannulation

5 Arterial cannulation for aortic arch procedures can be quite variable. If ACP is used or if significant atherosclerotic disease is present in the arch or major brachiocephalic vessels, then axillary/subclavian artery cannulation is an excellent choice and is used by many surgeons. Direct distal ascending aortic cannulation, into the aneurysmal component of the aorta, can also be performed for chronic dissections and atherosclerotic aneurysmal disease. Using this cannulation technique, the surgeon avoids any femoral or axillary incision. The patient is cooled in the standard fashion, and the cannula is removed when HCA is initiated. Additionally, femoral artery cannulation is often used for aortic arch aneurysm surgery as well. However, if the thoracoabdominal aorta has significant atherosclerotic disease, laminated thrombus, or both, then a substantial theoretical risk exists for increased CVA using femoral artery cannulation. The decision regarding which arterial cannulation method is best is individualized for each patient and is based on the overall assessment of aortic anatomy and the planned operative procedure.

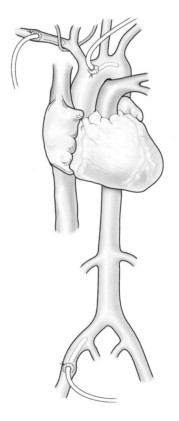

5

Complete aortic arch repair

After median sternotomy and mobilization of the aortic arch and initiation of cardiopulmonary bypass, the patient is cooled to profound hypothermia. At the completion of cooling, the circulation is arrested, and HCA is initiated. A second adjunct such as RCP or ACP can be used at this point (see circulation management).

6 The aorta is then opened. Visualization of the aortic arch at this level is improved by placing the patient in a slight Trendelenburg position. The aorta is then cut to allow for a small Carrel patch of brachiocephalic vessels, including the innominate artery, left common carotid artery, and left subclavian artery. The brachiocephalic patch should be cut in such a way that minimizes residual aortic tissues. Next, the aortotomy is continued along the left lateral (lesser curve) aspect of the aortic arch to the level of the proximal descending aorta where the distal anastomosis will be constructed. This spot is usually defined by the caliber and quality of aorta at this level and the extent of the desired resection. A satisfactory 'neck' is most optimal. Once this area is selected, the aorta is transected. Complete transection of the aorta usually allows for an easier and more visible distal anastomosis. However, to perform once off a 360 degree transection of the aorta at this level is often technically difficult, and a 180 degree or 270 degree transection suffices in many cases. The remainder of the aorta can be sutured using an inclusion technique.

6

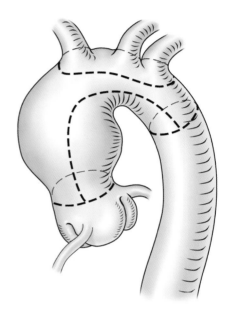

7a–c At this point, the distal anastomosis can be completed with a direct anastomosis using a 3/0 prolene suture with an SH or MH needle. An elephant trunk procedure can be used for the distal anastomosis, which the author prefers regardless of eventual distal operation. If an elephant trunk is desired, the Dacron graft is intussuscepted into itself. The intussusception is done to allow for an approximate 6–8 cm length of elephant trunk distally. A black silk stitch is placed at the end of the intussusception so that the graft can be easily pulled out after completion of the distal anastomosis. The graft is then fitted into the descending aorta, and the distal arch anastomosis is completed using a running 3/0 prolene suture with an SH or MH needle. The elephant trunk technique allows for excellent visualization of the distal anastomosis, as the graft itself is not obscuring any view. Of note, the sutures are placed through the aortic tissue as well as two layers of graft.

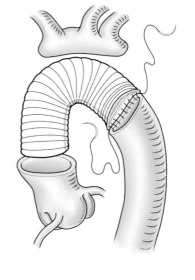

7a

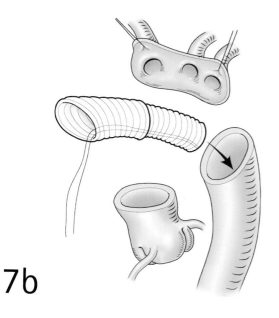

7b

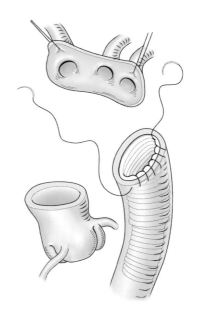

7c

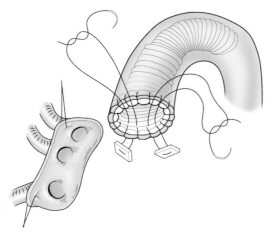

7d

7d This area will be very difficult to see again; therefore, pledgeted patch sutures are placed at this time to reinforce the suture line as necessary.

8a After examination of the distal anastomosis, the graft is then pulled up and marked in the appropriate area, along the greater curve, for brachiocephalic Carrel patch implantation. The arch graft is then cut for side-to-side anastomosis. The brachiocephalic patch is then sutured onto the graft using 3/0 or 4/0 suture. The anastomosis is begun distally at the level of the subclavian artery, running along the posterior row to the level of the innominate artery. The anterior row is then completed. Once the brachiocephalic vessel patch anastomosis is completed, it is checked, especially at the level of the subclavian artery because this area is difficult to see once the reconstruction is completed.

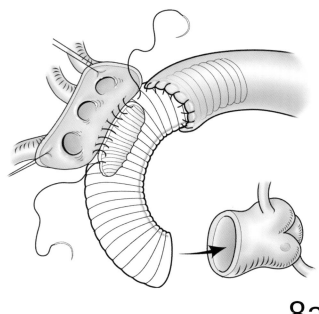

8a

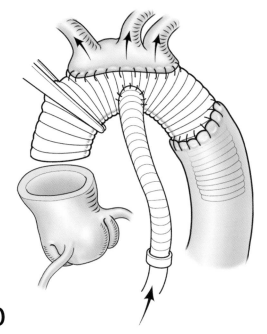

8b

8b After completion of the aortic arch anastomosis, the patient is prepared for cerebral deairing. The operating table is placed into a Trendelenburg position, and the arterial circulation is deaired. If RCP is used as the circulatory adjunct, then full deairing of the systemic arterial circuit can be performed by allowing the entire aorta and arch graft to fill via retrograde perfusion. This is an excellent deairing system for an open aortic arch. If ACP techniques are used, the aorta is easily filled, and the aorta and complete arterial circulation is deaired using this technique. Some surgeons prefer an ACP technique for most aortic arch cases but then switch to RCP at the very end to achieve optimal deairing of the open arch. At the completion of deairing, the cross-clamp is placed on the aortic arch graft, proximal to the innominate artery, and the arch procedure is complete. On many occasions, a transfer of the systemic aortic cannula is made to the arch graft to provide for 'antegrade' graft perfusion.

Once the arch graft is cannulated, the cross-clamp is placed, cardiopulmonary bypass is reinitiated, and rewarming is begun. The patient is taken out of the Trendelenburg position at this time.

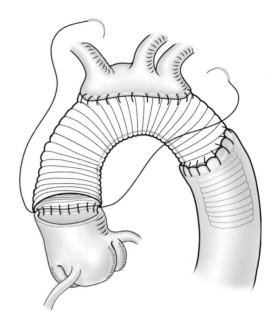

9a

9a, b Attention is directed more proximally, and the proximal anastomosis is completed. This anastomosis is done between the distal ascending aorta and graft. If additional proximal aortic reconstruction is necessary, such as an ascending aneurysm aortic root procedure, a Dacron graft-to-graft anastomosis is eventually completed. The graft-to-graft anastomosis should be completed with a 2/0 SH prolene suture because an intrathoracic graft-to-graft anastomosis always requires the strength of the suture itself for life, as no tissue ingrowth or significant healing occurs between two grafts.

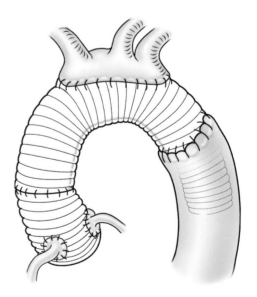

9b

Hemi-arch reconstruction

The hemi-arch procedure is widely used. This procedure is relatively straightforward and allows for extensive resection of the aortic arch and a single running suture line. Additionally, many surgeons believe that the 'better' operation for a subsequent distal thoracic aortic procedure is to use an 'open proximal anastomosis' routinely and, therefore, they do not need an elephant trunk reconstruction to facilitate sequential operations.

As in the previous description, once cardiopulmonary bypass has been initiated and cooling is completed, the circulation is interrupted and HCA is initiated. Use of circulatory adjuncts such as RCP or ACP are then instituted as necessary.

10a, b The aorta is then cut in the fashion as shown. The graft is then cut in the mirror image, and the anastomosis can be started. Again, the posterior suture line is completed first, beginning at the most distal portion of the resected aortic arch and followed by an anterior row. A technical note should be mentioned: After completion of the posterior row, if any patch sutures are necessary, they should be placed before completion of the anterior row. These sutures can be placed on the inside using pledgeted or nonpledgeted sutures as deemed necessary. The posterior row is not easily visualized after the completion of the anastomosis, and therefore caution is necessary because a strong distal anastomosis is desirable.

After completion of the 'hemi-arch' anastomosis, the patient is prepared for cerebral deairing. The bed is placed into a Trendelenburg position and the arterial circulation is deaired. If RCP is used as the circulatory adjunct, then full deairing of the systemic arterial circuit can be performed by allowing the entire aorta and arch graft to fill via retrograde perfusion. This is an excellent deairing system for an open aortic arch. If ACP techniques are used, the aorta is easily filled, and the aorta and complete arterial circulation can be deaired using this technique. Some surgeons prefer an ACP technique for most aortic arch cases but will then switch to RCP at the very end to achieve optimal deairing of the open arch. At the completion of deairing, the cross-clamp is placed on the aortic arch graft and the arch procedure is complete. On many occasions, a transfer of the systemic aortic cannula is made to the arch graft to provide for 'antegrade' graft perfusion.

Once the arch graft is cannulated, the cross-clamp is placed and rewarming is begun. The patient is taken out of the Trendelenburg position.

10c Once the distal hemi-arch anastomosis is completed, then attention is directed to the proximal anastomosis. Hemi-arch procedures are most often associated with a concomitant aortic root or ascending aortic reconstruction. The proximal aortic arch anastomosis is usually a graft-to-graft anastomosis cut and beveled in the appropriate fashion to simulate the normal curvature of the ascending aorta.

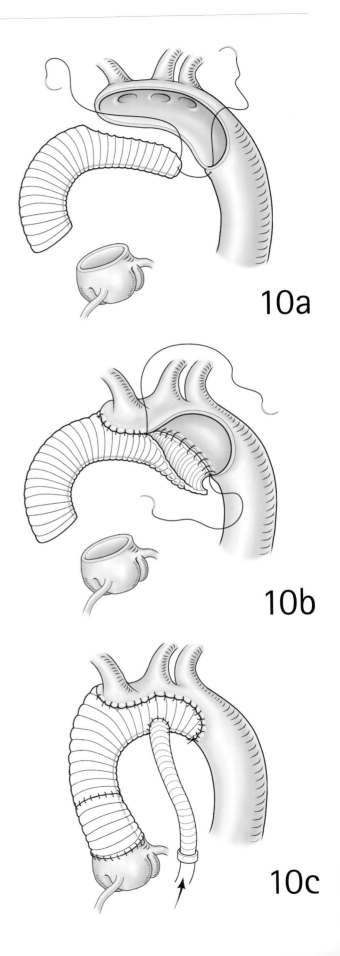

10a

10b

10c

Repair of distal aortic arch aneurysms via the left chest

11a On many occasions, distal aortic arch aneurysms cannot be adequately approached via a median sternotomy or an anterior approach. This situation usually occurs with true distal arch aneurysms involving the isthmus of the aortic arch, the subclavian artery, and often the proximal descending thoracic aorta. The approach to these aneurysms is via a posterolateral thoracotomy. Circulation management techniques used in these cases include initiation of full cardiopulmonary bypass via the left chest. This technique usually entails a femoral venous cannulation using a long femoral venous drainage cannula placed into the right atrium. Vacuum-assisted drainage is advantageous in this circumstance. Arterial cannulation usually consists of femoral artery cannulation or direct descending thoracic aortic cannulation. A left ventricular vent catheter is placed via the left inferior pulmonary vein. Full cardiopulmonary bypass is initiated, and profound hypothermia is achieved. The heart usually fibrillates at between 28° and 32°C, and intraoperative inspection as well as intraoperative TEE can facilitate observation of the left ventricle. Adequate left ventricular venting and a competent aortic valve are important under these conditions. This circulation management technique is hazardous under conditions of considerable aortic valve insufficiency. Cooling is continued for the prescribed time. This approach usually means a flat-line EEG or a specified amount of cooling time or a target nasopharyngeal temperature.

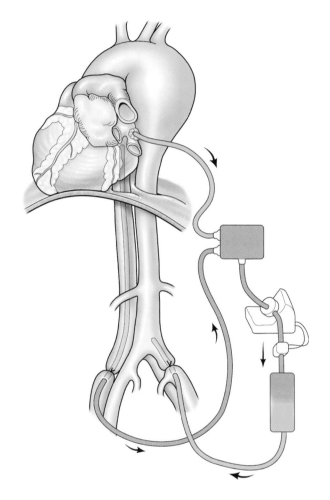

11a

11b–d

Once cooling has been completed, the circulation is terminated and HCA is begun. If the anticipated proximal aortic reconstructive time at the aortic arch is short, then RCP via the right atrium (or SVC) may not be necessary. However, if RCP is used, then 'total body retrograde perfusion' via the right atrium/SVC at a target CVP of approximately 15 mm Hg is usually quite adequate to allow for continual retrograde blood to emanate from the 'open proximal aortic arch.' The aorta is then cut and beveled in the appropriate fashion for distal arch resection and subsequent arch repair. The Dacron graft is then sewn to the aortic arch after resection of the aneurysmal component in a standard fashion. Once the anastomosis is completed, the entire open aortic arch is deaired. This procedure is optimally performed using RCP. Once deairing is completed, the graft is cannulated, and a cross-clamp is placed on the graft distal to this new cannulation site. Arterial perfusion of the proximal circulation is then initiated via the arch graft, and rewarming is begun. After adequate cardiac rewarming, the heart is defibrillated to allow for pulsatile perfusion and cardiac ejection as early as possible. At this point, the distal anastomosis at the appropriate level in the descending thoracic aorta is completed.

POSTOPERATIVE CARE

Prophylactic antibiotics are normally used and discontinued after approximately 72 hours or when the last remaining chest tubes are withdrawn. The use of postoperative neuro-

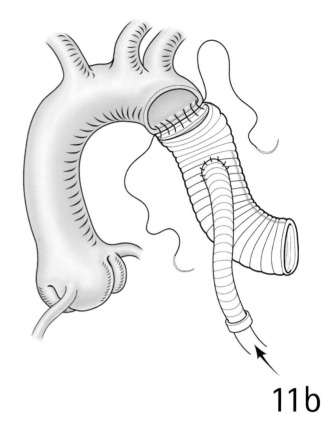

11b

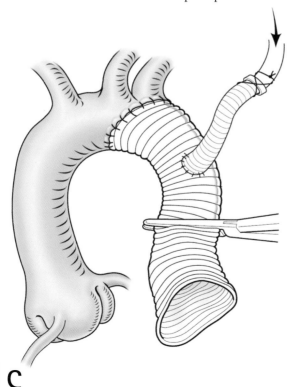

11c

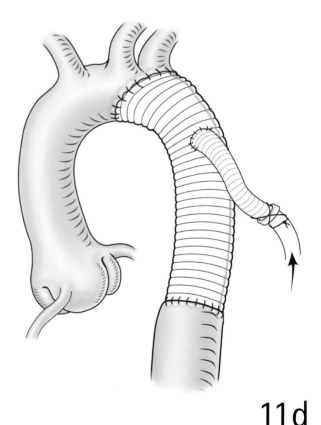

11d

protective agents is controversial, and this author uses these agents perioperatively but not postoperatively. The Swan-Ganz catheter is removed in a standard fashion and postoperative extubation is done using standard weaning protocols. However, the surgeon needs to remember that these patients are at higher risk for recurrent laryngeal nerve dysfunction secondary to distal aortic arch manipulation and anastomosis. Recurrent laryngeal nerve dysfunction can contribute to aspiration and subsequent pneumonia. Therefore, all patients undergoing a complete aortic arch procedure should be on aspiration precautions and avoid the supine position. By mouth intake should only begin after a careful examination of vocal chord function and competent swallowing.

Frequent neurological examinations by intensive care unit nursing staff and physicians are important. Focal stroke as well as global ischemic dysfunction, characterized by temporary neurological dysfunction, is relatively common. These complications can contribute to a stormy postoperative course and should be recognized as earlier as possible. Additionally, therapeutic maneuvers such as control of blood pressure and possible anticoagulation can be instituted early if perioperative neurological dysfunction occurs.

In the immediate postoperative period, bleeding is associated with all types of thoracic aortic surgery and aortic arch procedures in particular. Therefore, strict attention to the postoperative coagulation profile and correction of all abnormalities is paramount

Long-term follow-up care of patients with aortic arch aneurysms is important. These patients are best managed long term in a multidisciplinary thoracic aortic surgery clinic as additional aneurysmal formation, antihypertensive management, and abnormalities of aortic anatomy are best understood by the operative team.

Perioperative mortality is often associated with focal stroke. Generally, 50 per cent of perioperative deaths after aortic arch aneurysm surgery are associated with a concomitant CVA. Hence, any decrease in CVA rates substantially decreases mortality rates as well. Additionally, perioperative mortality is associated with advanced age, poor pulmonary function, and the presence of significant atheromatous disease of the arch and brachiocephalic orifices. Hemorrhage is still a cause for perioperative mortality as many of these procedures are extremely complex requiring deep hypothermia and long cardiopulmonary bypass times. With the recent addition of more sophisticated intraoperative circulation management techniques and neurocerebral monitoring, focal CVA and temporary neurological ischemic events have decreased in incidence.

In summary, overall morbidity and mortality after aortic arch aneurysm surgery has improved over the past decade. The introduction of more sophisticated circulation management techniques to protect the brain during an open aortic arch procedure have evolved. These techniques include RCP as an adjunct to HCA. Additionally, especially for anticipated HCA times of greater than 50 minutes, ACP techniques are being increasingly used. This method offers excellent results for increasingly complex aortic arch reconstruction. Additionally, better preparation and understanding of the different approaches and specific aortic arch reconstructive techniques have improved the results of aortic arch surgery. Technological advances including impregnated vascular grafts as well as a more sophisticated understanding of neurocerebral monitoring and perioperative neurological dysfunction have contributed to improved results by decreasing the previously dreaded bleeding complications and decreased overall neurological dysfunction.

OUTCOME

The mortality rate after aortic arch aneurysm resection has diminished significantly in recent years, although morbidity remains high. More recent outcomes reveal an approximate 5–10 per cent in-hospital mortality and 5–15 per cent incidence of perioperative neurological dysfunction. These complications include combined focal CVA and global, nonfocal, temporary neurological dysfunction. These results represent a significant improvement in mortality and overall neurological dysfunction compared to procedures performed 10–15 years earlier. Operations on atherosclerotic aortic arch aneurysms via the left chest remain a significant challenge and have the highest incidence of perioperative neurological dysfunction of all aortic arch aneurysm cases in most series. Some reports, from high-volume thoracic aortic surgery centers, evaluating aortic arch aneurysm repair via median sternotomy, report a combined neurological morbidity and overall mortality of less than 10 per cent. Most of these procedures have concomitant ascending aorta or aortic root reconstructive procedures.

FURTHER READING

Bavaria, J.E., Pochettino, A., Brinster, D.R., *et al.* 2001. New paradigms and improved results for the surgical treatment of acute Type A dissection. *Annals of Surgery* 234(3), 336–42.

Bavaria, J.E., Woo, Y.J., Hall, R.A., *et al.* 1995. Retrograde cerebral and distal aortic perfusion during ascending and thoracoabdominal aortic operations. *Annals of Thoracic Surgery* 60(2), 345–53.

Coady, M.A., Rizzo, J.A., Hammond, G.L., *et al.* 1997. What is the appropriate size criterion for resection of thoracic aortic aneurysms? *Journal of Thoracic and Cardiovascular Surgery* 113, 476–91.

Kazi, T., Washiyama, N., Mahammad, B.A., *et al.* 2001. Improved results of atherosclerotic arch aneurysm operations with a refined technique. *Journal of Thoracic and Cardiovascular Surgery* 121(3), 491–99.

Stecker, M.M., Cheung, A.T., Bavaria, J.E., *et al.* 2001. Deep hypothermic circulatory arrest: I. Effects of cooling on electroencephalogram and evoked potentials. *Annals of Thoracic Surgery* 70, 14–21.

Svensson, L.G., Crawford, E.S., Hess, K.R., *et al.* 1993. Deep hypothermia with circulatory arrest: determinants of stroke and early mortality in 656 patients. *Journal of Thoracic and Cardiovascular Surgery* 106, 19–31.

32

Ascending aortic aneurysm

BRUCE W. LYTLE MD
Surgeon, Department of Thoracic and Cardiovascular Surgery, The Cleveland Clinic Foundation, Cleveland, Ohio, USA

PRINCIPLES AND JUSTIFICATION

The indications for resection of ascending aortic aneurysms usually fall into one of four categories. First, the aneurysm is associated with aortic valve dysfunction that constitutes the indication for surgery. The aortic valve leaflets may be fundamentally normal, but enlargement of the sinotubular junction by the aneurysm may prevent coaptation and cause valve insufficiency, or the aortic valve leaflets may be intrinsically abnormal (such as a bicuspid aortic valve) and associated with an enlarged ascending aorta. When performing operations for aortic valve dysfunction or coronary surgery as the primary indication for operation, we usually replace the ascending aorta if it is larger than 5 cm in diameter. Second, an aneurysm of the ascending aorta may reach a size for which the time-related risk of a catastrophic aortic complication exceeds the risk of surgery. For patients without connective tissue disorders or severe hypertension, 5.5 cm is the diameter for which ascending aortic complications begin to constitute a significant risk. Third, large aneurysms may reach a size for which symptoms of dyspnea may be caused by occupation of the mediastinal space and/or bronchial compression. These aneurysms have usually reached the size for which operation is also indicated for prognostic reasons. Fourth, for patients with previous ascending aortic surgery, reoperation may be indicated by false aneurysms that are less than 5.5 cm but are expanding, or by the presence of ascending aortic infections.

The treatment of aortic dissection, aneurysms associated with connective tissue disorders, and valve-sparing operations for patients with aortic root aneurysms are described in Chapters 31, 33 and 34 and we will not focus our attention on these entities.

The majority of ascending aortic aneurysms occurs in older patients who have a substantial prevalence of coronary artery and noncoronary atherosclerosis and other comorbid conditions, such as chronic obstructive pulmonary disease and renal impairment. In addition to comorbid conditions, the risks of operation for ascending aortic aneurysms are related to stroke, myocardial infarction, embolization of atherosclerotic debris, and bleeding. Therefore, the preoperative evaluation and the details of operation must be designed to avoid those complications.

PREOPERATIVE ASSESSMENT

Preoperative studies should include coronary angiography, echocardiography, and either computed tomography (CT) scanning or magnetic resonance imaging (MRI) study of the entire aorta. Significantly stenotic coronary lesions are usually treated with concomitant bypass grafting at the time of operation. Echocardiography defines the status of the aortic and mitral valves and left ventricular function. Patients with an aneurysm in one location are at increased risk of having others, and aortic imaging is necessary to define not only the ascending aorta and arch, but also the presence of aneurysms or atherosclerosis in other areas of the aorta. Also, the identification of inflammatory changes in the aneurysm by MRI or CT scanning may be an indication of aneurysmal changes based on giant cell arteritis.

OPERATION

1 Most ascending aortic aneurysms are approached through a median sternotomy. For most patients with degenerative aneurysms, the entire ascending aorta is abnormal, and if aortic arterial cannulation is to be used this step must be accomplished in the aortic arch. More commonly, we use axillary artery arterial cannulation. Traditionally, femoral artery cannulation has often been used, but many older patients may have significant femoral artery atherosclerosis. Furthermore, retrograde femoral artery perfusion may be a potential source of cerebral embolization from a descending aorta that is atherosclerotic or aneurysmal.

The axillary artery is exposed through an incision parallel to and 1.5–2.0 cm inferior to the clavicle and usually can be palpated in the angle between the clavicle and the chest wall. Muscular layers are divided, and crossing venous branches (usually 1 to 2) are ligated and divided. The vein is retracted superiorly, and the artery is identified and dissected from the brachial plexus. At this point, heparin is given, and femoral clamps are used to clamp the axillary artery proximally and distally. A 4/0 monofilament suture is used to sew an 8-mm woven Dacron graft in end-to-side fashion to the axillary artery. A #21 or #22 arterial cannula may then be placed in the graft and tied into place with umbilical tapes. The axillary artery may also be directly cannulated, but if it is small or atherosclerotic, direct cannulation may be difficult. Sewing a graft to the artery and then cannulating that graft decreases the risk of local arterial complications, and we now use this approach preferentially. In addition to avoiding retrograde systemic arterial perfusion, axillary artery cannulation makes antegrade cerebral perfusion during systemic circulatory arrest possible via occlusion of the innominate artery. In obese patients, exposure of the axillary artery may be difficult, and direct cannulation of the innominate artery is another choice. However, atherosclerosis and calcification of the innominate artery are fairly common, creating an impediment to cannulation.

We use bicaval venous cannulation in patients undergoing ascending aortic resection to allow retrograde cerebral perfusion via the superior vena cava (SVC). Wire-reinforced cannulae (22-Fr) are placed into the cavae, and an SVC snare is placed. A transatrial, self-inflating balloon is placed through the right atrium into the coronary sinus to allow delivery of retrograde cardioplegia. Once cardiopulmonary bypass is initiated, a left atrial-ventricular vent is placed through the right superior pulmonary vein, through the mitral valve, and into the left ventricle for patients with significant aortic insufficiency.

In the majority of cases, we use circulatory arrest during the construction of the distal ascending aorta or arch anasto-

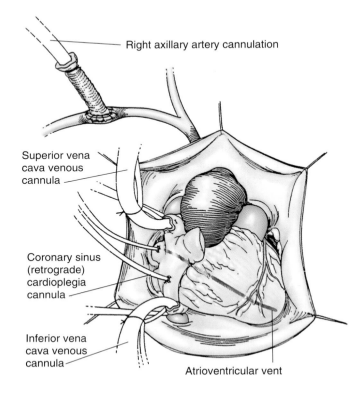

Right axillary artery cannulation

Superior vena cava venous cannula

Coronary sinus (retrograde) cardioplegia cannula

Inferior vena cava venous cannula

Atrioventricular vent

1

mosis because the abnormal aorta usually extends into the aortic arch or very close to it. Once cardiopulmonary bypass is established, systemic cooling is undertaken. If the patient has severe aortic insufficiency, cross-clamping of the aorta is usually necessary once the heart is cold enough to fibrillate. Although clamping a large aneurysm may be difficult, this goal usually can be accomplished if the pump flow is lowered to 200 cc/minute for a few seconds. After aortic cross-clamping, cold blood retrograde and antegrade cardioplegia (usually directly into the coronary orifices) are given for a total of 4 minutes at the time of induction of arrest, and 2 minutes of cold cardioplegia is repeated intermittently at 15- to 20-minute intervals throughout the case. Effective myocardial protection is critical. If no aortic insufficiency exists, systemic cooling can proceed without aortic clamping, and avoidance of aortic occlusion entirely probably decreases the risk of atherosclerotic embolization.

Proximal reconstruction

2a–c The aorta is clamped and then is opened vertically. Techniques for aortic root reconstruction are tailored to the pathology and based on the status of the aortic valve, the aortic sinuses, and the coronary orifices. If the aortic valve leaflets are normal and the aortic sinuses are normal, replacement of the ascending aorta with a supracoronary graft is indicated and usually effective in treating coexisting aortic insufficiency (Figure 2a). If the sinuses are normal and the aortic valve leaflets are abnormal, then aortic valve replacement combined with placement of a supracoronary graft is usually the best approach (Figure 2b). The advantage of this strategy versus total aortic root replacement is that reoperation for aortic valve re-replacement is straightforward, and

little disadvantage exists in using a bioprosthesis for valve replacement, thus avoiding the risk of taking anticoagulants. Also, if the aortic sinuses are normal and the coronary arteries are not displaced from the annulus, replantment of the coronary arteries into a composite graft is not always easy. This strategy is used most commonly for elderly patients and for patients with bicuspid aortic valves without significant dilatation of the aortic valve sinuses. If the aortic sinuses and the aortic valve leaflets are both abnormal, then aortic root replacement (Bentall operation) is indicated (Figure 2c). In situations in which the aortic sinuses are abnormal and the aortic valve leaflets are normal, then valve-sparing aortic root replacement, described in other chapters, may be possible.

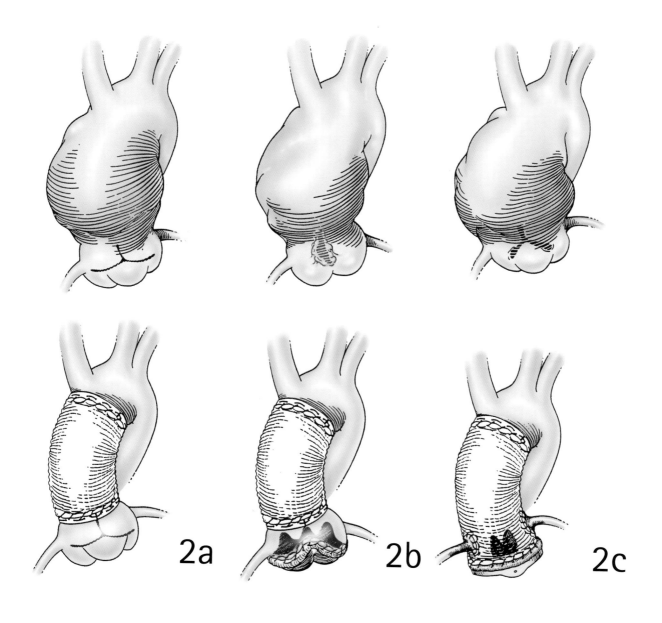

2a   2b   2c

3a

For patients with normal aortic valve leaflets and sinuses who have aortic insufficiency based on dilatation of the sinotubular junction by the aneurysm (Figure 3a), the ascending aortic replacement is designed to both replace the aneurysm and to correct the aortic insufficiency by reconstructing the sinotubular junction at its correct size. The 'correct size' for the sinotubular junction is approximately that of the aortic annulus. Therefore, aortic valve sizers are used to determine the annulus size, and an appropriately sized graft is selected. For example, for a 23-mm annulus, a 24-mm graft is selected. This graft is then cut at a slight bevel (this slightly increases the size of the graft), but it is everted as it is sewn into the aortic root (this slightly decreases the size of the graft).

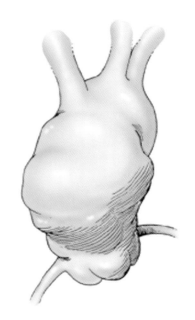

3a

3b–d

A Teflon felt strip is used outside the aorta, and the first suture line is started with a horizontal mattress stitch of 4/0 Prolene placed through the graft and tied on the outside of the felt in the middle of the left coronary sinus (Figure 3b). This step begins to evert the graft. To achieve the correct spacing, this suture is then run in a horizontal mattress fashion along each side of the sinotubular junction to a point just above the junction of the right and noncoronary aortic valve cusps (Figure 3c). This suture line everts the graft around the circumference of the anastomosis and establishes spacing. This suture line is then tied, and a second over-and-over layer of 4/0 Prolene is run from posterior to anterior to secure hemostasis (Figure 3d).

When the aortic valve is replaced along with the supracoronary graft, preservation of the sinotubular junction is not important. Excess aortic tissue distal to the coronary orifices is removed, and the graft is fashioned to fit the remaining aorta, then sewn into place with continuous 4/0 Prolene suture material.

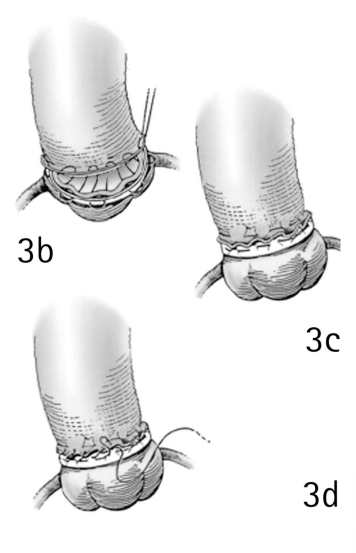

3b

3c

3d

4a, b Total aortic root replacement (Bentall operation) with a composite valve-graft prosthesis is usually reserved for situations in which all the aortic root components are abnormal, and the coronary arteries are usually clearly displaced from the aortic annulus. In previous years we often used an 'inclusion' type technique in which the aorta and coronary arteries were left intact, and the coronary arteries were reimplanted into the graft without separation from the aorta (Figure 4a). The aorta was then completely closed around the valve-graft composite (Figure 4b). This type of technique was of value during an era when bleeding through graft intercicies was often a problem. However, modern graft materials and the use of component coagulation therapy have greatly reduced the problem of bleeding during ascending aortic replacement and decreased the usefulness of inclusion techniques. The disadvantage of inclusion techniques has been a slight increase in the incidence of false aneurysm formation associated with the coronary-to-graft anastomoses. However, we still use inclusion techniques during operations for members of the Jehovah's Witness faith who will not accept any transfusion of blood products.

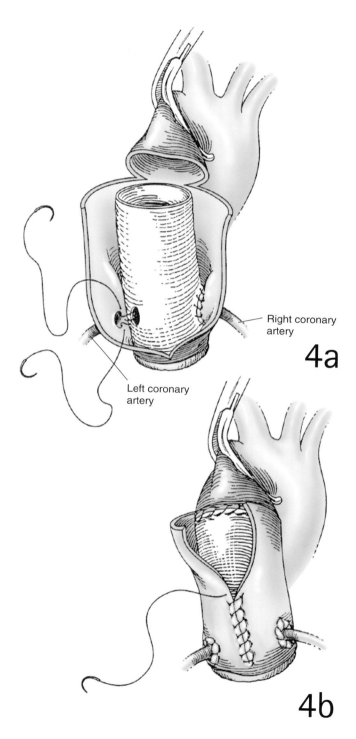

Right coronary artery

Left coronary artery

4a

4b

5 Today, for composite graft replacement of the aortic root, we more commonly use a technique that involves 'skeletonization' of the aortic root with the creation of coronary buttons that are separate from the aortic wall. With the skeletonization technique, once the aortic valve is excised and the coronary buttons are created, horizontal mattress sutures of 2/0 braided suture backed with small Teflon pledgets are placed through the annulus with the pledgets left on the aortic side, thus everting the annulus. These sutures are then placed through the sewing ring of the composite valve prosthesis and should be placed in the superior portion of the valve sewing ring. When these sutures are then tied, the valve is forced down into the outflow tract of the left ventricle, which provides a good hemostatic seal and also prevents the sewing ring from remaining above the level of the annulus and presenting a barrier to implantation of the coronary arteries into the graft. In performing this type of operation, the composite graft should not be too large relative to the annulus.

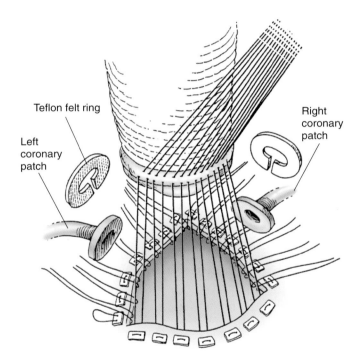

Teflon felt ring

Left coronary patch

Right coronary patch

5

6 Once the graft-to-aortic annular anastomosis is completed, the coronary button-to-graft anastomoses are constructed, beginning with the left coronary. Identification of the site of the left coronary anastomosis is made by allowing the aortic valve annulus to sink back into the diastolic position and using a marking pen to mark the location of the anastomosis. A button of graft slightly larger than the coronary artery diameter is then removed with a graft-cutting cautery. Many patients needing an aortic root replacement have a fundamental abnormality of aortic tissue, and the graft opening should be only slightly larger than the coronary artery diameter to avoid aneurysmal dilatation of the coronary button in the future. The coronary anastomosis is constructed with a continuous 4/0 or 5/0 Prolene suture through all the layers of the coronary artery and backed with a ring of Teflon felt on the adventitial side of the coronary artery. When that anastomosis has been completed, any gaps in the suture line are corrected by placing 4/0 double-ended silk sutures from the inside to the outside of both the graft and the coronary artery.

With mobilization of the coronary arteries, direct implantation of the coronary buttons into the composite graft is usually possible. Occasionally, usually during a reoperation, mobilization may be difficult due to the fixed position of the coronary arteries, and an 8-mm or 10-mm Dacron graft is used to connect the coronary orifices with the aortic graft, as has been suggested by Cabral. Also, if the left coronary orifice is greatly displaced from the aortic annulus, drawing the left coronary artery up to the graft may kink the takeoff of the anterior descending coronary artery at its bifurcation with the circumflex coronary artery. This problem is uncommon, but the surgeon must be alert to this possibility.

When the left coronary orifice is completed, the graft is filled with cardioplegic solution to distend it, and the right heart is filled with blood from the pump to mimic the right ventricular position during identification of the right coronary artery implantation location. A button is then cut out of the graft, and the right coronary artery anastomosis is carried out in a similar fashion to the left. Once the coronary anastomoses are completed, the graft is pressurized by placing a clamp across a rigid cardioplegia cannula and infusing into the aortic root to check for leaks.

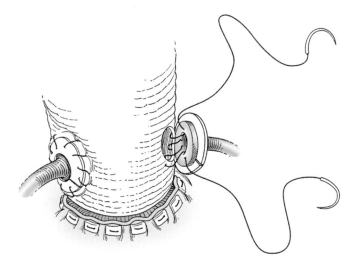

6

Distal reconstruction

Once the desired temperature for circulatory arrest is recorded, the process of proximal reconstruction is interrupted to construct the distal anastomosis. During systemic cooling, we measure bladder temperature, nasopharyngeal temperature, the temperature of arterial blood from the pump, and the temperature of the venous blood returning to the pump oxygenator. If the preoperative imaging studies clearly show that the aortic arch is normal and the distal anastomosis is being carried out at the level of the innominate artery, then the period of circulatory arrest is short (less than 15 minutes) and we cool only to a bladder temperature of 24°C. At that point, the blood temperature is often 18°C and the nasopharyngeal temperature is approximately 20°–22°C. However, if a more extensive reconstruction is to be carried out, we cool to the point at which the nasopharyngeal temperature and the bladder temperature are both 18°C, a process that usually takes approximately 30 minutes. In addition, plastic bags containing ice are placed around the head to create a cold environment and to insulate the head against heat loss.

7 The pump-oxygenator circuit is modified to allow perfusion of oxygenated blood into the SVC. Separate roller pumps are used for the SVC and systemic (axillary artery) arterial perfusion so that the oxygenated perfusion may be shifted back and forth from one to the other, or they may be run simultaneously. Once we have reached the desired systemic temperature, the systemic perfusion flow is lowered to 100 cc/minute, the SVC snare is placed down to prevent blood from leaking back into the right atrium, and the perfusion of oxygenated blood is started through the SVC cannula at 200 cc/minute. The central venous pressure usually rises to around 20 mm Hg. Antegrade systemic perfusion is then stopped. We usually maintain the central venous pressure between 20 and 30 mm Hg, which produces a consistent efflux of deoxygenated blood from the cerebral arteries. If this blood in the field is an impediment to completing the anastomoses, the retrograde cerebral perfusion can be slowed. However, perfusion is never completely stopped to avoid creation of a vacuum within the system and to prevent air from being sucked into the system. The temperature of the blood perfused into the SVC is 14°C. If flow into the SVC fails to elevate the central venous pressure, the possibility of a persistent left SVC should be considered. If a persistent left SVC is present, encircling and occluding this vessel is usually possible, thus allowing both retrograde SVC perfusion and a retrograde cardioplegia to be used effectively.

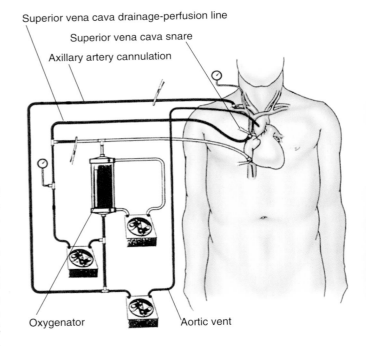

Superior vena cava drainage-perfusion line

Superior vena cava snare

Axillary artery cannulation

Oxygenator

Aortic vent

7

8a, b If the aneurysm extends to, but does not include, the aortic arch, the anastomosis is constructed at the level of the innominate artery. The area of the aorta is sized, and the graft is beveled if needed. A horizontal mattress suture of 4/0 Prolene is placed from the graft through the aorta and through a strip of Teflon felt, and it is tied. This step begins the eversion of the graft within the aorta. A suction catheter returning blood to the pump-oxygenator is placed through the graft to keep the field clear. Each limb of the suture is then run along each side of the anastomosis to meet anteriorly, and they are tied, completing the anastomosis. Once this anastomosis is completed, the graft is elevated, and the desaturated blood coming from the cerebral vessels is allowed to fill the graft, eliminating air.

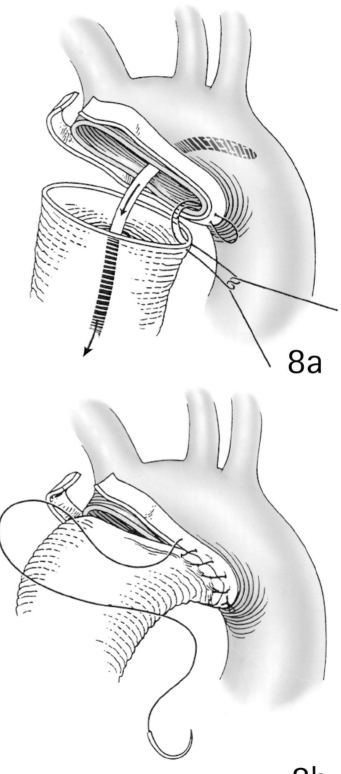

8a

8b

9 The systemic arterial perfusion is then restarted slowly, the cross-clamp is replaced (this time to the graft), and the retrograde cerebral perfusion is discontinued. Any bleeding sites in the anastomosis are identified. Because the anastomosis is everted, areas of bleeding can be controlled with 4/0 sutures that are external to the fundamental suture line.

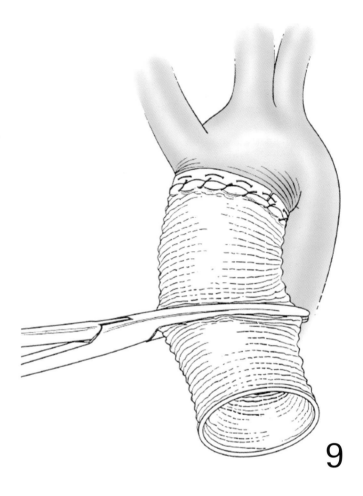

9

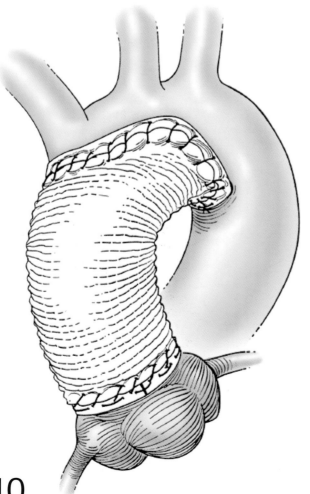

10

10 Aneurysms that involve the proximal aortic arch in addition to the ascending aorta, but that do not extend to the level of the left subclavian artery, may often be treated by creating a tongue for the cerebral vessels and beveling the graft to include this tongue, a 'hemiarch' replacement. This procedure requires more extensive beveling of the graft, and that bevel points the graft in a right lateral direction. Therefore, use of the same graft for the proximal anastomosis without kinking it is often difficult. In this situation, the proximal and distal reconstructions are done with two separate grafts that are then beveled appropriately and joined together to complete the procedure.

11a–c If the entire aortic arch is aneurysmal, then formal replacement of the entire arch must be accomplished. Often this procedure is done in conjunction with an 'elephant trunk'-type operation in which the anastomosis is created in the proximal descending aorta, but a segment of graft is left to dangle in the descending aorta to aid in the future treatment of a descending aortic aneurysm. To accomplish this maneuver, the proximal graft is folded inside of the elephant-trunk portion of the graft to create a double layer of graft, and both segments are placed into the descending aorta (Figure 11a). The circumferential anastomosis of the graft to the descending aorta is then completed through the two layers of the graft with a 3/0 or 4/0 monofilament suture (Figure 11a). The graft segment to replace the arch is then retrieved from within the elephant-trunk segment (Figure 11b), an oblong button is cut out of the graft, and the arch vessels are replanted into the graft (Figure 11c). Again, the direction of the graft is usually such that a separate graft must be used for the aortic root reconstruction to prevent kinking.

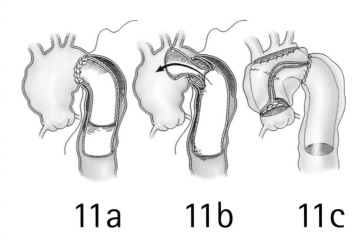

11a   11b   11c

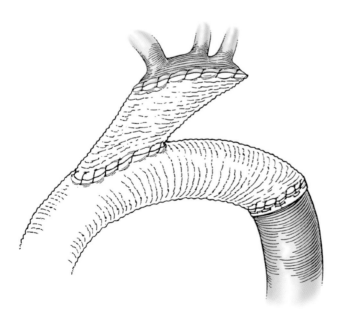

12

12 Another alternative, often used when a substantial distance exists between the cerebral vessels and the point of the descending aortic anastomosis, is to sew a beveled 18- or 20-mm graft to the cerebral vessels as the first maneuver. If a right axillary artery cannulation has been used, then antegrade cerebral perfusion can be restarted at that time, greatly decreasing the period of cerebral circulatory arrest. The descending aortic anastomosis is then completed in end-to-end fashion, and the two grafts are joined. This approach is more difficult if not much distance exists between the left subclavian artery and the point of anastomosis to the descending thoracic aorta.

After completion of the distal aortic anastomosis, attention is returned to the proximal reconstruction, which is finished while the patient is being warmed. Unfortunately, rewarming is often a prolonged process, as we do not take the temperature over 38°C and have a maximum difference between the patient temperature and the ingoing blood temperature of 10°C.

When all aortic anastomoses have been completed, any venous coronary bypass grafts that have been constructed are anastomosed to oblong orifices cut from the graft with a graft cautery using 5/0 Prolene suture material. With removal of the cross-clamp, the ascending aortic graft usually moves slightly to the patient's right, so left-sided bypass grafts must be long enough to tolerate that change.

Once all anastomoses have been completed, a 3-minute dose of warm reperfusion cardioplegia is given, and the cross-clamp is removed from the graft. When the patient has been rewarmed and the air has been removed from the cardiac chambers and from the graft, cardiopulmonary bypass is discontinued, and ventricular and valve function is assessed with transesophageal echo and inspection.

Once coronary bypass is discontinued, protamine is given and hemostasis is obtained. If possible, the old aneurysm is closed around the graft to protect it if reoperation is needed in the future.

REOPERATION

A repeat median sternotomy for a patient with an aortic aneurysm usually occurs after an operation for coronary bypass grafting, aortic valve replacement, ascending aortic replacement, or some combination of those operations. A repeat median sternotomy represents some danger, the degree of which may be evident by MRI or CT scanning. The specific dangers are usually an aortic injury or an injury to previously constructed bypass grafts.

13, 14 Before repeat median sternotomy, access for cardiopulmonary bypass should be established by preparation of the axillary or femoral artery and the femoral vein. If the patient does not have aortic insufficiency, the safest way to reopen the sternum is to use deep hypothermia and circulatory arrest. However, if aortic insufficiency is present, that strategy may cause serious left ventricular distention. In the presence of significant aortic insufficiency, a small right anterior thoracotomy (Figure 13) may aid in dissecting the aorta and right ventricle away from the sternum, and a small left thoracotomy (Figure 14) allows placement of a left ventricular vent through the apex to keep the ventricle clear if hypothermia is needed before opening the sternum.

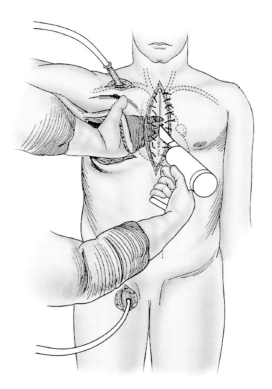

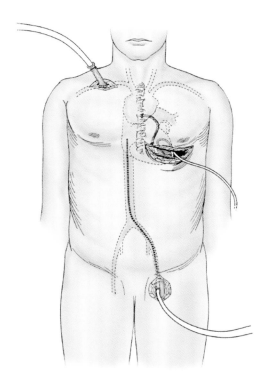

13

14

OUTCOME

Although coronary artery disease is rarely the primary indication for surgery for patients with aneurysms, myocardial ischemia – often because of anatomical reasons – is a major cause of morbidity and mortality associated with surgery for ascending aortic aneurysms. The myocardial protection achieved with modern methods of blood cardioplegia is reliable, and ventricular dysfunction after aneurysm surgery should be assumed to be based on a negative change in coronary anatomy, until proven otherwise.

The most benign cause of ventricular dysfunction is intracoronary air. Intracoronary air is difficult to completely avoid during aneurysm surgery, although intraoperative echo greatly aids in removing intracardiac air and appreciating that which is remaining. We treat ventricular dysfunction suspected to be based on air with a high perfusion pressure and coronary vasodilators. However, if ventricular dysfunction is based on intracoronary air, bubbles can often be visualized within the coronary vessels or within the left ventricle by echo, and this problem should quickly resolve. Ventricular dysfunction that does not quickly resolve must be taken seriously.

Among the reasons for ventricular dysfunction based on coronary anatomy are unappreciated pre-existing coronary stenoses, embolization of atherosclerotic debris into the coronaries, technical error or kinking of a coronary artery replanted into the graft, coronary artery dissection, and failed bypass grafts. Intraoperative echo helps to identify the area of the myocardium that is dysfunctional; and if the anatomical reason for the problem does not become readily apparent, the safest course is usually to perform a bypass graft to the coronary vessels subtending the dysfunctional area. Even relatively small vessels, such as a nondominant right coronary artery, can cause serious hemodynamic problems if acutely occluded during operation. The surgeon should not leave the operating room if any doubt exists about the integrity of the coronary anatomy.

FURTHER READING

Andrus, B.W., O'Rourke, D.J., Dacey, L.J., *et al.* 2003. Stability of ascending aortic dilatation following aortic valve replacement. *Circulation* **108 Suppl 1**, II295–9.

Coady, M.A., Rizzo, J.A., Hammond, G.L., *et al.* 1999. Surgical intervention criteria for thoracic aortic aneurysms: a study of growth rates and complications. *Annals of Thoracic Surgery* **67**, 1922–6; discussion 1953–8.

Elefteriades, J.A. 2002. Natural history of thoracic aortic aneurysms: indications for surgery, and surgical versus nonsurgical risks. *Annals of Thoracic Surgery* **74**, S1877–80; discussion S1892–8.

Ergin, M.A., Spielvogel, D., Apaydin, A., *et al.* 1999. Surgical treatment of the dilated ascending aorta: when and how? *Annals of Thoracic Surgery* **67**, 1834–9; discussion 1853–6.

Sundt, T.M. 3rd, Mora, B.N., Moon, M.R., *et al.* 2000. Options for repair of a bicuspid aortic valve and ascending aortic aneurysm. *Annals of Thoracic Surgery* **69**, 1333–7.

Yun, K.L., Miller, D.C. 1997. Ascending aortic aneurysm and aortic valve disease: what is the most optimal surgical technique? *Seminars in Thoracic and Cardiovascular Surgery* **9**, 233–45.

33

Ascending aortic dissection

D. CRAIG MILLER MD
Thelma and Henry Doelger Professor of Cardiovascular Surgery, Department of Cardiothoracic Surgery, Stanford University School of Medicine, Stanford, California, USA

DAVID T. M. LAI FRACS
Carl and Leah McConnell Cardiovascular Surgical Research Fellow, Department of Cardiothoracic and Vascular Surgery, Stanford University School of Medicine, Stanford, California, USA

HISTORY

A patient with an acute type A aortic dissection requires emergent surgical treatment to prevent the expected sequelae of ascending aortic rupture with cardiac tamponade, acute aortic regurgitation caused by loss of leaflet commissural suspension, myocardial infarction caused by coronary artery compromise, or infarction of distal end organs due to malperfusion. Operation may be contraindicated if irreversible injury has occurred to the central nervous system or if underlying systemic or terminal illness renders any intervention ill advised. The early operative mortality for patients with acute type A aortic dissection surprisingly still remains high (upwards of 15–40 per cent) despite many advances made in myocardial protection, anesthesia, cardiopulmonary bypass (CPB) circuits, suture materials, vascular clamps, antihemorrhagic and antifibrinolytic agents, prosthetic grafts, and improved valve substitutes since the first successful surgical procedures for patients with acute type A aortic dissections were performed in the 1960s. Even in centers with special interest and expertise in thoracic aortic surgery, the mortality still remains in the 10–20 per cent range in most reports. Indeed, the most recent collective experience, published in the year 2000 from 12 referral centers worldwide with special expertise in thoracic aortic disease (the International Registry of Acute Aortic Dissection, or IRAD, group) showed that the mortality was 26 per cent between 1996 and 1998.

The description of hypothermic circulatory arrest (HCA) by Griepp in 1975 marked a milestone in the history of the surgical treatment of patients with aortic dissection and opened up new surgical vistas for repair of the aortic arch. Since the 1980s, HCA has been used increasingly often for an 'open distal anastomosis' or hemiarch replacement in patients with acute type A dissections, and surgeons have become more aggressive about repairing or excising primary tears in the arch or arch extension of the ascending aortic tear. Nonetheless, the risk associated with concomitant arch repair remained formidably high until the 1990s. Subsequent efforts focused on methods to extend the safe period for circulatory arrest by using cold retrograde cerebral perfusion (RCP) or selective anterograde cerebral perfusion (SACP), thereby enabling more complex and time-consuming arch reconstructions to be undertaken safely. The incidence of stroke has fallen appreciably but still can unexpectedly thwart an otherwise perfect operation, perhaps as a result of malperfusion of the brain during the cooling phase if femoral arterial perfusion is used.

Concern about the friability of dissected aortic tissue for holding sutures led to the development of better tissue adhesives such as the gelatin resorcine formol (GRF) or 'French' glue, but anecdotal cases of late aortic necrosis and pseudoaneurysm formation after GRF glue have been reported. Other problems include a persistently patent distal aortic false lumen, which can rupture postoperatively or evolve into a false aneurysm later. The avoidance of aortic cross-clamping during cooling, better arterial cannulation sites for CPB perfusion, and the use of anterograde CPB reperfusion for rewarming have been advocated as methods to avoid pressurization of the aortic false lumen and may minimize the likelihood of a persistent and patent false lumen in the distal aorta. To avoid the long-term morbidity of a prosthetic valve substitute and indefinite anticoagulation in young patients, techniques for valve-preserving aortic root replacement (Yacoub or T. David–I procedures) have emerged. Despite these many advances, the operative mortality around the world has remained frustratingly high. Whether persistent high operative mortality is due to not enough operation (e.g. bleeding from the preserved aortic root and sinuses, postoperative rupture of the arch, or other causes) that might be avoided with a more radical operation or occurs because of too much of an initial operation (e.g. high stroke rate if concomitant total arch replacement is added, postoperative left ventricular [LV] pump failure, or excessive bleeding) remains unclear. In light of this rhetorical question, we present our current surgical approach to aortic repair for acute type A dissection, based on the pool of knowledge established by the surgical pioneers and on our cumulative institutional experience, which encompasses 320 patients with an acute type A aortic dissection between 1972 and 2000.

PRINCIPLES AND JUSTIFICATION

1a–c *Aortic dissection* is defined as separation of the layers of the aortic wall that begins at the site of a primary intimal tear, leading to the propagation of pulsatile blood flow in a false lumen that can extend proximally or distally, or both, and usually re-enters the true lumen. In the Stanford classification of aortic dissection, *type A dissection* is defined by any dissection that involves the ascending aorta, irrespective of the site of intimal tear and regardless of the distal extent of dissection. Descending thoracic aortic dissections are termed *type B dissections*, implying that the ascending aorta (proximal to the innominate artery) is not involved. In the DeBakey classification, *type I dissection* is defined by dissection that extends from the proximal aorta to involve most of the aorta; as modified in 1982, the tear does not necessarily have to be located in the ascending aorta. When the dissection is confined just to the ascending aorta, it is called a *DeBakey type II dissection*. Dissection of the descending thoracic aorta constitutes what is termed *DeBakey type III dissections*, which are subdivided into type IIIa (a dissection that involves the proximal descending aorta) and type IIIb (dissection that extends caudally to involve the suprarenal and abdominal aorta).

The acute phase of aortic dissections is defined arbitrarily by a time period of less than 14 days since the onset of symptoms related to the dissection; chronic aortic dissections are older than 14 days. Diagnosis of acute type A aortic dissection mandates immediate surgery to resect the diseased portion of the ascending aorta or arch, or both, in the absence of any major contraindications, as more than 50 per cent of patients with untreated acute type A aortic dissection are dead within the first 48 hours, largely as a result of intrapericardial aortic rupture. Ninety per cent of these patients die within 3 months without treatment. Therefore, very prompt and accurate diagnosis and expeditious transfer to the operating room are critical. Patients with acute type A dissections typically present with the acute onset of sharp, tearing chest pain, which radiates through to the back and can migrate downward. Other symptoms may be the result of secondary malperfusion related to obstruction of downstream aortic branches, resulting in stroke, myocardial infarction, spinal cord injury, visceral ischemia, kidney failure, or ischemic limbs. Abdominal malperfusion *per se*, however, does not constitute a contraindication to surgical repair.

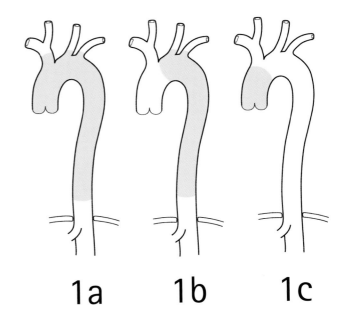

1a 1b 1c

PREOPERATIVE ASSESSMENT AND PREPARATION

Initial therapy of the patient with acute type A dissection centers on stringent blood pressure control with antihypertensive agents and reduction of LV contractility force with negative inotropic drugs to minimize aortic wall shear stress and the risk of rupture and possibly to limit the extent of distal propagation. Transesophageal echocardiography (TEE) constitutes the gold standard today for confirming the diagnosis of type A dissection and can also provide valuable ancillary information concerning aortic valve competence and LV systolic wall motion, size, and perfusion status of the true and false lumens at various levels; the presence and size of distal flap fenestrations or secondary intimal tears; and perfusion to aortic tributaries. The patient must be adequately sedated to minimize agitation and potential blood pressure swings. Before the widespread availability of TEE, dynamic computed tomography (CT) scanning with contrast was the primary diagnostic modality, as it was less invasive, more precise, and quicker than catheter aortography. CT scanning has excellent diagnostic sensitivity and specificity rates (although not as good as with TEE) and may provide additional useful information regarding the distal extent of the aortic dissection and abdominal end-organ perfusion. Magnetic resonance imaging (MRI) scanning also is very accurate, but given the potentially unstable status of these patients, it is used only rarely in our center for patients with acute aortic dissections. An MRI study, however, can help distinguish between aortic intramural hematoma, aortic penetrating ulcer, and a dissection with a thrombosed false lumen.

Speedy air transport from the hospital where the patient presents, prompt confirmation of the diagnosis, avoidance of additional unnecessary and time-consuming tests, and rapid transfer to the operating room have reduced the time between presentation and operation.

The patient's blood pressure is monitored continuously via a radial arterial catheter (left or right, but frequently both). The blood pressure and heart rate are strictly controlled to avoid hypertension and tachycardia. Large-bore venous access and level 1 rapid transfusion pumps facilitate rapid volume infusion if required. Baseline full blood counts, serum electrolytes, and arterial blood gases are obtained to detect thrombocytopenia, coagulopathy, acidosis, or azotemia and pulmonary problems. The patient undergoes general anesthesia with endotracheal intubation. Bladder temperature is used to monitor core body temperature. Cerebral temperatures are measured by using bilateral tympanic membrane temperature probes. Blood products are available to improve coagulation. Aprotinin is not used routinely because of the potential risk of thrombosis that is associated with HCA. A loading dose of epsilon–aminocaproic acid is administered, however, followed by an intravenous infusion to minimize intravascular fibrinolysis. Intraoperative TEE is mandatory; the probe should be passed early to avoid the risk of injury-induced hematoma of the esophagus after systemic heparinization.

OPERATION

The surgical goal in patients with acute type A aortic dissection is to exclude all portions of the dissected aorta, but this goal is often not attainable due to extension of the aortic dissection beyond the arch. Although one-stage total thoracic aortic replacement (ascending aorta, transverse arch, and descending thoracic aorta) using a clamshell, bilateral, anterior chest incision can be done, we reserve its use for exceptional circumstances. Our preferred approach is to resect all of the tubular portion of the ascending aorta along with the undersurface of the transverse arch, within which is located the primary intimal tear in most instances. A more radical approach to address the entire aortic root is indicated if severe annuloaortic ectasia, gross destruction of the aortic sinuses, or persistent aortic valve incompetence is present. In most patients with Marfan's syndrome in whom acute type A aortic dissection develops, the entire root and ascending aorta should be replaced using either a composite valve graft (CVG) or a valve-sparing root replacement technique. Resection of the transverse arch may be necessary when the intimal tear is located distally in the arch, when the dissection is superimposed on a pre-existing arch aneurysm, or, rarely, in selected young, low-risk patients following severe trauma to the arch.

2 Before sternotomy, the femoral or axillary artery is exposed, after which the sternotomy is performed. A branched CPB arterial line is added for ease of secondary anterograde reperfusion after the aortic graft is anastomosed distally. In addition, another perfusion circuit connected between the CPB arterial and venous lines allows for RCP with oxygenated blood to be directed up the venous line into the superior vena cava cannula. Arterial cannulation in the distal arch can be used in patients in whom the dissection is limited to the ascending aorta (DeBakey type II). In all other patients, in the past we cannulated the femoral artery with the weaker or absent pulse for CPB, which is usually in continuity with the true aortic lumen proximally; if distal pulses are equal, we prefer the right femoral artery. If peripheral venous cannulation becomes necessary, the right femoral vein affords a more reliable direct route to the inferior vena cava for passage of the femoral venous cannula into the right atrium, because the left common iliac vein passes under the right common iliac artery and joins the inferior vena cava at an abrupt angle.

More recently, we have frequently been using the right axillary artery for arterial cannulation and to achieve anterograde perfusion. This artery is seldom dissected; if it is challenging to isolate in a large patient and direct cannulation is judged to be hazardous, a short 6- to 8-mm Dacron graft can be anastomosed end to side to facilitate cannulation. Using the axillary artery increases the likelihood that the CPB flow will perfuse the aortic true lumen and may decrease the risk of thoracoabdominal or cerebral malperfusion or cerebral embolization, or both, that is associated with retrograde femoral arterial perfusion through a dissected and diseased thoracic aorta. This approach also facilitates brain perfusion during the circulatory arrest period using SACP without the need for additional arterial catheters. The right carotid artery is perfused at low flow rates by this CPB cannula when the innominate artery is clamped. Axillary cannulation is contraindicated when this artery is diseased with atherosclerosis and when the innominate artery appears to be dissected from the aortic true lumen.

When neither peripheral arterial site is available or when initiation of CPB produces abrupt malperfusion of the head, heart, or abdominal viscera, we cannulate the LV apex with a long, 7-Fr soft flow arterial cannula placed across the native aortic valve and into the true lumen of the ascending aorta. We place a 3/0 Prolene pursestring suture with interrupted Teflon felt pledgets around the LV apex, incise the apex with a No. 11 blade, dilate the incision gently, and introduce the cannula, taking special care to deair the cannula. The LV apical cannula is directed through the native aortic valve into the proximal aorta using TEE guidance; its position in the aorta can also be confirmed by palpation. Continuous manual compression of the heart is usually required once the heart fibrillates during cooling to combat distention of the left ventricle.

Through a median sternotomy, the pericardium is opened in an inverted Y-incision, and the pericardial edges are hitched to the retractor with heavy sutures to form a pericar-

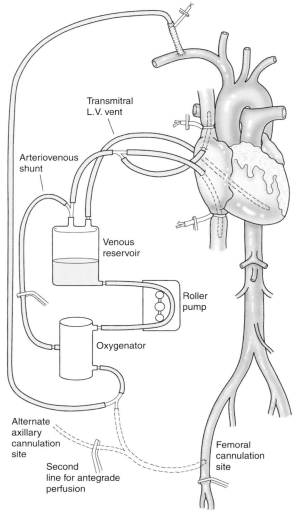

Transmitral L.V. vent

Arteriovenous shunt

Venous reservoir

Roller pump

Oxygenator

Alternate axillary cannulation site

Second line for antegrade perfusion

Femoral cannulation site

2

dial well. We prefer to cannulate the right atrium for venous drainage with two crossing cannulae (32-Fr straight and right-angle venous cannulae), and we use caval tourniquets to achieve total CPB. Peripheral venous cannulation via the femoral vein is only rarely required, for example, for ease of sternal re-entry in the setting of a prior sternotomy, in patients who have sustained cardiac arrest preoperatively, in individuals with false aneurysms in whom the sternotomy must be done after circulatory arrest has been established, and in those with a dextrorotated heart with inaccessible atria for cannulation. In these instances, a 28-Fr multi-fenestrated venous cannula is placed at the right atrial-superior vena cava junction under echocardiographic guidance, and a centrifugal pump system is used to augment venous drainage. Femoral-axillary or femoral-femoral CPB is carried out before the median sternotomy only when there is pericardial tamponade from aortic rupture or cardiac arrest or the redo sternotomy needs to be performed after HCA is induced.

CPB is established starting at a low arterial flow rate and maintained between 60 and 80 mL/kg per minute during systemic cooling, keeping the systemic blood pressure at approximately 50 mm Hg. All available arterial pressures, including those opposite the femoral cannulation site, are carefully monitored as CPB is commenced. In addition, TEE monitoring of the pump flow in the dissected descending and ascending thoracic aorta is very valuable to ensure that no collapse of the aortic true lumen and no thoracoabdominal malperfusion occurs. If any question exists about compromised perfusion of the aortic arch vessels, bilateral radial or even superficial temporal arterial monitoring lines are placed. When bypass is satisfactory, the patient is systemically cooled rapidly toward either 15°C (total arch) or 20°C (hemiarch), as assessed by bladder temperature. The tympanic membrane temperatures are monitored closely to ensure that both sides of the brain are being perfused and are cooling at an equal rate. Systemic core cooling should progress at a rate of 1°C per minute and usually takes 30–45 minutes. Systemic venous return to the right ventricle is minimized with caval tourniquets, and bronchial flow to the left ventricle is removed with a pulmonary artery or transmitral LV sump vent inserted via the right superior pulmonary vein. If access is difficult in redo cases, we occasionally vent the LV apex instead. If an LV arterial CPB perfusion cannula is used for cooling, this cannula is changed to an apical LV vent when the pump is turned off. A 15-Fr self-inflating coronary sinus catheter is inserted through an atrial purse-string with 4/0 polypropylene suture for retrograde cardioplegia.

Preparation for circulatory arrest

In principle, we advocate a no-clamp technique during cooling on CPB to avoid pressurization or malperfusion of the aortic false lumen that might result by interrupting mixing of blood between the aortic false and true lumens when placing an aortic clamp across the ascending aorta. Pressurization of the false lumen may predispose to new re-entry tears, which would favor a persistently patent distal aortic false lumen. While the patient is being cooled, the aorta is freed from the pulmonary artery down below the level of the sinotubular ridge to the annulus. This step involves mobilizing the right and left main coronary arteries, after the pericardial reflection across the top of the transverse sinus is divided. The proximal transverse arch is mobilized. Surgical dissection is kept close to the main and right pulmonary arteries, leaving all the aortic adventitia on the aortic root. As the patient is cooled, the heart fibrillates, usually at approximately 23–25°C, which may result in excessive LV distention if a substantial amount of aortic regurgitation is present. This situation occurs in at least 30 per cent of patients with acute type A aortic dissection. Under these circumstances, we place an aortic clamp down low across the proximal ascending aorta so that the aorta where the clamp is applied is subsequently resected. The heart is arrested with cold blood cardioplegia when the aorta is clamped, as prolonged ventricular fibrillation and LV distention must be avoided.

When early aortic clamping is required, we completely mobilize the proximal aortic root, by which time the patient should be sufficiently cool for HCA. If the heart fibrillates at a much warmer temperature, coronary malperfusion on CPB should be suspected immediately and appropriate alternative arterial cannulation performed quickly, for example, subclavian artery or LV apical cannulation. Immediate aortic clamping and cardioplegia should also be considered.

Before circulatory arrest, phenobarbital (1–2 mg/kg IV), dexamethasone (10 mg IV), and furosemide (20–40 mg) are administered, and ice is packed continuously around the patient's head to enhance cerebral hypothermia and to delay rewarming of the brain. The patient is placed in a steep Trendelenburg's position, the pump is turned off, 1000 mL cold blood cardioplegia is infused retrograde in the coronary sinus, the caval tourniquets are cinched down, and a myocardial cooling jacket is wrapped around the ventricles. A gauze pack is placed between the cooling jacket and pericardium to protect the left phrenic nerve. We use an alpha-stat regimen for blood gas monitoring. Myocardial temperature is kept below 10°C, and retrograde cardioplegia is reinfused every 20–30 minutes. We do not monitor the electroencephalogram.

During circulatory arrest, we rely solely on systemic and brain hypothermia if the arch component of the procedure is expected to be brief; our usual hemiarch repair can usually be accomplished in less than 15 minutes; if Bioglue (see following section) is used in an acutely dissected aorta, this procedure adds approximately 5–10 minutes to cement all the aortic layers together on both ends. A few minutes of RCP at the end is added for flushing and to fill the arch graft with blood. When the circulation will be arrested longer, we prefer to use some sort of SACP. This procedure is most easily established using the axillary artery CPB cannula with the innominate artery clamped or through the arch graft (see strategies for distal aorta – Figure 5, Chapter 34) at 10–12°C at low flow rates of 5–7 mL/kg per minute (500–800 mL/minute for most patients). If all three arch vessels are being perfused, the total SACP flow rate can be as high as 10 mL/kg. Back bleeding from the left carotid and subclavian artery orifices in the former and left radial artery pressure of approximately 50 mm Hg in the latter indicate adequate flow. Absence of back bleeding from the left common carotid artery indicates that the circle of Willis is possibly incomplete and may call for insertion of a separate supplemental cerebral perfusion catheter into the left common carotid artery if the time of circulatory arrest is going to be prolonged.

In the past, we used intermittent, low-pressure, low-flow RCP via the superior vena caval venous catheter to flush air and particulate matter from the brain. RCP was initiated at 100–500 mL/minute to keep the innominate vein pressure less than 20 mm Hg, and the cardiotomy reservoir volume was maintained using blood collected from the aorta and the field by cardiotomy suckers. Although RCP can be effective as a 'flush,' we were never convinced that it provides metabolic protection for the brain for long intervals of HCA.

3 Under HCA, the proximal ascending aorta is opened longitudinally, the true and false lumens identified, and the dissection septum resected. We then inspect the ascending aorta and arch for aortic tears, presence of annuloaortic ectasia with cephalad migration of the coronary orifices, and extent of the dissection and ascertain the status of the aortic valve leaflets. We do not use anterograde cardioplegia, to avoid iatrogenic injury to the coronary ostia, particularly when they may be rendered friable by acute aortic dissection.

Open distal aortic anastomosis with 'open distal anastomosis' and 'hemiarch' repair

For many years, we have advocated using a brief period of HCA such that the inside of the transverse arch can be inspected and a technically sound 'open distal anastomosis' can be constructed. Because little extra surgical effort and negligible additional risk are imposed, we believe that a formal 'hemiarch' distal repair is better than a simple end-to-end anastomosis in the distal ascending aorta. This step results in more extensive resection of friable dissected aorta and should lead to fewer late false aneurysms in the distal ascending aorta and proximal arch. Although we present operative techniques for both procedures, which are similar, we favor the more aggressive approach.

The inner surface of the aortic arch is inspected to ensure that no additional tears are downstream and that the great vessels arise from the true lumen of the aortic arch. The aorta is completely transected just proximal to the innominate artery down to the ligamentum arteriosum on the lesser curve of the distal arch; a beveled, full-thickness 'open distal anastomosis' is constructed at this level in the absence of any arch tears (called a *hemiarch repair*). Griepp's method, in which the 'tongue' or longer aspect of the beveled graft is attached to the greater curve of the arch at the innominate artery and the 'heel' is placed at the ligamentum (i.e. rotating the graft 180 degrees) works well, as it tucks the graft into the natural curve of the ascending aorta. In other words, the tongue of the beveled graft is orientated so that it lies upstream, contrary to conventional practice. This maneuver improves the lie of the graft and avoids undue kinking or angulation of the graft to the right when the reconstruction is completed.

In past years, when the aorta was very friable, the transected end at the ascending aorta and arch was reconstructed with a strip of Teflon felt or knitted, double-velour Dacron graft material sandwiched in the false lumen between the intimal and adventitial layers using a whip stitch of long (137 cm) 4/0 SH-1 polypropylene suture. If the tissues were particularly friable (e.g. in patients with Marfan's syndrome) or severely damaged by the dissection, the distal aortic cuff could be externally reinforced with another strip of felt or fabric in the same suture line. Since 1999, we have used Bioglue, which is injected for a depth of 2 cm down into the false lumen and around the adventitia (thickness of 2 mm);

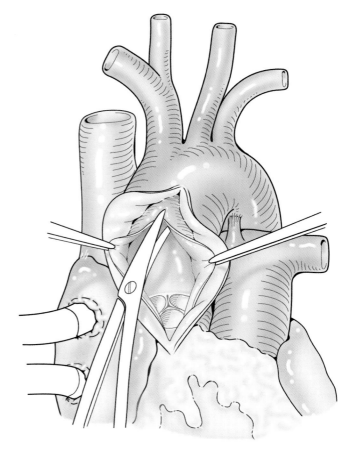

3

the aortic layers are held apposed for 2 minutes. This maneuver reconstitutes the layers of the dissected aortic wall solidly and avoids the need for any reinforcing fabric strips, but the operative field has to be kept absolutely dry. We have been very impressed with the effectiveness of Bioglue, and indeed, we have seen cases of patients with acute type A dissections who have generous sinuses of Valsalva treated successfully with Bioglue that otherwise would have required aortic root replacement. Long-term durability data are lacking, however, and therefore, more information is needed. We have no personal experience with GRF glue but have reoperated on patients years after it was used. We are concerned about the aortic wall necrosis that GRF glue can induce. Others have reported false aneurysm formation after the use of GRF glue. Other authorities, however, believe that this potential problem is overstated and probably due to using excessive amounts of formaldehyde when the glue is mixed on the table.

4 Following gluing to reconstruct the dissected distal aorta, the distal aortic cuff is sewn to the end of a woven double-velour, collagen-impregnated (Hemashield) vascular Dacron graft. The graft diameter is based on the dimension of the proximal sinotubular ridge, as even a small graft can be beveled easily to accommodate the longer oblique distal arch anastomosis. Using a 137-cm 3/0 SH or 4/0 SH-1 polypropylene suture, the anastomosis is started at the left posterior corner near the ligamentum arteriosum, running first along the posterior wall inside the aorta in a rightward direction toward the surgeon. The initial suture bites are placed loosely, the graft is parachuted down, and a fine nerve hook is used to ensure that sutures are evenly positioned and secured snugly. Extreme care is taken to ensure that the suture needle is passed along the arc of the needle curvature to prevent intimal needle hole tears. The first assistant needs to be attentive when following the suture to avoid excessive traction and tearing of the fragile aortic tissue while maintaining satisfactory tension on the suture. The anterior aspect of the distal hemiarch anastomosis is then completed using the other arm of the suture from the outside. We have never used – and do not recommend – any type of 'wrap inclusion' technique where the suture lines are not full thickness.

The arch vessels are deaired by using low-flow RCP or anterograde cerebral perfusion, placing the patient in a steep Trendelenburg's position and digitally manipulating the carotid arteries while the descending aorta and arch graft are allowed to fill with blood. The aortic graft is clamped. If axillary CPB perfusion is used, the innominate clamp is simply removed and anterograde systemic reperfusion re-established.

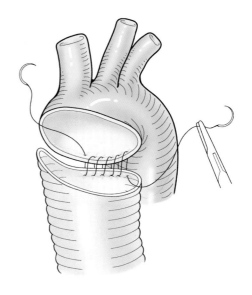

4

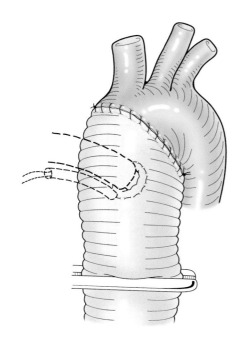

5

5 If axillary CPB perfusion is not used, a second arterial cannula is inserted directly into the arch graft near the distal anastomosis for anterograde reperfusion and rewarming. Reperfusion should always be commenced in an anterograde manner, and rewarming is not started until after 5 minutes of cold reperfusion to enhance brain protection. Immediately after CPB flow is recommenced, it is important that TEE be used to examine the flow patterns and the morphology of the dissection flap in the descending aorta to make certain that the aortic true lumen is being reperfused and that it is not collapsed by pressure or clot in the false lumen. If these situations are observed, double arterial perfusion with a second femoral artery cannula is instituted immediately. Depending on the circumstances, the distal anastomosis may have to be redone (either excising a long segment of flap to reperfuse both lumens or perhaps using an elephant trunk graft) or a distal aortic fenestration procedure or stent-graft may be required.

Total arch replacement

The need for concomitant total arch replacement in patients with acute type A aortic dissections has arisen rarely in our experience. This procedure is necessary only when severe disruption of the arch is encountered; that is, the arch branches are only tenuously attached due to rupture, the dissection flap is prolapsed distally up into one or more arch vessels causing obstruction, an extensive arch tear that extends down into the descending thoracic aorta is present, or acute dissection is superimposed on a pre-existent arch aneurysm.

Although one or more of the arch branches (frequently the innominate artery) can be involved with the dissecting process, the brachiocephalic arteries still usually communicate with the aortic true lumen and can be reimplanted as a single-island Carrel patch, formed by leaving a 5- to 10-mm rim of aorta around their ostia. If the arch vessels are severely dissected, obstructed, or diseased, they are amputated, and the dissected layers are reconstituted with Bioglue for later anastomosis to a small Dacron graft, which is subsequently sewn to the new arch graft. Total arch replacement using a branched aortic prosthesis that includes individual branch graft limbs has been reported. The distal arch and proximal descending thoracic aorta are mobilized to allow for a full-thickness distal anastomosis, and care is taken to avoid injury to the phrenic and vagus nerves during division of the ligamentum arteriosum. The previously described techniques for cerebral protection are used.

When total arch replacement is deemed necessary, the first step is complete transection of the proximal descending thoracic aorta just beyond the left subclavian artery takeoff, followed by creation of a full-thickness large island of arch that contains the branch vessels. A woven, double-velour Dacron Hemashield graft of appropriate size is anastomosed to the distal aorta (as described in the following section) using 3/0 SH or 4/0 SH-1 polypropylene suture, with or without Teflon felt reinforcement.

6 The dissected layers of the dissected aortic arch are repaired with Bioglue, if necessary. After an elliptical hole in the arch graft is created, the arch anastomosis is started distal to the left subclavian artery, progressing along the posterior wall and then anteriorly to complete the arch island. The graft and great vessels are deaired, using a combination of retrograde and anterograde cerebral perfusion, and the graft is clamped proximal to the arch island anastomosis.

Complex aortic arch reconstruction

In the rare circumstance in which a more complex arch procedure is necessary or when a long HCA time is expected, we sew a separate tubular graft to the arch vessels to allow anterograde cerebral perfusion to all three arch branches while the distal arch work is completed. Although this situation is not common when dealing with acute dissections, it is often necessary in cases of chronic type A dissection. The reconstructed arch cuff is first sewn to the beveled end of a smaller (16- to 20-mm) collagen-impregnated (Hemashield), woven, double-velour vascular graft as a long beveled end-to side anastomosis using a 137-cm 3/0 SH or 4/0 SH-1 polypropylene suture.

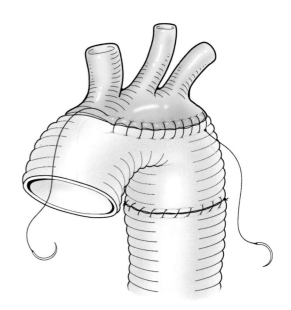

6

7 The anastomosis is started distal to the left subclavian artery orifice, running first along the posterior wall. The initial 5–10 suture bites are placed loosely, and then the graft is parachuted down to allow better visualization of the posterior suture line. A nerve hook is used to ensure that the sutures are evenly placed and pulled tight. The posterior suture line is continued anterior to the innominate artery, and the anastomosis is then completed by running the other arm of the suture anteriorly. The arch vessels are deaired using a brief period of low-flow RCP, steep Trendelenburg's position, and digital manipulation of the carotid and subclavian arteries.

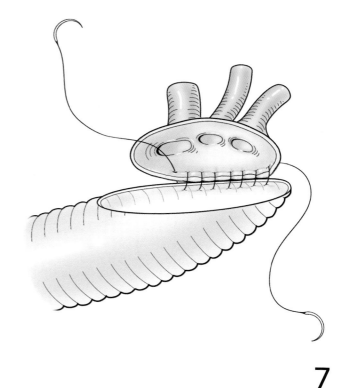

7

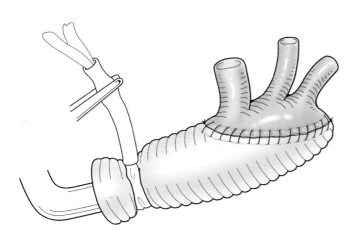

8

8 An arterial cannula is then inserted into the proximal end of the arch graft, RCP is discontinued, and SACP is started to the arch vessels at 15–20°C to keep the radial artery pressure at approximately 50 mmHg; usually, flow rates of 500–900 mL/minute are sufficient. The distal aortic anastomosis can then be performed carefully without undue time constraints.

9 If the descending thoracic aorta is markedly dilated or is aneurysmal distally, which is uncommon in patients with acute type A aortic dissections in our experience, it may be prudent to perform a total arch replacement along with a distal 'dangling' elephant trunk in younger and otherwise low-risk patients. The proximal descending thoracic aorta is prepared for an end-to-end, full-thickness distal anastomosis. Two long stay sutures are attached to the proximal end of a slightly undersized, woven, double-velour Dacron Hemashield graft. The future arch segment of the graft is invaginated inside the outer tube, which will become the elephant trunk. The elephant trunk segment should only measure 5–10 cm long (when stretched) to avoid inadvertent occlusion of downstream intercostal artery orifices (or, in cases of chronic dissection, the trunk graft becomes entrapped in either the distal aortic true or false lumen when the flap septectomy is not long enough).

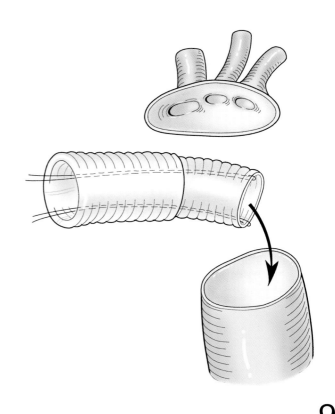

9

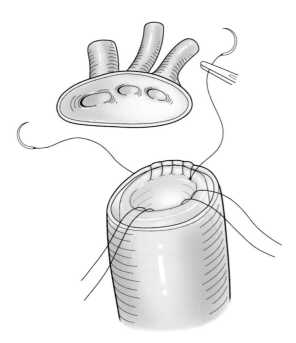

10

10 The doubled-up graft is inserted into the descending aorta such that the distal aortic anastomosis is located at the fold of the graft and the Bioglue-reinforced cuff of the descending thoracic aorta. Starting in the inferior corner, the posteromedial aspect of the anastomosis is completed with a 137-cm 3/0 polypropylene suture on an SH needle, taking deep bites through the double layer of graft material going inside to outside the aorta. The posterior suture line is tightened with a nerve hook at this stage. The distal aortic anastomosis is then completed anterolaterally by running the other arm of the suture upward. The stay stitches are then pulled out to extract the invaginated portion of the graft, and the inside of the elephant trunk graft distally is visually inspected to make sure it is fully deployed and not kinked.

11 Selective anterograde cerebral cold perfusion through the previously attached great vessel graft is discontinued, with the patient in Trendelenburg's position. Equal-sized small (4 cm × 1 cm) ellipses are excised from the inferior portion of the great vessel graft and the superior portion of the main arch graft, and a side-to-side anastomosis between the two grafts is completed using 4/0 SH-1 polypropylene suture. Intermittent RCP can be used during this graft-to-graft suturing. The distal aorta is allowed to fill passively during this anastomosis to remove air, which is aided by the return of dark blood backward down the arch branches. The head vessels are again deaired, and a cross-clamp is placed on the proximal aortic arch graft. If axillary CPB perfusion is used, simply turning up the CPB pump flow then re-establishes systemic perfusion to the entire body except the heart. If axillary artery cannulation was not used, a second arterial cannula is inserted directly into the new arch graft, and anterograde reperfusion and rewarming are started. Alternatively, a single 'branched' arch graft (woven double-velour Hemashield) is now available that can be used for the CPB arterial cannula. Attention is then turned to the proximal aorta. Following separation from bypass, the cannula in the open end of the arch vessel graft is subsequently removed, and the stump of the small branch graft is divided and oversewn.

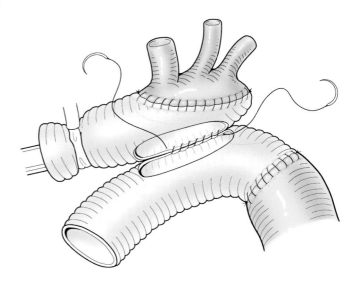

11

Aortic valve resuspension

Resuspension of the aortic valve commissures and tube graft replacement of the ascending aorta represent the most commonly performed technique that is used for patients with acute type A aortic dissection. We strive to preserve the patient's native aortic valve whenever feasible, but one needs to be confident that the valve repair is durable and that the sinuses of Valsalva do not dilate over time and become aneurysmal. When simple graft replacement of the tubular ascending aorta is performed (so-called supracoronary aortic grafting), one has to be certain that the retained aortic sinuses are not involved with any underlying pathological process and that the dissected proximal aortic root can be reconstructed in a durable fashion. If the sinuses of Valsalva are excessively dilated (e.g. annuloaortic ectasia), pathologically diseased (e.g. Marfan's syndrome), or damaged by the acute dissecting process, aortic root replacement should be considered. The availability of Bioglue has enabled us to preserve aortic roots that in previous years would have required replacement; however, whether this represents the best option for the patient will remain unknown until long-term follow-up data in patients who receive Bioglue become available. Restoration of the valve to functional competency is critical; the presence of advanced valve pathology or leaflet calcification usually is an indication for valve replacement, although normally functioning, noncalcified bicuspid valves can be preserved in selected cases. In certain circumstances, a separate valve and ascending aortic graft replacement proce-

dure can be used (not illustrated here), in which the bulk of the sinuses of Valsalva are resected but tongues of aorta that surround the coronary ostia are left intact and sutured to a scalloped aortic graft. This older technique is remarkably durable if used in properly selected patients and performed correctly. This procedure effectively excludes all of the residual sinus of Valsalva tissue. Its tactical advantage over a CVG or valve-sparing aortic root replacement is not having to reimplant the coronary ostia into the graft.

The entire aortic root is dissected out and mobilized. A veil of pericardial reflection characteristically covers the roof of the transverse sinus just caudad of the right and main pulmonary artery. Once this layer is divided, the left main coronary artery and its bifurcation can be readily identified. Complete mobilization of the main pulmonary artery, pulmonary valve annulus, right ventricular outflow tract, and ceiling of the left atrium off the aortic root down to close to the annular level is performed.

After complete transection of the aorta just above the sinotubular junction, circumferential reconstitution of the proximal full-thickness aortic cuff with Bioglue resuspends the aortic valve commissures and restores valvular competence.

Bioglue is injected to obliterate the space in the dissected proximal aortic wall (as described previously) and around the external layer of the aortic root, which really is the visceral epicardium. This maneuver creates a sturdy substrate for subsequent graft suturing. The size of the graft is determined before the distal arch anastomosis is performed based on the diameter of the aorta at the level of the sinotubular ridge, aiming to restore this dimension to the normal 90 per cent of aortic annular diameter.

12 If a single graft is used, the proximal end of the graft may need to be beveled to maintain the normal relationship between the greater and lesser curvatures of the ascending aorta and arch, which requires that a graft smaller than the sinotubular junction diameter be used. We most often use a single graft to avoid the need for a separate proximal graft and an extra suture line. Using two separate grafts (followed by a graft-to-graft anastomosis) is occasionally useful, however, especially when the sinotubular junction is dilated (and associated with pre-existent aortic regurgitation) and needs to be reduced in diameter to restore aortic valve competency. The proximal graft-to-aorta anastomosis is then constructed using a running 4/0 SH-1 or 3/0 SH polypropylene suture, as described below.

Partial disruption of the coronary ostia can be repaired with the use of Bioglue, taking care that no glue intrudes into the coronary arteries. If the aortic dissection involves the entire coronary ostium and the tissue is very friable, it is preferable to excise a full-thickness button of aortic wall circumferentially around the coronary and to reconstruct the dissected layers with 5/0 Bioglue, followed by a valve-sparing aortic root replacement using either the original David reimplantation technique or Yacoub's remodeling method. Coronary artery bypass grafting is less desirable (given the limited patency of venous grafts anastomosed to a Dacron graft) but is carried out when necessary. If time permits for taking down the internal mammary artery, this alternative is superior for coronary revascularization, but in the emergency circumstances of an acute type A aortic dissection, this procedure frequently is not practical.

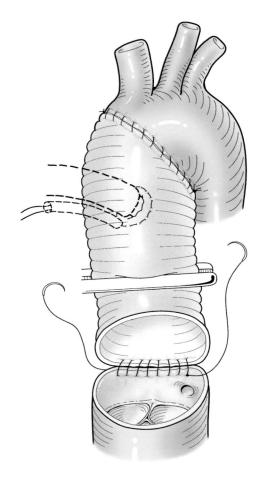

12

Aortic root replacement with a composite valve graft

Complete aortic root replacement with a CVG or a valve-preserving root replacement technique (see the section 'Valve-sparing aortic root replacement') is required only when gross annuloaortic ectasia (associated with pronounced cephalad migration of the coronary ostia and marked dilatation of the aortic annulus) or disruption of the aortic root with or without irreparable compromise of the coronary arteries by severe dissection damage is encountered. If attempts at commissural resuspension do not result in valvular competency, aortic valve replacement using either the separate valve graft or CVG approach is necessary. The aortotomy is extended down into the noncoronary sinus, the limits of the dissection flap are identified, and the valve leaflets are removed. Annular size is verified with appropriate valve obturators. The entire aortic root is dissected out and completely mobilized. A veil of pericardial reflection characteristically covers the roof of the transverse sinus just caudad of the right and main pulmonary artery. Once this layer is divided, the left main coronary artery and its main bifurcation can be readily identified. The takeoff of the right coronary artery, any large conus branch, and the left main coronary artery are identified and dissected free. Complete mobilization of the main pulmonary artery, pulmonary valve annulus, right ventricular outflow tract, and ceiling of the left atrium off the aortic root facilitates subsequent reimplantation of the coronary ostia without tension. When a valve-sparing root replacement is performed, this step is essential. In some patients, however, complete mobilization of the base of the aortic root can be impossible, including reoperations, especially in individuals who have previously undergone some type of ascending aortic surgical procedure in which the native aorta was not replaced.

The sinuses of Valsalva are excised, the coronary buttons fashioned, and the main coronary arteries mobilized. A mechanical CVG that includes a woven, double-velour Hemashield-coated Dacron graft and a bileaflet valve is used in younger individuals. It is important to undersize the CVG that is selected to permit maximal 'countersinking' down into the aortic annulus. In elderly patients and those in whom anticoagulation is either contraindicated or impractical, a bioprosthetic CVG is an attractive alternative in that it avoids the need for indefinite anticoagulation in the face of persistent downstream chronic aortic dissection. In such cases, a FreeStyle porcine bioprosthetic aortic root prosthesis works nicely. Alternatively, a suitable biological CVG can be fabricated in the operating room using any type of porcine or bovine pericardial prosthesis sewn to the end of an appropriately sized, woven, double-velour Hemashield graft. The Dacron graft is mounted onto the inner perimeter of the bioprosthetic valve sewing ring with polypropylene sutures using a running vertical mattress technique, thereby leaving the bulk of the sewing ring free for placement of the annular sutures.

13 Approximately 18 interrupted 2/0 nonabsorbable horizontal mattress sutures are reinforced with small Teflon felt pledgets taken from the aortic to the ventricular aspect; these sutures are placed in a 'subannular' planar configuration. This step starts at the junction of the left and noncoronary sinuses and proceeds counterclockwise. Such an everting technique ensures maximal countersinking of the CVG into the aortic annulus and maximizes the distance between the valve prosthesis and sites where the coronary artery ostia will be reimplanted. Tacking 5/0 polypropylene stay sutures are used to keep the coronary ostial buttons appropriately oriented and retracted out of the operative area during this stage. The CVG is then anchored to the aorto-ventricular junction, tying the sutures down but leaving cut ends sufficiently long (except under the coronary buttons) to allow them to serve as traction 'handles' in the event that the proximal suture line needs to be checked for hemostasis.

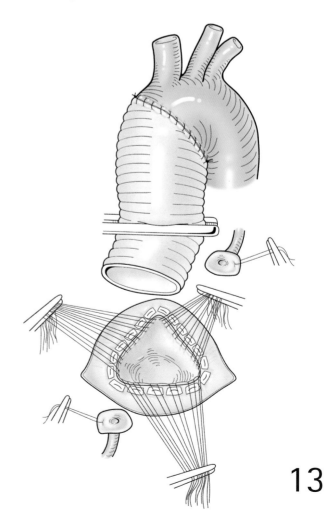

13

14 A hole is made in the graft with a No. 11 blade in the appropriate location, followed by creation of a 10- to 12-mm aperture in the graft using an ophthalmic loop cautery. It is important to ensure that the size of the aperture does not exceed the diameter of the coronary ostia to exclude as much of the diseased aortic wall as possible from the circulation. The posterior left coronary button is reimplanted first. A continuous 4/0 RB-1 or 5/0 RB-1 polypropylene suture is used, starting in the inferior posterior corner on the left side. The inferior rim is done first, taking bites from the graft to the button from the 'inside' and running rightward. The suture line is then tightened very gently with a fine nerve hook. The right side and one half of the superior rim are then done, continuing with the first needle working on the outside. Lastly, the other needle is used to complete the left lateral aspect and the remainder of the superior rim, as always taking care in passing the needle on its full curve or arc so as not to tear the coronary intima. Further mobilization of the main coronary artery may be necessary to relieve any tension on the coronary ostial suture line. It is seldom necessary in cases of acute aortic dissection to use an interposition graft to relieve tension on the coronary buttons if they are mobilized adequately; however, if the coronary tissue is damaged severely by the dissection, a short (1-cm) reversed saphenous vein interposition graft between the left main ostium and the defect in the aortic graft can be a lifesaving maneuver.

The right coronary reimplantation is performed after completion of the distal aortic anastomosis to know precisely where it should be placed. To judge the proper position for the right coronary ostial anastomosis, the aortic graft is filled with blood by momentarily releasing the cross-clamp on the graft with the head steeply down. After the correct position is determined, a suitably sized aperture is created with an ophthalmic cautery. Again, it is important to avoid tension and any twisting or angulation of the main coronary artery. Finally, the CVG is pressurized with warm blood cardioplegia before clamp removal to test for anastomotic leaks around the reimplanted coronary buttons.

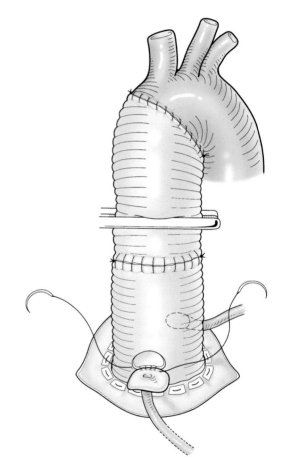

14

Valve-sparing aortic root replacement

Valve-preserving aortic root replacement is gaining in popularity in selected patients to avoid the requirement for lifelong anticoagulation. Patients with acute type A aortic dissections who are suitable candidates for this approach are quite rare in our experience but might include younger patients, those who cannot or will not be safely anticoagulated and otherwise need a CVG, and others who have a severely destroyed aortic root due to the dissecting process. We do not recommend this approach in patients with severe annuloaortic ectasia in whom the aortic annulus is markedly dilated and in those who have bicuspid aortic valves. We strongly prefer the David-I aortic valve reimplantation procedure, as this technique eliminates all dissected proximal aortic remnants from the systemic circulation, as the proximal graft suture line is constructed through healthy 'subannular' tissue. The native aortic annulus cannot dilate later on, and it is more hemostatic than Yacoub's remodeling method of valve-sparing aortic root replacement. The remodeling procedure popularized by Yacoub carries more short-term risk in terms of postoperative bleeding and a higher long-term risk of subsequent annular dilatation, causing recurrent aortic valvular regurgitation. More potential also exists for late false aneurysm formation within the rim of the dissected proximal aortic remnant to which the graft is sewn proximally. One theoretical drawback of the David reimplantation technique is that Dacron 'pseudosinuses' are not created, as they are with a remodeling procedure; these pseudosinuses theoretically minimize leaflet closing stresses, which should serve to prolong leaflet durability. David currently prefers his reimplantation technique, especially in patients with aortic dissection, over the remodeling approach; his current reimplantation technique calls for selecting a larger tube graft size than otherwise, which is plicated externally in a circumferential direction at the level of the tops of the commissures to create bulges in the Dacron graft that are analogous to pseudosinuses. More clinical data are necessary before one can decide if one method is superior to the other.

Relatively simple supracoronary graft replacement of the ascending aorta will suffice (as described in the section 'Aortic valve resuspension') if the sinuses were not severely damaged by the dissection. When proximal dissection has occurred, the noncoronary sinus usually is involved, as the coronary ostia tend to limit the circumferential propagation of the dissecting process around the aortic root. If the noncoronary sinus is severely damaged or nearly destroyed, this single sinus can be resected and replaced by a Dacron tongue in continuity with the aortic graft, which is analogous to Yacoub's 'unisinus' remodeling root replacement procedure with preservation of the valve. In general, one should err on the side of resecting more rather than less of the dissected proximal aortic remnant to avoid the possibility of potential anastomotic disruption.

An important step when using the David technique is adequate mobilization of the entire aortic root so as to expose the ventricle beneath the aortoventricular junction for placement of the proximal sutures (as described in Chapter 16) within the LV outflow tract. The proximal aorta is transected at the sinotubular ridge and dissected free from the anterior fat pad associated with the right coronary artery and atrioventricular groove down to the interventricular septum, the right ventricular outflow tract, the pulmonary valve annulus, and the main pulmonary artery. Specifically, the posterior band (or 'veil') of tissue, which actually is a thin, visceral pericardial reflection that tethers the proximal aortic root above the roof of the left atrium and left main coronary artery, needs to be divided. The mobilized proximal aorta can be lifted upward, enabling a direct view of where the leaflets attach to the ventriculoaortic junction, which normally is shaped like a coronet. A deeply countersunk aortic annulus that is abnormally located at the level of the tricuspid annulus cannot be safely mobilized, but this situation is rare. In such cases, conversion to a Yacoub remodeling root replacement should be considered.

15 For the David procedure, all three aortic sinuses are excised, leaving approximately 5 mm of aortic wall remaining around the leaflet hinge lines and the coronary ostia. The left coronary artery is dissected free as described previously, and the right coronary artery is also mobilized, taking care to avoid injury to any large conal branches. The left and right coronary buttons are trimmed down to appropriate size. Next, 12–15 interrupted horizontal mattress 2/0 nonabsorbable sutures are placed transmurally beneath the ventriculoaortic junction (leaflet hinges), trying to maintain a planar orientation except under the muscular interventricular septum beneath the commissure between the right and left cusps, starting along the anterior mitral valve leaflet and across the membranous interventricular septum. The graft is sized according to David's original formula, that is, multiplying the average height of all three leaflets by 2 and then multiplying this product by 0.67; to this number is added twice the thickness of the aortic wall (usually totaling 2–4 mm). Ideally, this formula results in a graft size (external diameter) of 26–28 mm if the leaflet heights average 15 mm or slightly more. A shallow smooth scallop is cut from the graft, corresponding to the junction of the right and left leaflets where the subannular sutures must be passed closer to the 'annulus.' The proximal mattress sutures are then passed through the graft, compensating for any asymmetry of the aortic annulus. The noncoronary sinus is normally the largest, the left is the smallest, and the right sinus subtends approximately 120 degrees. The sutures are tied and cut, with care taken to ensure that all the aortic commissural tissue and leaflets are inside the graft before these sutures are tied. In some cases, the native aortic valve is inverted temporarily down into the ventricle to keep it out of the way during this stage.

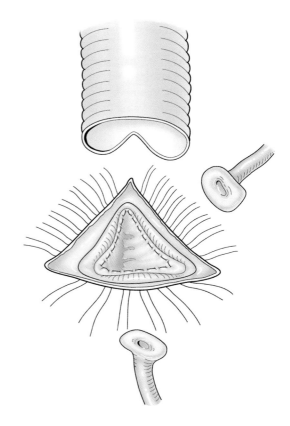

15

16 The valve commissures are anchored with 4/0 polypropylene mattress sutures at the appropriate locations, making sure that the graft is stretched out longitudinally when doing so, pulled up within the graft, and temporarily secured. It is important to ensure that the distances between the commissural pillars are spaced in similar proportion to the size of the leaflets and that the commissures are placed on tension. When the height and the angular orientation of the three new commissural locations within the graft are judged to be satisfactory, these commissural sutures can be tied. The graft is then cut approximately 1–2 cm above the top of the aortic valve commissures for easier visibility and suturing of the distal suture valve line. Beginning on the left sinus, one arm of the 4/0 polypropylene suture is passed in and out through the aortic wall close to the leaflet hinge lines and the graft, attaching the sinus remnants to the graft fabric, advanced to the next commissural pillar, and tied down. Care must be taken not to injure the leaflets with the suture needles inadvertently. The coronary ostial buttons are connected to holes in the ascending aortic graft as described previously. The graft is filled with saline as a preliminary test for possible cusp malcoaptation. If one or more leaflets appear to prolapse, a temporary 'Frater stitch' is used to align the three noduli of Aranti between all leaflets to identify which cusp needs further attention, which most commonly is the right or noncoronary leaflet. The free margin of this prolapsing leaflet can then be shortened by running a fine 6/0 or 5/0 nonabsorbable suture across the center of the cusp, incorporating the nodulus of Aranti to raise the leaflet coaptation plane of that leaflet to match the other two. When completing coronary reimplantation, disrupted right or left coronary arteries can be bypassed, using a short interposition vein graft and attaching the graft to the Dacron graft. In younger patients, it may be preferable to use a left internal mammary artery graft for the left anterior descending coronary artery.

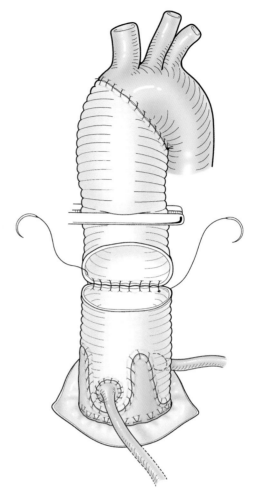

16

Completion of the proximal aortic anastomosis

Following reconstruction of the proximal aorta using whichever technique is chosen, the final step is suturing the proximal graft to the distal aortic graft. Before constructing the distal anastomosis, it is important to inspect the retroaortic mediastinal tissues for hemostasis and lymph leaks around the tracheal bifurcation. Determining proper graft length is critical, as too long a graft angulates the final repair and displaces it to the right and possibly will not restore adequate cephalad tension on the commissures such that native valve competency may be jeopardized. As was mentioned previously, the distal end of the graft should be beveled, with the 'toe' going to the greater curve of the arch near the innominate artery to foreshorten the graft, which helps prevent kinking or bowing of the graft to the patient's right. Any discrepancy between the diameters of the proximal and distal grafts is overcome by making small suture advances on the

smaller graft and larger advances on the larger one. After completion of the repair, 500–100 mL of warm blood cardioplegia is infused through a large-bore needle inserted directly into the aortic Dacron graft. During this controlled reperfusion period, the coronary ostial anastomoses are checked for hemostasis. At this time, we use a thin layer of Bioglue to cover the external surface of all the anastomoses.

Rewarming

Before removal of the cross-clamp, the pulmonary artery or LV vent is clamped, the vena cava tourniquets are released, and the heart is filled with blood from the CPB circuit to expel air. The lungs are then ventilated, the left atrial appendage is inverted, the LV apex is needle aspirated, and the heart is manually agitated. A cardiotomy suction vent is placed into the ascending aortic graft, and the heart is again meticulously deaired, after which the cross-clamp is finally removed.

Systemic rewarming usually takes about twice the time required for systemic cooling. CPB rewarming is started 5–10 minutes after the end of the circulatory arrest period and progresses at approximately 1°C every 3–5 minutes. The temperature gradient between arterial infusion and venous return blood should not exceed 10°C. In addition, the arterial blood temperature should not exceed 37°C to avoid exacerbating any neurological injury. After resuscitation of the heart and rewarming of the patient to 37°C, CPB is discontinued in the usual fashion. One needs to ensure that the coronary arteries are not compromised, either due to dissection or to the chance of intrinsic coronary artery disease. If one is in doubt, prophylactic grafting of the coronary arteries may be required, particularly if regional LV systolic wall motion abnormalities are seen at this time on the TEE.

Hemostasis

Bleeding can be a major problem, as these patients are often coagulopathic before the operation begins. Two to four units of fresh frozen plasma can be added to the pump during rewarming to replenish clotting factors. We also use our standard high-dose antifibrinolytic regimen on patients with acute type A aortic dissections, which is an initial loading dose of epsilon–aminocaproic acid at the start of the operation followed by an infusion for a total of 30 g. Following reversal of heparin, platelets, cryoprecipitate, and more fresh frozen plasma are added if required. We avoid the use of aprotinin because of the possibility of systemic thrombosis during HCA. When excessive suture hole bleeding occurs, the passage of time, patience, pressure with packs, and attention to replenishing clotting factors usually are successful. Avoiding swings of hypertension and having the patient fully rewarmed are helpful. Before Bioglue was available, we occasionally resorted to the topical application of a homemade 'fibrin glue' (consisting of 10 units of cryoprecipitate, bovine thrombin, and calcium) for persistent needle hole bleeding.

POSTOPERATIVE CARE

One should be cognizant of the potential for cerebral or thoracoabdominal malperfusion syndromes that occur postoperatively. If suspicion arises, an emergency CT angiogram is indicated; if malperfusion of an important end organ is confirmed, some sort of catheter fenestration or true lumen stenting, or both, by the interventional radiological team can be lifesaving. Pulses in all four limbs and the carotid arteries, neurological status, and urine output should be regularly monitored. Peritoneal signs and metabolic acidosis may herald impending visceral ischemia and should prompt suspicion of abdominal aortic malperfusion. Stringent blood pressure control is mandatory immediately and over the long term, particularly the use of beta-blockers to lower arterial dP/dt. This maneuver is especially important in patients with Marfan's syndrome, even if their blood pressure is normal. A discharge echocardiogram is recommended to assess baseline aortic valve competency. A CT angiogram of the chest and abdomen is performed before hospital discharge to ensure that the aortic repair is technically sound and to establish a baseline of downstream aortic pathology. Serial scans should be carried out thereafter every 6–12 months indefinitely.

OUTCOME

Using the surgical procedures described in this chapter, which have evolved substantially over the decades, the 30-day, 1-year, and 5-year survival estimates in 307 patients (up to 1999) with acute type A aortic dissection who were treated surgically at our institution are 82 per cent, 74 per cent, and 63 per cent, respectively. A great deal of progress has been achieved over the years, but the authors hope the reader appreciates that major clinical challenges still exist in this field.

FURTHER READING

Crawford, E.S., Svensson, L.G., Coselli, J.S., Safi, H.J., Hess, K.R. 1989. Surgical treatment of aneurysm and/or dissection of the ascending aorta, transverse aortic arch, and ascending aorta and transverse aortic arch. Factors influencing survival in 717 patients. *Journal of Thoracic and Cardiovascular Surgery* **98**, 659–74.

Fann, J.I., Smith, J.A., Miller, D.C., *et al.* 1995. Surgical management of aortic dissection during a 30-year period. *Circulation* **92**, 9 Suppl.: II-113–21.

Griepp, R.B., Ergin, M.A., McCullough, J.N., *et al.* 1997. Use of the hypothermic circulatory arrest for cerebral protection during aortic surgery. *Journal of Cardiac Surgery* **12**, 2 Suppl.: 312–21.

Kazui, T., Washiyama, N., Muhammad, B.A., *et al.* 2000. Extended total arch replacement for acute type A aortic dissection: experience with seventy patients. *Journal of Thoracic and Cardiovascular Surgery* **119**, 558–65.

Usui, A., Abe, T., Murase, M. Early clinical results of retrograde cerebral perfusion for aortic arch operations in Japan. *Annals of Thoracic Surgery* **62**, 94–104.

Yun, K.L., Miller, D.C., Fann, J.I., *et al.* 1997. Composite valve graft versus separate aortic valve and ascending aortic replacement: is there still a role for the separate procedure? *Circulation* **96**, 9 Suppl.: II-368–75.

34

Thoracic aortic aneurysm including dissection

G. MICHAEL DEEB MD
Professor of Surgery, Section of Cardiac Surgery, University of Michigan, Ann Arbor, Michigan, USA

DAVID M. WILLIAMS MD
Professor of Radiology , University of Michigan School of Medicine, and Director, Vascular and Interventional Radiology,
University of Michigan Medical Center, Ann Arbor, Michigan, USA

HISTORY

The perspective of surgical treatment for descending thoracic aortic aneurysms has changed over the past several years with the onset of clinical trials that use self-expanding endovascular stent-grafts (endografts). Although the use of endografts appears to be a promising modality of treatment for descending thoracic aortic aneurysms, anatomical limitations restrict their applicability, and few intermediate or long-term data are available for clinical outcome analysis. In our practice, patients who are anatomically unsuitable for endografts or who are in good general health with a life expectancy that exceeds 20 years continue to have open aortic reconstruction.

PREOPERATIVE ASSESSMENT

Several concerns exist in dealing with patients who have descending thoracic aneurysms, but the predominant concerns are the prevention of stroke as well as spinal cord and visceral ischemia. The main etiology for stroke is believed to be embolic, which may be secondary to retrograde showering from femoral cannulation or showering at the time of arch or proximal descending aortic cross-clamping. Analysis of the type (ectatic vs. atherosclerotic) and extent of the aortic disease has to be taken into consideration when planning the optimal surgical procedure for each patient. The necessary information is readily available with high-resolution spiral computed tomography (CT) scanning, magnetic resonance angiography, and transesophageal echocardiography (TEE). If the patient has significant intraluminal clot and atheromatous debris, ascending aortic or subclavian artery cannulation may be preferable to femoral or iliac cannulation. If the disease process does not allow safe proximal cross-clamping without a significant risk of embolic stroke, hypothermic circulatory arrest (HCA) with open proximal anastomosis is recommended. For spinal cord protection, several possible approaches are based on sound logic and excellent results. All of the various approaches are based on prevention of ischemia during the procedure and adequate perfusion to the spinal cord following repair. We generally use two open approaches for descending aortic aneurysm repair based on two factors: (1) the ability to cross-clamp the aorta proximal to the aneurysm safely and (2) the extent of the aneurysm and the number of intercostal vessels at risk with the repair.

OPERATION BY OPEN RECONSTRUCTION

Clamp technique using left heart bypass

For proximal aneurysms that have no contraindication to proximal aortic cross-clamping and the extent of which is limited to the T-6 level, we use proximal and distal aortic cross-clamping with distal perfusion of the spinal vessels and visceral organs using left heart bypass (LHB) with a centrifugal pump.

1 Patient preparation includes the insertion of right radial and femoral arterial lines as well as a Swan-Ganz catheter for hemodynamic monitoring. A double-lumen endotracheal tube is used for selective right lung ventilation. The patient is positioned for a left posterolateral incision. If the distal descending aorta has minimal disease and can be used for cannulation, this technicque is preferable to femoral arterial cannulation. If this approach is not an option, the hips are rotated back to the left to allow for femoral vascular access. A posterolateral incision is made, and the chest is entered through the fourth intercostal space, providing access to the arch and subclavian artery. If selective right lung ventilation is not tolerated because of oxygen desaturation secondary to ventilation perfusion mismatch, the left main pulmonary artery can be clamped to eliminate left lung perfusion. The phrenic and vagus nerves are identified and freed from the aneurysm. The left subclavian artery is dissected from the surrounding tissues, and a vessel loop is passed around the artery for control. Proximal access is gained around the aortic arch between the left carotid and the left subclavian arteries. This maneuver is performed by initiating dissection on the greater curvature of the arch between the carotid and subclavian and extending the dissection plane down to the trachea. Blunt dissection is used posteriorly on the arch by placing the tip of the forefinger on the anterior surface of the trachea and dragging the finger down the trachea, separating tissue off the trachea toward the aorta. Circumferential access is completed by sharply dissecting along the lesser curvature of the arch between the arch and the extrapericardial surface of the pulmonary artery back to the anterior surface of the trachea. Care is taken to identify the vagus and the recurrent laryngeal branch of the vagus and to protect them from injury during this dissection. An umbilical tape is then passed around the arch and brought out between the phrenic and vagus nerves.

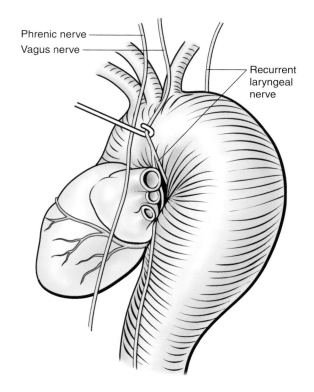

Phrenic nerve

Vagus nerve

Recurrent laryngeal nerve

1

2 Finally, access is gained circumferentially around the aorta distal to the aneurysm. Arterial inflow is obtained by left atrial cannulation either using the left atrial appendage or a left pulmonary vein. Distal perfusion is obtained either by distal descending aortic cannulation below the aneurysm if accessible or via direct insertion into the femoral artery.

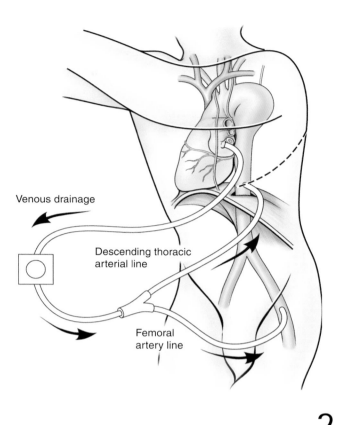

Venous drainage

Descending thoracic arterial line

Femoral artery line

2

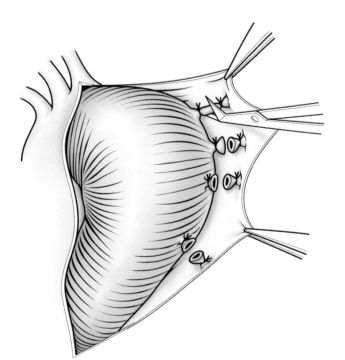

3 LHB with a centrifugal pump can be accomplished with heparin-coated tubing, thereby avoiding anticoagulation, or with standard pump tubing and systemic heparinization. Once low flow is established with LHB, the parietal pleura along the greater curvature of the aneurysm is incised, and the intercostal vessels that originate from the aneurysm are ligated or clipped.

3

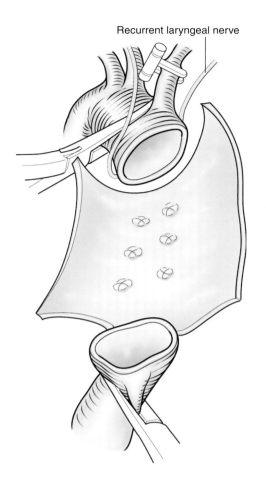

Recurrent laryngeal nerve

4 The aortic arch is carefully cross-clamped proximal to the aneurysm between the left carotid and subclavian arteries to avoid damage to the nerves. The right radial and femoral arterial pressure lines are used to monitor pressure and direct flow through the LHB. The left subclavian artery and the aorta distal to the aneurysm are cross-clamped. The aneurysm is incised in a longitudinal fashion, with this incision carried the entire length of the aneurysm. The aorta is then carefully transected at the proximal and the distal necks to avoid injury to surrounding structures and to retain adventitia circumferentially to allow for full-thickness anastomosis. Special care needs to be taken to identify the recurrent laryngeal nerve along the proximal neck and to be certain that, while transecting the aorta along the posterior wall, the nerve is identified and preserved. The bed of the aneurysm is now inspected for bleeding intercostal arteries, which are suture ligated with figure-of-eight 2/0 silk ligatures.

4

Recurrent nerve

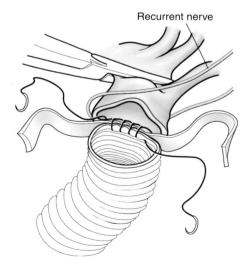

5 The proximal transected aorta is examined for extent of disease and the suitability for suturing. If the aortic tissue is friable, a strip of Teflon felt can be used to buttress the suture line. A collagen-impregnated, woven Dacron graft is used for aortic replacement and is anastomosed to the transected aorta using a continuous running 3/0 or 4/0 polypropylene suture, depending on the thickness of the anastomotic tissues.

5

6 On completion of the proximal anastomosis, a clamp is placed across the graft, and the arch clamp is removed to test the intactness of the anastomosis. Once good hemostasis is confirmed, the arch is reclamped, and the second clamp is removed from the graft. This proximal reclamping is particularly important if the patient has received no heparin, because leaving a clamp on the graft leads to thrombus formation from stasis in the graft proximal to the clamp site. Thrombin glue can be applied onto the proximal anastomosis to enhance hemostasis. The open graft is then irrigated to eliminate blood and clot prior to measuring and transecting it at the proper length prior to constructing the distal anastomosis. The graft should be measured under tension and then transected two to three additional rings proximal to obtain the best length. Next, the distal anastomosis is constructed using the same principles as for the proximal anastomosis. Before finishing the anastomosis, the graft is purged of air by removal of the distal clamp, and the anastomosis is completed. On completion, the proximal aortic clamp is removed, along with the subclavian clamp. After good hemostasis is assured, the graft can be covered with bovine pericardium to keep the separate adjacent lung from the graft and to reduce the possibility of a bronchoaortic fistula.

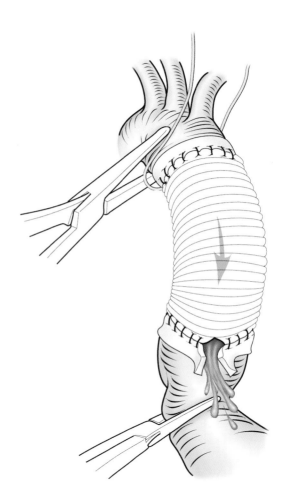

6

Hypothermic circulatory arrest technique

7 For patients with aneurysms that originate in the distal arch, have pathology that prohibits proximal cross-clamping, or extend distally and encompass intercostals at the level of T-6 through the lumbars, HCA can be used for repair. The intercostal arteries from T-6 through the lumbar vessels should be reimplanted whenever possible. Access for cardiopulmonary bypass (CPB) can be accomplished either via the femoral vessels or within the thorax using the proximal arch for arterial cannulation and the main pulmonary artery for venous drainage. We prefer femoral cannulation unless the risk of stroke from intraluminal debris is substantial, so that we can selectively perfuse the upper and lower halves of the body throughout the case. When femoral arterial cannulation is performed, a flexible wire-reinforced cannula, either 22 or 24 mm in size, is used. Venous access is obtained using a cannula, which is fed over a guide wire with an introducer and positioned in the right atrium using echo guidance.

For intrathoracic cannulation, a standard, flexible, wire-reinforced aortic cannula is placed through a double-pledgeted purse-string suture in the proximal arch or the ascending aorta. If access to normal aorta proximal to the cannula is difficult and it is known from CT scan and TEE that the aneurysm has minimal debris, the aneurysm itself can be cannulated. Venous access in the chest is accomplished with a large 30- or 32-mm right-angled, flexible reinforced cannula positioned through a pledgeted purse-string suture in the main pulmonary artery. Intrathoracic cannulation may necessitate anterior extension of the posterolateral incision to the sternal edge without sacrificing the internal mammary arteries. CPB is instituted, and the patient is cooled to 18°C. During cooling, the left heart is decompressed with a vent through a purse-string suture in the left superior pulmonary vein.

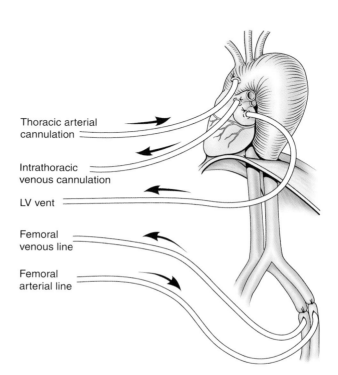

Thoracic arterial cannulation

Intrathoracic venous cannulation

LV vent

Femoral venous line

Femoral arterial line

7

8 While cooling, the vagus nerve is identified and mobilized from the aneurysmal tissue, the recurrent laryngeal branch of the vagus is also located, and care is taken not to damage the nerve as it courses around the lesser curvature of the distal arch and passes cephalad along the posterior surface of the arch back. The phrenic nerve is also located, mobilized off the aneurysm, and preserved. As cooling continues, the patient is placed in Trendelenburg's position, and the head is packed in ice. If the aneurysm extends distally to the crux of the diaphragm, the aorta is mobilized circumferentially, dissecting the tissues at the diaphragmatic hiatus, with care to avoid damage to the thoracic duct and the esophagus. A suitable area in the aneurysm above the level of the sixth thoracic vertebra is located (if possible) for distal cross-clamping and subsequent perfusion of the spine and lower body while the distal arch is repaired under HCA. The final maneuver during cooling is to choose the proper-sized replacement graft and to suture an 8-mm side graft to the replacement graft in an end-to-side fashion using a running 4/0 polypropylene suture. Once the temperature reaches 19°C, 1 g thiopental, 1 g methylprednisolone sodium succinate (Solu-Medrol), 25 g mannitol, and 5000 units heparin are given intravenously for cerebral protection. When 17°C is reached, a bolus of 40 mEq potassium chloride is given intravenously to arrest the heart. After CPB flow is reduced, and if the aneurysm is suitable, without calcification and thrombus debris, the aorta is cross-clamped above the T-6 level of the descending aorta to allow perfusion of the spine and visceral organs during HCA of the head and heart. If the aneurysm is atherosclerotic with calcification and debris, aortic cross-clamping is avoided, and the entire procedure is completed under HCA. The aneurysm is incised longitudinally and extended proximal to the level of the subclavian artery. Care is taken to observe the course of the vagus nerve as it moves over the anterior surface of the aorta at the level of the subclavian artery. The aorta is transected at this level, with great care given to preserve the recurrent laryngeal nerve as it courses around the lesser curvature of the aortic arch and ascends within the chest posterior and lateral to the left subclavian artery. The arch is inspected, and all aneurysmal tissue in the distal arch is resected, with care taken to preserve the vagus and phrenic nerves.

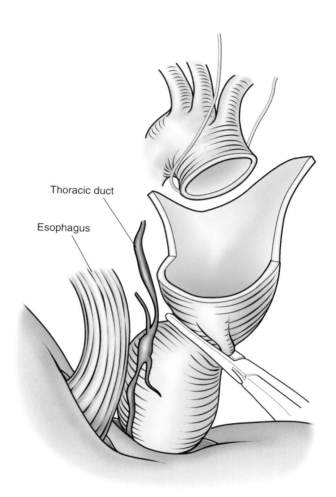

Thoracic duct

Esophagus

8

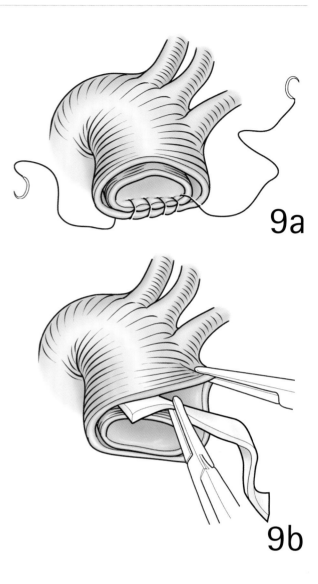

9a, b If the aneurysm surgery is being undertaken to treat acute type B dissection, the arch is examined for retrograde dissection and re-entry points. If a re-entry point is noted, this portion of the arch must be excised, and the distal arch is reconstructed with brachiocephalic artery implantation. If no re-entry point exists, the dissected layers of the distal arch are reapproximated either with glue and a continuous, running, 4/0 polypropylene stitch or with a continuous suture alone (Figure 9a). If the patient is being operated on for a chronic dissection and a blind pouch is present from retrograde dissection, this pouch is either resected or obliterated using a piece of Dacron felt sandwiched between the aortic layers and held securely with a running 4/0 polypropylene suture line (Figure 9b).

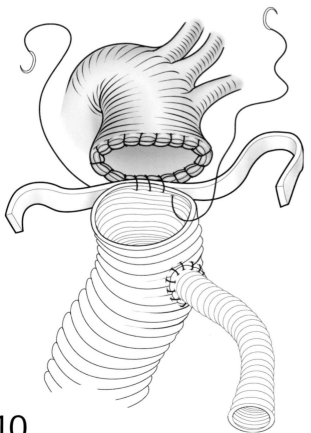

10 Once the distal arch has been prepared for the proximal anastomosis, an appropriate-sized collagen-impregnated Dacron graft with a size 8-mm side arm graft is anastomosed to the aortic edge with a continuous 3/0 or 4/0 polypropylene suture, depending on the thickness of the aorta and whether a strip of Teflon felt is used to buttress the suture line.

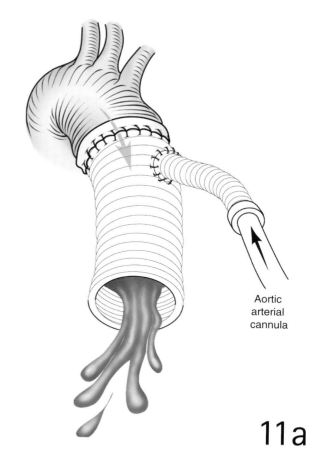

Aortic
arterial
cannula

11a

11a, b On completion, glue is placed around the anastomosis externally to enhance hemostasis. The side arm graft is then cannulated with a No. 8 French wire-reinforced aortic cannula, which is connected to the bifurcated line on the arterial limb of the CPB circuit. Flow is instituted through this line with the patient in Trendelenburg's position, and air and debris are evacuated through the distal end of the graft (Figure 11a). A soft-tipped clamp is placed on the graft distal to the cannula, and total bypass is now reinstituted (Figure 11b).

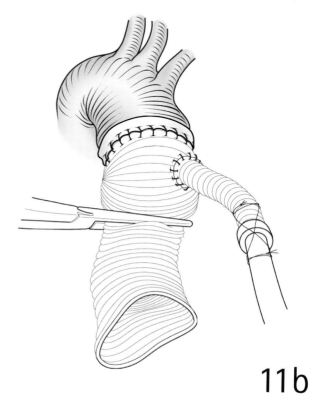

11b

12 Attention is next focused on the distal anastomosis. This anastomosis is made in a closed fashion, when distal clamping is possible, thus allowing for continuous perfusion to the visceral organs. The distal clamp is now moved down beyond the aneurysm, thereby allowing flow to the visceral organs through the femoral cannula. If a good distal anastomosis cannot be accomplished with a distal cross-clamp in place, the anastomosis is completed in an open fashion. The arterial line to the femoral cannula is clamped, and bypass flow is lowered to approximately a third of total calculated flow to accommodate flow into the cannula placed in the 8-mm side arm graft of the aortic graft that perfuses the upper half of the body. This selective perfusion limits the HCA arrest times for the two halves of the body. The aorta is split in a longitudinal fashion down to the level of the planned distal anastomosis. The distal aorta is tapered to allow for a long tail of the posterior aortic wall, with the distal intercostal vessels to be incorporated into the distal anastomosis whenever possible. If this approach is not possible, the intercostals are implanted as a separate island of aorta into the back of the graft. Every effort is made to implant the intercostals from T-6 through the lumbars.

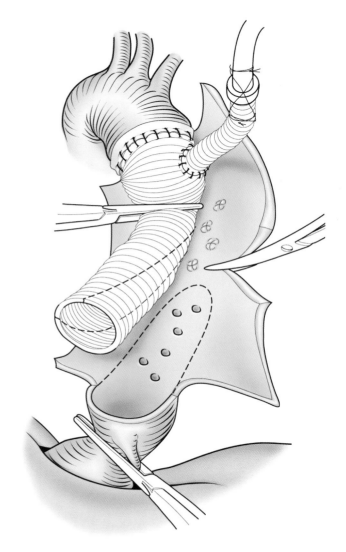

12

13 If the aneurysm is secondary to a chronic dissection, the tail of intercostals is formed by trimming the adventitia down to match the intima-media layer. The separated layers are then approximated with a running 4/0 polypropylene suture to form a full-thickness tail. The distal aorta in a chronic dissection cannot have the layers circumferentially reapproximated unless it is clear from CT scan or magnetic resonance angiography that the visceral organs and limbs are perfused by the true lumen or a re-entry tear exists in the abdomen. If neither of these situations is present, the flap of the true lumen needs to be incised longitudinally for 5 cm, and a wedge of this wall needs to be resected to allow for continuous flow into both lumens distally. The remainder of the wall of the true lumen is then folded back and approximated to the wall of the adventitia before the distal anastomosis with the graft is completed.

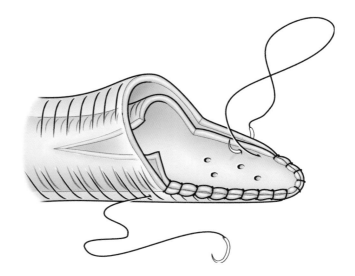

13

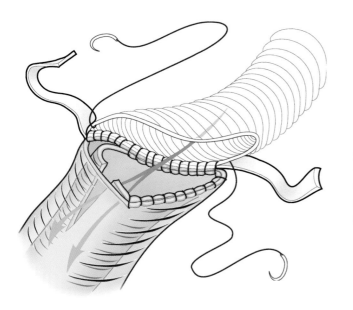

14

14 When the intercostals and the distal aorta are incorporated in one anastomosis, the collagen-impregnated graft is measured for appropriate length and tapered to the proper shape to accommodate the aorta. The distal anastomosis is made with running 3/0 polypropylene using felt reinforcement, if necessary, beginning just off the heel of the graft corresponding to just off the tip of the tail of the aorta.

15, 16 On completion of the distal anastomosis and before the sutures are tied down, air and blood are evacuated from the graft at the most superior portion of the suture line by back flushing the graft from the femoral cannula and forward flushing the graft from the cannula in the 8-mm side arm graft (Figure 15). If separate intercostal artery and distal anastomoses are performed, an appropriate-sized aperture is made in the back wall of the graft, and the intercostal vessel pedicle is constructed with continuous 3/0 or 4/0 polypropylene suture. The distal anas-

tomosis is then constructed in an end-to-end fashion and flushed as described previously (Figure 16). On completion of the distal anastomosis and restoration of flow, the patient is warmed to 37°C. If the cardiac rhythm does not return spontaneously, the patient is cardioverted. Ventilation is resumed, and the heart is evacuated of air with TEE guidance before the left atrial vent is removed. The patient is then weaned from CPB and decannulated, and the thorax is closed.

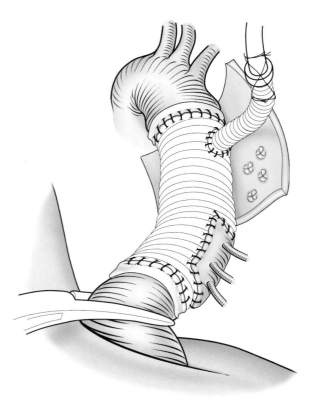

16

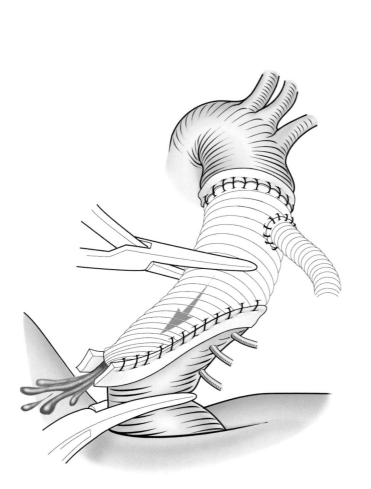

15

OUTCOME FOR OPEN REPAIR

From July 1994 to 1999, 91 patients at the University of Michigan underwent thoracic aortic surgery using LHB for aneurysms and traumatic transections, as well as for acute and chronic dissection. Eight (8.8 per cent) died during hospitalization (regardless of length of stay) or within 30 days of the procedure (regardless of location of death). Three patients (3 per cent) had a stroke, and two patients (2 per cent), both with traumatic transection, had lower extremity weakness and paresthesias but were able to ambulate and function without major disability. Fifty-three patients had surgery for the same indications but underwent HCA. Six (11 per cent) deaths, three (5 per cent) permanent strokes, two (4 per cent) transient neurological events, and three (5 per cent) paraplegias occurred. Two of the patients with paraplegia could not have reimplantation of the intercostals because of the poor quality of the aortic tissue.

OPERATION BY ENDOGRAFT

17 Treatment of thoracic aortic aneurysms by endografts requires close attention to the condition of the iliac arteries and to the configuration of the aorta proximal and distal to the aneurysm. Currently available thoracic aortic endografts depend for their hemostatic integrity on a friction seal between the device and the aortic wall. Consequently, a major requirement is a suitably long and narrow neck of aorta proximal and distal to the aneurysm. The neck should be long enough to allow safe deployment between the aneurysm and the brachiocephalic arteries proximally or the celiac artery distally and narrow enough to accommodate a self-expanding device with a resting diameter that is 10–20 per cent larger than the aortic lumen.

The exact length of neck segment and aortic diameter that are required for precise device deployment vary, as do the range of device diameters available from the manufacturer. Most devices require a segment of neck at least 2.0 cm in length and no more than 3.8 cm in diameter. Endografts of this large size require fairly stiff delivery catheters that are between 0.7 and 0.8 cm in diameter. This size limits the minimum diameter and tortuosity of the iliac arteries that are suitable as access conduits to the aorta.

Imaging

The imaging evaluation of a patient with a thoracic aortic aneurysm is important for operative treatment and absolutely crucial for endograft treatment. During surgical repair of an aneurysm, a graft can be appropriately sized during the procedure, and up to 5-mm diameter discrepancies between graft and aortic diameters can be accommodated. The graft can be tailored at the time of constructing the distal anastomosis. Inaccurate sizing of the diameter or the length of an endograft can result in device migration, with failure to exclude the aneurysm and possible occlusion of adjacent aortic branches. Imaging begins with a contrast-enhanced helical CT. When the aneurysm is in the vertical portion of the

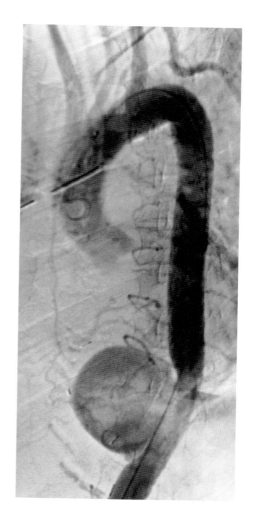

17

descending aorta, accurate aortic diameters can be measured from the axial slices. When the aorta passes obliquely from slice to slice, it takes on an elliptical cross-section, and care must be taken in this situation to measure the short axis of the aortic cross-section. When the aneurysm neck is adjacent to the anatomical arch or near the aortic hiatus, accurate aortic diameters may require three-dimensional reconstruction using a computer workstation. To determine accurate dimensions of the aneurysm and the proximal and distal necks, aortography may be required using a graduated catheter or three-dimensional reconstruction of the CT study. Pelvic arteriography in bilateral oblique projections is obtained to determine whether the external iliac arteries can accommodate the delivery catheter.

Endografts – aneurysms

Patient preparation includes securing arterial access for the delivery catheter into the distalmost iliofemoral segment, which is large enough to be accommodated. Percutaneous placement of a No. 7 French sheath into the opposite femoral artery is performed to allow contrast-aortography and/or intravascular ultrasound during the procedure. The patient is systemically heparinized as the artery distal to the arteriotomy is clamped. In men, the diameter of the femoral artery is sufficient to allow passage of the delivery catheter. In women, however, the common femoral artery may be too small, and access to the external iliac artery or even the distal aorta may be required. Focal iliac stenoses can be expanded by balloon angioplasty or stretched ('dottered') by serial dilators to allow for advancement of the deployment catheter. In preparation for deployment, landmarks for important side branches are determined. If a crucial aortic branch artery is at jeopardy during deployment, and reliable bony landmarks are not available, a catheter can be placed at the left subclavian origin from a brachial artery approach, or in the celiac trunk from a femoral artery approach. An intravascular ultrasound catheter can also be poised in the aorta immediately adjacent to the critical origin.

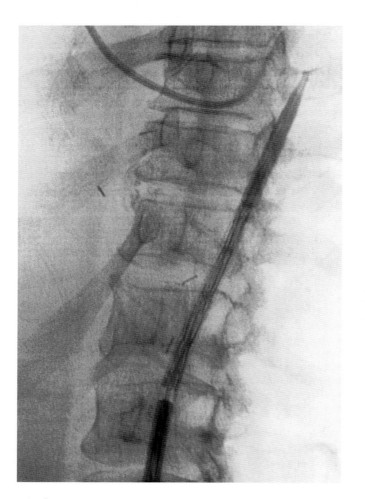

18 The deployment catheter is advanced from the entry site in the femoral or iliac artery or distal aortic conduit to just proximal to the thoracic aortic aneurysm over an extra-stiff guide wire. Our current wire of choice is the Lunderquist super-stiff wire (Cook, Bloomfield, IN). Passage of the delivery catheter, which can be as large as 0.87 cm in outer diameter, is scrupulously observed throughout the course of the iliac artery, with careful attention to areas of resistance at calcified stenoses and tortuous segments. Once the device is poised alongside the aneurysm, a final survey of landmarks is performed. If, during deployment in the aorta, the device is expected to be occlusive for more than a few seconds, systemic blood pressure is lowered pharmacologically.

18

19 The endograft is then deployed; the details of deployment vary from one device to another. The home-made endograft is extruded from a delivery sheath; using the inner coaxial blunt pusher-catheter to fix the distal end of the endograft, the operator retracts the outer sheath distally, allowing passive expansion of the endograft against the aortic wall. In contrast, the Gore Thoracic Excluder (WL Gore & Associates, Inc., Medical Products Division, Flagstaff, Arizona, USA) is rapidly released from a constraining jacket by retracting a chain stitch zipper. Accurate deployment of the endograft is documented by aortography and consists of exclusion of the aneurysm with sparing of major aortic branches.

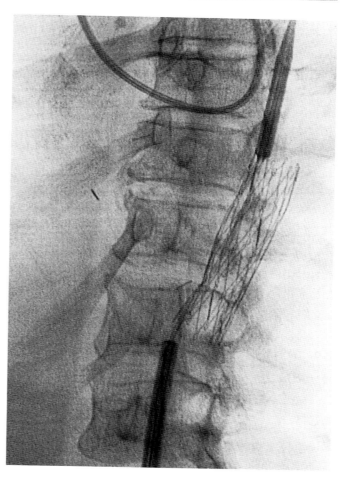

19

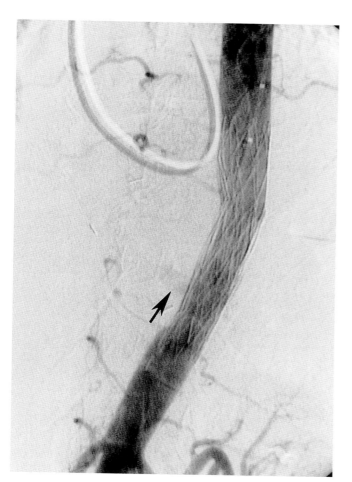

20

20 Leakage of contrast past the endograft into the aneurysm is called an *endoleak*. When an endoleak arises because of poor apposition of the endograft to the aortic wall (due to an error in measurement, deployment, mural calcification, thrombus, or excessive tortuosity), the leak can be sealed by deployment of an additional endograft overlapping the first, as long as no critical aortic branch is covered. Occasionally, contrast material accumulates in the aneurysm even though no discrete leak can be detected (*arrow* in Figure 20). In our experience, these slow diffuse leaks, presumably due to the porosity of the graft material, seal spontaneously.

OUTCOME FOR ENDOGRAFTS

Short-term results of endograft treatment of thoracic aortic aneurysms are encouraging. Endografts successfully exclude the aneurysm in approximately 80–90 per cent of cases. Thirty-day mortality is 10–30 per cent, depending on the mix of elective and urgent treatment. The rate of migration of endografts from their deployment position is in the range of 10–15 per cent. Paraplegia rates are less than 5 per cent and reflect the length of aorta covered and prior aortic surgery.

The endograft deployment procedure described previously applies to a nondissected thoracic aortic aneurysm with long proximal and distal necks. In appropriate circumstances, the proximal touch-down site, or neck, can be functionally lengthened by means of a carotid-subclavian artery bypass, so that the endograft is deployed over the origin of the left subclavian artery up to the left common carotid origin. Distally, the celiac artery can be sacrificed by proximal occlusion using Gianturco coils (Cook), allowing the endograft to be deployed down to the origin of the superior mesenteric artery.

Endografts – dissections

Aortic dissections are life threatening due to potential rupture of the false lumen or due to malperfusion. Prolonged malperfusion of the abdominal organs and lower extremities presents a relative contraindication to open aortic reconstruction with cardiac bypass or HCA. Infradiaphragmatic malperfusion can be treated nonoperatively by means of percutaneous balloon fenestration and deployment of uncovered stents. Rupture of the false lumen of an aortic dissection acutely or later in the course of the disease can still occur.

Treatment of aortic dissection by an endograft presents additional challenges over and above those presented by nondissected aneurysms. Complete exclusion of the false lumen requires the sealing of all entry and re-entry tears. Most entry tears are in the ascending aorta, for which current devices are not suitable, or in the proximal descending aorta, where endografts may be feasible. When a suitable neck is present between the subclavian artery and the entry tear, an endograft can be deployed across the entry tear to seal it. Whether sealing the entry tear translates into false-lumen thrombosis and true-lumen expansion depends on the size and proximity of re-entry tears in the brachiocephalic arteries and distal aorta.

Several small preliminary series of patients who have had placement of a thoracic endograft for acute or chronic aortic dissection have been reported with good short-term results. These results include a 30-day mortality of under 20 per cent, variable relief of malperfusion syndromes with 75 per cent reflow into previously obstructed vessels, and thrombosis of the false lumen in up to 80 per cent of patients. Chronic dissections with large proximal entry tears, aneurysmal false lumens that exceed 4.0 cm in diameter, and multiple re-entry tears present technical difficulties and have not been elucidated by clinical experience to date.

SUMMARY

In the thoracic aortic aneurysms and dissections that have been treated by endografts and reported to date, few intermediate and long-term data are available on several important issues: device integrity, hemostasis, and biocompatibility. Will the metal skeleton of the endograft resist fatigue and fracture? Will it continue to exclude the aneurysm despite changes in the aortic wall at the endograft anastomoses? Will the oversized endograft cause pressure necrosis in the underlying aortic wall? Because of these uncertainties, long-term clinical and imaging follow-up is required following endograft placement. Our current practice is to obtain contrast-enhanced helical CTs and renal function, at 3, 6, and 12 months after deployment and annually thereafter.

FURTHER READING

Cambria, R.P., Davison, J.K. 1998. Regional hypothermia for prevention of spinal cord ischemic complications after thoracoabdominal aortic surgery: experience with epidural cooling. *Seminars in Thoracic and Cardiovascular Surgery* 10(1), 61–5.

Dake, M.D., Kato, N., Mitchell, R.S., *et al.* 1999. Endovascular stent-graft placement for the treatment of acute aortic dissection. *New England Journal of Medicine* 340, 1546–52.

Kouchoukos, N.T., Rokkas, C.K. 1999. Hypothermic cardiopulmonary bypass for spinal cord protection: rationale and clinical results. *Annals of Thoracic Surgery* 67, 1940–2.

Mitchell, R.S., Miller, D.C., Dake, M.D. 1997. Stent-graft repair of thoracic aortic aneurysms. *Seminars in Vascular Surgery* 10(4), 257–71.

Safi, H.J., Miller, C.C. III. 1999. Spinal cord protection in descending thoracic and thoracoabdominal aortic repair. *Annals of Thoracic Surgery* 67, 1937–9.

Svensson, L.G. 1998. Management of segmental intercostal and lumbar arteries during descending and thoracoabdominal aneurysm repairs. *Seminars in Thoracic and Cardiovascular Surgery* 10(1), 45–9.

35

Thoracoabdominal aortic aneurysm

JOSEPH S. COSELLI MD
Professor and Chief, Division of Cardiothoracic Surgery, Michael E. DeBakey Department of Surgery, Baylor College of Medicine,
The Methodist DeBakey Heart Center, Houston, Texas, USA

SCOTT A. LEMAIRE MD
Assistant Professor, Division of Cardiothoracic Surgery, Michael E. DeBakey Department of Surgery, Baylor College of Medicine,
The Methodist DeBakey Heart Center, Houston, Texas, USA

JAY K. BHAMA MD
Surgical Resident, Division of General Surgery, Michael E. DeBakey Department of Surgery, Baylor College of Medicine, The Methodist DeBakey
Heart Center, Houston, Texas, USA

INTRODUCTION

Thoracoabdominal aortic aneurysms (TAAAs) involve the aorta at the diaphragmatic hiatus and, therefore, require thoracic aortic control for repair. These aneurysms can extend proximally to the transverse aortic arch and distally to the abdominal aortic bifurcation.

1 The Crawford classification of TAAAs is based on the extent of aortic involvement. Accurate classification of TAAAs is important because the operative strategy, risks, and results vary based upon the extent of aortic replacement. Despite recent advances in endovascular approaches to localized aortic aneurysms, open graft replacement remains the procedure of choice for successful management of these extensive aneurysms. While improvements in anesthesia, surgical technique, and critical care have allowed these operations to be performed successfully, they remain a formidable technical challenge. Variable pathology, extensive aortic involvement, frequent comorbid conditions, and unparalleled invasiveness have contributed to this challenge. As this disease entity becomes more common in the aging population, the need for therapeutic intervention will continue to increase.

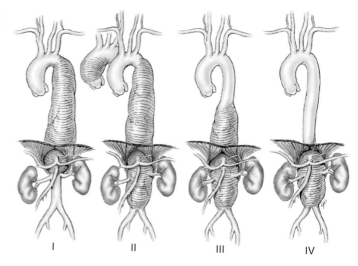

I   II   III   IV

HISTORY

In 1955, Etheredge reported successful replacement of a large aneurysm of the upper abdominal aorta involving the celiac and superior mesenteric arteries using an aortic homograft and temporary aortic bypass with a polyethylene tube. That same year, Rob reported surgical correction of six aortic aneurysms involving the upper abdominal aorta. In 1965, Crawford revolutionized TAAA repair by introducing the graft inclusion technique. Refinements in this technique over the subsequent 35 years form the basis for our current surgical strategy.

PRINCIPLES AND JUSTIFICATION

The two most common disease processes that affect the thoracoabdominal aorta are medial degeneration and aortic dissection. While both processes may exist separately, they serve as risk factors for one another, and thus often coexist. Dissection of the thoracoabdominal aorta can occur with (DeBakey type I) or without (DeBakey type III) involvement of the ascending and transverse arch segments. Infection and aortitis may also lead to disease of the thoracoabdominal aorta. Each of these mechanisms produces weakness and dilatation of the aortic wall, ultimately resulting in rupture.

PREOPERATIVE ASSESSMENT AND PREPARATION

Presentation

Patients with TAAAs often remain asymptomatic until the aneurysm becomes large enough to compress surrounding structures or weak enough to dissect or rupture. Therefore, TAAAs are commonly discovered serendipitously during imaging studies obtained for unrelated problems. The onset of symptoms is generally considered an indication of imminent rupture. The most common symptom is pain located in the chest, abdomen, flank, or back, often due to pressure from the aneurysm on adjacent structures, or the initiation of dissection or rupture. Wheezing, coughing, and pneumonitis may result from compression of the trachea or a segmental bronchus. Erosion of the aneurysm into the airway or pulmonary parenchyma may lead to hemoptysis, while similar compression or erosion of the esophagus may lead to dysphagia or hematemesis. Impingement of the left recurrent laryngeal nerve causes vocal cord paralysis and hoarseness.

Diagnosis

The diagnosis of thoracoabdominal aortic pathology is heavily dependent upon radiographic imaging.

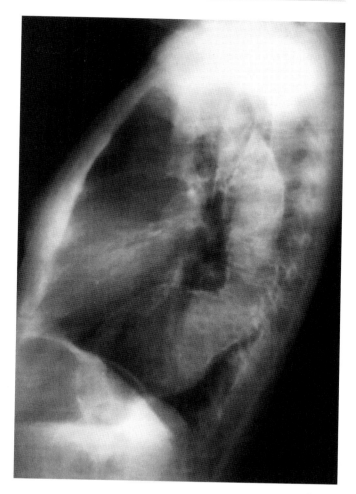

2a Plain chest roentgenograms may reveal widening of the descending thoracic aortic shadow that is often emphasized by calcification that outlines the dilated aneurysmal wall. The precise diagnosis of aneurysm, including its location and extent, can be determined noninvasively using computed tomography (CT) scanning or magnetic resonance imaging (MRI).

2a

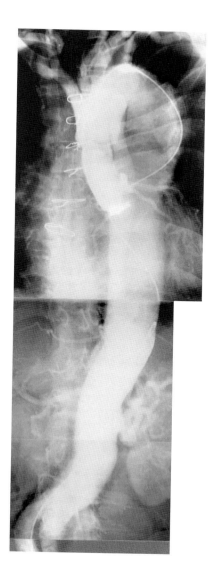

2b Contrast aortography is rarely required, but may be necessary for evaluation of patients with evidence of visceral or iliac arterial stenosis.

2b

Indications for repair

Indications for surgical repair of TAAAs are primarily based upon the presence of symptoms and the size of the aneurysm. For asymptomatic patients, we recommend elective repair when the aneurysm diameter exceeds 5.0–6.0 cm or when the rate of expansion exceeds 1 cm per year. The development of any symptom, regardless of how mild or uncharacteristic, is carefully evaluated and attributed to the aneurysm until proven otherwise. Signs of impending rupture, such as acute pain or hypotension, are clear indications for immediate surgical repair. Acute aortic dissection superimposed on a preexisting TAAA is a particularly unstable situation that is generally treated with urgent operation.

Preoperative evaluation

In the elective setting, assessment of physiologic reserve is a critical step in preoperative patient evaluation. Evaluation of the cardiac, pulmonary, and renal systems is necessary to ascertain the patient's potential operative risk and to determine their candidacy for surgery. We routinely employ transthoracic echocardiography to assess ventricular and valvular function. Additional testing is obtained in patients with a left ventricular ejection fraction of less than 30 per cent or other evidence of myocardial ischemia. Whenever possible, patients with significant coronary artery disease undergo either angioplasty or operative revascularization prior to aneurysm repair. Importantly, patients with previous coronary artery bypass using the left internal mammary artery may require left carotid–subclavian bypass before extent I or II TAAA repair to avoid cardiac ischemia if the aortic clamp is placed proximal to the left subclavian artery. Preoperative pulmonary function is assessed by routinely performing pulmonary function studies. Patients with a diminished forced expiratory volume in 1 second (FEV_1) or a blood carbon dioxide partial pressure greater than 45 mmHg undergo preoperative optimization of respiratory function with smoking cessation, an exercise regimen, and bronchodilators. Assessment of preoperative renal function is important because preoperative renal insufficiency is a strong predictor of early postoperative mortality. Patients undergoing arteriography are adequately hydrated prior to the procedure. In patients with borderline renal function, we administer an intravenous infusion of 5 per cent dextrose and Ringer's lactate solution with 25 g/L mannitol and 1 amp/L sodium bicarbonate prior to aortography. Acetylcysteine is often administered before and after aortography in an effort to further reduce the risk of contrast nephropathy. After the study, serum creatinine levels are followed; surgery is performed once renal function has returned to baseline.

ANESTHESIA AND SPINAL CORD PROTECTION

Anesthesia

In preparation for surgery, patients undergo placement of a right radial arterial line, a pulmonary artery catheter, and a large bore central venous access catheter to allow rapid fluid administration. Anesthesia is induced with agents that do not impair cardiac function, such as diazepam and fentanyl. Muscle relaxation is achieved with pancuronium bromide. Because deflation of the left lung is necessary for optimal exposure of the aorta, a double lumen endobronchial tube is inserted, allowing selective right lung ventilation. Arterial blood gas and serum electrolyte measurements are monitored closely and appropriate adjustments are made as needed. Broad-spectrum antibiotics are administered preoperatively. Steroids are given at the onset of the operation.

Vigilant attention to volume status is imperative during TAAA repair to avoid wide fluctuations in blood pressure. Crystalloid administration begins prior to the operation. Central venous pressure and pulmonary arterial pressures are maintained at normal or preanesthetic levels. At the time of induction of anesthesia, mannitol is administered to promote vigorous diuresis. During periods of aortic cross-clamping, we use sodium nitroprusside in conjunction with replacement of fluid and blood losses to keep blood pressure within acceptable limits. Prior to release of the aortic clamp, the nitroprusside is discontinued and blood components and crystalloid are administered rapidly to avoid declamping hypotension. Acidosis during aortic clamping is prevented with a continuous intravenous sodium bicarbonate infusion.

Often, fresh frozen plasma is given throughout the operation, and 10–16 units of platelet concentrate are administered after aortic declamping, as needed. The use of routine autotransfusion of washed red cells has led to a significant reduction in banked blood transfusion requirements. As some large aneurysms may contain up to 2 000 mL of blood within them, autotransfusion during surgical repair is of paramount importance. Because we prefer to use citrate rather than heparin in the autotransfusion device, intermittent monitoring of the serum calcium is necessary.

Spinal cord protection

Spinal cord protection during TAAA repair continues to be a major focus of investigation. Our approach to spinal cord protection is based on the extent of the aneurysm being repaired. All TAAAs, regardless of extent, are repaired with the use of permissive mild hypothermia (32–34°C) and moderate heparinization (1 mg/kg). We also advocate aggressive reattachment of patent segmental intercostal and lumbar arteries, particularly those between T8 and L1, as well as sequential aortic clamping whenever possible.

Additional adjuncts are used in patients with extensive TAAAs. In a retrospective analysis of 695 patients undergoing repair of extent I or II TAAAs, we found that the use of left heart bypass significantly reduced the risk of paraplegia. More recently, we studied the efficacy of cerebrospinal fluid (CSF) drainage on spinal cord protection. In this randomized clinical trial of 145 patients with extent I and II TAAAs, we found that CSF drainage significantly reduced the rate of paraplegia. Therefore, we advocate using both left heart bypass and CSF drainage, whenever possible, in patients undergoing repair of extent I and II TAAAs.

OPERATION

Operative strategies and techniques vary considerably depending upon the extent and characteristics of the aneurysm. The following description focuses primarily on extent II TAAAs, which require the most extensive graft repairs.

Preparation and exposure

3a, b Using a deflatable beanbag, the patient is held in position with the right side down, the shoulders at 60 degrees, and the hips at 30 degrees (3a). Draping allows access to the entire left chest, abdomen, and both groins. A curvilinear thoracoabdominal incision is used (3b). The level of the incision is based upon the proximal extent of the aneurysm in the thoracic aorta. Lesions beginning near the diaphragm (extent IV) are exposed through the eighth or ninth interspace, while those extending more proximally (extents I, II, and III) are usually approached through the sixth interspace. Proximal exposure may require division or resection of the sixth rib. The incision is gently curved and extended obliquely across the costal arch and left abdomen to the level of the umbilicus. The incision is occasionally extended in the midline to the pubis when access to the iliac arteries is required. Acute angulations near the costal margin are avoided to prevent tissue necrosis.

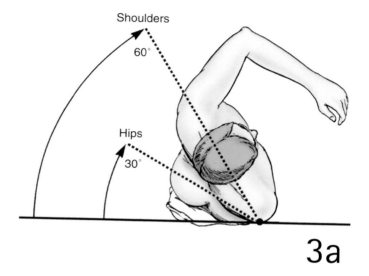

Shoulders

60°

Hips

30°

3a

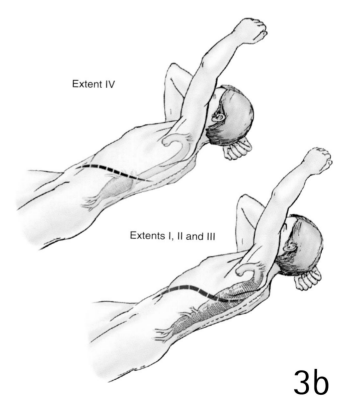

Extent IV

Extents I, II and III

3b

4 Prior to entering the chest, the left lung is deflated and single lung ventilation is initiated. The diaphragm is divided in a circumferential fashion to protect the phrenic nerve. A 3–4 cm cuff of diaphragmatic tissue is left intact on the chest wall, preserving the bulk of central musculature and allowing secure closure upon completion of the procedure. Self-retaining retractors provide stable exposure. A transperitoneal approach is used to allow assessment of visceral perfusion after aortic repair. Exposure of the abdominal aorta is accomplished by entering the retroperitoneum lateral to the left colon and developing the avascular plane anterior to the psoas muscle and posterior to the left kidney. The diaphragmatic crus is divided. The left renal artery is identified and exposed. The superior mesenteric and celiac arteries are not specifically identified externally. In preparation for placement of the proximal aortic clamp, the distal aortic arch is gently mobilized by dividing the remnant of the ductus arteriosus. The vagus and recurrent laryngeal nerves are identified and protected. The vagus nerve may be divided distal to the take-off of the recurrent laryngeal nerve if additional mobilization is required. Circumferential dissection of the distal transverse aortic arch allows its separation from the adjacent pulmonary artery and esophagus. The left subclavian artery is also mobilized circumferentially if the need for more proximal clamping – between the left common carotid and left subclavian arteries – is anticipated.

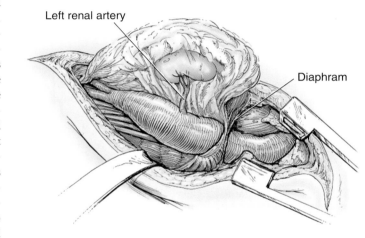

Left renal artery

Diaphram

4

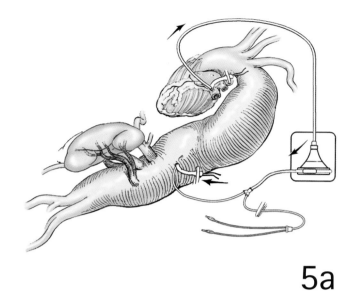

5a

Left heart bypass and preparation of the proximal aorta

5a, b In patients with extent I and II TAAAs, left heart bypass with a closed circuit in-line centrifugal pump is used to provide distal perfusion during the proximal portion of aortic repair. Heparin is administered intravenously and cannulae are usually placed in the left inferior pulmonary vein and distal descending thoracic aorta (5a). The left atrium and left femoral artery can be used as respective alternatives. Following institution of left heart bypass, the proximal portion of the aneurysm is isolated by placing clamps distal to the left subclavian artery and across the upper mid-descending thoracic aorta between T4 and T7. Occasionally, if the aneurysm extends more proximally, the aorta is clamped between the left common carotid and left subclavian arteries and a separate bulldog clamp is placed on the left subclavian artery. The isolated aortic segment is then opened using electrocautery and cleared of any intraluminal thrombus (5b).

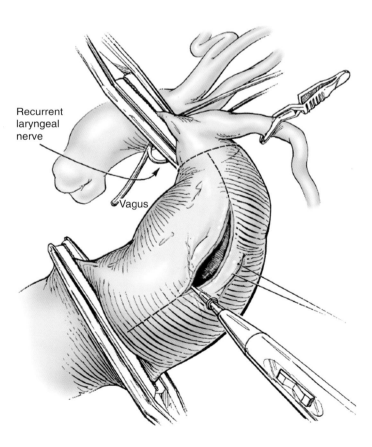

Recurrent laryngeal nerve

Vagus

5b

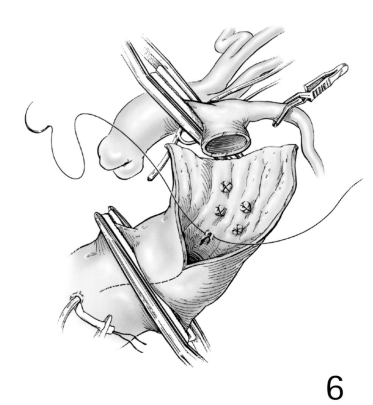

6 Meticulous anastomotic technique is critical to achieve hemostatic suture lines. In preparation for the proximal anastomosis, the aorta is transected at least 2 cm distal to the proximal clamp and separated from the esophagus to allow for full-thickness suturing of the aortic wall. This maneuver minimizes the risk of esophageal injury. In cases of aortic dissection, the dissecting membrane is usually excised. Intimal calcifications at the site of the anastomosis should be adequately debrided in order to create a supple, pliable aortic wall. Bleeding intercostal arteries at this level are ligated using 2-0 silk suture.

6

Proximal anastomosis and intercostal reattachment

7 An appropriately sized gelatin impregnated woven Dacron graft is selected; the diameter usually ranges from 20 to 24 mm. The proximal anastomosis is carried out using running 3-0 polypropylene suture. Alternatively, in patients with fragile aortic tissue, such as those with Marfan syndrome, 4-0 polypropylene suture is utilized. Teflon strips are generally not used to reinforce the anastomosis. In cases of aortic dissection, the false lumen is obliterated within the suture line. Similar principles are employed for the remaining anastomoses. The anastomosis is often reinforced with pledgeted mattress sutures.

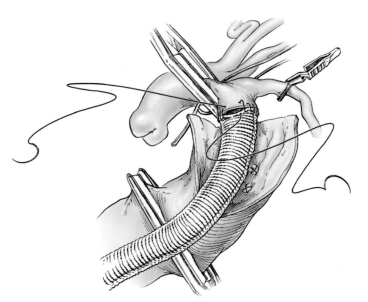

7

8a, b If the main proximal aortic clamp was positioned between the left common carotid and left subclavian arteries, the main proximal aortic clamp is repositioned onto the graft and the left subclavian artery is unclamped allowing its reperfusion. Distal aortic perfusion is discontinued at this time and the aneurysm is opened longitudinally to its distal extent, staying posterior to the left renal artery origin (8a). A distal clamp is not used. Residual chronic thrombus is removed, and in cases of aortic dissection the dissecting membrane is completely resected (8b).

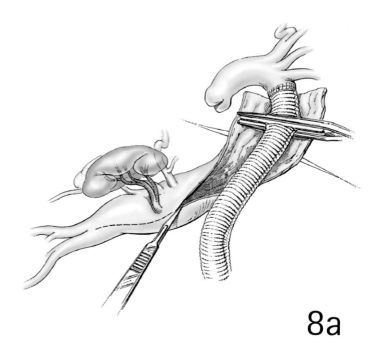

8a

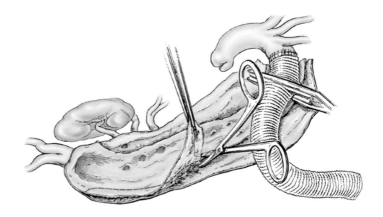

8b

Visceral vessel attachment and distal anastamosis

9a, b Perfusion of the viscera is maintained by individual 9-French balloon perfusion catheters placed within the origins of the celiac and superior mesenteric arteries. These are attached to a **Y**-line off of the arterial return tubing allowing continued delivery of oxygenated blood from the pump circuit to the abdominal viscera. Intermittent cold crystalloid perfusion of the kidneys is delivered by placement of 9-French balloon perfusion catheters within the origins of the renal arteries. Following initiation of visceral and renal perfusion, the aortic graft is placed under appropriate tension and one or more oval openings are made for reattachment of selected patent intercostal arteries from T7 to L2 (9a). The opening is then sutured around the origins of these arteries in a circumferential pattern. Following completion of this anastomosis, if anatomically feasible, the aortic clamp can be repositioned beyond the anastomosis allowing for reperfusion of the intercostal arteries. Attention is then directed to the visceral vessels. A similar oval opening is made in the graft and an island of native aorta around these vessels is incorporated into a circumferential anastomosis. Ideally, selective visceral and intermittent cold renal perfusion continues until reattachment is nearly complete. Often the left renal artery requires separate reattachment due to excessive separation from the other vessels, as is commonly seen in cases of chronic dissection (9b).

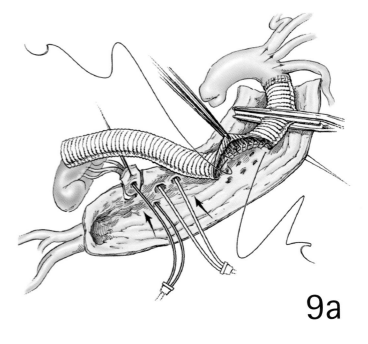

9a

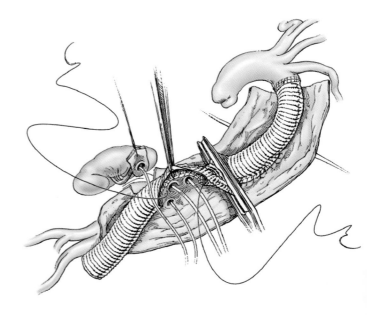

9b

10 After completion of the anastomosis, the aortic clamp may be repositioned distal to these vessels allowing their reperfusion. Aneurysm repair is completed by end-to-end anastomosis of the graft to the distal aorta at the level of the bifurcation. We routinely employ an 'open-distal' technique without placing a distal cross-clamp. The distal aorta is opened at least halfway in circumference. Complete division is generally not necessary, but may be required in cases of dissection if uncertainty exists as to the location of the true and false lumens. Because vital organs may depend upon perfusion of the false lumen in cases of chronic dissection, the dissecting membrane is fenestrated prior to carrying out the distal anastomosis. Conversely, with acute dissection, the distal false lumen is obliterated within the suture line, directing blood flow into the true lumen. Following aortic reconstruction, heparin is reversed with protamine sulfate. Meticulous hemostasis must be achieved and secured at all suture lines and cannulation sites. Renal, visceral, and peripheral perfusion are assessed. The remaining aneurysm wall is then wrapped around the aortic reconstruction and secured with a running suture. Two thoracic drainage tubes are positioned in the posterior thorax, and a closed suction drain is placed in the retroperitoneum. The diaphragm is reapproximated with a running #1 polypropylene suture. The thoracotomy is closed using both heavy braided polyester suture and stainless steel wires around the ribs.

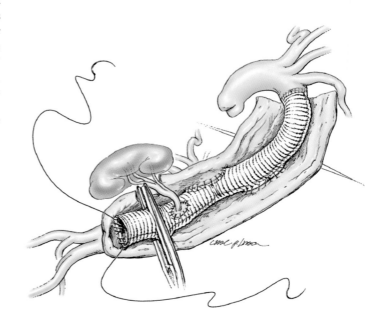

10

POSTOPERATIVE CARE

Meticulous control of blood pressure is important during the initial 24–48 hours postoperatively, as even brief periods of hypertension may disrupt fresh suture lines. Nitroprusside and β-antagonists are used during this period to maintain the mean arterial blood pressure between 80 and 90 mmHg. A lower target may be selected in patients with particularly fragile tissue (i.e. Marfan syndrome, acute aortic dissection). In patients with a CSF drain, fluid is drained as needed to maintain CSF pressure between 10–12 mmHg. The CSF drain is usually removed in 48 hours if the patient is neurologically intact. In most cases, the ventilator is weaned and the patient is able to be extubated within 24 hours. To stimulate and maintain renal function, a low-dose dopamine infusion is administered for at least 48 hours. The retroperitoneal closed suction drain is removed after 24 hours. Thoracic drainage tubes are removed once drainage is less that 300 mL/day, commonly within 48–72 hours. Ambulation is initiated on the second or third postoperative day and aggressive physical rehabilitation is emphasized early during convalescence. Broad-spectrum parenteral antibiotics are administered throughout the postoperative course until all drains and central venous catheters are removed.

OUTCOMES

Table 35.1 presents the results of TAAA repair in 1914 consecutive patients who underwent surgery between 11 January, 1986, and 31 July, 2002. The causes of the aneurysms were chronic medial degeneration (nondissection) in 1401 patients (73.4 per cent), chronic dissection in 439 patients (22.9 per cent), and acute aortic dissection in 71 (3.7 per cent). Marfan syndrome was present in 131 patients (6.8 per cent), and 109 patients (5.7 per cent) were treated for rupture.

Table 35.1 *Results of thoracoabdominal aortic aneurysm repair in 1914 consecutive patients*

Extent of aneurysm	No. of patients	30-day survival	Paraplegia or paraparesis*	Renal failure[†]
I	615 (32.1%)	581 (94.5%)	22 (3.9%)	15 (2.5%)
II	635 (33.2%)	592 (93.2%)	46 (7.3%)	56 (9.0%)
III	315 (16.5%)	298 (94.6%)	9 (2.9%)	21 (6.8%)
IV	349 (18.2%)	337 (96.6%)	6 (1.7%)	22 (6.5%)
Total	1 914 (100%)	1 808 (94.5%)	83 (4.4%)	114 (6.1%)

* Excludes six patients who died during operation and 12 patients with preoperative paraplegia.
[†] Excludes six patients who died during operation and 27 patients on hemodialysis preoperatively.

FURTHER READING

Coselli, J.S., Conklin, L.D., LeMaire, S.A. 2002. Thoracoabdominal aortic aneurysm repair: review and update of current strategies. *Annals of Thoracic Surgery* **74**, S1881–4.

Coselli, J.S., LeMaire, S.A. 1999. Left heart bypass reduces paraplegia rates following thoracoabdominal aortic aneurysm repair. *Annals of Thoracic Surgery* **67**, 1931–4.

Coselli, J.S., LeMaire, S.A., Köksoy, C. 2000. Thoracic aortic anastomoses. *Operative Techniques in Thoracic and Cardiovascular Surgery* **5**, 259–75.

Coselli, J.S., LeMaire, S.A., Köksoy, C., *et al.* 2002. Cerebrospinal fluid drainage reduces paraplegia after thoracoabdominal aortic aneurysm repair: results of a randomized clinical trial. *Journal of Vascular Surgery* **35**, 635–9.

Coselli, J.S., LeMaire, S.A., Miller, C.C. III, *et al.* 2000. Mortality and paraplegia after thoracoabdominal aortic aneurysm repair: a risk factor analysis. *Annals of Thoracic Surgery* **69**, 404–14.

Köksoy, C., LeMaire, S.A., Curling, P.E., *et al.* 2002. Renal perfusion during thoracoabdominal aortic operations: cold crystalloid is superior to normothermic blood. *Annals of Thoracic Surgery* **73**, 30–8.

Svensson, L.G., Crawford, E.S., Hess, K.R., *et al.* 1993. Experience with 1509 patients undergoing thoracoabdominal aortic operations. *Journal of Vascular Surgery* **17**, 236–48.

SECTION VI

Surgery for Cardiac Rhythm Disorders and Tumors

36

Bradyarrhythmias/pacemakers

CHARLES R. BRIDGES MD, SCD
Assistant Professor of Surgery, University of Pennsylvania School of Medicine; Chief, Division of Cardiothoracic Surgery, Pennsylvania Hospital, Philadelphia, Pennsylvania, USA

MICHAEL S. HANNA MD, FACC
Assistant Clinical Professor of Medicine, Director, Electrophysiology Laboratory, Pennsylvania Hospital, Philadelphia, Pennsylvania, USA

HISTORY

The historical beginnings of pacemakers for the treatment of bradyarrhythmias were predated by the recognition of heart block as one etiology for syncope. Patients with extremely slow pulse rates were noted to be prone to 'epileptic' seizures and dizziness. Between 1826 and 1846, several cases of the Stokes-Adams syndrome were described, clearly implicating profound bradycardia as the *cause* of syncope. An understanding of the physiological basis for heart block awaited the discovery by Wilhelm His in 1895 of a bundle of conduction tissue that resulted in atrioventricular (AV) block when cut.

Several investigators, including Benjamin Franklin in the eighteenth century and others in the early nineteenth century, used electrical stimulation therapeutically to treat a variety of illnesses. The development of clinical cardiac pacing paralleled the emergence of cardiac surgery as a clinical reality. The iatrogenic complication of complete heart block after the repair of congenital cardiac defects galvanized the development of the techniques for pacing the heart through the intact chest wall. The development of an implantable pacemaker was made possible by the invention of the transistor in 1947 and the diode in 1949 at Bell laboratories making circuit miniaturization possible. The earliest implantable pacemaker was based on the rechargeable nickel-cadmium battery. These early, implantable pacemakers required that a coil be placed around the patient to recharge the batteries by induction. Within the next few years, several groups developed implantable pacemakers based on the mercury-zinc battery. In 1960, Wilson Grabatch, an electrical engineer, and Drs. William Chardack and Andrew Cage accomplished the first complete implantation of a pulse generator with a self-contained power supply suitable for long-term use on 6 June 1960, ushering in the modern era of cardiac pacing.

PRINCIPLES AND JUSTIFICATION

Surgical anatomy of the conduction system

1a, b The topography of the conduction system from the viewpoint of the cardiac surgeon is unique. As discussed previously, one of the earliest indications for pacemaker insertion was surgical injury to the conduction system. Such injuries may occur during aortic, mitral, or tricuspid valve repair or during replacement or repair of atrial or ventricular septal defects. The surgical anatomy of the aortic valve reveals the close proximity of the membranous septum to the noncoronary and right coronary leaflets. Placement of excessively deep sutures below the level of the annulus during aortic valve replacement can result in postoperative AV block. In mitral valvular surgery, the bundle of His lies in the interventricular septum anteromedial to the right fibrous trigone and posterior commissure. Sutures in this area that traverse the interatrial septum or are placed deeply into the ventricular septum may damage the AV node or the His bundle. During tricuspid valve surgery or closure of atrial septal defects, the incision in the right atrium to gain access to the interior of the chamber is important. The sinoatrial node lies in the lateral (rightward) portion of the superior cavoatrial junction in the superior portion of the terminal groove of the right atrium. Incisions that cross the cavoatrial junction (e.g. repair of sinus venosus defects with high-lying anomalous pulmonary veins) should be placed toward the left (medial) side to avoid direct injury to the sinoatrial node. During closure of atrial septal defects, tricuspid valve surgery, or mitral valve surgery via a transseptal approach, the proximity of the AV node to the tricuspid annulus must be appreciated. The bundle of His arises from the AV node in the distal aspect of the triangle of Koch, and it enters the septum on the leftward aspect of the septal crest adjacent to the posteroinferior rim of ventricular septal defects of the perimembranous type. In repair of ventricular septal defects of this type, care must be taken to place the sutures on the right ventricular aspect of the defect several millimeters inferior to the rim of the defect.

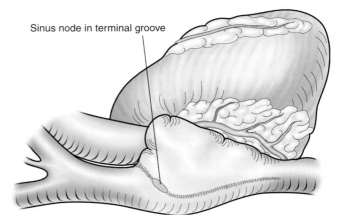

Sinus node in terminal groove

1a

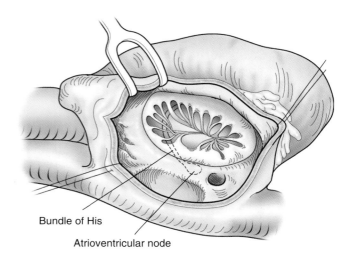

Bundle of His

Atrioventricular node

1b

Physiology

RESTING POTENTIAL

The cardiac cell in its resting state is polarized (i.e. the interior of the cell has a *negative* electrical potential). The electronegativity of the cell is a direct consequence of the Nernst equilibrium. Large macromolecules, such as proteins and organic phosphates, are *negatively* charged at physiological pH. Thus, to maintain overall electroneutrality of the cell interior, there is a relative abundance of positively charged species dominated by potassium ions. In contrast to the steric restriction of large impermeable anions, the sarcolemma is relatively permeable to potassium ions, as most potassium channels are open in the polarized state. A negative intracellular potential then arises so that an equilibrium occurs such that potassium efflux (from diffusion) exactly counterbalances potassium influx (due to the negative electrical potential). Maintenance of this 'equilibrium' is an energy-requiring process, and adenosine triphosphate is expended as the sodium-potassium adenosine triphosphate–dependent pump exchanges potassium for sodium ions. The reason that the potassium concentration gradient dominates the resting electrical potential of the cell is that its permeability is two orders of magnitude greater than that of sodium and other ions in diastole.

DEPOLARIZATION AND ACTION POTENTIAL PROPAGATION

An action potential occurs when an electrical current travels across the myocyte membrane that is sufficient to depolarize the cell interior to a threshold potential of approximately –60 mV. Depolarization of this magnitude triggers opening of the fast sodium channel and an increased permeability to sodium ions. Within a few milliseconds, the result is complete depolarization of the cell. During any given systole, the earliest depolarizing cells ordinarily reside in the sinoatrial node, and the heart rate is determined by the rate of spontaneous depolarization of these cells. Internodal pathways in the atrium, AV node, bundle of His, and Purkinje fibers constitute the specialized conduction tissue that facilitate rapid conduction of these impulses to all regions of the myocardium. Alternatively, the earliest depolarizing current can arise from an electrical pacemaker. The depolarization is then conducted throughout the myocardium by cell-to-cell propagation, which is slower, generally resulting in slower ventricular activation than that resulting from impulses originating in the specialized conduction pathways.

ATRIOVENTRICULAR BLOCK

AV block is classified as first degree, second degree, or third degree. *First-degree block* refers to prolongation of the PR interval beyond 200 ms. *Third-degree block* is defined as interruption of the conduction pathways resulting in complete dissociation of atrial depolarization from ventricular depolarization, allowing for independent rates of contraction. The hallmark of complete AV dissociation is that P waves are seen 'marching through' the QRS complexes. *Second-degree block* is intermediate between first-degree and third-degree block in that some, but not all, impulses originating in the atrium are conducted to the ventricles. Second-degree block is divided into Mobitz I, also called *Wenckebach*, in which there is a progressive prolongation in the PR interval until a P wave is not conducted, and Mobitz II, in which there is no prolongation of the PR interval before the dropped beat. In general, Mobitz I results from impaired conduction in the AV node and is associated with a narrow QRS. Mobitz II implies disease in the infranodal conduction system and is generally associated with a wide QRS (e.g. left bundle branch block). Distal to the bundle of His, the Purkinje system bifurcates into the left and right bundle branches. The left bundle branch further subdivides into anterior and posterior fascicles. Specific electrocardiogram (ECG) patterns exist to identify right and left bundle branch blocks as well as left anterior and posterior hemiblock. Delayed conduction through two of the three fascicles (right, left anterior, and left posterior) is referred to as *bifascicular block*. AV block can be congenital or acquired. Patients with congenital AV block usually have escape pacemakers located in the AV node or His bundle, whereas in acquired AV block, nodal escape rhythms are less reliable. The common causes of AV nodal–His block include cardiac surgical procedures, idiopathic fibrosis, myocardial infarction, sclerodegenerative processes (e.g. Lev's disease), Lyme disease, aortic valve endocarditis, lupus erythematosus, medications, and hyperkalemia.

AV block with two atrial beats for each ventricular beat (2:1) may be either nodal or infranodal and is best judged by 'the company it keeps.' A narrow QRS and occasional periods of Wenckebach suggests Mobitz I, whereas a wide QRS suggests infranodal (Mobitz II) disease. Mobitz I and 2:1 AV block associated with a narrow QRS typically carry a benign prognosis and seldom require permanent pacing. Mobitz II and other AV conduction disturbances associated with infranodal disease are more ominous, with frequent and unpredictable progression to complete heart block, and usually indicate the need for permanent pacing.

SINUS NODE DYSFUNCTION

Sinus node dysfunction is often a degenerative process and is the most common indication for permanent pacing in the United States. Significant sinus node dysfunction occurs when sinus bradycardia is profound or when periods of sinus arrest result in pauses of duration sufficient to cause symptoms. In normal individuals, sinus pauses of up to 30 seconds have been observed. Sinus arrest of this magnitude in normal individuals usually occurs during periods of high vagal tone such as vomiting, micturition, or deglutition.

The 'tachy-brady' or sick sinus syndrome is characterized by periods of sinus bradycardia alternating with supraventricular tachyarrhythmias, including atrial fibrillation or atrial flutter and AV nodal re-entry tachycardia. This syndrome is a common indication for pacemaker placement, particularly in elderly patients. Effective treatment of the tachyarrhythmias is often precluded, as effective therapy increases the severity of the sinus bradycardia when it occurs. With placement of a dual-chamber pacemaker, AV synchrony can be maintained while normal sinus rhythm can be preserved (when present), and the supraventricular arrhythmias can be treated with agents that prolong AV conduction or suppress atrial irritability without risking potentially dangerous bradyarrhythmias.

PACEMAKERS

INTERNATIONAL PACING CODE

A five-letter code is used to provide a working description of both permanent, implantable, and temporary external pacemakers currently in use and is the essential clinical language of cardiac pacing. The North American Society of Pacing and Electrophysiology and the British Pacing and Electrophysiology Group endorse the code. The first letter refers to the chambers paced, the second is the chambers sensed, and the third represents the response to sensed activity. The fourth letter refers to the programmability and rate modulation features of the pacemaker, and the fifth letter refers to the antitachyarrhythmic functions of the pacemaker. The pacemaker code is summarized in Table 36.1. The pacemakers/modes most commonly used include VVIR, AAIR, and DDDR. These pacemakers pace the ventricle only, the atrium only, or both the atrium and the ventricle. The earliest pacemakers were of the VOO type. In general, pacemakers of the DDD type can be programmed into any mode that can be derived by substituting "O," "V," "A," or "I" for "D." Thus, DDD pacemakers can be programmed to VVI, AOO, DOO, DVI, or AAI modes as the clinical situation dictates. Similarly, rate-responsive pacemakers such as DDDR can be programmed to any of these modes with rate response enabled or disabled. In specific clinical situations, particularly in the early postoperative or intraoperative periods after cardiopulmonary bypass, DOO, AAO, or AAI pacing may have

advantages over DDD pacing. Unfortunately, the external temporary pacemaker may be programmed in the DDD mode by default. This practice frequently results in suboptimal performance due to inhibition by mechanical or electrical stimuli (e.g. the surgeon's hand or electrocautery) at times when there is no appreciable intrinsic cardiac activity (e.g. immediately postarrest), and it occasionally potentiates atrial or ventricular arrhythmias due to inadequate sensing.

DUAL-CHAMBER PACING

In the normal heart at rest, the contribution of AV synchrony to cardiac output at rest is 20–30 per cent. The relative contribution of AV synchrony to cardiac output depends on heart rate, left ventricular (LV) systolic and diastolic function, LV filling pressure, the presence of vascular disease, left atrial size, contractility, compliance, retrograde ventriculoatrial conduction, and the timing between atrial and ventricular systole. In the presence of mitral stenosis or decreased LV compliance (e.g. diastolic dysfunction as occurs with LV hypertrophy), AV synchrony may contribute as much as 30–40 per cent to cardiac output. Conversely, during exercise, most of the increase in cardiac output is controlled primarily by the increase in ventricular rate, and rate-responsiveness is more important than AV synchrony. The PR interval normally shortens with exercise, and dual-chamber pacemakers with rate-adaptive modulation of the PR interval are associated with better exercise performance. Even in situations in which AV synchrony contributes little to cardiac output, by preventing ventriculoatrial conduction and the resultant increase in systemic and pulmonary pressures associated with inappropriately timed atrial contraction, dual-chamber pacing may provide significant symptomatic relief.

RATE-RESPONSIVENESS

With exercise, an appropriate increase in heart rate is critical to the maintenance of cardiac output. During exercise, cardiac output may increase 300 per cent or more. Most of the increase in cardiac output is due to an increase in heart rate. Therefore, single-chamber VVIR pacing is superior to VVI pacing. Chronotropic incompetence occurs when AV con-

Table 36.1 *The North American Society of Pacing and Electrophysiology and the British Pacing and Electrophysiology Group generic pacemaker code*

Position	I	II	III	IV	V
Category	Chamber(s) paced	Chamber(s) sensed	Response to sensing	Programmability, rate modulation	Antitachyarrhythmic function(s)
	0, none	0, none	0, none	0, none	0, none
	A, atrium	A, atrium	T, triggered	P, simple programmable	P, pacing (antitachyarrhythmia)
	V, ventricle	V, ventricle	I, inhibited	M, multi-programmable	S, shock
	D, dual (A + V)	D, dual (A + V)	D, dual (T + I)	C, communicating	D, dual (P + S)
Manufacturer's designation only	S, single (A or V)	S, single (A or V)	—	R, rate modulation	—

duction is maintained but the sinus node does not increase its rate appropriately to meet increased metabolic demand. Currently available rate-responsive pacemakers use a variety of techniques to estimate metabolic demands. Piezoelectric crystals can detect direct mechanical pressure on the pacemaker. Piezoelectric accelerometers measure acceleration and are thought to reflect body motion more accurately. Transthoracic impedance sensors measure impedance changes across the torso as a function of respiration that are correlated with minute ventilation; QT-interval sensors measure the QT interval, which correlates with metabolic activity independent of the actual heart rate. Intracardiac impedance sensors measure changes in impedance as a function of heart rate that are correlated with stroke volume and myocardial contractility. Other sensors have been developed using mixed venous oxygen saturation, central venous temperature, and right ventricular pressure relationships to estimate metabolic activity. All of these sensors are subject to errors in estimating metabolic demands under certain circumstances. Dual-chamber pacemakers combining QT-interval and piezoelectric activity sensors in a single pacemaker allow for sensor cross-checking. This feature combines the rapid, early rate-responsiveness of the activity sensor with the more robust QT-interval sensor, allowing excellent overall correlation with metabolic demand and relative insensitivity to unphysiological motion–induced pacing rate increases.

Indications for pacemaker placement

The indications for permanent pacemaker implantation are summarized in Table 36.2. Permanent or temporary cardiac pacing is indicated for bradycardic rhythms that result in symptoms of cerebral hypoperfusion or hemodynamic instability or for rhythm disturbances likely to progress to significant bradycardia. Permanent pacemaker insertion is generally not warranted in asymptomatic patients with

Mobitz I second-degree block, asymptomatic sinus bradycardia, sinus pauses of less than two seconds, and left or right bundle branch blocks. A careful review of the guidelines in Table 2 indicates that implantation of a permanent pacemaker is indicated even when the signs and symptoms result from necessary medication to treat angina, supraventricular arrhythmias, ventricular arrhythmias, or hypertension. Newer indications for permanent pacemaker insertion include hypertrophic obstructive cardiomyopathy. In patients with hypertrophic obstructive cardiomyopathy and significant LV outflow obstruction, dual-chamber pacing may reduce symptoms and outflow tract gradient. The mechanism of this beneficial effect relates, in part, to disruption of the normal activation sequence, resulting in a decrease in the mean LV–aortic pressure gradient.

SELECTION OF PACING MODE

The selection of the programmed mode of pacing is related to the selection of the type of pacemaker implanted. As discussed previously, excluding antitachycardia pacing, DDDR pacemakers can be programmed to function in any mode. VVIR pacemakers can only be programmed in modes that do not require pacing or sensing of atrial activity. Thus, by selecting one of these two types of pacemakers, essentially all necessary pacing functions can be achieved. An exception to this general rule are VDDR pacemakers that pace only the ventricle but sense atrial and ventricular activity. The ventricular pacing is synchronized with atrial activity, and the ventricle is paced after a preset AV delay after atrial contraction. Upper and lower rates can be specified. Originally, this type of system required both atrial and ventricular leads and offered no important technical advantages over DDDR pacemaker implantation. More recently, however, single-lead VDDR systems have become available that allow for atrial sensing and ventricular pacing with a single lead and may have significant advantages over other single-lead ventricular pacemakers, as well as technical advantages over dual-

Table 36.2 *Common indications for permanent cardiac pacemaker implantation*

Sinus node dysfunction
    With symptoms of cerebral hypoperfusion or chronotropic incompetence, with or without symptoms, but with escape rates less
    than 40 beats/min, regardless of whether due to necessary medications
Acquired atrioventricular block
    Complete or high grade
        With symptoms, regardless of whether the symptoms are due to necessary medications
        With asystolic pauses exceeding 3 sec
        With escape pacemaker rates less than 40 beats/min
    Second degree
        Mobitz Type I or II, with symptoms
Neutrally mediated ('vasovagal') syndromes
    With recurrent syncope or presyncope, bradycardia, and hypotension during head–up tilt testing
Carotid sinus hypersensitivity
    With symptoms due to bradycardia provoked by carotid sinus massage in patients with recurrent syncope or presyncope
    With asystolic pauses in rhythm exceeding 3 sec in response to carotid sinus massage in patients with recurrent syncope

chamber pacemakers. The role of these pacemakers is still questionable, however, as, in contrast to DDDR systems, pacemaker syndrome may occur in the presence of atrial chronotropic incompetence. Therefore, most implanted pacemakers today are of the DDDR variety. These pacemakers offer access to all pacing modes and minimize the incidence of pacemaker syndrome. The added risk of implanting a second (atrial) lead is negligible with appropriate technique, and the added benefits of AV synchrony and rate-responsiveness generally outweigh the risks. There are a few situations in which single-chamber pacemakers are still the most reasonable choice for implantation. These situations include the use of VVIR pacemakers in patients with chronic atrial fibrillation and AV block and the use of AAI pacemakers in cardiac transplant patients with sinus node dysfunction.

PREOPERATIVE ASSESSMENT AND PREPARATION

The procedure is usually performed in either a cardiac catheterization laboratory specifically suited for electrophysiology or in an operating room. Typically, cardiologists perform the procedure in the electrophysiology laboratory, and cardiac surgeons perform the procedure in the operating room. Electrophysiology laboratories often have superior radiological imaging and electrical recording capabilities that may be important for gaining venous access or documenting lead position. In contrast, the operating room usually has superior lighting and technical and anesthesia support. A variety of sheaths and specialized wires are also often available. Regardless of the setting, the keys to successful performance of the procedure are (1) maintenance of sterile technique at all times, (2) assurance of hemostasis, and (3) having all equipment and technical assistance necessary to perform the procedure. It is assumed that the room is equipped with fluoroscopy or that a fluoroscopy machine and table will be available when needed. A single person can perform the circulating-nurse/anesthetist/pacemaker-analyst function, but we prefer to have a separate individual committed for each of these tasks. Most pacemaker representatives are happy to perform the analyst function. Their input is often valuable as they may offer technical suggestions and are experienced at trouble-shooting device-related issues. Because each brand of pacemaker can generally only be interrogated by programmers manufactured by the same company, familiarity with the products of a given manufacturer is often required. If electrical measurements are inconsistent, contradictory, or otherwise inappropriate, the cables should be inspected and the leads retested using new cables. The cables are the 'Achilles' heal' in this system, and one must maintain a high degree of vigilance as to their quality control. Changing cables is easy and can be accomplished quickly, allowing one to avoid wasting operative time and increasing risk by unnecessarily repositioning leads. Similarly, the function of the programmer/analyzer must be periodically checked. If two programmer/analyzers are available, the substitution of one analyzer for another may also help in trouble-shooting the source of a problem.

Necessary equipment/personnel for pacemaker implantation

2 The pacemaker surgical instrument tray should consist of a selection of forceps and scissors, Weitlaner retractors, Senn retractors, fine mosquito clamps, a No. 15 scalpel and knife handle, 2/0 silk suture for lead fixation, and 4/0 Vicryl suture for closing the skin.

Pacemaker supplies consist of pacemaker generator, atrial and ventricular leads, programmer/analyzer, an assortment of lead stylets of various lengths and degrees of stiffness; screwdriver set, Allen wrenches, silicone glue, lead connector caps, wire cutter, sterile plastic sleeves for placement of the programmer head on the field for interrogation/programming of the pacemaker, and two sets of (atrial and ventricular) cables for connecting the programmer/analyzer to the implanted leads.

Personnel should consist of a surgeon, scrub nurse, circulating nurse/anesthetist/pacemaker analyst, and radiology technician.

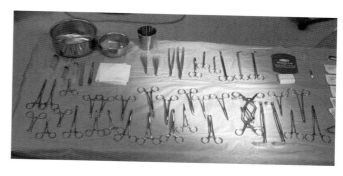

2

ANESTHESIA

3 For transvenous pacemaker lead implantation, the patients are prepared and draped using standard techniques for skin disinfection. An adhesive drape is used to minimize the contamination of the incision by adjacent skin bacteria. Monitoring includes an ECG rhythm monitor with at least two leads displayed at all times, a pulse oximeter, and an automatic blood pressure cuff/monitor. Access to a ventilator and equipment for emergency endotracheal intubation should be available at the head of the table. A 'roll' is placed parallel to the spine that allows the shoulders to fall backward toward the table, opening the space between the first rib and clavicle, allowing for easier and safer access to the subclavian vein. Prophylactic antibiotics are used in every case. Our practice is to use cefazolin, 500 mg to 1 g i.v., given immediately before the skin incision. Patients who are allergic to cephalosporins or those with penicillin allergy receive vancomycin, 1 g i.v. Anesthesia usually consists of local 1 per cent lidocaine, up to 20 cc, along with conscious sedation. The lidocaine must be administered subcutaneously to anesthetize the area of the skin incision, typically using a 25-gauge needle. A larger, 19-gauge or 21-gauge, 1.5- to 2-in. needle is used to infiltrate the subcutaneous tissue in the region of the pacemaker pocket and to inject directly the periosteum on the underside of the clavicle for subclavian punctures. In our institution, a combination of a short-acting narcotic such as fentanyl, a short-acting benzodiazepine such as midazolam, and, occasionally, a short-acting hypnotic such as propofol is used for conscious sedation.

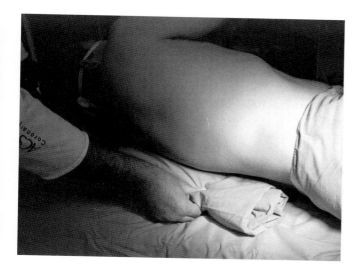

3

OPERATION

Temporary pacing

For cardiac surgeons, the primary indication for temporary pacing is in the postoperative period. After the completion of cardiopulmonary bypass, both atrial and ventricular temporary epicardial leads are usually placed. The ventricular leads are placed on the posterior/inferior or anterior surfaces of the right ventricle and brought out through the chest wall, inferior and lateral to the sternotomy incision. The atrial leads are placed on the right atrial surface and may be secured carefully with 5/0 or 6/0 Prolene suture. A pair of these leads functions as a bipolar lead system. If concern exists that placement of the lead will cause bleeding, or if only a small part of the epicardial surface is visible (e.g. minimally invasive incisions), it is only necessary to place one lead in the atrium and ventricle, respectively. In each case, the other lead can be placed conveniently in the pericardium or on the interior of the chest wall. The leads then function as a unipolar system. In the unipolar configuration, the pacing threshold may be a strong function of the polarity of the two leads. Both leads are brought out of the chest under the costal margin for attachment to an external pacemaker. Some temporary pacing wires are manufactured with a plastic flange on the insulation, designed to prevent premature dislodgment of the pacing wire from the epicardium. Other temporary pacing wires are designed without such a flange with the 'bare' (Teflon-coated) wire exposed. We prefer the bare wire–type leads. These leads may have a slightly higher incidence of dislodgment than the flange-type leads. However, when these leads are removed, typically on postoperative day three, less force is transferred to the myocardium, decreasing the risk of myocardial injury and tamponade, a rare but occasionally fatal complication. In fact, we prefer to convert the flange-type leads to the bare-type, simply by cutting off the flange and removing the insulation from the end of the wire for a distance of 1–2 cm. Patients' vital signs should be monitored frequently, and they should receive bedrest for 1 hour after removal of temporary pacing wires. In the event of tamponade, emergency thoracotomy may occasionally be necessary without time for transport to the operating room.

External pacemakers used today are predominately DDD stimulators, many of which have rapid atrial overdrive pacing capabilities. Both the anesthesiologist and the surgeon should resist the temptation to use routinely the DDD pacing mode unless they perform appropriate measurements of ventricular and atrial thresholds and P-wave and R-wave amplitudes. Otherwise, use of the external pacemaker in the DDD mode with the 'default' settings often leads to failure to capture and over- or undersensing. For patients with sinus bradycardia but intact AV conduction, AAI pacing is often most appropriate. Overdrive atrial pacing at 20–30 per cent faster than the patient's own sinus rate for 72–96 hours postoperatively exclusively may significantly decrease the incidence of atrial fibrillation. For patients with atrial fibrillation, VVI pacing is most appropriate. For patients immediately post-cardiopulmonary bypass with little or no intrinsic atrial or ventricular activity, DOO pacing may be most appropriate. This pacing mode should be changed to DVI, AAI, VVI, or DDD, depending on the situation as electrical activity returns. If one of two pacing wires becomes dislodged, a new pacing wire can be placed using the skin of the chest wall as a ground.

Atrial leads, whether in bipolar or unipolar configuration, can be used to diagnose a variety of supraventricular arrhythmias. An atrial electrogram is easily performed by connecting each atrial lead to one of the arm leads of a standard ECG machine. Lead I shows the atrial electrogram best. For atrial flutter, the atrial leads can be used therapeutically to overdrive-pace the atrium. As flutter rates are typically 275–325 beats per minute, atrial pacing at 350–400 will allow conversion of a significant fraction of cases of atrial flutter to sinus rhythm. Many postoperative patients have Swan-Ganz catheters, and some have continuous mixed venous oxygen saturation monitors. Optimizing the external pacing algorithm, by adjusting the pacing mode, rate, and AV delay, can result in significant increases in cardiac output and blood pressure. These factors may be critically important in patients with poor ventricular function postoperatively.

Selection of permanent pacemaker generators

4 The current generation of permanent pacemaker devices is quite remarkable. Soon, it seems, they will actually insert themselves without our help! We have not arrived at that ideal yet, but today's dual-chamber pacemakers offer numerous standard features that were only introduced within the last several years. Currently available dual-chamber devices include (clockwise from the top left) the Medtronic Kappa 700 series (Medtronic, Minneapolis, MN), the Biotronik Actros DR devices, Berlin, Germany, the St. Jude Integrity AFx, St Paul, Minnesota, and the Guidant Pulser MCX DR, Indianapolis, Indiana. For all of these DDDR devices, required programming parameters include the lower rate, upper rate, AV delay, ventricular and atrial output (mV) and pulse width (ms), and atrial and ventricular sensitivity (mV).

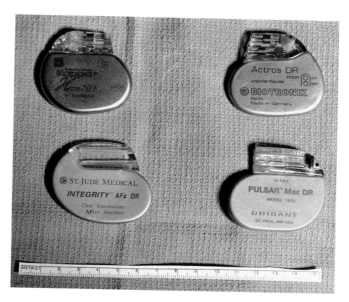

4

These pacers function by sensing atrial activity, tracking atrial beats, and following sensed atrial beats by stimulating the ventricle after the programmed AV delay if no ventricular beat is sensed. If the atrial rate falls below the lower rate, the atrium is paced. If the atrial rate exceeds the upper rate, then AV synchrony is lost, and upper rate behavior is complex. Usually, a Wenckebach mechanism is used to avoid 2:1 block. Most dual-chamber pacemakers today are sophisticated enough to differentiate between sinus tachycardia and atrial fibrillation, usually by measuring atrial rate and regularity (e.g. atrial fibrillation greater than 225 beats/minute and irregular). In the latter condition, instead of pacing the ventricle at the upper rate, 'mode switching' occurs, and the ventricle is paced at a lower rate. This rate need not be fixed, but may be rate-responsive (usually DDIR or VVIR mode). Newer features incorporated into some of these devices include the following:

- Rate-drop response – The device recognizes sudden (inappropriate) decreases in heart rate in patients with carotid sinus syndrome or vasovagal syncope. Thus, rather than pacing at the programmed *lower rate* in these circumstances, pacing occurs at the (higher) *intervention rate* (Medtronic Kappa 700 series, Guidant Discovery II).
- Sensing assurance – The pacemaker automatically measures/adjusts the atrial and ventricular sensitivity to prevent oversensing or undersensing (Medtronic Kappa 700 series, St. Jude Integrity AFx).
- Ventricular capture management – The pacemaker automatically and periodically performs a pacing threshold search and adjusts the amplitude to ensure capture while maximizing longevity (St. Jude Integrity AFx, Medtronic Kappa 700 series).
- Measuring myocardial impedance – The pacemaker measures myocardial impedance, an index of myocardial contractility, which increases in situations of increased metabolic demand independent of intrinsic heart rate. The pacemaker then adjusts rate appropriately (Biotronik Inos^{2+} CLS).

- Dual chamber pacing (DDDR) with a single lead – The use of overlapping biphasic stimulation allows for efficient stimulation and sensing of the atrium using the intravascular atrial portion of the single (ventricular) lead (Biotronik Eikos SLD).
- Continuous monitoring of ventricular evoked response and monophasic action potential – Monitoring of these two parameters of cellular function allows for sensitive and specific diagnosis of allograft rejection after heart transplantation (Biotronik Physios CTM).
- Automatic AV delay adjustment – In addition to rate-sensitive adjustment of the AV interval, the pacemaker periodically measures the patient's intrinsic AV delay and automatically adjusts the programmed AV delay to maximize conduction through the native conduction system. In addition to the physiological advantages of intrinsic AV conduction, this feature increases device longevity (Medtronic Kappa 700 series).

In general, any of the above pacemaker generators will suffice for the most common pacing indications. Individual features may lead one to prefer a specific pacemaker for specialized circumstances.

Selection of pacing leads

5a, b Pacemaker leads serve as the electrical interface between the pacemaker generator and the heart. The earliest implementation of an implantable pacemaker system by Senning used epicardial leads placed via a right thoracotomy incision. Epicardial leads may also be placed via a subxiphoid incision or via a median sternotomy incision when permanent pacing is indicated and a median sternotomy has been performed for another procedure. Permanent epicardial leads are rarely used today for permanent pacing. Endocardial leads are preferred because they can be inserted transvenously and have other advantages over epicardial permanent leads. Due to a larger surface contact area, epicardial leads are associated with a higher incidence of fatigue-related fracture, higher pacing thresholds, and a greater degree of myocardial trauma. Epicardial leads are an important part of the pacing armamentarium, however. In infants and children with congenital heart disease with left-to-right shunts, single-ventricle physiology, or in patients with subclavian or innominate vein thrombosis or SVC occlusion, the use of epicardial leads may be the preferred approach.

Endocardial leads are either bipolar or unipolar. Both lead types have a cathode positioned at the tip of the lead. In unipolar leads, the pacemaker generator functions as the anode. In bipolar leads, the anode is incorporated into the distal end of the lead, several millimeters proximal to the cathode. Previously, bipolar leads were somewhat cumbersome, less malleable, and required use of a larger introducer when placed transvenously than unipolar leads. Current designs minimize these concerns, and unipolar and bipolar leads can be inserted safely and easily.

Repair of unipolar leads, however, is easier. The portion of the lead outside the vascular system can be cut, and a lead repair kit can be used. Bipolar leads cannot generally be repaired in this manner if fractures occur. Bipolar leads have a clear advantage in terms of sensing, however, as the electrical signal is measured between two closely spaced electrodes near the tip of the lead. Occasionally, ventricular electrical activity can be missensed as atrial activity, due to 'far-field R-wave' sensing. This problem is essentially eliminated with bipolar pacing, because the amplitude of far-field ventricular electrical signals is substantially reduced. *Crosstalk* is sensing in one chamber of a pacing stimulus from another chamber. This phenomenon is much less common with bipolar leads as well. Similarly, skeletal muscle myopotential oversensing and undesirable skeletal muscle stimulation are complications that are minimized by using bipolar leads. Right ventricular perforation is rare with the current generation of bipolar and unipolar leads. The use of newer leads with flexible tips and silicone rubber or polyurethane insulation has dramatically reduced the incidence of this complication. Some of the newer bipolar leads use a coaxial design that allows for minimization of overall lead diameter and stiffness.

Lead fixation is either passive or active. The most common

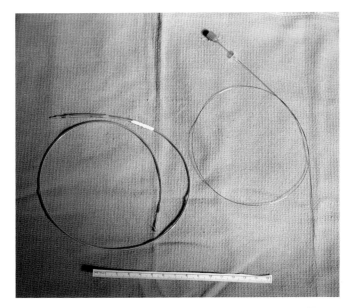

5a

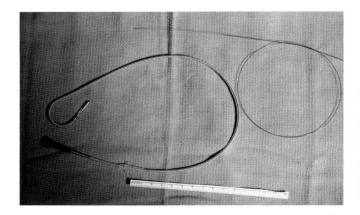

5b

design of passive fixation leads incorporates 'tines' (small plastic hooks) positioned immediately behind the electrode. These tines become entrapped in the myocardial trabeculae and are unlikely to become dislodged once properly positioned. Active fixation or 'screw-in' leads use a retractable screw that is withdrawn into the lead tip during positioning. Once the lead is in a good position with acceptable threshold and R-wave and P-wave amplitudes and impedance, the screw is deployed to fix the electrode at the lead tip to the myocardium. Typically, the lead is retracted or extended by rotating a component of the end of the lead that will subsequently be inserted into the pacemaker generator. The tip of the lead is designed so that deployment of the screw can easily be recognized fluoroscopically. Screw-in leads cause more myocardial injury than tined leads. The resulting scar formation may result in significantly higher thresholds 1–2 months after implantation. A significant advance in lead technology was the development of steroid-eluting leads. Steroid-eluting leads were developed to decrease inflammation at the electrode-tissue interface. As a result of the inflammatory process, lead thresholds increase to a maximum value within the first 6 weeks after implantation and then decrease to a chronic value. Steroid-eluting leads have been shown to maintain long-term stable stimulation thresholds in both the ventricle and atrium, avoiding early postimplantation unpredictable increases in thresholds.

Screw-in leads are often slightly larger in diameter than tined leads and may require a larger introducer. For patients who previously have undergone cardiac surgery, screw-in leads are often preferred. In many adult and congenital cardiac procedures, the right atrial appendage is amputated. In patients who retain their entire right atrium, the right atrial appendage is an excellent site for lead fixation. Secure, passive fixation can be achieved in the majority of cases due to the abundance of trabeculae and the morphology of this area. For patients who need permanent pacing after cardiac surgery, active fixation leads are clearly preferred in the atrium. In the right ventricular apex (RVA), tined passive fixation leads can usually be used with a high degree of success, regardless of previous cardiac surgical procedures. Fixation to less common locations, such as the lateral atrial wall or the right ventricular outflow tract, generally requires screw-in leads, and some operators prefer to use screw-in leads routinely.

Technique of pacemaker implantation

OBTAINING VENOUS ACCESS

6a, b For transvenous pacemaker insertions, obtaining venous access efficiently, reliably, and safely are the hallmarks of a proficient pacemaker surgeon. Knowledge of the anatomy of the upper thorax, upper extremities, and neck is necessary for successful pacemaker implantation. A precise knowledge of the location and relationships of the internal jugular, external jugular, subclavian, and cephalic veins is essential to obtaining venous access. An understanding of the relationships of each of these structures to surrounding structures, particularly the lung, subclavian artery, and carotid artery, is necessary to avoid the common complications of pacemaker insertion.

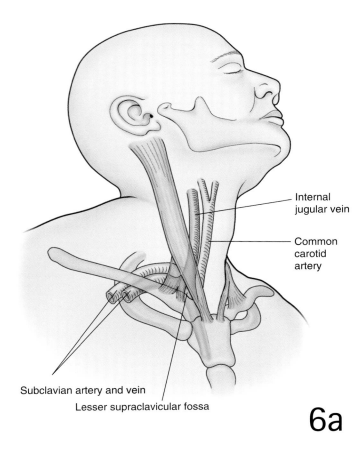

Internal jugular vein

Common carotid artery

Subclavian artery and vein

Lesser supraclavicular fossa

6a

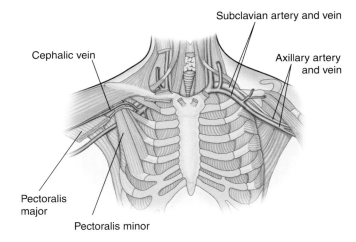

Subclavian artery and vein

Axillary artery and vein

Cephalic vein

Pectoralis major

Pectoralis minor

6b

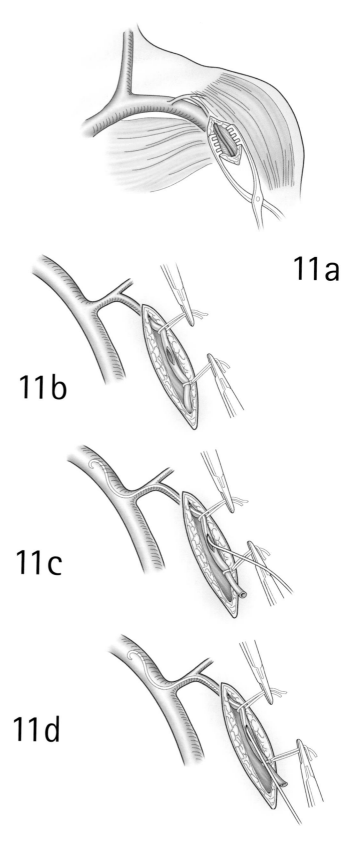

11a–d The cephalic vein may also be cannulated directly via the lateral end of the incision by exposing the vein in the deltopectoral groove. Additional lidocaine should be infiltrated directly into this area. For single-lead pacemaker systems with cephalic vein cutdown, the lead can be placed directly via the vein as illustrated. An 11 blade is used to incise the anterior 50 per cent of the vein cross section. A small plastic dilator is advanced into the vein. A mosquito clamp is opened gently to further dilate the vein, and the lead is inserted into the vein and passed into the heart. In some cases, the lead will not pass into the subclavian vein, even though there is good blood return. In these cases, the cephalic vein is used for passage of a wire into the subclavian vein and centrally. A dilator is advanced over the wire, and lead placement then proceeds in direct analogy to lead placement via the subclavian or internal jugular routes. If the diameter of the cephalic vein is inadequate to accommodate the dilator, the dilator tip is inserted into the cephalic vein. The vein is then retracted, and the vein is incised for a distance of approximately 1 cm on top of the dilator. The dilator is advanced further. These steps are repeated as many times as necessary to pass the introducer centrally.

12 After an introducer/peel-away catheter has been passed centrally, the guide wire is removed, and the lead is inserted. For ventricular leads, a gentle curve is created in the distal 10 cm or so of the guide wire. Creation of this curve is somewhat of an art, as a different configuration will be used for left subclavian than for right subclavian access. The spiral curve is designed to allow for negotiation of the innominate-SVC junction while promoting passage of the lead/stylet from the right atrium, across the tricuspid valve, into the right ventricle, and subsequently into the pulmonary artery. The stylet is then removed, and it is replaced by a less stiff stylet that will be used to position the tip of the lead in the RVA. This stylet will either be straight or have a tiny curve subtending approximately 45 degrees over a distance of 1–2 cm. It is important that this stylet be less stiff than the first stylet to decrease the risk of perforation. The first stylet is removed while maintaining the position of the lead in the pulmonary artery. The second stylet is then advanced again, maintaining lead position. The lead and stylet are then withdrawn slowly. Once the lead crosses the pulmonary valve and enters the right ventricular outflow tract, it is quickly but gently advanced inward toward the RVA. Placement in the right ventricle is confirmed by development of premature ventricular contractions, by the fluoroscopic appearance in the right anterior oblique view, or by pacing and confirming a wide QRS morphology with deep QS waves in the inferior leads. Although the previously described procedure is usually satisfactory, passage of the ventricular lead into the pulmonary artery or right ventricular outflow tract is not required for lead placement. In the alternative procedure, the operator puts a slight curve in the stylet with the stylet slightly withdrawn. The lead is advanced into the right atrium. Often, the lead will catch inferiorly and will prolapse into the right ventricle, minimizing the risk of perforation. Once placement into the right ventricle is confirmed, it may be necessary to advance the lead toward the apex. Then, a soft, straight stylet is placed into the lead, and the lead is withdrawn 1 cm or so and advanced toward the apex. The same procedure is followed for both screw-in and tined leads.

For screw-in leads, we prefer to test the lead before fixing it to the myocardium. Newer leads permit measurement of pacing thresholds and impedance before deploying the screw. Otherwise, the risk of perforation and unnecessary myocardial injury is incurred with a lead position that may be unacceptable. If the parameters indicate an acceptable lead position, then the lead is screwed into position. Six to ten clockwise turns of the lead shaft will result in extension of the screw into the myocardium. A one-half to three-quarter turn on the lead body often helps to seat the screw and abut the lead tip against the endocardium. Usually, extension of the screw can be confirmed fluoroscopically. To ensure adequate fixation of ventricular or, particularly, atrial leads, the lead is advanced and then withdrawn so that the operator can feel just a little resistance while observing the lead fluoroscopically. If the lead tip resists the gentle traction, this situation suggests that it is appropriately fixed into position.

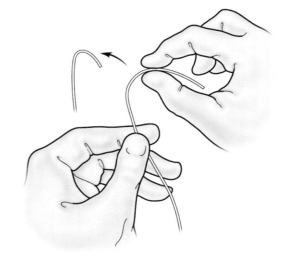

12

13a–e

The passage of a ventricular pacing lead is depicted in the series of fluoroscopic images. In Figure 13a, an anteroposterior (AP) view, the lead has been inadvertently advanced into the coronary sinus. The ventricular pacing lead is labeled VPL, and an external defibrillator lead is labeled EDL. Confirmation of this situation was obtained by viewing the lead in the left anterior oblique 30-degree view (not shown), and by demonstrating atrial capture during pacing threshold determination. To cross the tricuspid annulus, the lead was gently withdrawn so that its tip remained in the coronary sinus os, whereupon the stylet was withdrawn approximately 12 cm to 'soften' the tip. The lead was then carefully advanced, causing it to prolapse a leading edge into the right ventricle. This position is shown in Figure 13b, also an AP view. Note that this technique has two advantages: first, the prolapsing bend of the lead is unlikely to perforate the relatively thin-walled right ventricle; second, it is too large to enter the coronary sinus ostium. Next, the stylet was advanced a few centimeters and the lead gently torqued in a clockwise direction. This moved the tip of the lead anteriorly and freed it from the coronary sinus os. The lead was then smoothly and continuously advanced into the right ventricular outflow tract as shown in the AP view in Figure 13c. At this point, the stylet was advanced to the lead tip and the lead itself was gently withdrawn, causing it to 'fall' into the RVA. This step is depicted in Figure 13d. Note that in this AP view, the lead appears to be only modestly advanced into the apex. The AP view often foreshortens the lead position in the apex, especially if the heart is rotated. For this reason, confirmation of the lead position should be obtained by viewing in the right anterior oblique 30-degree projection. This position is shown in Figure 13e, in which the tip of the lead is noted to be well out towards the RVA. At this point the screw was deployed and electrical measurements performed.

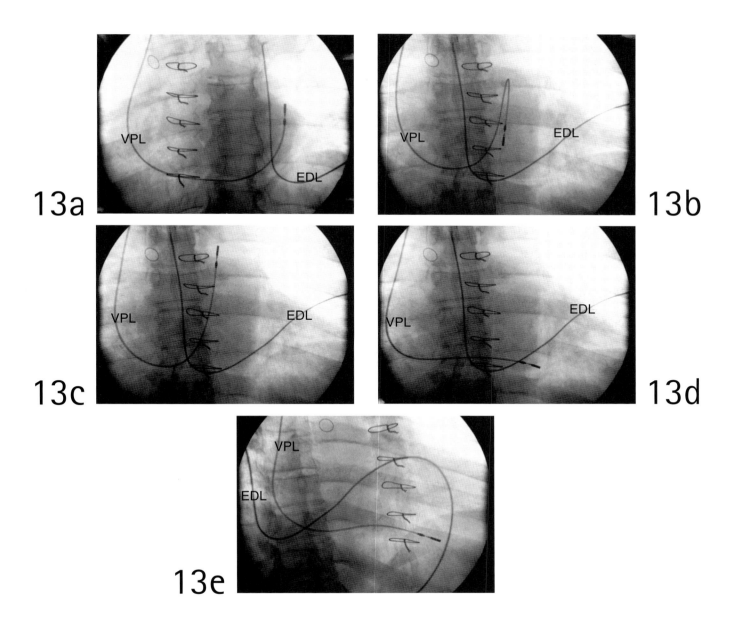

14a–c Atrial leads are typically placed with the goal of lodging the tip in the right atrial appendage. Both tined and screw-in atrial leads are available with and without a preformed 'J' configuration. Leads with a preformed 'J' have the distal 2–3 cm of the atrial lead configured to resemble the letter 'J.' This configuration makes it easier to get the tip of the lead to lodge in the right atrial appendage. The stylets for these leads are usually straight. For atrial leads without a preformed 'J' configuration, usually stylets are available with a 'J' configuration. Thus, with the stylet in place, the lead/stylet combination assumes the 'J' configuration. With passive-fixation tined leads, having the preformed 'J' configuration in the lead itself is important to obtain stable positioning in the right atrial appendage. For screw-in leads, having the preformed 'J' in the stylet alone is adequate, as the screw will be used to fix the lead in position in the atrium once the appropriate site has been contacted. In either case, the lead/stylet combinations are advanced into the right atrium just beyond the superior cavoatrial junction. The stylet is either advanced ('J' configuration in the stylet) or withdrawn ('J' configuration in the lead itself) until the lead attains sufficient 'J' configuration to allow positioning of its tip securely in the right atrial appendage. For tined leads, the stylet is gently withdrawn, whereas for screw-in leads, the screw is deployed, fixing the lead to the myocardium, after which the stylet is withdrawn. Once the tip of the lead is positioned in the appendage, fixation is assessed by gently withdrawing the lead. In the presence of adequate fixation, the tip of the 'J' stops moving, and catheter withdrawal opens the 'J.' The 'J' rocks back and forth rhythmically in synchrony with the atrial contraction. At full inspiration, downward movement of the heart bends the 'J' open to approximately 60–90 degrees. At full expiration, the 'J' closes, typically to 45 degrees or less, and is near the relaxed configuration. Further confirmation of the stability of atrial lead positioning is obtained by retesting the lead at the end of the implant procedure. Deflectable stylets are available to 'map' regions outside the appendage and secure good pacing sites in patients whose appendages have been amputated.

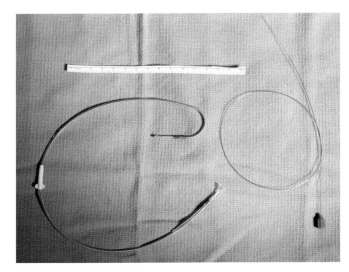

14a

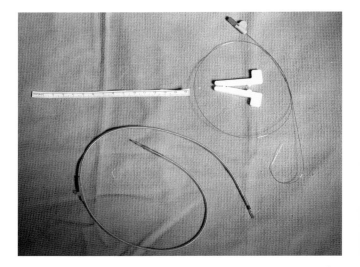

14b

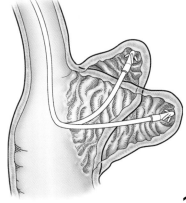

14c

SPECIAL TECHNIQUES FOR LEAD PLACEMENT

15a–c As previously outlined, the standard position for the ventricular lead is in the RVA. The standard position for the atrial lead is in the right atrial appendage. There are a variety of situations in which alternative lead positions should be considered. In these instances, active-fixation screw-in leads should generally be used. For ventricular pacing, the right ventricular outflow tract may also be used for lead fixation. The central portion of the right ventricular silhouette should be avoided, as the lead may become entangled in the chordae tendineae, occasionally interfering with tricuspid valve function. In patients with previous cardiac surgery, the atrial appendage is often absent, and screw-in leads should be used routinely. In these cases, and when thresholds or P-wave amplitudes are inadequate in other locations, the low lateral atrial wall near the inferior cavoatrial junction often provides acceptable pacing function, although care must be taken to avoid phrenic nerve pacing.

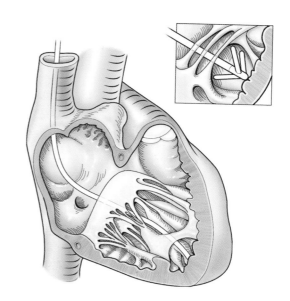

15a

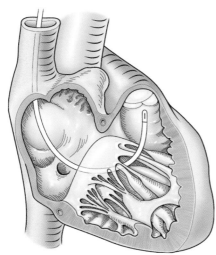

15b

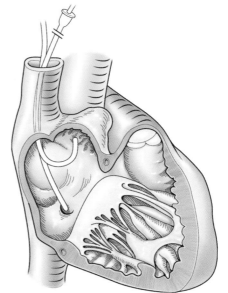

15c

EPICARDIAL LEAD PLACEMENT

Thoracotomy is rarely necessary today for implantation of permanent pacemaker leads. In the presence of severe anomalies of the tricuspid valve or a prosthetic tricuspid valve, epicardial lead placement may be required. Epicardial leads are more traumatic than current transvenous leads and generally have higher thresholds. The operative incisions for permanent epicardial lead placement include median sternotomy, subxiphoid approach, right paramedian incision, and right and left anterior thoracotomy. The advantage of the median sternotomy, right paramedian, and right anterior thoracotomy incisions is that the right atrium and right ventricle can be accessed for dual-chamber lead placement. The most common approaches, however, are the subxiphoid and left thoracotomy approaches, which are useful primarily for ventricular lead placement only and are illustrated.

16a–c

For a subxiphoid approach, the patient is placed on the table in the supine position and draped as for a median sternotomy. A midline incision is made directly over the xiphoid. The xiphoid is resected for additional exposure. The pericardium is identified and opened on its inferior surface. Gentle traction on the pericardium will allow exposure of a sufficient portion of the inferior right ventricular surface to allow placement of two corkscrew epicardial leads. The leads are tunneled to a subcutaneous pocket in the left upper abdominal wall and connected to the pacemaker generator.

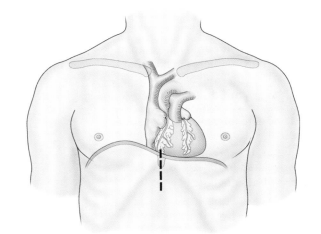

16a

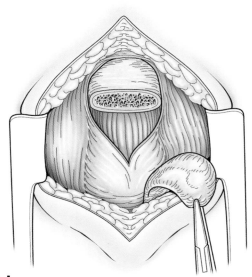

16b

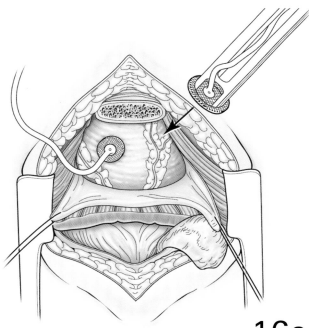

16c

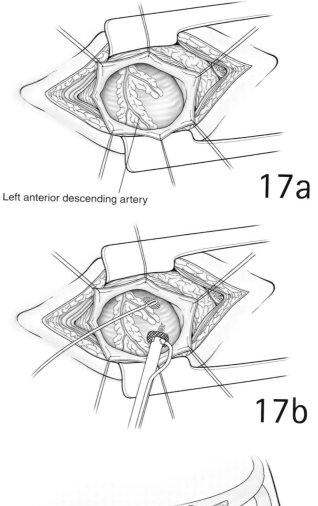

Left anterior descending artery

17a

17a–c In the left anterior thoracotomy approach, a 10–15 cm incision is made in the fifth or sixth intercostal space. The pericardium is opened, and two sites are selected that are free of coronary vessels. The left anterior descending coronary artery is identified, and the leads are placed to the left of the artery on the LV wall. Two corkscrew leads are fastened to the ventricular surface. As in the subxiphoid approach, the leads are tunneled to a subcutaneous pocket on the left upper abdominal wall and connected to the pacemaker generator in the standard fashion.

17b

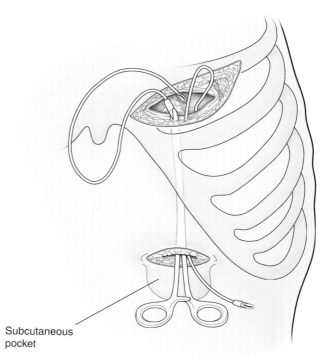

Subcutaneous pocket

17c

EVALUATION OF LEAD FUNCTION

The first requirement for successful lead placement is good radiographical position and stability. Atrial and ventricular lead function must be assessed by measuring three basic parameters: (1) pacing threshold, (2) P-wave and R-wave amplitude, and (3) lead impedance. Each of these parameters is discussed in the following sections.

Pacing Threshold

The output of the ventricular and atrial channels of most available pacemakers allows specification of voltage (V) and pulse width (ms). The 'pacing threshold' is actually a combination of these two variables and is most closely related to their product. When the pacing threshold is specified in terms of voltage, it is commonly assumed that the pulse width is set at a default value of 0.4–0.5 ms. Under these circumstances, acceptable ventricular thresholds are 1.0 V at time of implant and 2.0 V chronically. Similarly, the atrial channel pulse width is typically set at 0.4–0.5 ms. An acceptable atrial threshold is 2.0 V at the time of implant and 3.0 V chronically. Both atrial and ventricular leads are connected via cables to the programmer/analyzer. The ventricular threshold is measured by increasing the heart rate to a value that exceeds the patient's rate, starting with an amplitude of 5 V and decreasing the output in a stepwise manner until loss of capture is observed. The minimum output that results in reliable ventricular capture is the threshold value.

Measuring the atrial threshold is often less straightforward. Capture of the atrium is unambiguous in patients with sick sinus syndrome and intact intrinsic AV conduction. Under these circumstances, one simply increases the atrial pacing rate above the patient's intrinsic rate. Atrial capture is indicated when the patient's heart rate corresponds to the set rate. The output of the atrial channel of the analyzer/programmer is then decreased from 5 V to determine the threshold value in direct analogy to the ventricular lead. In cases in which there is complete AV block, the ventricular rate on the ECG monitor supplies no information about atrial capture. Under these circumstances, two alternatives exist. Ideally, the programmer/analyzer is sophisticated enough to pace, sense, and display the atrial electrogram. This function allows unambiguous determination of atrial capture. In the presence of atrial capture, the pacing spike and the P wave appear on the electrogram. In the absence of capture, only the pacing spike appears. If the programmer/analyzer does not have the capacity to display ventricular and atrial electrograms, and complete AV block is present, the ECG must be inspected to determine whether a P wave occurs after each atrial pacemaker spike, which is occasionally difficult. The pacemaker spike itself may be difficult to see, and visibility may be enhanced by using the unipolar mode. Here, the anode (red insulation) cable is connected to the wound while the cathode cable (black insulation) is connected to the end of the pacemaker lead. Alternatively, atrial capture may be observed flu-oroscopically, and loss of capture may be determined by changes in the atrial contraction pattern.

P-wave and R-wave amplitude

P-wave amplitudes should be greater than 1.5 mV, and R-wave amplitudes should be greater than 5 mV. The slow rate is also measured by most programmer/analyzers and should be greater than 0.5 V/second. The slow rate is the first derivative of the electrogram (dV/dt). In the majority of cases, if the amplitude is in the acceptable range, the slow rate is also. However, if the slow rate is not in the acceptable range, the pacemaker often does not sense atrial or ventricular activity adequately.

Impedance

Typically, atrial and ventricular lead impedance should be in the 300–1300 ohm range. If both the pacing threshold and the R-wave and P-wave amplitude are in the acceptable range, the impedance is usually acceptable as well. Rarely, however, the lead may be defective or the insulation or conductor damaged during the implantation process. For chronic leads, relative changes in lead impedance are the best indicators of lead integrity. Fracture of a lead conductor increases impedance, whereas breakage of insulation may decrease impedance. For bipolar leads, if only one conductor or insulator is affected, switching from a bipolar to a unipolar mode may restore effective pacing. Pacemakers with automatic lead configuration–switching will perform this function automatically. Higher impedance may indicate failure to deploy the screw adequately (extracardiac lead position) or adapter failure. Lower impedance often indicates trauma to the lead insulation during placement or coaxial breakdown.

Pacemaker generator replacement

The most common indication for pacemaker generator replacement is battery depletion at end-of-life. Other indications include sensing malfunction, need for generator upgrade to include rate-responsiveness or dual-chamber pacing, device recall, infection, erosion, generator migration, or hematoma. The administration of preoperative antibiotics and preparation and draping of the patient for generator change is identical to first-time pacemaker insertion. If pacemaker infection is the indication for generator change, then antibiotics specifically directed against the offending organism should be used. If interrogation of the pacemaker has indicated acceptable thresholds, P-wave and R-wave amplitudes, and lead impedances, only the pacemaker generator must be changed. In this case, anticoagulation need not be completely reversed before generator change, although meticulous attention to hemostasis is required. If lead replacement is necessary, nearly normal coagulation parameters are required. Lead replacement with venous access via the subclavian route should only be performed with the international normalized ratio less than 1.7 and prothrombin time less than 15 seconds.

Generally, the original pacemaker incision is used. Bipolar electrocautery is useful for incising the pacemaker capsule. Before delivering the old generator from the wound, atrial and ventricular pacing cables should be available on the field and connected to an appropriate programmer/analyzer. Using a sterile sleeve, the programmer/analyzer can be used to interrupt pacing function briefly to determine whether the patient has an acceptable escape rhythm. Alternatively, the original pacemaker can be reprogrammed to VVI mode at 40 beats/minute. Doing so may allow an escape rhythm to develop. If so, the generator replacement can be performed safely after electrical measurements have been made. If not, all members of the team should be prepared to move quickly

to ensure that effective pacing is never interrupted for more than a second or two. If the existing pacemaker generator is in a unipolar mode, the pacemaker cannot be delivered completely from the wound, as pacing would be interrupted. The programmer/analyzer should be set to pace the atrial and ventricular channels at an output that equals or exceeds that of the pacemaker being replaced. The ventricular lead should then be quickly disconnected from the generator and connected to the ventricular cables from the analyzer/programmer, and ventricular pacing should be re-established. Once effective ventricular pacing has been established, the atrial lead can be disconnected from the old generator and connected to the atrial set of cables. If, for some reason, effective pacing cannot be established, the old generator should be reconnected.

18 Once the pacemaker leads have been connected to the analyzer/programmer, the leads should be inspected to ensure that they are compatible with the new generator to be implanted. All newer bipolar pacemakers generally conform to the international pacemaker standard called the *International Standard–1* (IS-1), which uses IS-1 UNI for unipolar leads and IS-1 BI for bipolar leads. Both types of IS-1 connectors incorporate sealing rings into the design and are 3.2 mm in diameter. When changing generators, however, the surgeon may encounter older leads of a variety of designs. Most leads manufactured since 1985 conform to the Voluntary Standard–1 (VS-1), VS-1A, and VS-1B designs. Like IS-1 BI connectors, these connectors are also 3.2 mm in diameter, with varying lengths of the lead connector pin and with or without sealing rings. Owing to differences in the length of the connector pins, VS-1 and IS-1 leads may not be equally compatible with a given generator, due to improper alignment of the anode ring. Older bipolar leads have separate connector pins for the cathode and anode. Older unipolar and bipolar leads generally have 5-mm or 6-mm pin diameters. A selection of step-up and step-down adapters, as well as adapters for converting separate–pin design bipolar connectors to the IS-1 BI standard, should be available to ensure lead/generator compatibility. An adapter for converting separate–pin design bipolar connectors to the IS-1 BI standard is illustrated.

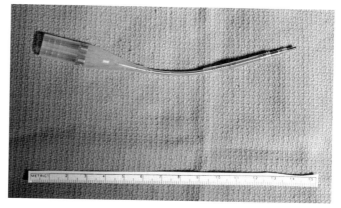

18

POSTOPERATIVE CARE

Not infrequently, the success of the implantation procedure depends in no small amount on the postoperative care. In general, the patient is awake and alert immediately after the procedure and able to receive instructions. First, the patient's arm on the side of the implantation is placed in a sling to remind him or her not to move it in an exaggerated fashion. If the patient is confused and unable to cooperate with this order, a mastectomy dressing may be applied. This dressing involves taking several lengths of ACE wrap bandages and stringing them together with safety pins, end to end. The first several meters of bandage are placed around the patient's trunk, and then the arm on the side of the implant is placed against the trunk. The ACE bandage is wrapped three to four times around the upper arm and secured with a safety pin. The advantage of this approach is that it reminds the patient to keep his or her arm close to his or her trunk, while not tying or restraining the patient in a way that may cause him or her to become confused and agitated. This is a successful approach in patients who are confused or have a poor mental status at baseline. A nursing report must be called to the floor to which the patient will return. A chest x-ray is obtained to exclude hemothorax or pneumothorax. Orders are written to continue prophylactic antibiotics for 24 hours after implantation. Pain medication orders, usually given orally, are written, and the patient's other medications and diet are resumed. The patient is maintained on telemetry for the following 24 hours, completing his or her antibiotic course.

On the following day, the patient is examined with particular attention to the wound. Any exudate, bleeding, or hematoma formation is noted. The presence of fever is determined. An ECG, with and without a magnet, is obtained. Frequently, the pacemaker is reinterrogated the following day, and the thresholds are checked. The chest x-ray is reviewed for pneumothorax and to ascertain whether lead migration has taken place. Hemothorax or pneumothorax greater than 10–15 per cent, or unstable pneumothorax, increasing in size on serial films, should be managed with a thoracostomy tube. Wound hematoma is usually managed conservatively, with antibiotics and warm compresses applied to the area. A liquefied wound hematoma may be aspirated once or twice on successive days using sterile technique followed by a compression dressing. Cultures of the aspirate should be obtained. Prophylactic antibiotic therapy is recommended in the presence of hematoma. Signs of infection, such as warmth, drainage, erythema, fever, or leukocytosis, generally require removal of the generator, while leaving the pocket open. For infections occurring in the early postoperative period, the leads may be removed safely. If pacemaker lead endocarditis is confirmed, extraction may be performed using a variety of techniques, including use of the eximer laser sheath. For late-occurring infections, the leads are generally capped and left in place. In patients who are pacemaker dependent, a new pacemaker can be placed on the other side at the same sitting, provided sterility of the operative site can be maintained. Alternatively, a temporary transvenous pacemaker can be used until local control of the infection has been obtained. In cases in which long-term pacing is required, an exteriorized, permanent lead may be used. When possible, the best results are obtained by exploration, 2 weeks on intravenous antibiotic therapy, and implantation on the contralateral side.

On the first postoperative day, once the aforementioned checks have been made and in the absence of any complications, the patient may be discharged with follow-up in 1 week's time for a wound check and reinterrogation. In 6 weeks, the patient returns for another wound check and reinterrogation, and final pacemaker settings are programmed to maximize battery life after the leads have had a chance to heal and assume their chronic pacing characteristics. At that time, rate response is assessed by reviewing the patient's heart rate histograms, and transtelephonic monitoring is arranged.

OUTCOME

In the past 40 years, advances in both technique and technology have improved cardiac pacing dramatically. It is now possible to implant both antibradycardia and antitachycardia devices transvenously using a nonthoracotomy approach. As a result, the majority of patients who present with rhythm disturbances amenable to pacing may be treated with very low morbidity and negligible mortality. Major complications are rare; these include perforation and tamponade, pneumothorax, air embolus, and infection. In our experience, combined rates for major complications should be less than 2 per cent. Perforation may be minimized by careful lead handling, especially by withdrawing the stylet ('softening the tip') before advancing the lead, particularly when entering the ventricle. In addition, the operator should resist the temptation to add too much slack or redundancy to the ventricular lead after positioning it successfully, as doing so increases the risk of perforation. In truth, many perforations are probably subclinical in presentation and do not result in tamponade. Features that increase the risk of tamponade include anticoagulation and pulmonary hypertension, both of which may result in increased hemorrhage at the perforation site.

Pneumothorax is a recognized complication of subclavian access. Patients with bullous lung disease and chest wall abnormalities (e.g. 'scalloped' clavicle) are more likely to develop pneumothorax and should be considered for cephalic vein access. Very obese patients may also have an increased risk of pneumothorax, but this complication can generally be reduced if the pocket is created first, and if access is obtained via the pocket, which permits the needle to be advanced parallel to the chest wall.

Air embolus is a greatly feared complication that is fortunately rare. Stroke may result from this complication if the patient has a patent foramen ovale or other intracardiac right-to-left shunt. The risk of air embolus is increased in confused patients who may take deep breaths unexpectedly, lowering intrathoracic pressure and sucking air into the vascular space through the introducer. The risk may be reduced by proper patient sedation, proper hydration and anesthetic technique, and the use of introducers with vascular clamps or, alternatively, by 'peeling away' the introducer immediately after the lead has been successfully passed into the vena cava.

Infection is a recognized and feared complication that requires constant vigilance. The implant suite must be carefully cycle-cleaned between cases, and care must be focused on the air-handling ducts and fluoroscopy equipment. Traffic in and out of the room must be kept to an absolute minimum, and prophylactic antibiotics must be used. The time that any implant hardware (i.e. leads or pulse generator) is exposed to the air should also be minimized by breaking packaging seals only as each item is to be used. Careful wound closure and follow-up care is mandatory. We prefer to bury knots fairly deeply and use glue for the skin closure, as these steps reduce the incidence of suture abscess. A wound check performed one week after implantation often identifies problems early, when they can be corrected in an outpatient setting by suture removal and oral antibiotics, before they advance to the point at which a pocket infection results. With these measures, we have managed to keep our infection rate at below 0.5 per cent. Any cluster of infections that is noted should be investigated thoroughly, with particular attention to room cleanliness, staff training, and infection-control inquiry into any possible contaminants in consumable supplies.

Lead migration may be a vexing problem, particularly for atrial leads. The incidence of migration is higher in patients who have had previous surgery in which the right atrial appendage was amputated. Placement of an atrial screw-in lead along the lateral right atrium is generally a better option in such patients.

Hematoma formation is a common problem that is, fortunately, self-limited. Careful attention to hemostasis and pocket formation reduces the risk of hematoma. Generally, conservative management is successful with frequent wound checks. As long as the suture line remains intact, even fairly large hematomas resolve without sequelae. We make it a practice not to aspirate hematomas, as doing so increases the risk of infection. Should a hematoma require evacuation, this task is best accomplished in the operating suite under sterile conditions.

In summary, improved technology and careful technique have made pacemaker implantation a safe procedure for even the sickest patients with rhythm disturbances. Proper attention to lead positioning and surgical technique make it possible to restore normal chronotropy and AV synchrony to such patients. Device lifespans of 10 years are not unusual – the equivalent of half a billion heart beats.

FURTHER READING

Bernstein, A.D., Camm, A.J., Fletcher, R.D., et al. 1987. The NASPE/BPEG generic pacemaker code for antibradyarrhythmia and adaptive-rate pacing and antitachyarrhythmia devices. PACE 10, 794–9.

Chardack, W.M., Gage, A.A., Greatbach, W. 1960. A transistorized, self-contained, implantable pacemaker for the long-term correction of complete heart block. Surgery 48, 643–54.

Furman, S. 2000: Introduction: history of cardiac pacing. In Ellenbogen, K.A., Kay, G.N., Wilkoff, B.L. (eds.), Clinical cardiac pacing and defibrillation. 2nd ed. Philadelphia: W.B. Saunders, 1–13.

Guyton, R.A. 1997: A synopsis of cardiac physiology. In Edmunds, L.H. (ed.). Adult cardiac surgery. New York: McGraw-Hill, 59–83.

Kutalek, S.P., Kantheria, B.K., Maquilan, M. 2000. Approach to generator change. In Ellenbogen, K.A., Kay, G.N., Wilkoff, B.L. (eds.), Clinical cardiac pacing and defibrillation. 2nd ed. Philadelphia: W.B. Saunders, 645–68.

37

Cardiac tumors

GABRIEL S. ALDEA MD
Professor and Chief of Adult Cardiac Surgery, Department of Cardiothoracic Surgery, University of Washington School of Medicine, Seattle, Washington, USA

EDWARD D. VERRIER MD
Vice Chairman of Surgery and Chief of Cardiothoracic Surgery, Department of Surgery, University of Washington Medical Center, Seattle, Washington, USA

PRINCIPLES AND JUSTIFICATION

Primary tumors of the heart are much less common than metastatic tumors, with an incidence of less than 0.3 per cent in large autopsy series. Over 75 per cent of cardiac tumors are benign and present with a variety of nonspecific clinical signs and symptoms that overlap many other cardiovascular and systemic disorders. The types and distribution of benign and malignant primary tumors of the heart are strikingly different in adults and children (Tables 37.1 and 37.2).

Of all primary cardiac tumors, approximately 25 per cent are malignant. In adults, almost all malignant cardiac tumors are sarcomas, most commonly angiosarcomas, as shown in Table 37.2. Malignant tumors occur in adults most commonly in the fourth decade of life and have a similar incidence in men and women. The right atrium is most commonly involved. Patients present with symptoms of congestive heart failure, hemopericardium with or without tamponade, myocardial ischemia, or arrhythmias. In children and infants, the most common primary cardiac malignancy is a rhabdomyosarcoma. Children are more likely to present with complications resulting from intracavitary extension.

Clinically, patients with sarcomas display a rapid downhill course, and most patients die within the first year of diagnosis, despite adjunctive multi-modality chemotherapy and radiation therapy, because of hematogenous spread. The role of surgery in the management of primary malignant cardiac neoplasms is generally to establish a definitive diagnosis and guide multi-modality adjunctive therapy. Rare longer-term survivals have been reported in some patients with primary cardiac lymphomas.

Neoplasia of the heart and pericardium is much more likely to be secondary, or metastatic, than primary. Reports of prevalence derived from large autopsy studies of patients with known malignancies demonstrate cardiac and/or pericardial involvement in up to one in five patients. The valves and endocardium are rarely involved. Although leukemias and melanomas are particularly likely to metastasize to the heart, thyroid, lung, esophagus, kidney, and breast metastases may be seen. The mode of extension can be either direct invasion and extension (such as lung cancer and mesothelioma), through lymphatic channels (such as Hodgkin's or large cell lymphoma), or via hematogenous routes (such as breast, melanoma, pancreatic, or gastric malignancies).

Table 37.1 *Incidence of benign cardiac tumors*

Tumor type	% Adults (*n* = 241)	% Children (*n* = 78)
Myxoma	49	15.5
Lipoma	19	–
Papillary fibroelastoma	17	–
Hemangioma	5	5
Rhabdomyoma	<1	45
Teratoma	1	14
Fibroma	2	15.5
Atrioventricular node mesothelioma	4	4
Other	2	1

Modified with permission from McAllister *et al.* 1996. Primary cardiac tumors. In Goldhaber, S, Braunwald, E (eds). *Atlas of Heart Diseases*, Philadelphia, Current Medicine 15: 1–15.

Table 37.2 *Incidence of primary malignant cardiac tumors*

Tumor type	% Adults (*n* = 117)	% Children (*n* = 9)
Angiosarcoma	33	–
Rhabdomyosarcoma	21	33
Mesothelioma	16	–
Fibrosarcoma	11	11
Malignant lymphoma	6	–
Osteosarcoma	4	–
Thymoma	3	–
Neurogenic sarcoma	3	11
Other	3	44

PRIMARY BENIGN TUMORS OF THE HEART

Myxoma

Myxomas are the most common primary tumors of the heart and represent 30–50 per cent of all primary cardiac tumors in adults. Any cardiac tumor, particularly a myxoma, may present with systemic manifestations and can be confused with collagen vascular diseases. Signs and symptoms include fever, cachexia, malaise, arthralgias, rash, clubbing, and atrial fibrillation. Laboratory evaluation may indicate elevated sedimentation rate, thrombocytopenia, and circulating antimyocardial antibodies. The systemic constitutional symptoms are thought to result from secretion by the tumor cells of interleukin-6, a cytokine known to be a major promoter of acute-phase response that leads to the activation and amplification of the inflammatory, complement, and clotting cascades. Although originally thought to represent myxomatous degeneration of organized thrombi, most experts recognize atrial myxomas as true neoplasms. Neuroendocrine markers have been identified in over 60 per cent of these tumors, suggesting an endocardial nerve tissue origin.

Myxomatous tumors arise from the endocardium and are often pedunculated, gelatinous, and friable, extending into the cardiac chamber. Embolization of tumor fragments and thrombi from the tumor surface is frequent. Over 80 per cent of myxomas arise from the left atrium, and more than 90 per cent occur as a solitary tumor. Systemic embolization may result in infarction and hemorrhage of viscera, heart, brain, and extremities. These peripheral emboli sometimes mimic and may be confused with the presentation of infectious endocarditis or vasculitis. A biopsy of the skin may demonstrate intravascular tumor emboli. Right-sided tumors can also result in tumor emboli with secondary pulmonary hypertension and, rarely, in cor pulmonale. Pedunculated left atrial myxomas are mobile, with the stalk often originating near the limbus of the fossa ovale. These tumors often prolapse across the orifice of the mitral valve, obstructing flow across the valve orifice and presenting with signs and symptoms of mitral stenosis or insufficiency.

Patients with a myxoma often present with symptoms including dyspnea, orthopnea, paroxysmal nocturnal dyspnea, pulmonary edema, cough, hemoptysis, and fatigue. Typically, symptoms are intermittent in nature and are characteristically elicited or accentuated by change in body position. On physical examination, a loud S_1 is noted, with S_4 (denoting congestive heart failure) and a systolic or diastolic murmur heard best at the apex, consistent with mitral (or tricuspid with right-sided tumors) stenosis or regurgitation. Right atrial tumors frequently present with signs of right heart failure, including peripheral edema, ascites, hepatomegaly, prominent jugular venous pulse a-waves, and murmurs consistent with obstruction to tricuspid valve flow. Familial cardiac myxomas constitute 10 per cent of all myxomas and have an autosomal dominant transmission. The familial myxoma pattern is referred to as *Carney syndrome* and consists of a cluster of symptoms including multiple spotty pigmentation, peripheral myxomas (breast and skin), and endocrine hyperactivity (pigmented adrenocortical disease with Cushing's syndrome, testicular Sertoli cell tumors, or pituitary adenomas).

Lipoma

Lipomas are the second most common primary cardiac tumor occurring in adults. These tumors are often encapsulated and occur in the subendocardium or subepicardium. Subendocardial tumors are frequently located in the interatrial septum. Symptoms result from the specific tumor size and configuration that can cause intracavitary obstruction or rhythm disturbance.

Papillary fibroelastoma

Papillary fibroelastomas are smaller, pedunculated tumors with frond-like projections emanating from a short stalk, which share with myxomas a high incidence (greater than 30 per cent) of systemic embolization, thought to be a consequence of thrombus formation on the tumor surface. They frequently arise from valves (typically the aortic valve) without any associated valve dysfunction or involvement of the papillary muscles, chords, or endocardium.

Rhabdomyoma

Rhabdomyomas are the most common primary cardiac tumors in children and infants. They occur in equal frequency in the right ventricular, left ventricular, and septal myocardium, and they nearly always occur as multiple lesions. These tumors are frequently intracavitary and result in obstructive symptoms. Cardiac rhabdomyomas are frequently associated with tuberous sclerosis, a familial syndrome presenting with diffuse hamartomas, epilepsy, mental retardation, and adenoma sebaceum.

Fibroma

Fibromas are the second most common primary cardiac tumor seen in children. The tumors frequently involve the anterior free wall of the left ventricle and have a biological behavior similar to fibromatous tumors at other sites.

PREOPERATIVE ASSESSMENT

The diagnosis of a primary cardiac tumor is most definitively confirmed by echocardiography, either transthoracic or transesophageal. This technique not only demonstrates the specific lesion, its appearance, size, and location (e.g. chamber, relation to valves, septum), but also gives very important anatomical information to plan the appropriate surgical approach. Occasionally, a magnetic resonance imaging scan or spiral ultrafast computed tomographic scan may be helpful to delineate other associated mediastinal pathology. Lipomas can be further identified by the tumor's characteristic density (Hodenshield units) on magnetic resonance imaging. Definitive diagnosis is made by histology and immunohistochemistry.

The diagnosis of myxoma is confirmed postoperatively by identifying patterns of 'lipidic' cells embedded in myxoid stroma rich in glycosaminoglycans. The histological appearance of a fibroelastoma demonstrates multiple papillary columns with a collagen core surrounded by elastic fibers and endocardial endothelium. Rhabdomyomas are grossly yellow-gray and well circumscribed, and they microscopically differ from normal myocardium by clusters of abnormal large cells, 'spider cells,' with a central cytoplasmic cell, suspended in fine fibrillar processes radiating to the periphery. The cytoplasm is rich in glycogen. These tumors are myocardial hamartomatous malformations rather than true neoplasms. Fibromas are typically encapsulated with a whorled appearance, and they microscopically demonstrate fibroblasts admixed with fibrous tissue and collagen. Lipomas are encapsulated as well and microscopically are composed of mature fat cells admixed with connective tissue and, occasionally, muscle.

OPERATION

Although histologically benign, most cardiac tumors are potentially lethal as a result of intracavitary and valvular obstruction, embolization, or rhythm disturbances. Operative excision is the treatment of choice for most cardiac tumors. Although some rare epicardial tumors can be excised without extracorporeal circulation, the removal of most tumors is done using the heart-lung machine. The major surgical considerations are avoiding manipulation and inadvertent embolization, along with complete excision, while trying to preserve adequate ventricular myocardium, the conduction system and valve function.

Left atrial myxoma

1, 2 A myxoma should be resected with its stalk and with at least a 1-cm portion of surrounding fossa ovale or atrial wall to minimize risk of recurrence from a pretumorous focus. With the patient on full cardiopulmonary bypass using bicaval cannulation, and with the aorta cross-clamped, the left atrium is opened just anterior to the right pulmonary veins. The myxoma is carefully visualized and partially retracted through the atriotomy, exposing its base or stalk, which is resected with a small margin of normal atrial septal tissue or atrial wall. Especially in the case of a myxoma with a broad, sessile base, partial-thickness excision of the septum may be adequate. After excision of the myxoma and repair of the atrial septum or wall is completed, the atrial and ventricular cavities are irrigated to ensure that no residual tumor fragments remain in the heart. The left atriotomy is then closed in the usual fashion, with left-heart deairing maneuvers undertaken as the aortic cross-clamp is removed.

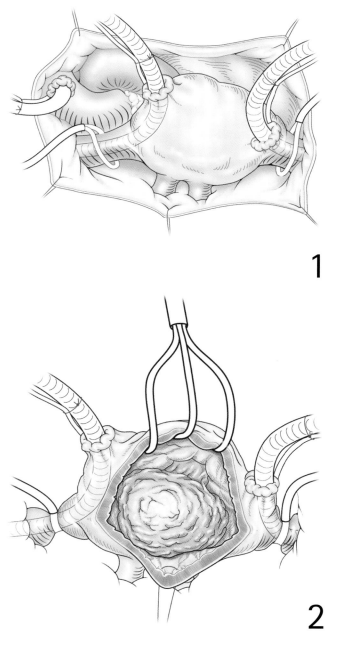

1

2

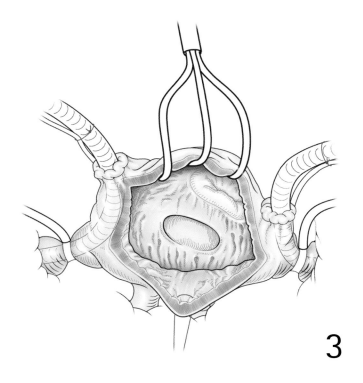

3

3, 4 Alternate exposure for a particularly large left atrial myxoma can be achieved via a right atrial approach. Although this approach facilitates examination of the left atrium for residual tumor fragments and multicentric tumors, the transatrial septal incision may increase the occurrence of postoperative atrial arrhythmias. After establishing full cardiopulmonary bypass, the right atrium is opened and the right atrial cavity carefully examined for tumor involvement. A septal incision is made anterior to the fossa ovalis, and the left atrium is entered. Myxoma excision then proceeds as described previously.

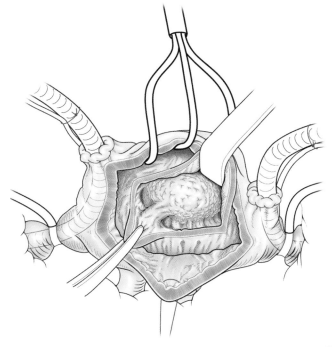

4

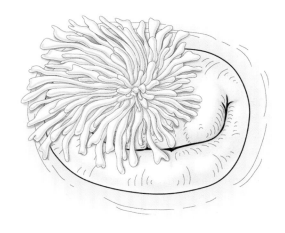

5

Papillary fibroelastoma

5, 6 A papillary fibroelastoma arising on the anterior leaflet of the mitral valve is shown in Figures 5 and 6. This tumor resembles a sea anemone with multiple papillary fronds. As shown, the tumor is attached to the anterior mitral valve leaflet by a relatively short pedicle. After resection of the tumor with a portion of the leaflet, autologous or bovine pericardial patch repair is performed to reconstruct the anterior mitral leaflet.

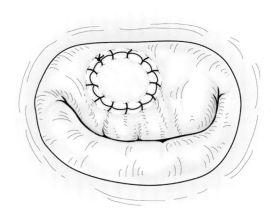

6

MANAGEMENT OF METASTATIC CARDIAC TUMORS

Most metastatic cardiac lesions are clinically silent and detected only at autopsy. Pericardial and cardiac metastases should be suspected, however, if a patient with known malignancy develops a new cardiac murmur, conductions delay, arrhythmia, congestive heart failure, or pericardial effusion. Metastatic disease may have to be differentiated in such patients from the effects of cardiac toxicity secondary to mediastinal radiation and chemotherapeutic agents, such as the anthracycline family of drugs. In addition, a patient with disseminated cancer may present with signs or symptoms of infectious endocarditis, which can occur in these immunosuppressed patients, especially in those with chronic indwelling central intravenous lines.

Cardiac compromise can arise in patients with advanced neoplastic disease for a variety of reasons, including the following:

- Extracardiac direct tumor extension from the lung and mediastinum into the pericardium can lead to pericardial effusion, tamponade, or regional compression of cardiac chambers or coronary vessels. Depending on the degree of pericardial involvement (regional or diffuse), myocardial invasion, and size and/or rapidity of the pericardial effusion, patients may present with either a restrictive or constrictive presentation with exertional dyspnea, tachycardia, cough, and chest pain (with or without evidence of pulsus paradoxus), and clinical signs of tamponade.

- Direct intramyocardial involvement may occur, either focal or diffuse, resulting in arrhythmia or conduction abnormalities.
- The tumor may grow into the cardiac chambers, resulting in obstruction to blood flow as well as systemic embolization. The patient may present with signs of congestive heart failure or vena caval obstruction, with associated facial edema, headaches, prominent venous collateral circulation, hepatic congestion, and peripheral edema.
- The presence of circulating tumor mediators may lead to complications such as hypercoagulability, which can present with nonbacterial thrombotic endocarditis manifesting with embolization in the absence of fever and leukocytosis.

Diagnostic evaluation of metastatic cardiac involvement

Most patients with thoracic and other disseminated malignancies can be evaluated by spiral, ultrafast computed tomography, magnetic resonance imaging, or positron emission tomography scanning, which can demonstrate associated pulmonary and mediastinal pathologies. The diagnosis of secondary cardiac involvement, however, may be best delineated by echocardiography, either transthoracic or transesophageal. This modality not only demonstrates the degree of pericardial and myocardial involvement but also allows for physiological assessment. The diagnosis of metastatic cardiac or pericardial involvement requires definitive confirmation by acquisition of tissue for diagnosis (cytology or biopsy) when appropriate.

Management of metastatic cardiac involvement

Initial treatment of malignant pericardial disease should address any significant hemodynamic compromise caused by a pericardial effusion with cardiac compression. Percutaneous echocardiographic-guided drainage should be effective in ameliorating acute symptoms. Whereas pericardial effusions from lymphomas frequently respond to chemotherapy, those caused by lung cancer usually require surgical drainage, either by a subxyphoid or video-assisted thoracoscopic surgery (anterior thoracotomy or thoracoscopy) approach. Although surgical resection of a solitary cardiac metastasis may prolong survival, the primary goal of surgical intervention for cases in which cardiac compromise is related to intramediastinal metastases is to establish a definitive diagnosis and palliate complications of advanced systemic disease.

OUTCOME

As noted previously, benign primary cardiac tumors rarely recur. Only rarely are myxomas multicentric. Malignant degeneration of myxomas and other benign primary cardiac tumors is very likely. Because progressive enlargement of even benign tumors may result in obstruction or systemic embolization, excision of any intracardiac tumor is recommended. Even complete excision of malignant primary cardiac tumors, sometimes facilitated by explanting the heart as in a transplant cardiectomy with back-table reconstruction, is rarely curative. These very aggressive malignancies may recur locally or metastasize systemically. Prognosis with such neoplasms is poor.

Invasive or metastatic secondary cardiac tumors likewise carry a very poor prognosis. Therapy directed at such malignancies should be diagnostic, and then palliative, in nature.

FURTHER READING

Allard, M.F., et al. 1996. Primary cardiac tumors. In Goldhaber S, and Braunwald, E. (eds) Atlas of Heart Diseases, Philadelphia: Current Medicine 15, 1–15.

Burke, A.P., Virmani, R. 1991. Cardiac rhabdomyoma: a clinicopathologic study. Modern Pathology 4, 70.

Chitwood, W.R. Jr,. 1988. Cardiac neoplasms: current diagnosis, pathology, and therapy. Journal of Cardiac Surgery 3, 119.

Jourdan, M., Bataile, R., Seguin, J., Zhang, X.G., Chaptal, P.A., Klein, B. 1990. Constitutive production of interleukin-6 and immunologic features in cardiac myxomas. Arthritis and Rheumatism 33, 398.

Kriekler, D.M., Rhode J., Davis M.J., et al. 1992. Atrial myxoma: a tumor in search of its origins. British Heart Journal 99, 1203.

Murphy, M.C., Sweeney, M.S., Putnam, J.B. Jr., et al. 1990. Surgical treatment of cardiac tumors: a 25-year experience. Annals of Thoracic Surgery 49, 612.

SECTION VII

Surgery for Congenital Heart Disease

38

The anatomy of congenital cardiac malformations

ROBERT H. ANDERSON BSC, MD, FRCPATH
Joseph Levy Professor of Paediatric Cardiac Morphology, Institute of Child Health, University College, London, United Kingdom

INTRODUCTION

Knowledge of detailed cardiac anatomy is a prerequisite for successful surgery. Nowhere is this more important than in the setting of congenital cardiac malformations. Although the anatomy displayed in these anomalies is often complex, it is not necessarily difficult to understand. In this chapter, the basic rules of cardiac anatomy which permit the surgeon to diagnose and recognize the arrangement of the cardiac chambers at surgery will be described, at the same time providing guidelines to the position of the vital conduction tissues. The basic layout of the heart should, of course, be established prior to commencement of intracardiac procedures. The diagnosis of even the most complex cases demands in the first instance only the distinction, in terms of morphology, of a right atrium from a left atrium, a right ventricle from a left ventricle, and an aorta from a pulmonary trunk. Distinction of these various chambers and vessels then provides the basis of the approach for simple sequential segmental analysis. Obviously, the anatomy of 'holes' and 'stenoses', and so on, are of equal, or even greater, significance, but this morphology will be described in the appropriate chapters. Here we are concerned specifically with setting the 'ground rules' for a systematic approach to cardiac anatomy.

APPROACHES TO THE HEART

When usually arranged, the heart lies in the mediastinum with its apex pointing to the left and two-thirds of its bulk to the left of the midline. An unusual location of the heart should alert the surgeon to the possibility of complex malformations, although these are not always present. When the heart is abnormally located, it is best to describe this finding in simple terms, such as heart mostly in the right chest with the apex pointing to the left, or as appropriate. Whatever its position, the heart and its great vessels can be approached either through the midline anteriorly or via the thoracic cavities.

A median sternotomy is used most frequently. The anterior mediastinum immediately behind the sternum is devoid of vital structures. This tissue plane is reached through separate incisions in the suprasternal notch and beneath the xiphoid process, the two being joined by blunt dissection. Splitting the sternum will then expose the pericardial sack between the pleural cavities. An important structure in this region in the infant is the thymus gland. This gland wraps itself over the anterolateral aspects of the pericardium in the area of the arterial pole. The gland itself is made up of two lateral lobes joined by a midline isthmus, which sometimes must be divided or partially excised to provide adequate exposure. Care must be taken with its arterial supply from the internal thoracic and inferior thyroid arteries. If divided, these arteries may retract beneath the sternum and produce troublesome bleeding. The thymic veins are also a potential problem, being fragile structures which often empty via a common trunk to the left brachiocephalic vein. This vein may be inadvertently damaged by undue traction.

Once the pericardium is exposed via a median sternotomy, access to the heart poses few problems. The vagus and phrenic nerves traverse the length of the pericardium well clear of the operative field, the phrenic nerves anterior and the vagus nerves posterior to the lung hilums, respectively. The phrenic nerves may be vulnerable when the pericardium is harvested for use as an intracardiac patch or baffle. Again, excessive traction on the pericardial cavity is to be avoided, since this can avulse the origin of the pericardiaco-phrenic arteries which accompany the phrenic nerves. The internal thoracic arteries themselves should not be at risk during exposure of the heart via a median sternotomy, but may be damaged when the incision is closed.

Lateral thoracotomies provide exposure either to the heart or great vessels via the pleural spaces. Most frequently these incisions are made in the fourth intercostal space, using the posterior bloodless triangle between the edges of the latissimus dorsi, trapezius and the teres major muscles. The floor of this triangle is the sixth space, but division of the latissimus posteriorly, together with serratus anteriorly, frees the scapula and provides access to the fourth space, which is identified by counting from above.

An incision midway between the ribs avoids the intercostal neurovascular bundle, which is protected beneath the lower margin of the fourth rib. Having entered the pleural space on the left side, retraction of the lung posteriorly exposes the middle mediastinum, with the left thymic lobe overlying the pericardium and the aortic arch with its associated nerves and vessels. If access is needed to the heart, this is usually achieved anterior to the phrenic nerve. More frequently, the aortic isthmus and descending aorta are approached and then the lung is retracted anteriorly, the parietal pleura being divided on its medial aspect posterior to the vagus nerve.

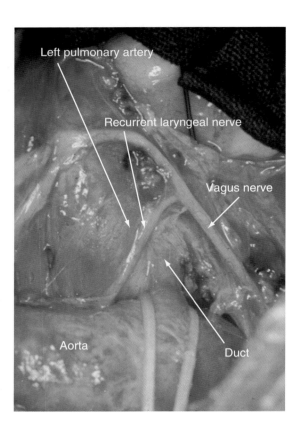

1 An important structure in this area is the left recurrent laryngeal nerve. This nerve takes origin from the vagus and curves round the inferior border of the arterial ligament, or duct if still patent. Excessive traction to the vagus can cause injury to this structure just as readily as direct trauma in the environs of the ligament. The thoracic duct ascends through this area to drain into the left jugular vein at its junction with the internal jugular vein. Accessory lymph channels draining into the duct can be troublesome when dissecting the origin of the left subclavian artery.

A right thoracotomy is performed in similar fashion, reaching the heart via the fifth interspace or the right-sided great vessels through the fourth interspace. When approaching the right pulmonary artery, it is sometimes useful to divide the azygos vein near its junction with the superior caval vein. On the right side, the recurrent laryngeal nerve passes round the subclavian artery as it courses medially from the vagus towards the larynx. Also encircling the artery on this side is the subclavian loop from the sympathetic trunk. Damage to this structure can result in Horner's syndrome.

Surface anatomy of the heart

2 Opening the pericardial cavity reveals the surface of the heart, which almost always is mostly in the left hemithorax with its apex pointing to the left. Important and readily recognizable landmarks enable the nature of the cardiac chambers to be determined with considerable accuracy by external inspection. Attention should first be directed to the atrial appendages. These antero-lateral outpouchings from the atrial chambers usually clasp the arterial pedicle. The finding of both appendages on the same side of the pedicle is itself an anomaly – so-called juxtaposition of the atrial appendages. Left-sided juxtaposition is almost always associated with abnormal connections of the cardiac segments, but right-sided juxtaposition, whilst much rarer, tends to be found with relatively simple malformations such as atrial septal defect. Juxtaposition in itself is a nuisance to the surgeon, since it will necessitate alterations in planning the cannulation, and so on. Juxtaposition can also markedly distort the architecture of atrial anatomy, and can produce problems unless properly recognized. Once recognized, nonetheless, the problems are readily surmountable.

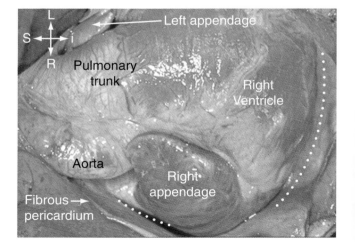

3a, b Having established the position of the appendages, the next step is to establish their morphological nature. When the terms 'right' and 'left' are used in this chapter, they are used to indicate morphology rather than position. Where position is also abnormal, this situation will be indicated separately. The shape of the appendage is a very good means of distinguishing the morphologically right from the morphologically left atrium, with the right appendage having a triangular shape (Figure 3a) in contrast to the tubular left appendage (Figure 3b). The most reliable method to distinguish between the appendages, however, is to examine the nature of their junctions with the remainder of the atrial chambers. The pectinate muscles in the triangular morphologically right appendage extend to the crux of the heart, whereas the morphologically left junction is smooth, with the pectinate muscles confined within the antero-superiorly located tubular appendage. These differences are best appreciated by inspection of the isolated heart but can easily be seen at straightforward surgical inspection. In most instances, the triangular appendage is right-sided, and the narrow, tubular, appendage is left-sided. This arrangement is the usual, so-called 'situs solitus'. Rarely, the tubular appendage is right-sided and the triangular one is left-sided. This situation is the mirror-image, or 'inverted', arrangement. It is better to describe mirror-imagery than 'inversus' because the appendages themselves are not turned upside down. More frequently, when the heart is complexly malformed, an arrangement will be found in which the appendages have comparable morphology.

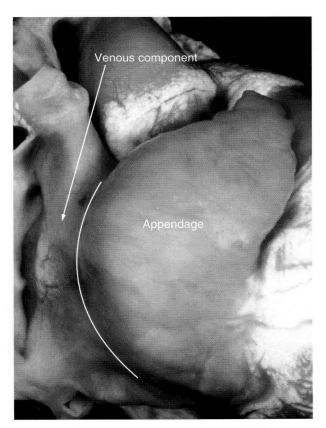

3a

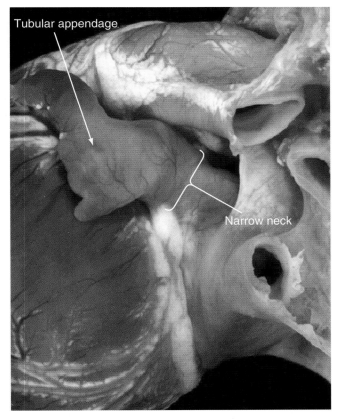

3b

4 Then, either each appendage is broad and triangular, with pectinate muscles extending all round the atrioventricular vestibules, or else each is tubular and narrow, with bilaterally smooth vestibules. The syndromes associated with this arrangement, which is one of isomerism, are also known as the 'splenic syndromes', or visceral heterotaxy. Interest in these constellations has usually been the province of the pathologist but, by the simple expedient of inspecting the appendages, the surgeon has the means of diagnosing these entities during life. This permits drawing all the inferences that go with the recognition of right isomerism ('asplenia'), or left isomerism ('polysplenia').

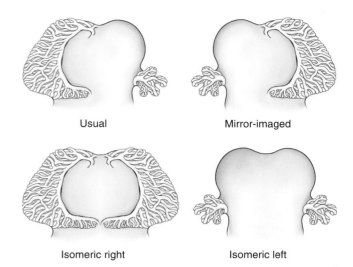

Usual   Mirror-imaged

Isomeric right   Isomeric left

4

5 While inspecting the appendages, the surgeon will at the same time examine their junctions with the venous components of the atriums. Here again, a vital difference exists between morphologically right and left sides. The right junction is the extensive terminal groove, marking the site of the terminal crest internally. Lying in the terminal groove, in an immediate subendocardial position, and usually lateral to the crest of the atrial appendage, is the sinus node. The left junction is not marked by any such prominent groove, and no conduction tissue is present at this junction. These findings complement the information gained from the location of the appendages. Thus, with the usual arrangement, the sinus node is right-sided, whereas in the setting of mirror-imagery, the node is a left-sided structure. In right isomerism, sinus nodes are present bilaterally, but in left isomerism the sinus node is hypoplastic and abnormally positioned, being variously located in the posterior atrial wall close to the atrioventricular junction.

Inspection of the appendages should lead attention directly to the venoatrial connections. Here, the important features to note are abnormal connections of either the pulmonary or the caval veins. Search should be made for a persistent left superior caval vein between the left appendage and the left pulmonary veins, while the finding of left isomerism should always alert the surgeon to the likelihood that the inferior caval vein is interrupted, being continued via the azygos or hemiazygos veins, which would be correspondingly enlarged.

Considerable information also can be derived from external inspection concerning the ventricular arrangement. Here, it is the descending branches of the coronary arteries that are the guide. In the usual situation, the anterior descending interventricular coronary artery, in reality a superior structure, arises from the main stem of the left coronary artery. It descends close to the obtuse margin of the ventricular mass.

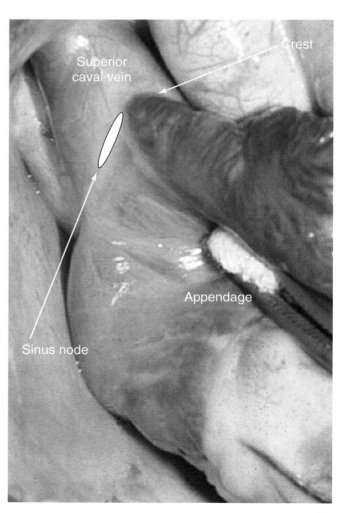

Superior caval vein

Crest

Appendage

Sinus node

5

When this anterior interventricular artery arises from the right-sided coronary artery, then almost always a mirror-imaged ventricular arrangement is present, with the left ventricle found on the right side. The precise connections between the atriums and ventricles will depend on the arrangement of the atrial appendages, but this coronary arterial pattern should alert the surgeon to the potential presence of congenitally corrected transposition (see below). The other abnormal arrangement of the coronary arteries to be sought by inspection is the presence of two 'delimiting' arteries on the anterior surface of the ventricular mass, rather than prominent interventricular arteries on the obtuse and diaphragmatic surfaces. This situation indicates a disproportion between the sizes of the ventricles. Usually, this finding suggests the presence of a dominant left ventricle and a small, rudimentary, right ventricle, such as is found in double inlet left ventricle or tricuspid atresia. Alternatively, absence of prominent interventricular arteries on the anterior ventricular surface should raise the suspicion of a solitary indeterminate ventricular chamber, or else a dominant right ventricle with a postero-inferior rudimentary left ventricle. The latter will be revealed by inspection of the diaphragmatic surface.

The final feature to be inspected, which will usually be studied at the same time as the ventricular mass, is the relationship of the arterial trunks. The first step is to confirm the presence of separate aortic and pulmonary trunks as opposed to a common trunk. When separate trunks are found, then almost always the aortic trunk is posterior and right-sided, with the pulmonary trunk spiralling around the aorta as it divides into right and left pulmonary arteries. Abnormal relationships of the great arterial trunks almost always indicate intracardiac malformations, but the connections of the cardiac chambers cannot be inferred from these abnormal relationships. At best, the anomalous arterial positions raise the suspicion of a given lesion. Most frequently, an anterior and right-sided aorta is found with discordant ventriculo-arterial connections, but can also be found with double outlet right ventricle. An anterior and left-sided aorta suggests congenitally corrected transposition, but it, too, can be found with double outlet right ventricle or, rarely, with concordant

atrioventricular and ventriculoarterial connections – so-called 'anatomically corrected malposition'. In similar fashion, it cannot be presumed that the ventriculo-arterial connections are normal simply because the arterial trunks are 'normally related'. Often there are 'normal' spiralling arterial relationships in the presence of double outlet right ventricle, and rarely this arrangement can be found when the arterial trunks are discordantly connected.

ANATOMY OF THE CARDIAC CHAMBERS

In the previous section, emphasis has been placed on the recognition of the morphology of the different chambers, whilst stressing also that these chambers are not always in their usual position, nor connected to their anticipated neighbors. Each chamber, nonetheless, has a relatively constant anatomy irrespective of its position or its connections, although subtle changes in morphology are found when the chambers are connected together in abnormal fashion. In this section, it is the anticipated normal morphology which receives attention, with additional remarks concerning abnormal structure where pertinent.

The right atrium

The right atrium has its extensive triangular appendage separated from the systemic venous sinus by the terminal groove (white line in Figure 3a). As usually seen by the surgeon, the superior caval vein enters the left-hand side, and the inferior caval vein the right-hand side, of the sleeve-like sinus, which is separated inferiorly by the interatrial groove from the right pulmonary veins. This groove, known also as Waterston's, or Sondergaard's, groove, is the extensive interatrial gulley produced by the deep infolding of the right and left atrial walls. As discussed above, the terminal groove is a vital surgical landmark, since immediately beneath its epicardial surface lies the sinus node.

6 Opening the right atrium with the freedom permitted the morphologist reveals the extensive terminal crest which underlies the groove (Figure 6 – anatomical position). This muscular crest swings round the orifices of both the superior and inferior caval veins. An extension from the inferior end of the terminal crest runs anteriorly towards the atrial septum, striking towards the vestibule of the tricuspid valve. This muscular ridge separates the orifice of the inferior caval vein from the mouth of the coronary sinus. Extending from it, as opposing sickle-shaped folds of varying dimensions, are the remnants of the Eustachian and Thebesian valves, which guard the venous orifices. The valves themselves are of varying dimensions in different hearts. Of more surgical significance is the fibrous commissure of these two valves, which buries itself in the musculature between the coronary sinus and the oval fossa and runs toward the left-hand margin of the tricuspid vestibule. This important structure is the tendon of Todaro, which forms one boundary of the triangle of Koch (see below).

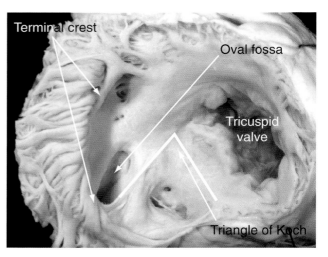

6

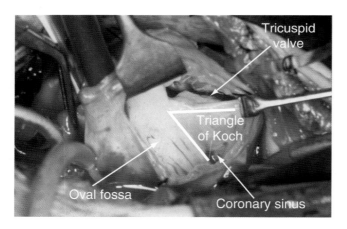

7

7 As seen by the surgeon, an extensive pouch is present above the orifice of the coronary sinus, located between the sinus, the hinge of the tricuspid valve, and the infero-anterior extension of the terminal crest. This sinus is the so-called sub-Eustachian, in reality sub-Thebesian with the heart viewed anatomically. A triangular area is then formed, with the sub-Eustachian sinus as its base. Its inferior border, as viewed in the operating room, is the site of the tendon of Todaro, and its superior border is the site of annular attachment of the septal leaflet of the tricuspid valve. This vital area is the triangle of Koch. The atrioventricular node is entirely contained within its confines, and the atrioventricular bundle penetrates towards the left ventricular outflow tract at its apex.

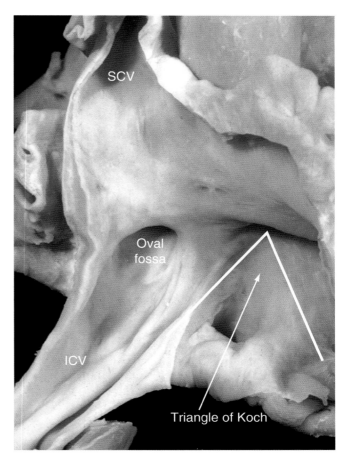

8a

8a, b
Between the triangle of Koch and the orifice of the superior caval vein (SCV) is the right atrial surface of the oval fossa. At first sight, this entire surface gives the impression of being interposed between the right and left atriums (Figure 8a). Sectioning shows that this is not the case (Figure 8b). The true septal area is confined to the floor of the fossa and its antero-inferior margin. The extensive mound to the left-hand side of the fossa as viewed by the surgeon is the atrial wall overlying the aortic root. The rim between the fossa and the superior caval orifice, seen in inferior position by the surgeon, is no more than the infolded walls of the interatrial groove. The right-hand margin is the wall of the inferior caval vein (ICV). The inferior margin, seen superiorly by the surgeon, is the tissue separating the fossa from the coronary sinus, which becomes continuous with the floor of the triangle of Koch.

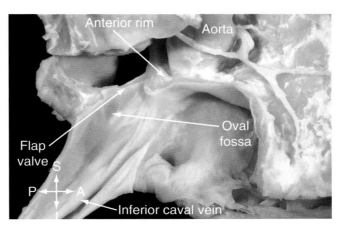

8b

The left atrium

9 The proportions of the left atrium formed by appendage and venous component are reversed compared to the right atrium, and overall the left atrium has a much simpler structure. The venous component, located posteriorly, receives the four pulmonary veins, one at each corner. This component leads directly into the anteriorly positioned mitral vestibule. As seen by the surgeon entering through the atrial roof, the narrow opening of the tubular appendage is to the left hand, while the septal surface is to the right. The sweep of muscular tissue above the mitral vestibule is the extensive anterior atrial wall related to the aortic root. The smooth inferior and posterior margin of the mitral vestibule overlies the coronary sinus as it runs round from the obtuse margin of the ventricular mass. The septal surface of the left atrium is much simpler than the right, being formed by the flap valve of the oval fossa. The left atrium also has a body of significant size, a fact that can be deduced from examination of hearts from patients having totally anomalous pulmonary venous connection. In these hearts, in which the left atrium lacks its pulmonary venous component, a substantial part of the chamber still cannot be accounted for in terms of the appendage, the vestibular, and the septum. This part is the atrial body.

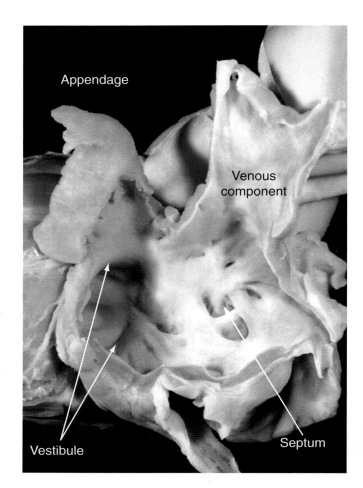

9

The atrioventricular junctions

The surgeon will never see the entirety of the atrioventricular junctions, although at different times he or she will be concerned with their various parts. Knowledge of the junctions in their entirety, nonetheless, is fundamental to the proper understanding of several congenital anomalies, particularly atrioventricular septal defects in the setting of common atrioventricular junctions.

10 In this section, therefore, the detailed anatomy of the entire junctions will be presented. This anatomy is best appreciated by removing the atrial chambers and great arteries from the ventricular base, and viewing it from the superior aspect as in Figure 10. The dominant feature is the 'wedged' position of the aortic valve. Equally significant is the oblique orientation of the mitral and tricuspid valvar orifices relative to the aortic root. Although we usually speak of the valvar annuluses, none of the four cardiac valves has a true and complete fibrous ring which supports its leaflets. The mitral annulus approximates most closely to the concept of a ring. In its parietal component, nonetheless, it is often the case that very little collagenous tissue supports the mural leaflet of the valve and, at the same time, separates the atrial and ventricular myocardial masses. In the tricuspid orifice, furthermore, a collagenous annulus is rarely found. Indeed, usually it is the fibro-fatty tissues of the atrioventricular groove which separate the right atrial muscle from the ventricular mass. When the arterial valves are considered, then the concept of a 'ring' becomes totally deficient. Rather, each of the semilunar valvar leaflets is attached in part to the arterial sinuses, and in part to the underlying ventricular structures. The subarterial roots are, therefore, formed in the shape of coronets, tenting up in the areas of attachment to the sinotubular junction, and sweeping down to the nadir of the attachments to the ventricular bases. These attachments in the pulmonary 'ring' are exclusively to right ventricular muscle – the free-standing subpulmonary infundibulum. In the case of the aortic valve, a good half of the circumference of the leaflets is supported by, and attached to, fibrous and collagenous tissues.

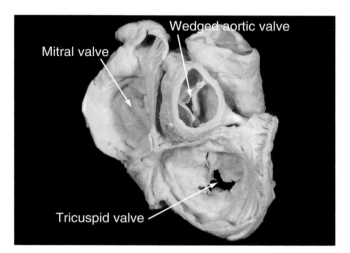

10

11 As a consequence of its wedged position, the aortic valve is in extensive fibrous continuity with the leaflets of both the mitral and tricuspid valves. The entirety of the aortic, or 'anterior', leaflet of the mitral valve is in fibrous continuity with two of the leaflets of the aortic valve (white line in Figure 11). For this reason alone, this leaflet of the mitral valve is best termed the aortic leaflet, differentiating it in this way from the mural leaflet. The two ends of the region of aortic-mitral valvar continuity are thickened to form the right and left fibrous trigones, respectively.

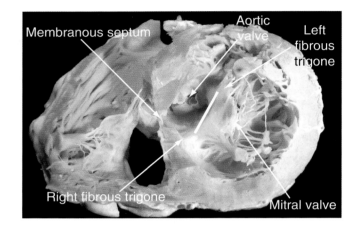

11

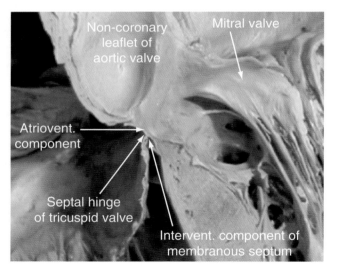

12

12 The right fibrous trigone is itself an integral part of the fibrous mass where the aortic root is continuous with the leaflets of the tricuspid valve. This whole area is usually called the central fibrous body. The part between the aortic root and the right side of the heart is the so-called membranous septum. This septum forms the medial wall of the subaortic outflow tract immediately beneath the zone of apposition between the right coronary and non-coronary leaflets of the aortic valve. Examination of long-axis sections taken at right angles to the septum through this region show that the leaflet of the tricuspid valve is attached to the right-sided aspect of this area. This attachment of the tricuspid valve divides the membranous septum into its atrioventricular and interventricular components (see arrows in Figure 14).

13 The obliquity of the mitral and tricuspid valvar orifices relative to each other is responsible for the unusual morphology of the muscular area immediately behind the central fibrous body. This area is the floor of the triangle of Koch (see above). Careful dissection of the region shows how the wedged aortic outflow tract 'lifts' the aortic leaflet of the mitral valve away from the muscular ventricular septum. Because of this, the two atrioventricular valves are attached to opposite sides of the septum, or 'facing' each other over only a short distance. In this short 'facing' area, the tricuspid valve is attached to the septum more towards the ventricular apex than is the mitral valve. By virtue of these differential levels of attachment (arrows in Figure 13), part of the ventricular septum interposes between the left ventricle and the right atrium, albeit with right atrial musculature on its atrial face. This area has previously been termed the 'atrioventricular muscular septum'. In reality, an extension of the fibrofatty inferior atrioventricular groove separates the atrial and ventricular musculatures between the valvar hinges, so that the area is better likened to a sandwich rather than a septum. Irrespective of such niceties, the area is short and shallow, because almost immediately inferior to the aortic root the two atrioventricular orifices diverge away from each other, the inferior 'swing' of the tricuspid orifice being more marked than that of the mitral valve. In this inferior bay the coronary sinus opens to the right atrium, having traversed the posterior and inferior aspect of the left atrioventricular junction.

The atrioventricular muscular sandwich is of particular importance to the surgeon because its atrial component contains the atrioventricular node. The cross-sectional cut (Figure 13) shows the oblique nature of the atrioventricular junction at this site. The atrioventricular node lies on the sloping atrial aspect of this junction. From the left atrial aspect, this point is marked by the inferomedial attachment of the zone of apposition of the leaflets of the mitral valve. By virtue of the extensive postero-inferior diverticulum of the aortic root, the atrioventricular bundle, having penetrated through the central fibrous body, passes directly into the left ventricular outflow tract. From the standpoint of the subaortic root, the landmark to the point of penetration is the zone of apposition between the right and non-coronary aortic valvar leaflets. Thus, the landmarks of the triangle of Koch delineate the site of the specialized atrioventricular junction as seen from the right atrium. Seen from the left atrium, it is the posteromedial attachment of the leaflets of the mitral valve which points to the danger area.

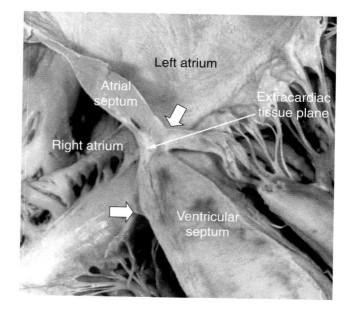

13

14 From the aorta, the junction of the non-coronary and right coronary valvar leaflets indicates the danger area. When seen from the right ventricle, it is the area immediately adjacent to the medial papillary muscle and the zone of apposition between the septal and antero-superior leaflets of the tricuspid valve that must be avoided.

Examination of the dissected atrioventricular junctions reveals other features of note. The encircling branches of the coronary arteries are an integral part of the junctions (see Figure 10). The right coronary artery has an extensive junctional course. In its first few centimetres or so, it lies directly within the inner curvature of the heart. The right margin of the ventriculoinfundibular fold, when viewed from the right ventricle, is seen as the supraventricular crest. The left coronary artery emerges into the inner curvature, and then immediately branches into its anterior descending and circumflex branches. The anterior descending branch immediately moves out of the junction to become interventricular. The circumflex artery, in contrast, becomes an integral part of the left junction. The extent of its intimate relationship to the junction varies markedly from heart to heart. Most frequently, it fades out at the obtuse margin, and the right coronary artery extends across the crux to supply the diaphragmatic surface of the left ventricle. In other cases, the right coronary turns down at the crux to become the posterior, or inferior, interventricular artery, while the circumflex artery supplies the diaphragmatic surface of the left ventricle. Least frequently, the circumflex artery supplies the diaphragmatic region, and continues to become the posterior interventricular artery. This highly significant variability cannot be expressed simply in terms of right and left 'dominance' of the coronary arteries. Instead, it is necessary to specify separately the origins of the posterior interventricular coronary artery, and the nature of the arteries that supply the diaphragmatic surface of the left ventricle.

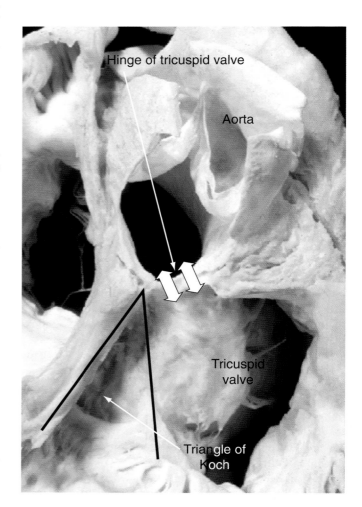

14

The right ventricle

Before going into specifics of ventricular morphology, a few remarks concerning ventricular division and valvar morphology are appropriate. Traditionally, ventricles have been divided simply into inlet and outlet parts, or sinus and conus, respectively. For the normal heart, this convention is adequate, although less than ideal. When abnormal hearts are considered, its deficiencies are soon evident. The incomplete and rudimentary right ventricle seen in tricuspid atresia, for example, lacks an inlet component. Nevertheless, it is unequivocally recognized as a right ventricle, because of the presence of the 'sinus' component. In tricuspid atresia, therefore, according to conventional wisdom, the 'sinus' is not the same thing as the ventricular inlet.

15a, b This potential controversy can be circumvented by assessing the ventricle from a different viewpoint. In terms of descriptive morphology, each ventricle can be considered to possess three rather than two components, namely the inlet, apical trabecular, and outlet portions. All ventricles, no matter how deformed, are readily described using this tripartite convention. Figure 15a shows these three components in the right ventricle, whilst the three components in the left ventricle are shown in Figure 15b. For instance, the problematic incomplete and rudimentary right ventricle in tricuspid atresia possesses outlet and apical trabecular components. It lacks its inlet portion.

When considering valvar morphology, it is important to have a convention which enables leaflets to be distinguished from one another, and from so-called 'scallops'. The best way of distinguishing between the leaflets is to view the valve in its closed position. This orientation permits recognition of the zones of apposition between adjacent leaflets. Such an approach is much better than taking as the criterion of division between leaflets the presence of a commissural cord arising from a prominent and easily recognized papillary muscle. It can be impossible to distinguish morphologically such 'commissural' cords from so-called 'cleft' cords – hence the problem of determining whether the mitral valve has two, four, or more leaflets. When viewed from the stance of the closed valve, no question exists that the mitral valve possesses two leaflets with a solitary zone of apposition between them. In similar fashion, the tricuspid valve closes in trifoliate fashion and, therefore, possesses three leaflets. The leaflets within the orifice of the tricuspid valve are located septally, anterosuperiorly, and inferiorly.

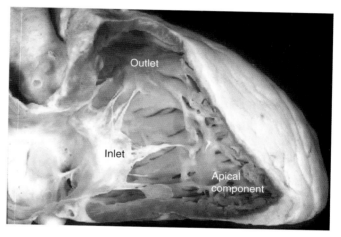

15a

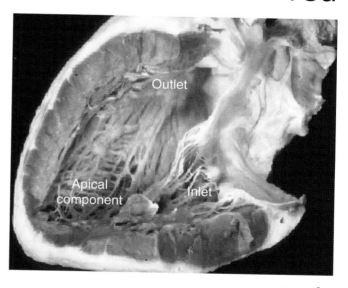

15b

16 Returning now to the right ventricle, this chamber, when normally constituted, possesses the tricuspid valve in its inlet portion. Its three leaflets are readily seen by the surgeon from the right atrium although Figure 16 shows the valve as seen from its ventricular aspect. The peripheral attachment of the zone of apposition between the septal and antero-superior leaflets, supported by the medial papillary muscle, is 'round the corner' from the area of the membranous septum. Often the septal leaflet is itself cloven to the level of the membranous septum. This area is intimately related to the site of penetration of the atrioventricular bundle.

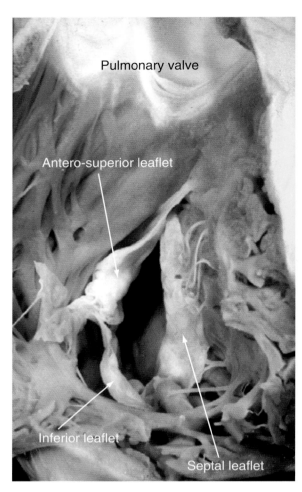

16

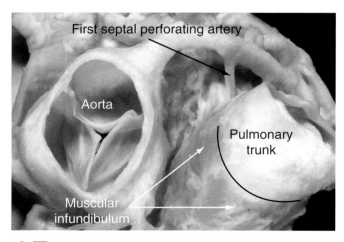

17

17 The apical trabecular component of the right ventricle has typically coarse trabeculations (see Figure 15a). It is on the basis of the nature of the apical trabeculations that the ventricle is most reliably differentiated from a left ventricle. Extending upwards and leftwards from the apical trabecular component is the outlet portion, supporting the leaflets of the pulmonary valve. In the normal right ventricle, this outlet component is a free-standing muscular sleeve. (The black line indicates the junction between the infundibular musculature of the right ventricle and the wall of the pulmonary trunk). The presence of this infundibulum provides another very characteristic feature of the right ventricle, namely, the muscular supraventricular crest which separates the attachments of the leaflets of the tricuspid and pulmonary valves. As can be appreciated from study of the atrioventricular junctions (see Figure 10), this apparently extensive muscle bundle as seen from inside the ventricle is no more than the inner aspect of the parietal ventricular wall. In other words, it is the ventriculoinfundibular fold.

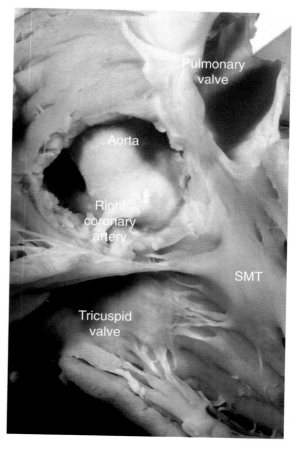

18 This observation is readily confirmed by dissection which, at the same time, shows the important relationship of the right coronary artery to the muscular fold. One further very characteristic anatomical feature of the right ventricle is the extensive septal muscle bundle which runs down into the apical trabecular component, then splitting into its various trabeculations, including the moderator band, the anterior papillary muscle, and various septoparietal trabeculations. The basal part of this prominent bundle itself divides into two limbs which embrace the supraventricular crest. The posterior of these two limbs gives rise to the medial papillary muscle, while the anterior limb runs up to the pulmonary valve.

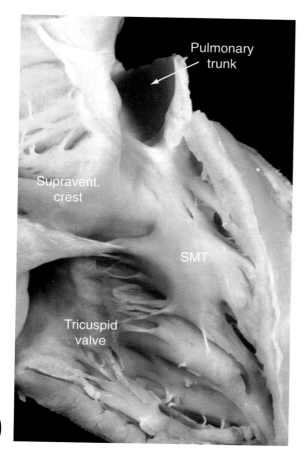

19 The extensive bundle is considered as part of the supraventricular crest. Because of this, it is frequently called the 'septal band'. Even the most cursory examination shows that this structure cannot, at the same time, be both septal and supraventricular. It is better to distinguish this important structure as the septomarginal trabeculation (SMT) distinguishing it in this way from both the ventriculoinfundibular fold, which forms the supraventricular crest, and from the outlet component of the ventricular septum. In the normal heart, in fact, it is not possible with certainty to distinguish the precise location of that small part of the muscular septum which interposes directly between the subaortic and subpulmonary outlet components. Although not directly visible, it is located between the two limbs of the septomarginal trabeculation. The atrioventricular conduction axis branches in relation to the posterior limb of the septomarginal trabeculation, but on the left ventricular aspect of the septum. The right bundle branch then penetrates through the septum, and surfaces beneath the medial papillary muscle. It then runs down towards the apex either on the surface of, or embedded within, the body of the septomarginal trabeculation.

The left ventricle

20a, b As with the right ventricle, the left ventricle can readily be divided into inlet, apical trabecular, and outlet components (see Figure 15b). The inlet component contains the mitral valve. When viewed from the atrial aspect, the ends of the solitary zone of apposition between the aortic and mural leaflets are in superolateral and inferomedial position (arrows in Figure 20a). By virtue of this position, the two leaflets themselves have grossly dissimilar annular attachments. The aortic leaflet has a relatively short attachment, guarding only about one-third of the circumference. As seen in the open valve, this leaflet has considerable depth, and is a well-defined sail-like structure (Figure 20b). In contrast, the mural leaflet, although having a much more extensive annular attachment, has much less depth, and is more curtain-like. In most hearts, this mural leaflet is further divided into a series of 'scallops'. Usually, three such scallops are present, but five or even six may be seen on occasion. The overall result of these dissimilar arrangements is that the two leaflets have more or less equal surface area. As discussed in the section on the atrioventricular junctions, it is the area around the inferomedial end of the zone of apposition which is related to the site of penetration of the atrioventricular bundle.

The apical trabecular component of the left ventricle is characterized by particularly fine trabeculations. The apex of the ventricle itself is remarkably thin, with often no more than 1 mm of myocardium between the epicardial and endocardial surfaces at this point. Unlike the right ventricle, the trabecular component of the left ventricle has a smooth septal surface, down which cascades the fan-like left bundle branch. The initial portion of the fan is an undivided fascicle; but having descended about one-third of the septum, the bundle divides into its interconnected anterior, septal, and posterior divisions.

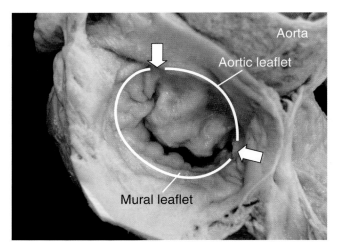

20a

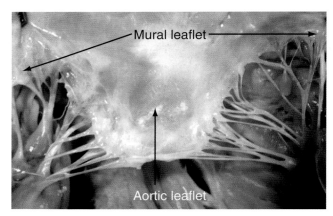

20b

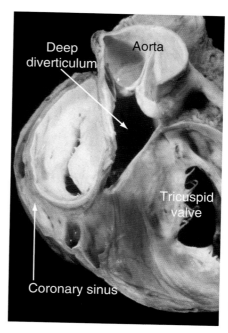

21a, b Although not a completely muscular structure as in the right ventricle, the outlet portion is well formed in the left ventricle. It has a particularly prominent deep infero-posterior diverticulum (Figure 21a). The outlet does not have completely muscular walls because of the fibrous continuity between the aortic and mitral valves, the ventriculoinfundibular fold being eradicated in this area (see Figure 10). The significant surgical feature of this area, in addition to the fact that the infero-posterior diverticulum is related to a considerable area of the right atrium, is the coronet-like attachment of the aortic valve leaflets (Figure 21b: RC, right coronary; LC, left coronary; NC, non-coronary). Thus, at the apexes of the zones of apposition between the leaflets, the aortic outflow tract is directly related to such structures as the anterior wall of the left atrium and the transverse sinus. Further important features are the descent over the midseptal surface of the outflow tract of the left bundle branch (arrow in Figure 21b), and the origin of the coronary arteries from two of the aortic sinuses. All of these features are highly significant when planning operations to enlarge the aortic root.

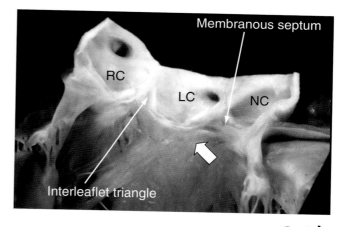

SEQUENTIAL SEGMENTAL ANALYSIS OF CONGENITAL HEART DISEASE

In the preceding paragraphs, the basic morphology of the cardiac chambers has been described, and I have indicated how it may be recognized by the surgeon. At the same time, I have emphasized how the basic disposition of the conduction tissues is dictated by this morphology. Thus far, anatomy has been considered mostly in the setting of the normal heart. Almost all patients with congenital cardiac lesions undergoing surgery will have these malformations in the setting of the normal heart. For example, persistent patency of the arterial duct, or a simple aortic coarctation, in no way alters the basic cardiac morphology. Similarly, the presence of simple atrial or ventricular septal defects, or even an atrioventricular septal defect with common atrioventricular junction, does not distort the basic arrangement to such an extent that the heart is not readily recognized as being normal. In a few cases, nonetheless, the anatomy can be exceedingly bizarre, often with the heart itself being abnormally positioned. Even in these complex cases, understanding can be simply achieved if attention is paid to the principles established in the previous paragraphs. The ways in which the atrial chambers themselves can be arranged are strictly limited, as are the ways in which the atrial chambers can connect to the ventricles, and the ventricles in turn connect to the great arteries. This chapter will be concluded, therefore, with a brief description of the principles and philosophy of sequential segmental analysis, concentrating once more on the vital information provided by these principles concerning the distribution of the atrioventricular conduction tissues.

Philosophy of sequential segmental analysis

When describing any given congenital cardiac malformation, it is necessary to account separately for the features of the morphology of the individual cardiac segments, the connections of the segments to each other, and the interrelationships of the chambers within each segment. It does not particularly matter how each of these features is described, provided that each is accounted for using mutually exclusive terms. A variety of terms have been used for this purpose, but the value of using simple everyday words in description has been appreciated, rather than having a vocabulary deeply rooted in classical etymology. The essential morphological features of each of the cardiac chambers have been described, but it is necessary to decide which of these features is taken as the final arbiter for identification of a given chamber. In this respect, it is best to follow the so-called 'morphological method'. This states that chambers, however deformed or abnormal, should always be identifiable in terms of their own intrinisic characteristics. This system means, for example, that venous connections cannot be used to identify an atrium, since the veins themselves may connect anomalously. An atrioventricular valve cannot be used as the final arbiter of the nature of a ventricle because some ventricles do not possess atrioventricular valves. Thus, the morphology of the atrial appendages turns out to be the most reliable feature for atrial recognition. For the ventricles, it is the nature of the apical trabeculations

which is most useful. The great arteries have no intrinsic features which permit their recognition, but almost always their patterns of branching are sufficiently discrete to permit distinction of an aorta from a pulmonary trunk, and a common trunk from a solitary arterial trunk. For full description, it is necessary to account separately for connections and relations. Ideally, each element should have equal weight in description. Practically, the surgeon is most concerned with the way the cardiac components are joined together. In this account, therefore, it is the connections between the parts that are given the pre-eminent position, with relationships relegated to a secondary role.

Atrial arrangement

The importance of inspecting the morphology of the atrial appendages has already been stressed, and the possible variations have received attention. Recognition of the arrangement of the appendages is doubly important in sequential analysis, since the remainder of the heart cannot be described adequately without knowledge of the morphology of the atrial segment. Only four ways exist in which the atrial appendages can be arranged (Figure 5). In the first two patterns, morphologically right and morphologically left appendages are both present. These two arrangements are lateralized. When the right appendage is right-sided, this usual arrangement is often called 'solitus'. When the right appendage is left-sided, then a mirror-image arrangement is frequently called 'inversus', despite the fact that the atriums are not upside down. The other two patterns are found when each appendage has comparable morphology, or in other words the two appendages are isomeric. Right isomerism then describes the existence of two appendages each having right morphology, while left isomerism exists when each appendage has left morphology. As discussed above, the disposition of the sinus node is dictated by the morphology of the atrial appendages, hence the importance of the surgeon of recognizing the isomeric arrangements.

Atrioventricular junctions

22 Analysis of the atrioventricular junctions demands knowledge of the nature of both the atrial appendages and the ventricular chambers. It is necessary to determine first, how the atriums are connected to the ventricles and, second, the morphology of the atrioventricular valves which guard the atrioventricular junctions. When each atrium connects to its own separate ventricle, then there are biventricular atrioventricular connections. This situation can occur either with lateralized or isomeric atrial appendages. With lateralized appendages, there are then two possibilities, which can exist either when the appendages themselves are usually arranged or mirror-imaged. The first is when the right atrium connects to the right ventricle, and the left atrium to the left ventricle. This gives concordant atrioventricular connections. The second is when the right atrium connects to the left ventricle, and the left atrium to the right ventricle. This situation produces discordant connections.

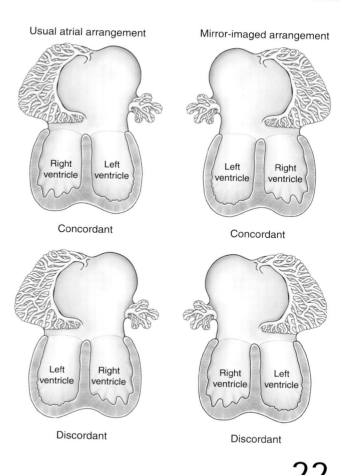

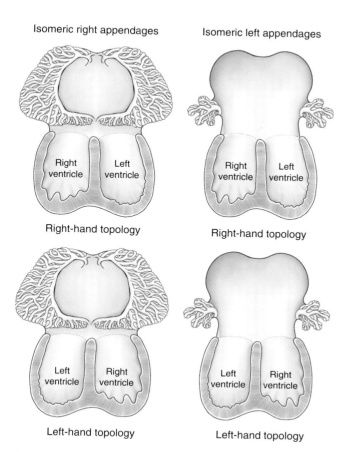

23 When the appendages are isomeric, then whatever the arrangement of the ventricles, the atrioventricular connections must perforce be ambiguous. In this situation, the topological arrangement of the ventricular mass is of vital importance.

22

23

24 Only two basic patterns of ventricular architecture exist. The usual pattern is seen in the normal heart with usual atrial arrangement and concordant atrioventricular connections. The right ventricle more-or-less wraps itself round the left ventricle in such a way that, figuratively speaking, the palmar surface of only the observer's right hand can be placed on the septal surface with the thumb in the inlet, the wrist in the apex, and fingers in the outlet. This arrangement, therefore, can be described as right-hand topology (Figure 24a). The second basic pattern is typically seen in the heart with usually arranged atrial appendages, but with discordant atrioventricular connections. It is also seen in the situation of mirror-imaged atrial arrangement and concordant atrioventricular connections (Figure 24b). With this topological arrangement, only the left hand can be placed upon the right ventricular septal surface, hence left-hand topology (Figure 24b).

Either of these two topological arrangements can exist with either right or left isomerism (Figure 23), and must be described so as to provide full categorization. This knowledge is important, because the topological arrangement dictates the disposition of the conduction tissues when biventricular atrioventricular connections are ambiguous (see below). Almost without exception, in patients with lateralized atrial appendages the ventricular topology is harmonious with the atrioventricular connections. Usually, the ventricular relationships are also as expected, with the right ventricle to the right with right-hand topology, and right ventricle to the left with left-hand topology. Sometimes, however, the ventricular relationships may be unexpected because of either rotation or tilting of the ventricular mass around its long axis. Such rotation or tilting produces the so-called 'criss-cross' or 'upstairs-downstairs' hearts. Providing that relations are described, and identified separately from connections and topology, these hearts should not give problems either in diagnosis or description.

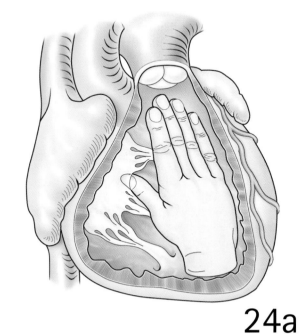

24a

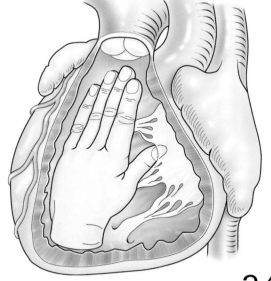

24b

25 A second group of hearts is different from those with biventricular connections. In this group, the atriums connect only to one ventricle, or in other words the hearts have a univentricular atrioventricular connection. These hearts can exist with either lateralized or isomeric atrial appendages. The specific connections to be found in the hearts making up this group are double inlet ventricle, together with absence of either the right or the left atrioventricular connection. These univentricular connections can be found when the atriums are connected to a dominant left ventricle, a dominant right ventricle, or to a solitary and indeterminate ventricle. Almost always when a univentricular connection to either a dominant left or a right ventricle exists, the complementary ventricle is present in hypoplastic and rudimentary form because it lacks at least its inlet portion. Rudimentary right ventricles, found with univentricular connection to a dominant left ventricle, are always in antero-superior position, although they may either be right-sided or left-sided. Rudimentary left ventricles, found with univentricular connection to a dominant right ventricle, are always posteroinferior, but again may be either right- or left-sided. By arguing from developmental principles, it is possible to account for the position of rudimentary and incomplete ventricles in terms of right-hand and left-hand topologic patterns. It is much simpler just to describe the position of the rudimentary ventricle using anterior/posterior, superior/

inferior and right/left coordinates. Solitary and indeterminate ventricles do not possess second rudimentary ventricles. Self-evidently, only these solitary ventricles, in morphological terms, are 'single ventricles', or 'univentricular hearts'.

The so-called mode of atrioventricular connection simply describes the arrangement of the atrioventricular valves. When concordant, discordant, ambiguous and double inlet connections exist, then both atriums are connected with the ventricular mass. The dual atrioventricular junctions can be guarded by two separate valves, or by a common atrioventricular valve. One of two valves, or rarely both, may straddle the ventricular septum when the tension apparatus is attached on both sides of the septum. When a valve straddles, then usually its junction also overrides the septum. The degree of this override determines the commitment of the valve to the two ventricles. It is well known that spectrums of degrees of override exist with different segmental combinations. These extend from the hearts having effectively biventricular to effectively univentricular atrioventricular connections. For the purposes of categorization of the precise connection in such hearts, in other words double inlet versus biventricular connections, the overriding valve is assigned to the ventricle connected to its greater part, the so-called '50 per cent law'. Common valves usually straddle, but not always. For instance, a common valve in the presence of double inlet connection can be exclusively connected to one ventricle. A common valve, nonetheless, always guards two atrioventricular

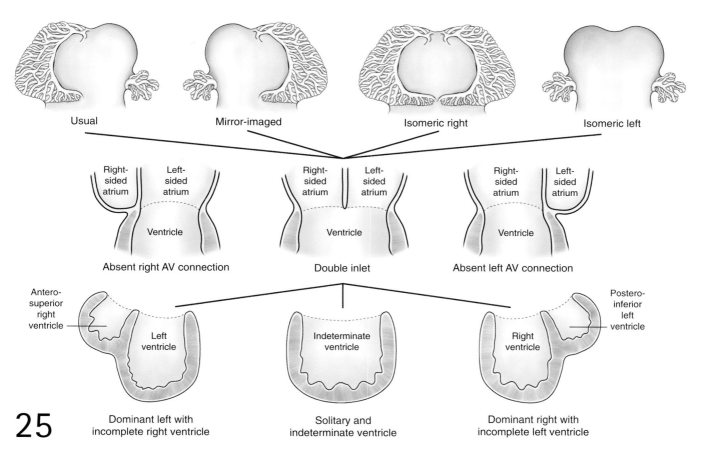

25

junctions, the right and the left, so this fact must be taken into account when assessing the degree of override. A further mode of connection when two valves exist is for one of the valves to be imperforate. This situation is different from absence of one atrioventricular connection, but both arrangements produce atrioventricular valvar atresia. Absence of one connection is probably the commonest cause of atrioventricular valvar atresia. When one atrioventricular connection is absent, then the modes of connection of the persisting junction are strictly limited. The atrioventricular valve may either be exclusively connected to one ventricle, or alternatively may straddle or override. The latter arrangement gives a connection which is uniatrial but biventricular.

Influence of ventricular topology on conduction tissues

In the section on the normal atrioventricular junctions, a description was provided for how the triangle of Koch provided the landmarks to the atrioventricular junctional area. In hearts with abnormal atrioventricular connections, in contrast, the regular atrioventricular node is not always the one which gives rise to the penetrating atrioventricular bundle. During fetal life, a complete ring of potential conduction tissue surrounds the atrioventricular junction. Remnants of this ring often persist into adult life, but then they are sequestrated on the atrial aspect of the fibrous annulus, and they do not give rise to atrioventricular conduction bundles. In the presence of abnormal connections between the atriums and ventricles, however, parts of this atrioventricular ring tissue can take over the role of the atrioventricular node. The rules which determine whether a regular or an anomalous node exists, or rarely both, are governed by several factors. The most important is whether good alignment exists between the atrial septum and the muscular ventricular septum. Almost always in hearts with concordant atrioventricular connections, good alignment and a regular conduction system exists. The exception is found when the straddling and overriding of the tricuspid valve occurs. In this setting, an anomalous node is formed at the point at which the muscular ventricular septum makes contact with the atrioventricular junction. In hearts with usual atrial arrangement and discordant atrioventricular connections, and in hearts with univentricular connection to dominant left and indeterminate ventricles, the normal septal alignment is lacking. In these hearts, therefore, an anomalous anterior atrioventricular node exists. In those with dominant left ventricles, the antero-superior position of the muscular ventricular septum dictates that there cannot be alignment with the atrial septum, so that an anterior node is the rule. With univentricular connection to a dominant right ventricle, in contrast, septal alignment is maintained when the rudimentary left ventricle is left-sided, so that regular conduction systems are found. Similarly, when discordant atrioventricular connections are found with mirror-imaged atrial chambers, again good septal alignment and a regular

conduction system usually exist. Ventricular topology, nonetheless, is also significant. Thus, abnormal systems are found most frequently when a left-handed ventricular topology is present. This rule holds good also when a univentricular connection is made to a dominant right ventricle, and when biventricular atrioventricular connections are also ambiguous. The exception is found when left-handed topology coexists with mirror-imaged atrial chambers, because almost always this situation means that the atrioventricular connections will be concordant. Thus, the atrioventricular connections are the best guide to disposition of the atrioventricular conduction axis, but the topological arrangement of the ventricular mass is also highly significant.

The ventriculoarterial junctions

At these junctions, it is again necessary to take account of the type and mode of connections. Additionally, attention should be paid to arterial relationships. The morphology of the ventricular outflow tracts, so-called infundibular or conal anatomy, is also variable but is rarely of surgical significance.

The ventriculoarterial connections are said to be concordant when the aorta is connected to the left ventricle, and the pulmonary trunk to the right ventricle. An aorta connected to a right ventricle, and a pulmonary trunk to a left ventricle, produces discordant connections. Both arteries connected to the same ventricle are described as double outlet, whereas single outlet of the heart is used for the situation in which only one patent arterial trunk can be traced to make contact with the ventricular mass. The latter may be a common trunk, or alternatively an aortic trunk with pulmonary atresia, a pulmonary trunk with aortic atresia, or a solitary arterial trunk when the intrapericardial pulmonary arteries are lacking. The modes of connection are more limited at the ventriculoarterial junctions. A common valve only exists with a common trunk. When two valves are present, then both may be patent. One or both may then override the septum. As with overriding atrioventricular valves, the precise connection is determined by using the 50 per cent law. One arterial valve may also be imperforate. In this situation, either the imperforate valve or the patent valve may override.

All of the above connections are determined irrespective of the arterial interrelationships. It is not possible to infer with complete accuracy the ventricular origin of the great arteries from their external relationships. This statement is not meant to say that relationships give no help in diagnosing connections. Certain basic arrangements are seen more frequently with one given connection, for example a right-sided and anterior aorta with concordant atrioventricular and discordant ventriculoarterial connections. Immutable laws, however, do not exist, and trends should be treated only as a guide to the possibility of abnormal connections. When describing the abnormal relationships, it is necessary to account for both the positions of the arterial valves and the orientation of the ascending portions of the arterial trunks. Valvar relationships are best described by accounting for the position of the aortic valve in comparison to the pulmonary valve in right/left and anterior/ posterior coordinates. When describing the orientation of the arterial trunks, two basic patterns occur. Either the pulmonary trunk spirals round the aorta towards its bifurcation, or else the trunks ascend in parallel fashion. By combining these two variables, it is an easy matter to describe all anticipated patterns of arterial interrelationships.

Although the morphology of the outflow tracts in itself is rarely of surgical significance, great emphasis has been placed in the past on the role of the bilateral conus, or bilateral infundibulum. Each arterial valve is potentially capable of being supported by a complete muscular infundibulum in the setting of any ventriculoarterial connection. These infundibulums have three basic components. One component separates the arterial valves, along with their subvalvar outflow tracts, from each other. This component is the muscular outlet, infundibular, or conal septum. The second part is the free parietal ventricular wall. The third part has given most problems in comprehension. This part represents the inner heart curvature between the antero-superior wall of the atriums, and the postero-inferior wall of the great arterial trunks. This curvature separates the arterial valves from the atrioventricular valves and is called the ventriculoinfundibular fold. The variability in morphology of the outflow tracts usually depends on the integrity of this fold. When it is intact, then discontinuity exists between the leaflets of the atrioventricular and arterial valves, and a complete muscular infundibulum usually is present. When the fold is deficient, then continuity exists between the leaflets of the atrioventricular and arterial valves, and part of the infundibulum is deficient. The term 'usually' is used above purposely, since it is possible for the ventriculoinfundibular fold to be intact, producing arterial-atrioventricular discontinuity, and yet for the outlet septum to be deficient, thus permitting valvar continuity between the leaflets of the aortic and pulmonary valves. In this setting, the muscular infundibulums would be incomplete. Obviously, therefore, the integrity of the ventricular outflow tracts depends on the morphology of both the ventriculoinfundibular fold and the outlet septum. It should also be noted that this discussion has made no mention of the septomarginal trabeculation. This latter muscular structure is an integral part of the right ventricle, and is not part of the subvalvar outflow tracts.

Subsequent steps in sequential analysis

The analysis described thus far accounts only for the segmental combination of the heart. In most instances, this will be normal. But it will have cost the surgeon nothing to prove this normality. Indeed, it is essential so to do. Having established the segmental pattern, analysis is concluded by assessing all the associated defects present. This assessment is also best done in segmental fashion, commencing by confirming the normality of the venoatrial connections. Attention can then be directed in turn to the atrial segment, the ventricular segment, and the arterial segment, at the same time looking for any junctional malformations that may not have been accounted for during the analysis of the connections. Then, the anatomy of the aortic and pulmonary pathways is assessed. In this way, any congenital cardiac lesion, or combination of lesions, however simple or complex, is accounted for and understood in the segmental setting of the heart itself. Separate description is then provided for the location of the heart, the direction of its apex, and the arrangement of the thoracic and abdominal organs, taking care to describe each system separately when discrepancies are encountered from the anticipated patterns.

ACKNOWLEDGMENTS

The work on which this chapter is based was supported by the British Heart Foundation, together with the Joseph Levy Foundation. It would not have been possible to prepare all the illustrations, nor to write the surgical aspects of this chapter, without the considerable help of, and intellectual input from, Dr Benson Wilcox, from the University of North Carolina, Chapel Hill. I have been indebted to him throughout my studies, and I thank him for his support and continuing collaboration. Figures 1, 2, 5 and 7 were photographed by him and are reproduced with his permission. Some of the illustrations were also prepared with the help of Yen Ho, Andrew Cook, Gemma Price, Nigel Brown, and Sandra Webb (Figure 12 photographed and reproduced by kind permission of NB and SW). I thank them all.

FUTHER READING

Anderson, R.H. 1996. How should we optimally describe complex congenitally malformed hearts? *Ann Thorac Surg* **62**, 710–16.

Anderson, R.H., Ho, S.Y. 1997. Sequential segmental analysis – description and categorisation for the millennium. *Cardiol Young* **7**, 98–116.

Anderson, R.H., Ho, S.Y., Becker, A.E. 2000. Anatomy of the human atrioventricular junctions revisited. *Anat Rec* **260**, 81–91.

Anderson, R.H., Webb, S., Brown, N.A. 1999. Clinical anatomy of the atrial septum with reference to its development components. *Clin Anat* **12**, 362–74.

Sutton, J.P. 3rd., Ho, S.Y., Anderson, R.H. 1995. The forgotten interleaflet triangles: a review of the surgical anatomy of the aortic valve. *Ann Thorac Surg* **59**, 419–27.

Uemura, H., Ho, S.Y., Devine, W.A., Kilpatrick, L.L., Anderson, R.H. 1995. Atrial appendages and venoatrial connections in hearts with patients with visceral heterotaxy. *Ann Thorac Surg* **60**, 561–9.

39

Palliative procedures: shunts and pulmonary artery banding

DAVID P. BICHELL MD
Director of Cardiovascular Surgery, Children's Hospital, San Diego, California, USA

HISTORY OF MODIFIED BLALOCK–TAUSSIG SHUNT

Introduced in 1945, the Blalock-Taussig shunt in its modified form has become a standard adjunct to the interim palliation of cyanotic heart defects. As neonatal and infant open heart procedures have been refined, the use of the Blalock-Taussig shunt or other interim systemic-to-pulmonary shunts for many defects has given way to early complete anatomical repair. The role for the modified Blalock-Taussig shunt, with the resultant risks inherent to parallel circulation, has become limited largely to short-term palliation in staged univentricular pathways.

PRINCIPLES AND JUSTIFICATION

In its current use, the modified Blalock-Taussig shunt is applied as a means of maintaining predictable pulmonary blood flow for defects of pulmonary hypoperfusion, or, most commonly, in univentricular physiology, where ventriculopulmonary continuity is disrupted to create exclusive and unobstructed ventriculosystemic continuity (the Norwood stage I). In this setting, the patent ductus arteriosus is divided, and the Blalock-Taussig shunt provides the exclusive source of pulmonary blood flow for 3–6 months, at which time pulmonary vascular resistance has fallen sufficiently to accept passive systemic venous flow by direct cavopulmonary anastomosis.

A successful shunt must be planned to conduct a narrow range of appropriate flow, providing pulmonary blood flow that is sufficient but not excessive, so as to avoid low cardiac output, pulmonary vascular damage, and excessive ventricular volume overload.

Some principles of hydrodynamics are integral to the planning and construction of the successful shunt. Assuming laminar flow, the volumetric flow rate through a regular cylindrical conduit is governed by the Hagen-Poiseuille equation,

$$Q = \Delta p \pi d^4 / 128 L \mu$$

in which Q = volumetric flow rate, Δp = pressure drop, d = diameter, L = length, and μ = fluid viscosity. This relationship illustrates the concept that a small change in shunt diameter results in a large change in resultant flow, relating to the diameter raised to the fourth power. For a great majority of newborns, a 3.0–3.5-mm polytetrafluoroethylene (PTFE) conduit provides an appropriate balance of systemic-to-pulmonary blood flow. Bulky anastomotic suture lines can diminish the effective diameter, with accordingly amplified effects on shunt flow. Shunt length has a much weaker influence on flow. Placing the origin of a Blalock-Taussig shunt anastomosis distally or proximally along the innominate or subclavian artery may modulate shunt flow, owing to the diameter of the vessel of origin, but the resulting small changes in shunt length with these maneuvers are of minor influence. Shunt length and angle of anastomosis are best planned to preserve, undistorted, the geometry of the innominate and pulmonary arteries. A shunt millimeters too long can efface its inflow; millimeters too short can place distorting tension on the pulmonary artery.

The modified Blalock-Taussig shunt can be constructed through a thoracotomy or sternotomy. In recent years, the sternotomy approach has gained favor at most institutions for a variety of reasons, particularly because the shunt is used usually as an interim palliation that will be followed by a subsequent sternotomy-requiring procedure. Other advantages of the sternotomy approach include technical ease, better shunt patency, more even distribution of flow bilaterally, better access to ligate the PDA or perform other concomitant procedures, and less pulmonary artery distortion.

PREOPERATIVE ASSESSMENT AND PREPARATION

Although a majority of newborns are appropriately served by a 3.5-mm PTFE shunt, smaller shunt diameters may better suit the infant weighing less than 2.5 kg. An arterial monitoring line, preferably not in the limb affected by the shunt, and venous access, are imperative before starting the case. Pulse oximetry aids in assessing the balance between pulmonary and systemic circulations and the patient's tolerance for partial pulmonary artery clamping.

OPERATION

1 A standard median sternotomy is performed. A subtotal thymectomy provides exposure and removes tissue that becomes adherent to adjacent structures, complicating subsequent re-entry sternotomies. The upper pericardium is incised, and pericardial suspension sutures assist in exposure of the upper mediastinal structures. The innominate artery is mobilized circumferentially beyond its bifurcation into subclavian and common carotid arteries. The innominate vein can be gently retracted with Silastic vessel loops. Between the aorta and superior vena cava (SVC), the right pulmonary artery is identified and mobilized circumferentially from its origin at the main pulmonary artery to beyond the origin of the upper lobe branch.

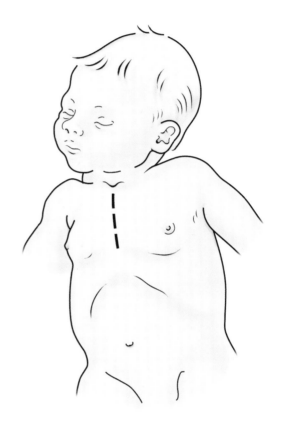

1

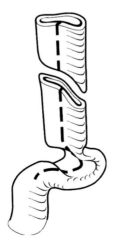

2

2 Before the placement of any clamp, a PTFE conduit is brought onto the field, and its end is cut on an angle corresponding to the angle of the innominate artery as it relates to the aorta.

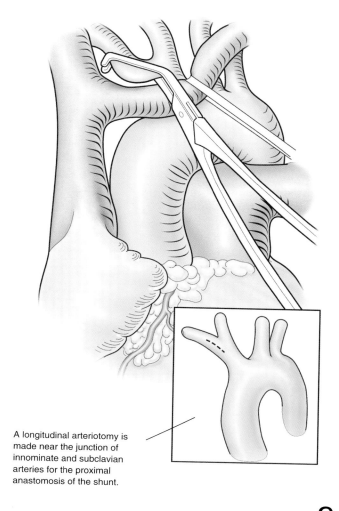

3 A forcep is used to grasp the point of intended anastomosis to the innominate artery. Caudad traction on this point during the application of a **C**-clamp centers the point of anastomosis within the jaws of the clamp.

A longitudinal arteriotomy is made near the junction of innominate and subclavian arteries for the proximal anastomosis of the shunt.

3

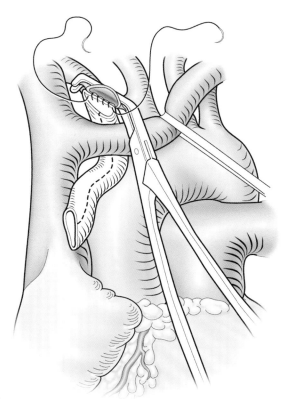

4 A 7/0 polypropylene suture is used to form the proximal anastomosis, with caution so as not to create a bulky, inverted, or distorted suture line. At the completion of the proximal anastomosis, the PTFE graft is clamped distally after passing it posterior to the innominate vein on its course toward the pulmonary artery.

4

5 As the graft is distended with blood, a point is chosen at which to divide it transversely, corresponding to the point of distal anastomosis to the right pulmonary artery. A neuroclip is placed proximally on the graft to block flow without compromising exposure for the distal anastomosis. Traction sutures on the ascending aorta can broaden exposure for this anastomosis significantly. The center point of the intended distal anastomosis on the right pulmonary artery is grasped and tented cephalad, to center it within a **C**-clamp. The patient's saturation and hemodynamics are observed during a trial pulmonary artery clamping before making the pulmonary arteriotomy. Care is taken to ensure that the clamp does not exert compression on the coronary arteries or aorta. A longitudinal pulmonary arteriotomy is made medial to the upper lobe branch, and a 7/0 polypropylene suture is used to complete the distal anastomosis.

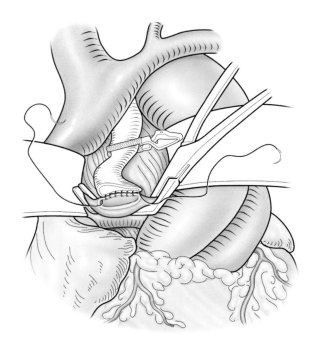

5

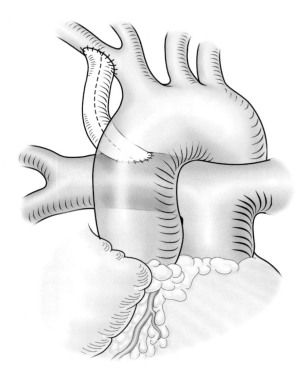

6

6 If the shunt is being created as an isolated procedure, the patent ductus is ligated and divided as the shunt is opened. Mobilization of a patent ductus before the shunt construction in ductal-dependent lesions is ill-advised, as ductal spasm induced by the dissection can render the patient unstable before the establishment of an alternative source of pulmonary blood flow. Briefly test-clamping the shunt demonstrates patency and runoff, and careful hemodynamic monitoring ensures the appropriate balance of pulmonary and systemic circulations. Rarely, pulmonary overcirculation requires tailoring the shunt before closure.

POSTOPERATIVE CARE

Pulmonary overcirculation from an inappropriately large shunt, high systemic vascular resistance, or low pulmonary vascular resistance can result in systemic hypoperfusion, excessive ventricular volume overload, acidosis, and arrest. Shunt thrombosis results in pulmonary hypoperfusion and cyanosis. Meticulous monitoring of hemodynamic data and arterial blood gas data must continue postoperatively, with a high index of suspicion and a low threshold for intervention to revise the shunt. In the presence of postcardiopulmonary bypass pulmonary edema or other comorbidities resulting in parenchymal lung disease, gas exchange may be inefficient, resulting in the phenomenon of low arterial oxygen saturation despite pulmonary overcirculation. The illusion of pulmonary undercirculation in this setting tempts a reaction to increase the FiO_2, thereby further lowering pulmonary resistance and exacerbating systemic hypoperfusion. Venous O_2 saturation and systemic acidosis are more sensitive indicators of the adequacy of systemic perfusion, and a proactive treatment of these findings with a low threshold for reoperating to adjust pulmonary overcirculation must be pursued. Residual arch obstruction is important to rule out as an indirect etiology for pulmonary overcirculation.

When postoperative bleeding is not a concern, a continuous heparin infusion may prevent early thrombosis. Many centers maintain shunted patients on daily aspirin.

OUTCOME

Perioperative complications after the construction of a modified Blalock-Taussig shunt include phrenic nerve injury, Horner's syndrome, shunt thrombosis, pericardial effusion, and chylothorax.

Hospital mortality for the isolated construction of a palliative modified Blalock-Taussig shunt is reported as 8–11 per cent. Shunt failure was a more prominent contributing factor to mortality in the thoracotomy group than in the sternotomy group, owing to pulmonary artery distortion. The majority of modified Blalock-Taussig shunts is created in conjunction with additional procedures, such as the Norwood stage I palliation, and outcome data depend on a variety of factors associated with the principle procedure. Worthy of note is the fact that the parallel circulation imparted by the systemic-to-pulmonary shunt causes systemic ventricular volume overload and labile shifts in circulation from pulmonary to systemic circuits. The morbidity and mortality associated with these factors reinforces the principle that the modified Blalock-Taussig shunt should be left in place for only the shortest possible period before the subsequent repair or palliation is performed.

HISTORY OF BIDIRECTIONAL CAVOPULMONARY ANASTOMOSIS (BIDIRECTIONAL GLENN SHUNT)

Experimentally induced severe right ventricular damage in a dog model, performed in the 1940s, demonstrated only a minimal resultant increase in systemic venous pressure and no demonstrable decrement in pulmonary blood flow. These experiments established the scientific substrate for the development of right heart bypass procedures commonly in use today to palliate the univentricular heart. Carlton, Mondini, and de Marchi first described the cavopulmonary anastomosis in cadaveric and animal feasibility studies in 1950. The first clinical application of the cavopulmonary shunt was reported by Shumacher, and the first clinically successful reported cavopulmonary anastomosis was performed in 1956 by Meshalkin et al. After several years of detailed animal studies of right heart bypass physiology, William Glenn, for whom the superior cavopulmonary anastomosis is most commonly named, reported its use in a 7-year-old progressively cyanotic boy with single ventricle physiology and pulmonary stenosis. The classic Glenn shunt, diverting SVC flow exclusively to the right lung, resulted in an uneven distribution of pulmonary blood flow and pulmonary artery distortion complicating a subsequent Fontan and contributed to the formation of pulmonary arteriovenous malformations. Experimentally developed by Haller et al., the first clinical application of the end-to-side bidirectional cavopulmonary anastomosis was reported by Azzolina et al. in 1972. The bidirectional cavopulmonary anastomosis is the only form in common clinical use today, mostly as a second stage in the three-staged palliation of the univentricular heart.

PRINCIPLES AND JUSTIFICATION

The prolonged volume load burdening the single ventricle with parallel circulation contributes to ventricular dilatation, atrioventricular valve regurgitation, ventricular dysfunction, and the resultant risk of a suboptimal Fontan outcome. The bidirectional cavopulmonary anastomosis augments pulmonary blood flow while reducing ventricular work. For infants, the SVC contributes 50 per cent of the total cardiac output, and so the bidirectional cavopulmonary anastomosis diverts a significant amount of volume load away from the ventricle. An early bidirectional cavopulmonary anastomosis in the univentricular heart may reduce the deleterious effects of prolonged hypoxia and volume overload. Early volume unloading has been shown to result in improved late exercise performance in Fontan patients when compared with those whose unloading procedures were performed later. Since the late 1980s, the bidirectional cavopulmonary anastomosis has become a routine interim stage for a majority of Fontan pathway patients. Additionally, the bidirectional cavopulmonary anastomosis is used as an adjunct to 1.5 ventricle palliations for lesions such as pulmonary atresia with intact ventricular septum or Ebstein's anomaly and unbalanced atrioventricular conduction in which a diminutive right ventricle or tricuspid valve is capable of conducting inferior vena caval flow, but not an entire cardiac output.

PREOPERATIVE ASSESSMENT AND PREPARATION

Age

Systemic venous-to-pulmonary artery blood flow without ventricular propulsion depends on a sufficiently low pulmonary vascular resistance to permit the passive transit of blood across the pulmonary circuit, and sufficiently low pulmonary artery pressures to avoid systemic venous hypertension. The newborn's pulmonary vascular resistance is too high to satisfy these criteria but falls in the first weeks or months of life, as the cross-sectional area of the pulmonary microvascular bed expands. A cavopulmonary anastomosis performed in the first weeks of life invariably results in prohibitive cyanosis and SVC hypertension. Although successful cavopulmonary shunts have been performed at 4 weeks of age, a majority are performed at or beyond 4 months. Within these constraints, several theoretical and practical advantages exist to performing the cavopulmonary anastomosis as early as reasonably possible.

Anatomical considerations

Every candidate for cavopulmonary anastomosis undergoes a preoperative diagnostic echocardiogram and cardiac catheterization. Anatomical details must be clarified to plan modifications of the procedure to accommodate such findings as left SVC, or interrupted inferior vena cava with azygos continuation. Although some atrioventricular valve regurgitation may resolve with ventricular volume load reduction, important structural atrioventricular valve regurgitation can complicate the postoperative course and deserves attention. This situation should prompt the con-sideration of a concomitant valvuloplasty. Pulmonary artery stenosis or distortion is mapped for concomitant repair. Present or incipient ventricular outflow obstruction might require a Damus-Kaye-Stansel anastomosis or an intracardiac procedure concomitantly with the cavopulmonary anastomosis. Important venous collateral vessels to the lower compartment can be identified and coil-occluded preoperatively. Pulmonary vein obstruction is ruled out.

Hemodynamic criteria

Pulmonary artery pressure determinations and/or pulmonary venous wedge pressure data, ventricular end-diastolic pressure data, and saturation data are imperative to assess the appropriateness of constructing the bidirectional cavopulmonary anastomosis. The omission of these determinations can result in postoperative cyanosis, systemic venous hypertension, poor cardiac output, and the need to disassemble the shunt. In general, and subject to exceptions, an indexed pulmonary vascular resistance greater than 2 U/m^2, a mean pulmonary artery pressure greater than 18 mm Hg, a transpulmonary gradient greater than 10 mm Hg, or ventricular end-diastolic pressure greater than 12 mm Hg are catheterization values above which the cavopulmonary anastomosis may fail. A reversible etiology should be sought for any of these findings to improve a patient's likelihood of sufficient pulmonary blood flow without systemic venous hypertension.

Monitoring

A peripheral arterial monitoring line and venous access are important, although central venous access can be placed intraoperatively. Although upper compartment percutaneous venous lines are routine in some institutions, an indwelling line left in a low flow system carries the disastrous risk of SVC thrombosis.

OPERATION

7 The SVC is mobilized circumferentially from its atrial attachment cephalad onto the innominate vein. The azygos vein is ligated and divided. The ipsilateral pulmonary artery is mobilized fully, beyond the origin of the upper lobe branch. Cardiopulmonary bypass is initiated with bicaval venous cannulation.

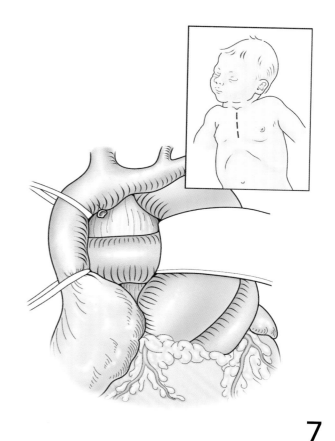

7

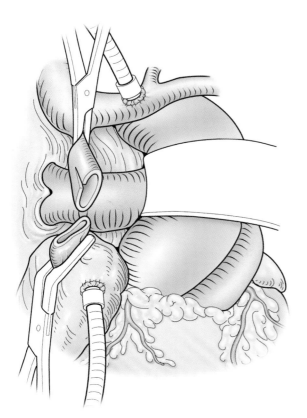

8 A vascular clamp is placed across the SVC just cephalad to the atriocaval junction. The SVC is divided and the atrial end oversewn, taking precaution not to clamp or sew adjacent atrial tissue where the sinoatrial node may reside. The orientation of the SVC is carefully preserved.

8

9 A spatulation of the lateral aspect of the SVC is performed.

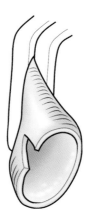

9

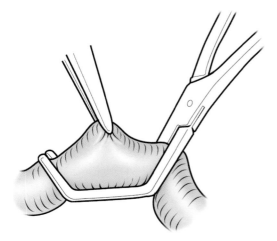

10

10 The mobilized pulmonary artery is grasped at a center point for the planned anastomosis, and a curved clamp is applied, taking care to not compress the coronary artery as it emerges from the adjacent aortic root.

11 A longitudinal pulmonary arteriotomy is made.

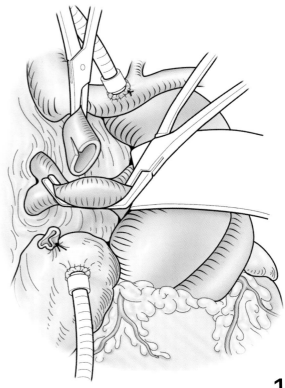

11

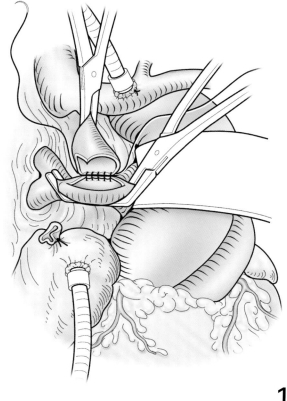

12 The anastomosis is carried out with a 7/0 Prolene continuous suture.

12

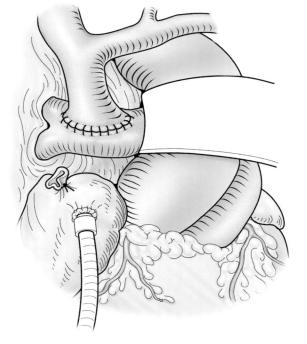

13 The completed anastomosis should result in a smooth transition from SVC to pulmonary artery, without any form of prepulmonary stenosis.

13

14 When necessary to ameliorate pulmonary artery stenosis, or to augment the cavopulmonary anastomosis to ensure no distortion, a pericardial patch is applied on the branch pulmonary artery before the completion of the SVC–pulmonary artery anastomosis.

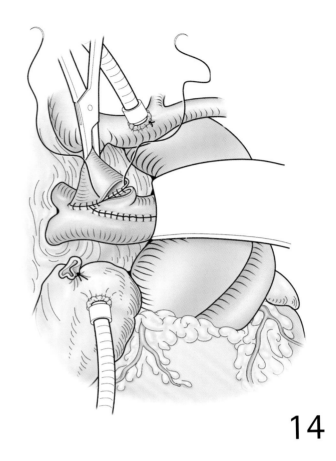

14

POSTOPERATIVE CARE

The perioperative management of patients after bidirectional cavopulmonary anastomosis requires a concerted effort to promote the transit of blood through the pulmonary circuit. Positive pressure ventilation may itself impede pulmonary blood flow. This effect is minimized if strategies of low inspiratory-to-expiratory ratio and early extubation are pursued. Hyperventilation impairs oxygenation even as it lowers pulmonary vascular resistance, possibly as a result of cerebrovascular resistance increasing in response to a decreasing PCO_2. An elevation of the patient's head may help minimize upper body edema.

Pharmacological maneuvers to optimize pulmonary blood flow include the routine use of phosphodiesterase inhibitors such as milrinone, which affects pulmonary as well as systemic vasodilatation. Nitric oxide may augment pulmonary blood flow, but it is seldom necessary in the postoperative period.

Postoperative hypoxia, despite the previously described maneuvers, prompts an aggressive investigation of possible etiologies. A high level of suspicion is maintained for pulmonary artery or prepulmonary stenosis that could require surgical revision. Decompressing venovenous collaterals

from the upper to lower compartment should be ruled out. Atrioventricular valve regurgitation or poor ventricular function results in elevated atrial and ventricular end-diastolic pressures, and these problems are addressed with appropriate inotropic support or surgical intervention. In rare instances hypoxia, it may be necessary to construct a second source of pulmonary blood flow in the form of an aortopulmonary shunt, although this strategy produces a volume-load to the ventricle, and can exacerbate upper compartment venous hypertension.

Other considerations in investigating an unstable postoperative course include acute geometric changes in the heart imparted by the acute reduction in volume load. A bulboventricular foramen, on which ventricular outflow depends, can become restrictive after ventricular unloading.

OUTCOME

Perioperative and late mortality from the construction of a bidirectional cavopulmonary anastomosis in the present era is less than 2 per cent. Fontan morbidity may be reduced when the interim cavopulmonary anastomosis is used. Late sequelae include progressive cyanosis secondary to growth, venovenous collateral formation, or the development of pulmonary arteriovenous malformations. The late development of pulmonary arteriovenous malformations has been reported to occur in 25–50 per cent of patients with bidirectional cavopulmonary shunts, especially in heterotaxy patients. Fontan completion to include hepatic venous effluent in the pulmonary vascular circuit contributes to their resolution. Aortopulmonary collateral formation may occur in two-thirds of patients, requiring coil embolization where possible.

HISTORY OF THE PULMONARY ARTERY BAND

The pulmonary artery band, originating as an animal model for the study of hypertrophy, was introduced as palliation for excessive pulmonary blood flow by Muller and Dammann in 1952. Pulmonary artery banding gained popularity for many years for the palliation of large ventricular septal defects (VSDs) and a variety of other defects associated with pulmonary overcirculation, permitting an infant to gain sufficient size for a safe anatomical correction or additional palliation. Advances in cardiac surgery for infants and newborns have resulted in the early anatomical correction of a majority of defects that constituted former indications for pulmonary artery banding, and the procedure is currently uncommon. The pulmonary artery band is presently reserved for the short-term palliation of infants with excessive pulmonary blood flow, such as that associated with tricuspid atresia, double-inlet left ventricle, double-outlet single ventricle, multiple VSDs, or large VSDs requiring interim palliation owing to other comorbidities that prohibit cardiopulmonary bypass. The pulmonary artery band is also used for the short-term conditioning of the left ventricle in preparation for the arterial switch procedure in patients not corrected as newborns.

PRINCIPLES AND JUSTIFICATION

In accordance with Poiseuille's equation, flow through a cylindrical constriction is proportional to its diameter raised to the fourth power, divided by the length of the constriction (band width). The diameter is such a powerful determinant of flow that a 1-mm change in band diameter can effect a threefold change in flow.

Plotting band circumference and weight, Trusler and Mustard examined the adequacy of empirically placed pulmonary artery bands for patients with VSD, based on the absence or persistence of congestive symptoms. A formula

was devised predicting the optimal band circumference to be 20 mm plus 1 mm for each kilogram of the patient's weight. Further analysis of survival data and anatomical features led to the following revised formula of band circumference: 20 mm + 1 mm/kg for simple defects without intracardiac bidirectional mixing, and 24 mm + 1 mm/kg for mixing lesions, with loosening only if cyanosis or bradycardia occurs. Infants weighing less than 2 kg were recommended to have bands measuring 1.0–1.5 mm smaller in circumference than Trusler's formula predicts. Taking into account the nonlinear growth of the pulmonary valve in infants, Kawahira et al. have derived a formula for determining the optimal pulmonary artery band circumference as 87 per cent of the normal (angiographically derived) pulmonary artery circumference ($51.81 \times [BSA]^{0.45}$), which applies more consistently to infants of any weight and correlates with Trusler's rule when applied to larger children. Using Trusler's rule as a starting point, most centers add pre- and postband direct pressure measurement and peripheral O_2 saturation measurement to fine adjust the band. The objective is to reduce the systolic pulmonary artery pressure as close as possible to 30 mm Hg or half of the systemic pressure, without causing bradycardia or systemic desaturation below 80 per cent.

PREOPERATIVE ASSESSMENT AND PREPARATION

Careful consideration of the patient's cardiac anatomy must be made to select appropriate candidates for a palliative pulmonary artery band, as deleterious – if not fatal – sequelae result from its inappropriate application.

Subaortic or aortic obstruction presents a relative contraindication to the placement of a pulmonary artery band, as a band creates physiological biventricular outflow obstruction, promoting myocardial hypertrophy and ischemia-fibrosis. When not already present, the tendency to form subaortic stenosis has been observed, especially in patients with double-inlet single ventricle or tricuspid atresia with transposed great vessels and a VSD-dependent aortic outlet. Pulmonary artery banding in these patients can accelerate aortic outflow obstruction by promoting muscular hypertrophy and a resultant bulboventricular foramen restriction. A bulboventricular foramen area index less than 2 cm^2/m^2 predicts an obstructive outflow unless bypassed as an initial palliation. This anatomy should prompt the consideration of a Norwood procedure as the initial palliation rather than a pulmonary artery band. As outflow obstruction and ventricular hypertrophy are both risk factors affecting Fontan survival, these anatomical presentations are relative contraindications to pulmonary artery banding.

OPERATION

Sternotomy approach

15 The sternotomy approach is used when concomitant aortic procedures that require a thoracotomy, such as coarctation repair, are not indicated. The median sternotomy provides a safer, more precise exposure of the main pulmonary artery and its branches for positioning of the band. As the median sternotomy is the incision most often needed for future staged palliations or anatomical repair, this approach has the additional advantage of leaving the patient with only one scar. The main pulmonary artery is mobilized circumferentially.

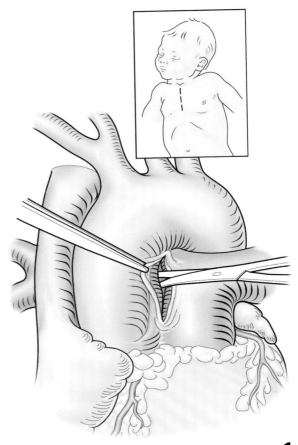

15

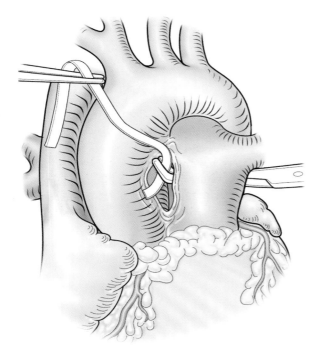

16 The pulmonary artery band material, premarked at a circumference estimated by Trusler's formula, is passed around the mobilized segment.

16

17 A Prolene suture is passed through the band at the premarked endpoints and tied.

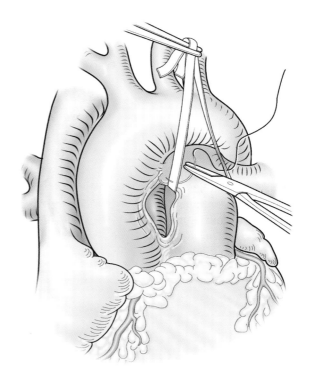

17

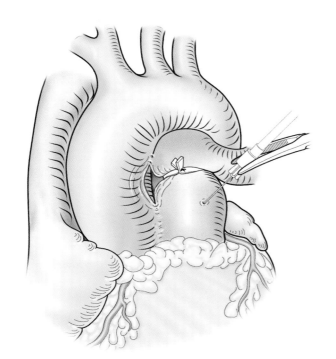

18

18 Direct pre- and postband pressure measurements are made, peripheral arterial line tracings and pulse oximetric determinations are observed. Additional mattress sutures are placed through the band to adjust its tightness to the goal of postband pulmonary artery pressure equal to half the systemic pressure, while preserving O_2 saturations greater than 80 per cent. Cyanosis or bradycardia suggests that the band should be loosened.

19 The band is positioned at a point sufficiently proximal to not impinge on the origin of the branch pulmonary arteries, approximately at the level of the sino-tubular junction of the main pulmonary artery. Adventitial sutures secure this position and prevent band migration.

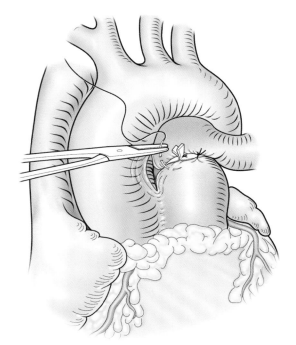

19

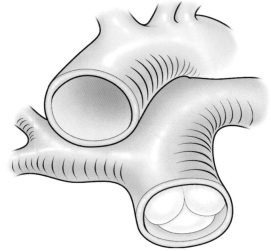

20

20 The right branch pulmonary artery typically originates proximal to, and at a more acute angle than, the left branch pulmonary artery.

21 Even a slight migration of the band can result in a partial or complete occlusion of the right branch pulmonary artery and insufficient limitation of flow to the left.

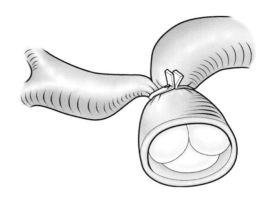

21

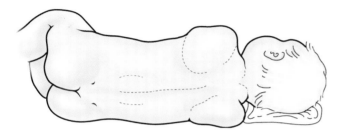

22

Pulmonary artery banding, thoracotomy

22 A left lateral thoracotomy is made in the third or fourth intercostal space to expose the juxtaductal aorta. A ductal ligation and/or concomitant aortic procedure is performed.

23 The pulmonary artery is exposed through an incision in the pericardium anterior to the phrenic nerve. Retraction sutures placed in the pericardium assist exposure of the main pulmonary artery and ascending aorta.

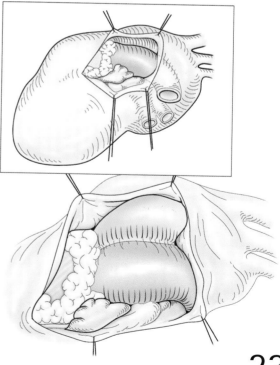

23

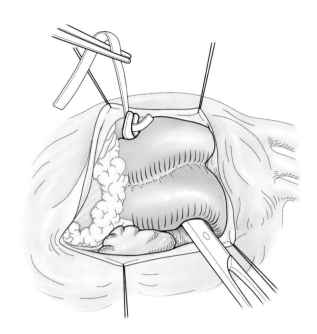

24 A curved clamp is passed through the transverse sinus, and a tape, premarked at the appropriate band circumference as estimated by Trusler's formula, is passed to encircle the aorta and the pulmonary arteries together.

24

25

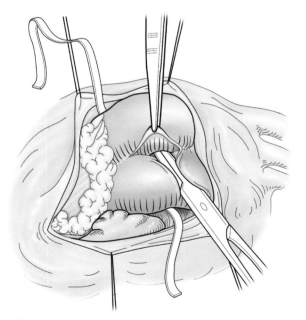

25 A plane is carefully dissected between the aorta and the main pulmonary artery, entering the transverse sinus under direct visualization. The dissection is carried out in a plane close to the back wall of the aorta, minimizing chances of injuring the right branch pulmonary artery as it passes in proximity to the posterior aorta.

26 The clamp is then insinuated around the aorta alone to grasp the tape and exclude the aorta.

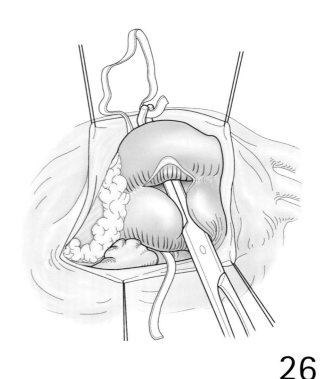

26

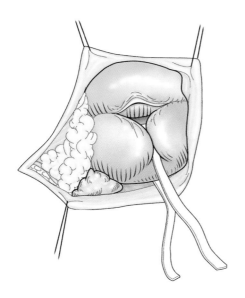

27

27 This technique results in an encirclement of the pulmonary artery without passing the clamp blindly around the thin-walled pulmonary artery itself.

28 A Prolene suture is then placed through the band material at the marked endpoints to draw the band tight. Direct pre- and postband pressure measurements are made, peripheral arterial line tracings, and pulse oximetric determinations are observed. Additional mattress sutures are placed through the band to adjust its tightness to the goal of postband pulmonary artery pressure equal to half the systemic pressure, while preserving O_2 saturations greater than 80 per cent. Cyanosis or bradycardia suggests that the band should be loosened.

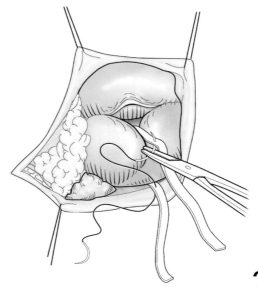

28

29 After a satisfactory adjustment, the band is fixed to the adventitia of the pulmonary artery with several sutures to prevent its migration. The pericardium is re-approximated, and the thoracotomy closed.

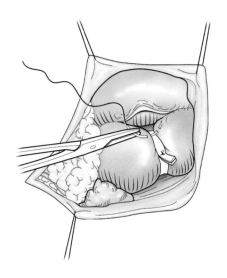

29

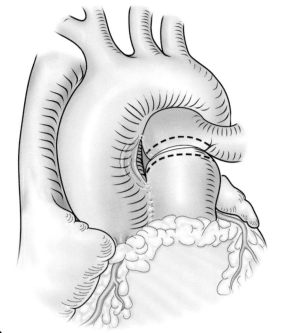

30

Pulmonary artery debanding and reconstruction

30 The pulmonary artery is exposed through re-operative sternotomy, and main and branch pulmonary arteries are mobilized. Cicatricial tissue around the pulmonary artery band site results in a circumferential intimal ridge, and a simple anterior patch plasty of the band site results in residual obstruction from the retained posterior ridge. The pulmonary artery band and a segment of affected main pulmonary artery must be segmentally resected for a complete relief of obstruction.

31 As a segmental resection of the main pulmonary artery is carried out, particular caution is exercised at its posterior wall, as the left main coronary artery usually lies immediately subjacent. Along the posterior wall, the pulmonary artery is only resected as the structures deep to it are clearly visualized, and safety sometimes dictates that a portion of back wall be retained. The pulmonary valve is inspected and repaired if necessary.

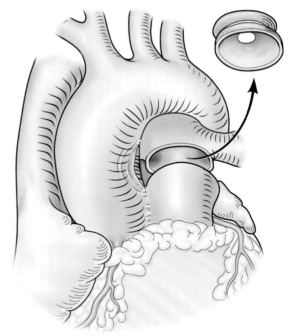

31

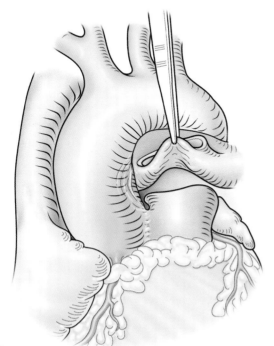

32

32 Further mobilization of the confluence and branch pulmonary arteries is carried out to minimize any distortion-producing tension on the planned anastomosis.

33 A circumferential native pulmonary artery–to–pulmonary artery anastomosis is carried out with a continuous polypropylene suture technique. Where tissue is deficient, a pericardial patch augmentation is indicated.

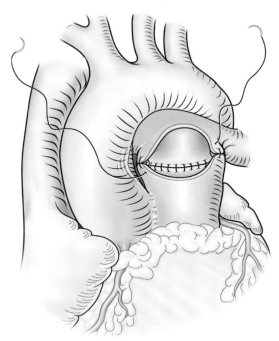

33

POSTOPERATIVE CARE

Early complications include phrenic or recurrent laryngeal nerve palsies, chylothorax, and coronary artery compromise. As ongoing congestive heart failure carries a significant associated mortality, attention must be paid to the possibility of an inadequately protected pulmonary vascular bed, either unilaterally or bilaterally, with a low threshold for returning to the operating room for band revision.

Late complications include congestive failure owing to an inadequate band, band migration resulting in right or bilateral branch pulmonary artery distortion, band erosion into the infundibulum, and pulmonary artery aneurysm or pulmonary valve distortion, precluding the use of the pulmonary valve in subsequent reparative or palliative procedures. Hypertrophy with exacerbation of subaortic obstruction from pulmonary artery banding is discussed, under preoperative assessment and preparation.

OUTCOME

As pulmonary artery banding is now largely reserved for patients with concurrent medical conditions that prohibit immediate corrective surgery, multiple factors contribute to survival risk. A recent retrospective study of pulmonary artery band outcomes reported an overall hospital mortality of 8.1 per cent for the palliative pulmonary artery band, deaths being largely among neonates, and almost 10 per cent of survivors either died before, or were unsuitable for, definitive repair, a mean 9.5 months after palliation. Many failures are due to a loose band and/or band migration with pulmonary artery distortion and unprotected pulmonary vasculature. The pulmonary artery band that is adequate at placement can fail with the remodeling of the bunched intima. Poststenotic dilatation can distort the distal pulmonary artery, and pulmonary valve distortion, with time, can render the valve incompetent, a result particularly problematic if the valve becomes systemic in a subsequent Damus-Kaye-Stansel construction. These findings support the strategy that, when used, the pulmonary artery band is safest when considered a very short-term palliation, with a definitive repair performed as early as possible.

FURTHER READING

Bernstein, H.S., Brook, M.M., Silverman, N.H., Bristow, J. 1995. Development of pulmonary arteriovenous fistulae in children after cavopulmonary shunt. *Circulation* **92[suppl II]**, II-309–314.

Bradley, S.M., Simsic, J.M., Mulvihill, D.M. 1998. Hyperventilation impairs oxygenation after bidirectional superior cavopulmonary connection. *Circulation* **98**, II-372–7.

Gladman, G., McCrindle, B.W., Williams, W.G., Freedom, R.M., Benson, L.N. 1997. The modified Blalock-Taussig shunt: clinical impact and morbidity in Fallot's tetralogy in the current era. *Journal of Thoracic and Cardiovascular Surgery* **114**, 25–30.

Mahle, W.T., Wernovsky, G., Bridges, N.D., Linton, A.B., Paridon, S.M. 1999. Impact of early ventricular unloading on exercise performance in preadolescents with single ventricle Fontan physiology. *Journal of the American College of Cardiology* **34**, 1637–43.

Odim, J., Portzky, M., Zurakowski, D., *et al.* 1995. Sternotomy approach for the modified Blalock-Taussig shunt. *Circulation* **92[suppl II]**, II-256–61.

Shah, M.J., Rychik, J., Fogel, M.A., Murphy, J.D., Jacobs, M.L. 1997. Pulmonary AV malformations after superior cavopulmonary connection: resolution after inclusion of hepatic veins in the pulmonary circulation. *Annals of Thoracic Surgery* **63**, 960–3.

40

Total anomalous pulmonary venous drainage and cor triatriatum

EDWARD L. BOVE MD
Professor of Surgery and Head, Section of Cardiac Surgery, University of Michigan Medical School; Director of Pediatric Cardiac Surgery, University of Michigan Medical Center, Ann Arbor, Michigan, USA

JENNIFER C. HIRSCH MD
Section of Cardiac Surgery, Department of Surgery, The University of Michigan School of Medicine, Ann Arbor, Michigan, USA

HISTORY

Total anomalous pulmonary venous connection (TAPVC) encompasses a group of anomalies in which the pulmonary veins drain into the systemic venous circulation via persistent splanchnic connections. The entity was first described in 1798 by Wilson. Muller performed the first partial correction at UCLA in 1951. The first complete correction was accomplished using inflow occlusion by Lewis and Varco in 1956.

TAPVC is a relatively uncommon congenital defect, representing approximately 2 percent of all congenital heart anomalies.

Cor triatriatum is a variant of TAPVC in which the common pulmonary vein fails to completely incorporate into the left atrium. Cor triatriatum is an uncommon entity, with only a few hundred cases reported since the initial description by Church in 1868.

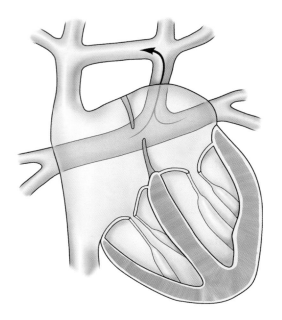

EMBRYOLOGY AND ANATOMY

1a, b *Total anomalous pulmonary venous connection* refers to the circulation of pulmonary venous flow into the systemic venous system. This abnormality results from failed transfer, in the normal developmental sequence, of pulmonary venous drainage from the splanchnic plexus to the left atrium. The lungs arise as buds of the foregut with initial vascular supply based on the foregut splanchnic circulation. The venous branches of the lung buds ultimately coalesce to become the common pulmonary vein, which, in the normal development, connect to the sinoatrial outpouching of the heart. This connection leads to pulmonary venous drainage entering the left atrium. After this connection is established, the primitive connections to the splanchnic circulation normally involute. However, in TAPVC, the connection with the left atrium fails to develop, and persistence of the splanchnic connections provides for venous drainage. Great variability in pulmonary venous connections can result from the many combinations of persistent splanchnic communications. The most common classification system was originally described by Darling and consists of four types: supracardiac, cardiac, infracardiac, and mixed. Supracardiac TAPVC occurs in approximately 45 per cent of patients. In this type, the common pulmonary vein drains superiorly into the left innominate vein or superior vena cava via an ascending vertical vein (Figure 1a). Cardiac TAPVC occurs in approximately 25 per cent of patients. In the cardiac form, the common pulmonary vein drains into the coronary sinus, or, on rare occasions, individual pulmonary veins connect directly into the right atrium (Figure 1b).

1a

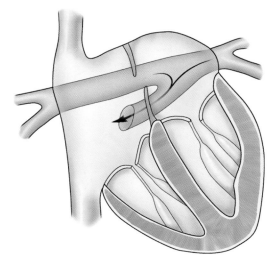

1b

1c In infracardiac TAPVC, which represents approximately 25 per cent of patients, the common pulmonary vein drains through the diaphragm into the portal vein or ductus venosus (Figure 1c). Finally, a mixed type of TAPVC occurs in approximately 5 per cent of patients and can involve any or all components of the previous three types.

In addition to the anatomical connections of the common pulmonary vein, TAPVC can be classified by the presence of obstruction. Impingement from surrounding structures or inadequate caliber of the draining pulmonary veins can result in obstruction of varying degrees. Obstruction in supracardiac TAPVC often occurs by compression of the ascending vertical vein between the left main stem bronchus and left pulmonary artery. Obstruction is always present in the infracardiac type, because the pulmonary venous blood must pass through the sinusoids of the liver. Obstruction is uncommon in the cardiac type.

Partial anomalous pulmonary venous connection defines patients in whom some, but not all, venous drainage enters the left atrium, while the remaining veins drain via one or more persistent splanchnic connections.

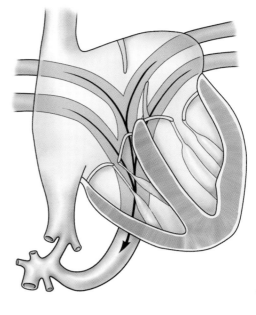

1c

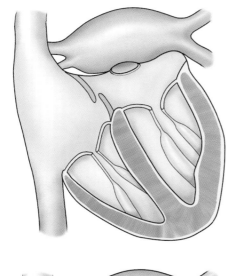

2a

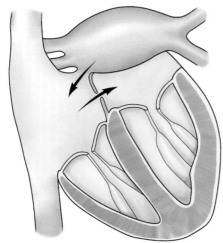

2b

2a, b Cor triatriatum results from failure of the common pulmonary vein to completely incorporate into the left atrium. The common pulmonary vein forms an accessory chamber, with a fibromuscular septum separating it from the left atrium. An orifice in this septum allows venous drainage to either enter the left atrium directly or enter the right atrium with flow into the left via an atrial septal defect (ASD) (Figures 2a, b). This entity can also be present with various persistent splanchnic connections. The orifice for pulmonary venous drainage from the accessory chamber may be inadequate, with resultant obstruction leading to symptoms in the early newborn period.

PATHOPHYSIOLOGY

TAPVC produces a mixing lesion, because oxygenated blood from the pulmonary system drains back into the systemic venous circulation. The size of the ASD dictates the distribution of blood flow. Thus, a restrictive ASD results in decreased venous return to the left side of the heart, decreased cardiac output, and increased right-sided pressures. Rarely, these patients present early in life with cardiovascular collapse. With a nonrestrictive ASD, the distribution of blood flow at the atrial level depends on the relative ventricular compliance, as well as the relative resistance of the systemic and pulmonary vasculature. Most patients with unobstructed TAPVC have few to no symptoms in infancy and present with signs and symptoms similar to those of an ASD (i.e. large, atrial-level left to right shunt). In the neonatal period, the distribution of blood flow varies as pulmonary vascular resistance falls, resulting in increased pulmonary blood flow. Patients with excessive pulmonary blood flow present later in life with symptoms of congestive heart failure or pulmonary artery hypertension. This increase in flow can produce vascular changes, leading to pulmonary vascular occlusive disease over time. Elevated pulmonary vascular resistance in the presence of a nonrestrictive ASD or patent ductus arteriosus can produce severe cyanosis from right to left shunting.

In the neonate with obstructed TAPVC, venous drainage from the pulmonary vasculature is impaired, leading to pulmonary venous hypertension and pulmonary edema. In severe cases, this increased pressure leads to reflexive vasoconstriction of the pulmonary vasculature with pulmonary hypertension and progressive cyanosis. Patients with obstruction present early in life with profound cyanosis.

PREOPERATIVE ASSESSMENT AND PREPARATION

Patients with TAPVC and significant obstruction present in the newborn period with pulmonary edema and, occasionally, right heart failure. Symptoms include poor feeding, tachypnea, and cyanosis. Physical examination demonstrates a loud second heart sound due to pulmonary hypertension and hepatomegaly from congestive heart failure. Electrocardiographic abnormalities include right ventricular hypertrophy and, occasionally, an enlarged P wave (P pulmonale). A chest roentgenogram demonstrates pulmonary edema with a normal heart size and represents a classic finding of obstructed TAPVC.

Patients with TAPVC in the absence of significant obstruction present later in life with symptoms of congestive heart failure, poor feeding, failure to thrive, and frequent respiratory infections. Physical examination demonstrates a hyperactive precordium with a widely split second heart sound and a systolic ejection murmur over the right ventricular outflow tract. Electrocardiogram findings of right ventricular enlargement are present. Chest roentgenogram shows increased pulmonary vascular markings along with cardiomegaly.

Diagnosis can be made with echocardiographic identification of the anomalous connection of the common pulmonary vein to the systemic venous system. The ASD can be delineated, as well as any other associated anomalies. Cardiac catheterization is rarely necessary, unless accurate measurement of pulmonary vascular resistance is needed.

The management of TAPVC is surgical repair. Medical management for stabilization and optimization of oxygenation and hemodynamics in patients with obstruction may be used, but they are often unsuccessful and should not delay surgical intervention. The use of prostaglandins to maintain ductal patency is generally not recommended in obstructed TAPVC in the newborn, because it results in a decrease in pulmonary blood flow as blood shunts from right to left across the duct.

OPERATION

The primary principles of operative repair are to establish a nonobstructed communication between the common pulmonary vein and the left atrium, to interrupt the connections with the systemic venous circulation, and to close the ASD. The specific repair is dependent on the type of anomalous connection.

The patient undergoes standard cardiac anesthesia. An umbilical or radial arterial line is placed for monitoring. Ventilatory measures to reduce pulmonary hypertension are used, including hyperventilation and 100 per cent oxygen. The chest is opened via a median sternotomy. The presence of thymic tissue should be noted. A portion of anterior pericardium can be harvested and fixed in glutaraldehyde. Standard hypothermic cardiopulmonary bypass can be established with an arterial cannula in the ascending aorta and a single venous cannula in the right atrial appendage. The ductus arteriosus should be identified and ligated after establishing cardiopulmonary bypass. The patient is cooled to a core temperature of 18°C. A dose of cold blood cardioplegia is administered at 30 mL/kg before circulatory arrest. Essential to successful repair is the proper identification of all four pulmonary veins and their anomalous connection before repair. Although preoperative studies are highly accurate, a mixed type of lesion may be missed.

3a–c For supracardiac connections, the optimal approach is to retract the pulmonary artery and ascending aorta laterally to expose the common pulmonary vein. The vertical vein can then be ligated outside the pericardium at the level of the innominate vein. Care should be taken to avoid the phrenic nerve, which travels along the lateral aspect of the vertical vein and the entry of the left upper pulmonary vein. The dome of the left atrium and the pulmonary venous confluence are optimally exposed between the aorta and the superior vena cava. This approach provides excellent exposure without distortion of the heart or venous structures. A transverse incision is made in the common pulmonary vein confluence, and a parallel incision is placed on the dome of the left atrium beginning at the base of the left atrial appendage. The common pulmonary vein is then anastomosed to the left atrium, taking care not to narrow the orifice (Figures 3a, b). The anastomosis may be performed with either continuous monofilament absorbable suture or polypropylene. A right atriotomy is then made to identify and repair the ASD. Use of a prosthetic or pericardial patch is often required. Attempts to enlarge the left atrium are rarely, if ever, needed.

An alternate approach uses a transverse right atriotomy that is extended across the atrial septum at the level of the ASD. The incision is then continued across the posterior aspect of the left atrium to the base of the left atrial appendage. A parallel incision is then made in the common pulmonary vein. The posterior wall of the left atrium can then be anastomosed to the common pulmonary vein, beginning at the most leftward extent of the atriotomy (Figure 3c). After the anastomosis is complete, the ASD is then closed with a prosthetic patch. Finally, the right atriotomy is closed with reinstitution of cardiopulmonary bypass and rewarming.

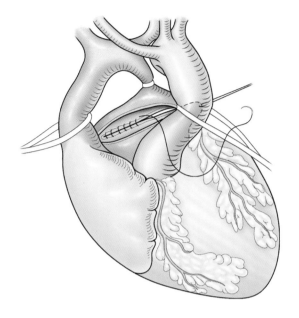

3a

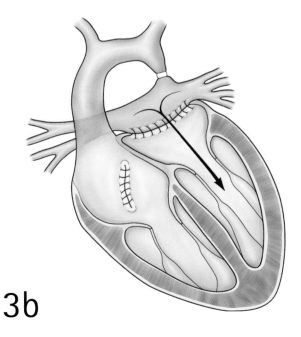

3b

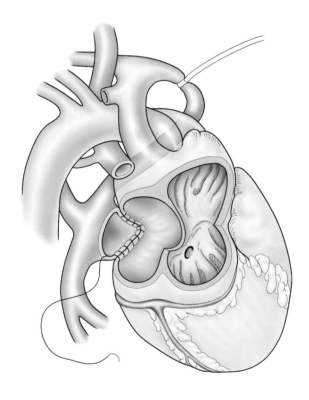

3c

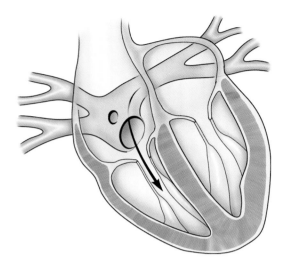

4a

4a–c For cardiac connections, a right atriotomy is performed with identification of the ASD and the orifice of the coronary sinus (Figure 4a). The roof of the coronary sinus is excised into the left atrium (Figure 4b). A patch of pericardium is then placed to close the enlarged ASD, effectively channeling the pulmonary venous return into the left atrium (Figure 4c). The conduction system travels in proximity to the coronary sinus; therefore, care must be taken while suturing the patch to avoid postoperative dysrhythmias.

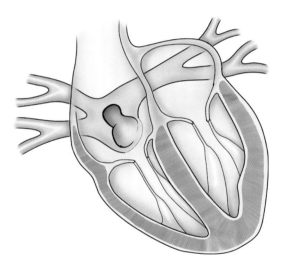

4b

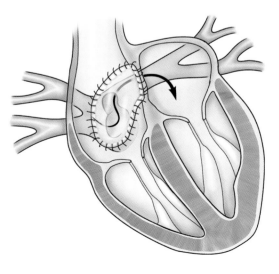

4c

5a, b

For infracardiac connections, the heart is rotated superiorly. The connection to the descending vertical vein is ligated at the level of the diaphragm. An incision is made along the length of the common pulmonary vein with a parallel incision on the posterior wall of the left atrium (Figure 5a). The common pulmonary vein is then anastomosed to the left atrium, taking care not to narrow the orifice (Figure 5b). The heart can then be returned to normal position. A right atriotomy can be performed, through which the ASD is closed.

The repair of mixed-type TAPVR involves a combination of the above approaches as dictated by the specific anatomy of the lesion.

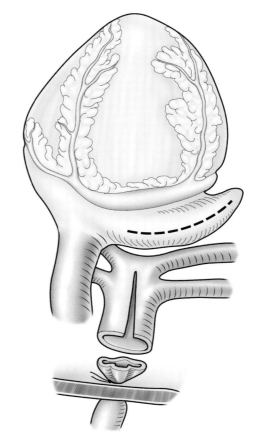

5a

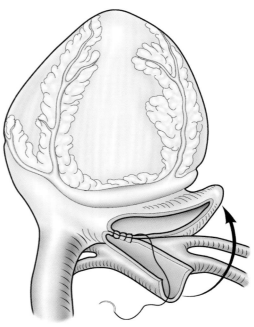

5b

6a–d Cor triatriatum with an accessory chamber in communication with the left atrium can be approached through a vertical incision in the accessory chamber (Figure 6a). The membrane separating the two chambers can be identified and excised to allow unobstructed communication (Figure 6b). The vertical incision in the accessory chamber is then closed.

Cor triatriatum with an accessory chamber in communication with the right atrium can be approached via a right atriotomy. The ASD can be enlarged into the orifice between the left atrium and the accessory chamber (Figure 6c). This step allows visualization and wide excision of the membrane (Figure 6d). The interatrial septum can then be reconstructed using a pericardial patch.

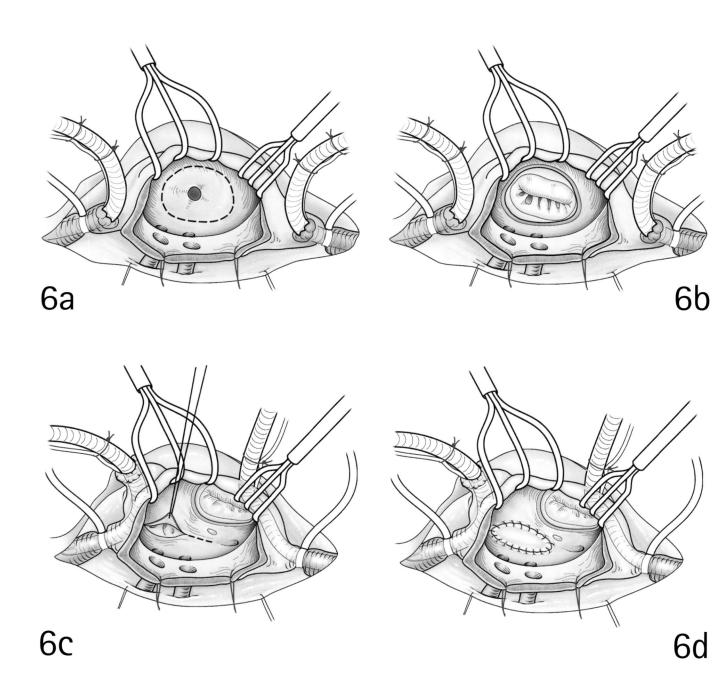

POSTOPERATIVE CARE

Cardiac output and systemic vascular resistance are optimized through the use of inotropes and afterload reducing agents. A pulmonary artery catheter should be placed for postoperative monitoring. Pulmonary vascular resistance is kept as low as possible with hyperventilation and nitric oxide as needed. Fluids are minimized with judicious use of diuretics to optimize the respiratory status. Preoperative pulmonary edema may take several days to resolve, requiring prolonged postoperative mechanical ventilation. In severe cases of respiratory failure, extracorporeal membrane oxygenation can be used while the pulmonary edema resolves.

Pulmonary hypertensive crises, manifested by sudden hypoxemia with rapid cardiovascular collapse and metabolic acidosis, can develop in patients with elevated preoperative pulmonary artery pressures. These crises can be precipitated by simple measures such as endotracheal suctioning. Measures to reduce the risk of such crises include fentanyl and/or paralysis for 24–48 hours. Interventions to circumvent a crisis include hyperventilation, maintenance of adequate oxygenation, and inhaled nitric oxide.

OUTCOME

Early mortality in patients undergoing repair of TAPVC is largely dependent on the initial degree of obstruction. The early mortality rate for initial repair was 4.9 per cent for all types in a review of 41 patients undergoing repair at the University of Michigan. Early diagnosis and repair, as well as optimal methods of postoperative management including extracorporeal membrane oxygenation as required, have resulted in a dramatic reduction in operative risk. For patients surviving the perioperative period, the long-term survival and functional status are good. In a recent review, survival at 15 years for all types was 84 per cent with a reoper-ation-free survival of 74 per cent. All patients were in New York Heart Association functional class I at the time of follow-up.

MANAGEMENT OF RECURRENT VENOUS OBSTRUCTION

An infrequent but challenging problem is the development of recurrent venous obstruction in 5–15 per cent of patients. Obstruction can develop at the anastomosis or at the individual pulmonary vein ostia in the common pulmonary vein. The obstruction usually develops within the first several months after initial repair and is believed by many to be the result of an exuberant inflammatory response. Repair of this lesion is technically challenging, and recurrent early stenoses remain a problem. The mortality associated with reoperation can be in excess of 50 per cent when bilateral stenoses are present.

The approach to recurrent venous obstruction is dependent on the level of obstruction. Isolated narrowing of the anastomosis between the common pulmonary vein and left atrium can often be repaired with revision of the anastomosis. Many efforts have been used to prevent inadequate growth at the suture line, including the use of absorbable sutures or interrupted sutures, without significant differences in the rate of stenosis.

Obstruction of the individual pulmonary venous ostia can be a greater challenge. Although the obstruction often appears to be limited to the ostium initially, recurrence is common, with progressive narrowing along the length of the vein into the hilum of the lung. Results after balloon angioplasty and/or stent insertion have been disappointing, and recurrent stenoses are the rule. Individual patch angioplasty of the ostia has also been used with poor long-term results. Lung transplantation has been considered in severe cases of extensive, bilateral disease.

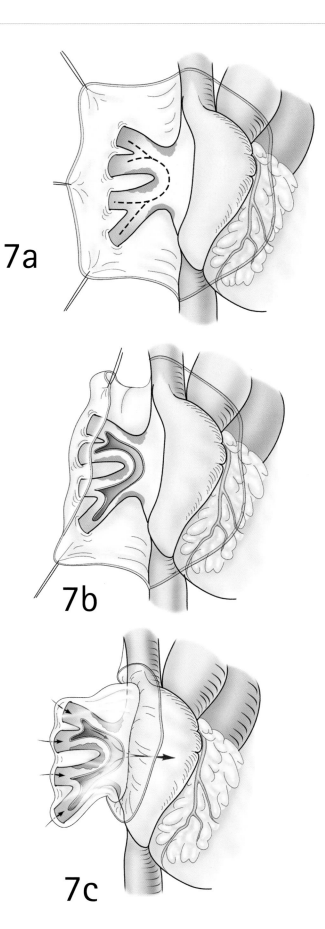

7a

7b

7c

7a–c A new approach to recurrent pulmonary vein stenosis after repair of TAPVC was reported by Lacour-Gayet. This technique uses a sutureless repair using *in situ* pericardium to create a neoatrium. The theory behind this repair is based on the concept that pulmonary venous obstruction results from inflammation induced locally by suture placement. Repair involves wide unroofing of the narrowed portion of each involved pulmonary vein from the left atrial anastomosis to the hilum (Figures 7a, b). A wide flap of pericardium is then elevated, with care taken to avoid disruption of posterior adhesions. The flap of pericardium is rotated over the unroofed pulmonary veins and sutured to the left atrial wall away from the venous ostia (Figure 7c). A large neoatrium is created into which pulmonary venous return can drain.

Two studies reviewing the use of the sutureless neoatrium for recurrent pulmonary vein stenosis have been reported. Lacour-Gayet and associates reviewed 14 patients with bilateral pulmonary vein obstruction undergoing reoperation. Pulmonary vein patch enlargement with or without endothelial debulking had a failure rate of 67 per cent, whereas the technique of *in situ* pericardial sutureless neoatrium had a failure rate of 29 per cent. Caldarone and colleagues reported nine patients with bilateral pulmonary vein obstruction of whom six died. Two of the three survivors were repaired with the creation of a sutureless neoatrium. Although these reports represent relatively few patients, this new procedure offers additional options for the treatment of a highly challenging and morbid condition.

FURTHER READING

Boger, A.J., Baak, R., Lee, P.C., *et al.* 1999. Early results and long-term follow-up after corrective surgery for total anomalous pulmonary venous return. *European Journal of Cardiothoracic Surgery* **16(3)**, 296–9.

Caldarone, C.A., Najm, H.K., Kadletz, M., *et al.* 1998. Relentless pulmonary vein stenosis after repair of total anomalous pulmonary venous drainage. *Annals of Thoracic Surgery* **66**, 1514–20.

Lacour-Gayet, F., Rey, C., Planché, C. 1996. Pulmonary vein stenosis: description of a sutureless surgical technique using the in situ pericardium. *Archives des Maladies du Coeur et des Vaisseaux* **89**, 633–6.

Lacour-Gayet, F., Zoghbi, J., Serraf, A., *et al.* 1999. Surgical management of progressive pulmonary venous obstruction after repair of total anomalous pulmonary venous connection. *Journal of Thoracic and Cardiovascular Surgery* **117**, 679–87.

Lupinetti, F.M., Kulik, T.J., Beekman, R.H., Crowley, D.C., Bove, E.L. 1993. Correction of total anomalous pulmonary venous connection in infancy. *Journal of Thoracic and Cardiovascular Surgery* **106**, 880–5.

Sano, S., Brawn, W.J., Mee, R.B.B. 1989. Total anomalous pulmonary venous drainage. *Journal of Thoracic and Cardiovascular Surgery* **97**, 886–92.

41

Atrial septal defect

PETER B. MANNING MD

Associate Professor of Pediatric Cardiothoracic Surgery, University of Cincinnati College of Medicine; Director of Cardiothoracic Surgery, Children's Hospital Medical Center, Cincinnati, Ohio, USA

HISTORY

The management of atrial septal defects (ASD) holds a special place in the history of congenital cardiac surgery and also serves as an example of current trends in treatment of congenital cardiac anomalies. Closure of a secundum ASD by Gibbon in 1952 was the first successful operation that was performed using cardiopulmonary bypass support. ASD closure is the most frequently performed open heart operation in children in most centers. In selected cases, closure using catheter-delivered devices is now performed, completely avoiding the need for surgical incision and cardiopulmonary bypass.

PRINCIPLES AND JUSTIFICATION

Occasionally, an ASD results in a large enough shunt to cause symptoms of congestive heart failure in young children. Most isolated atrial level shunts, however, are asymptomatic during childhood. Closure is indicated to prevent long-term sequelae of pulmonary hypertensive vascular disease, atrial arrhythmias, congestive heart failure, and cerebrovascular accident from paradoxical embolization.

The preschool years are generally chosen for closure of most secundum ASDs. Spontaneous closure beyond 2 years of age is exceedingly rare. If diagnosis is made early, delaying the procedure until the child is 2–3 years old (more than 12 kg) often allows it to be done without the need for any blood product transfusion. In older children the defect is repaired electively on discovery.

OPERATION

Surgical incisions

Median sternotomy is most commonly used. Adequate exposure can be obtained using partial sternotomy or limited thoracotomy, which may be chosen for cosmetic reasons.

Cannulation for bypass

1, 2 Standard ascending aortic cannulation is used for arterial inflow. Bicaval cannulation for secundum ASD closure can be most easily obtained using two cannulae placed via the right atrial (RA) appendage, which is typically enlarged due to chronic volume overload (Figure 1). For sinus venosus defects, the superior cannulation is best placed directly into the superior vena cava (SVC), well above the entrance of any pulmonary veins (Figure 2). Preliminary dissection of the SVC should be performed before a cannulation site is chosen. When a persistent left SVC is present, it can be directly cannulated, or its return can be controlled using cardiotomy suction. Rarely, a communicating vein to the right SVC exists, allowing tourniquet occlusion of the left SVC during repair.

Myocardial protection

Due to the short period of cardiac arrest that is needed for most repairs, systemic hypothermia can be avoided. Myocardial protection is most easily achieved using anterograde, cold blood cardioplegia with the addition of topical hypothermia.

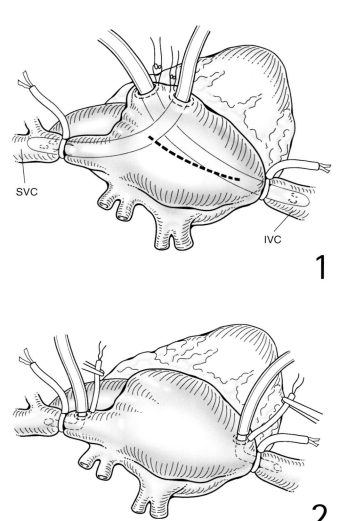

Secundum atrial septal defects

3 A limited right atriotomy typically affords excellent exposure of the defect. An anterior retractor can hold the inferior vena cava cannula out of the way if atrial appendage cannulation is used. Defects in the fossa ovalis are the most commonly encountered. If the defect seems more superior or posterior in the septum than is typical, a sinus venosus defect should be suspected, and confirmation of the entry of the right pulmonary veins to the left of the septum should be made. Often, thin multi-fenestrated remnants of septum primum partially cover the fossa ovalis. These can be resected to facilitate suture placement in stronger tissue. A left-sided vent is rarely needed, and care should be taken to avoid suction into the left atrium to prevent air entrapment after closure of the defect.

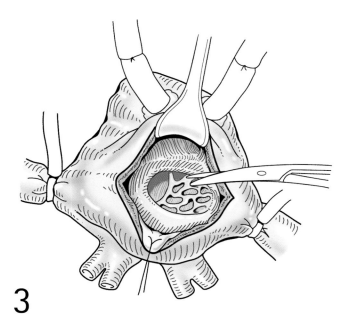

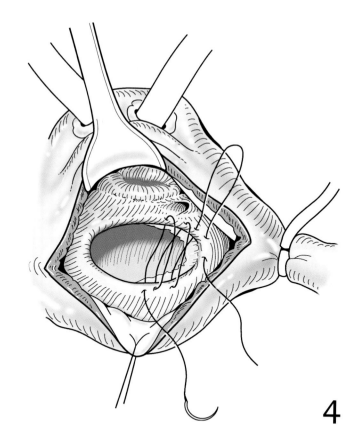

4

4, 5 Because of the oval shape of most secundum defects, 80 per cent can be closed by the primary suture technique. A double layer of polypropylene is begun at the inferior limit of the defect, as this margin is typically most difficult to define. Before complete closure of the defect, entrapped air should be evacuated from the left atrium.

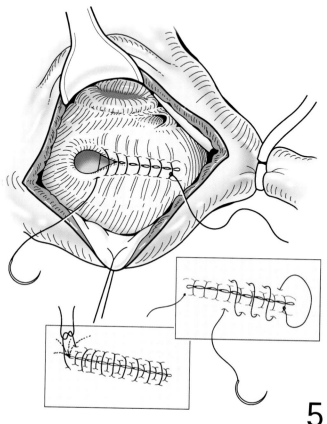

5

6 If the defect is large or rounder in shape, patch closure should be performed to avoid closure under tension and distortion of atrial anatomy. A patch of autologous pericardium that is slightly smaller than the relaxed size of the defect can be used, again beginning the suture line inferiorly. Polytetrafluoroethylene, Dacron, and bovine pericardium are also suitable patch materials.

With the septal defect securely closed, the aortic cross-clamp can be removed, and the atriotomy is closed using a double layer of polypropylene suture. Caval tourniquet snares are released after atriotomy closure, and cannulae that were placed via the right atrial appendage can be backed into the body of the atrium to improve venous drainage.

Maneuvers to evacuate any residual air from the left side of the heart using the left atrial vent (if used) or the cardioplegic site should be performed during rewarming. Generally, temporary pacing wires are not necessary unless the patient has exhibited evidence of arrhythmia or conduction delay during rewarming.

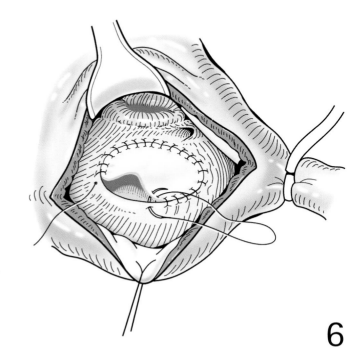

6

Sinus venosus atrial septal defect

The ASD is generally more superior and posterior than the typical secundum ASD. The right upper pulmonary veins typically drain into the junction of the SVC and right atrium. Occasionally, multiple veins drain the right upper lobe and may enter the SVC some distance from its atrial junction. Careful circumferential dissection of the SVC allows identification of these anomalous venous connections for cannulation site selection and planning of the repair. Injury to the right phrenic nerve must be avoided during dissection of the lateral aspect of the SVC.

If the pulmonary veins drain to the cavoatrial junction area, baffle repair of the defect using a pericardial patch is performed. If pulmonary veins enter some distance up the SVC, or if the right SVC is unusually small as seen in the presence of a persistent left SVC, the so-called Warden repair is performed, directing the lower SVC flow through the septal defect, with translocation of the upper SVC to the right atrial appendage.

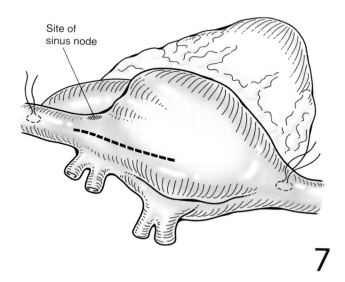

Site of
sinus node

7

BAFFLE REPAIR

7, 8 The right atrial incision is oriented longitudinally and is extended superiorly across the lateral aspect of the cavoatrial junction and up the SVC to the upper limit of any anomalously connected pulmonary veins. The lateral placement of this incision is important to avoid injury to the sinus node.

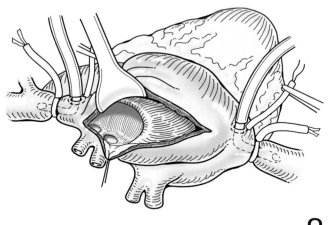

8

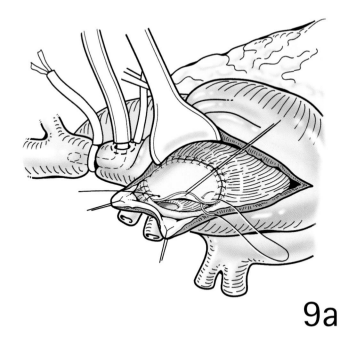

9a

9a, b The patch is sutured from the lower edge of the septal defect, transitioning up and around the superior edge of the highest pulmonary vein to direct the flow of pulmonary venous blood through the septal defect to the left atrium. The patch should be slightly redundant to avoid obstructing this pathway, especially when it is extended up the vena cava for more than a few millimeters. A single, small, pulmonary vein branch that drains high into the SVC can be ignored, as this amount of persistent left-to-right shunt is of little consequence. The atriotomy closure should be augmented with a patch superiorly to prevent stenosis of the SVC–right atrial junction.

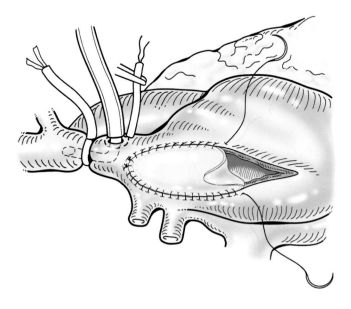

9b

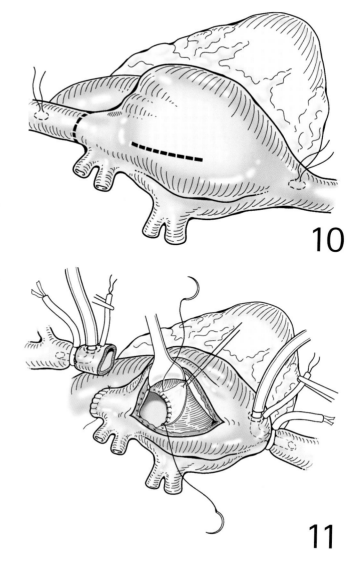

WARDEN REPAIR

10, 11 A limited, longitudinal right atriotomy allows exposure of the septal defect and the cavoatrial junction. The patch is sutured from the lower edge of the septal defect around the lateral aspect of the cavoatrial junction, directing all SVC flow through the defect to the left atrium. The SVC is then transected just at the upper level of the highest pulmonary vein.

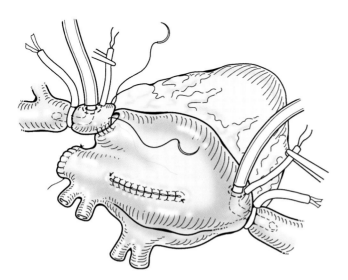

12 The cardiac end is oversewn, avoiding stenosis of the highest pulmonary vein. The cephalic end of the SVC is mobilized further, if necessary, and then anastomosed to a position on the right atrial appendage, where it reaches without tension or angulation using fine, absorbable monofilament suture. Care must be taken to avoid purse-stringing this anastomosis.

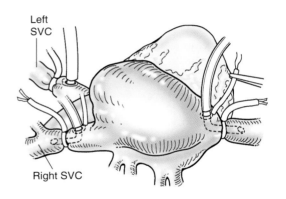

Left SVC

Right SVC

Coronary sinus septal defect – unroofed coronary sinus

13 The coronary sinus septal defect is associated with persistence of a left SVC, typically without a communicating innominate vein to the right SVC. The coronary sinus is often completely unroofed, with the left SVC draining to the roof of the left atrium just medial to the left atrial appendage. In the rare case in which the coronary sinus is partially unroofed, the defect can be closed either directly or with a patch. Care should be taken to avoid either narrowing the coronary sinus with direct closure or making the patch too redundant, obstructing left ventricular inflow.

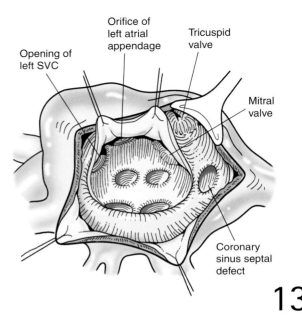

Orifice of left atrial appendage

Tricuspid valve

Opening of left SVC

Mitral valve

Coronary sinus septal defect

13

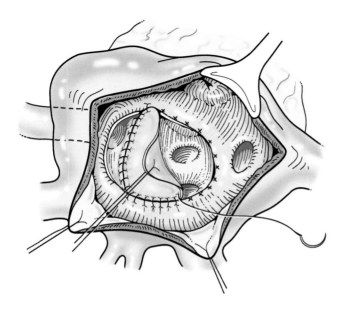

14

14 When the coronary sinus is completely unroofed, the anomaly is best repaired using a pericardial baffle to direct the left SVC blood across the roof of the left atrium to the secundum ASD. This approach avoids the need to sew near the pulmonary veins or the mitral valve annulus. The secundum ASD is enlarged superiorly to the roof of the atrium. An oblong patch is attached to the far side of the left SVC orifice, typically between this opening and the opening into the left atrial appendage. The first suture line is run above the superior pulmonary vein orifices to the posterior aspect of the ASD. The other end of the suture is run more anteriorly across the roof of the left atrium to the anterior edge of the ASD. The suture lines converge at the inferior aspect of the ASD, thus directing the left SVC blood to the right atrium and closing the secundum ASD. A second atrial defect may be present lower in the septum at the usual site of the coronary sinus orifice. This defect is closed separately, either directly or by patch, with care taken superiorly to avoid injury to the atrioventricular (AV) node.

Primum atrial septal defect

15 Venous cannulation should allow unobstructed exposure of the intra-atrial anatomy, especially in the smaller child. This goal is accomplished using direct cannulation of the inferior cavoatrial junction with a thin-walled, right-angle cannula. Superior caval cannulation may be via the right atrial appendage or directly into the SVC. Venting of the left side of the heart via the right superior pulmonary vein facilitates exposure by capturing pulmonary venous return.

Initial careful inspection of the intracardiac anatomy must be carried out after right atriotomy. The limits of the primum ASD should be defined, as well as the presence of an additional septal defect in the fossa ovalis region. The absence of interventricular communication should be confirmed by gentle inspection and probing of the subvalvular region using a fine right-angle clamp. Particular attention to the anatomy of the left-sided AV valve is crucial, as most postoperative complications relate to the function of this structure. The presence of the cleft in the anterior or septal leaflet is identified, the presence of two well-separated papillary muscles within the left ventricle is confirmed, and anomalies such as a double orifice or parachute valve configuration are excluded.

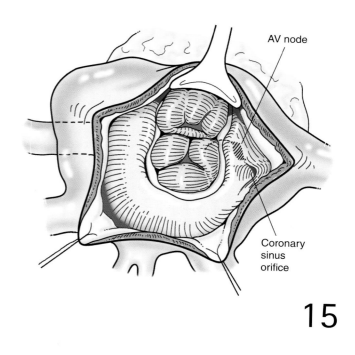

15

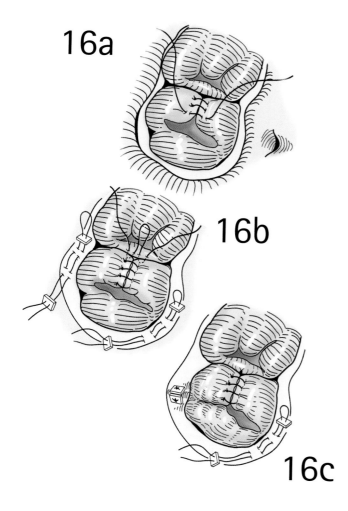

16a–c The cleft in the anterior left AV valve leaflet is closed, first using fine sutures with an interrupted simple or mattress technique. Testing of the valve by instilling iced saline into the ventricle confirms competence of the repair and identifies the need for the addition of any annuloplasty stitches.

17 The septal defect is closed with a pericardial patch. The use of a non-smooth-surfaced patch such as Dacron has been associated with postoperative hemolysis in the presence of even a small regurgitant jet directed against the septal patch. A pledgeted mattress suture is placed at the midpoint of the base of the reconstructed anterior leaflet, passing the suture through some of the ventricular septal crest from the right ventricular side. One edge of the patch is cut without a curve, and this edge is anchored to the heart using the mattress suture. A line of demarcation between the right- and left-sided components of the valve is usually easily appreciated, although this may be accentuated by traction on the mattress suture at the midpoint on the valve. Each end of the suture is run to the AV annulus, securing the straight edge of the patch to the demarcation line between right- and left-sided valve tissue. The patch is now trimmed to the appropriate size to match the septal defect, and the suture line is continued at each end, attaching the patch to the inferior free edge of the atrial septum. Inferiorly, care must be taken to avoid injury to the bundle of His. If the edge of the atrial septum is quite close to the site where the patch is attached to the valve leaflets, superficial bites can be used in this area. Alternatively, the patch can be cut with a projection to allow suturing directly toward the coronary sinus, then within the medial margin of the coronary sinus, and finally transitioning over to the free edge of the atrial septum.

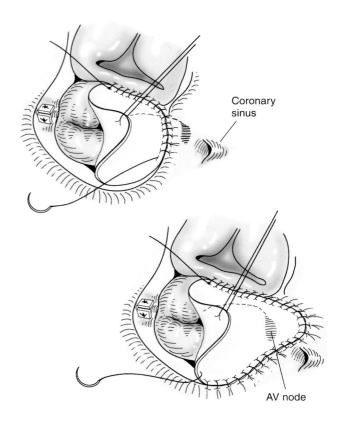

Coronary sinus

AV node

17

POSTOPERATIVE CARE

In most cases the patient can be extubated in the operating room. Close monitoring of the cardiac rhythm should be carried out, particularly after repair of sinus venosus defects (sinus node dysfunction) and partial AV canal (heart block or accelerated junctional rhythms). In many centers blood product transfusion can be completely avoided for ASD repair, even in children as small as 10 kg, using small volume circuits and blood conservation techniques. Postoperative anemia to a hematocrit level in the low 20s is usually well tolerated, although monitoring for signs of poor perfusion or acidosis should be carried out to ensure adequate tissue oxygen delivery in the face of this anemia.

OUTCOME

When repair is accomplished early in the patient's life, longevity and exercise capacity are no different from those of the general population. Although patients with isolated ASDs are not at increased risk for bacterial endocarditis, antibiotic prophylaxis is recommended postoperatively for a period of 6 months following closure of a secundum defect. In older patients, when atrial arrhythmias have developed before repair, closure of the defect often does not reverse the atrial dilation that has developed, and ongoing dysrhythmia management may be necessary.

FURTHER READING

Du, Z.D., Hijazi, Z.M., Kleinman, C.S., Silverman, N.H., Larntz, K. 2002 Amplatzer Investigators. Comparison between transcatheter and surgical closure of secundum atrial septal defect in children and adults: results of a multicenter nonrandomized trial. *J Am Coll Cardiol* 39, 1836–44.

Baskett, R.J., Tancock, E., Ross, D.B. 2003 The gold standard for atrial septal defect closure: current surgical results, with an emphasis on morbidity. *Pediatr Cardiol* 4, 444–7.

Horvath, K.A., Burke, R.P., Collins, J.J. Jr., Cohn, L.H. 1992 Surgical treatment of adult atrial septal defect: early and long-term results. *J Am Coll Cardiol* 20, 1156–9.

Meijboom, F., Hess, J., Szatmari, A., Utens, E.M., McGhie, J., Deckers, J.W., Roelandt, J.R., Bos, E. 1993 Long-term follow-up (9 to 20 years) after surgical closure of atrial septal defect at a young age. *Am J Cardiol* 72, 1431–4.

Gustafson, R.A., Warden, H.E., Murray, G.F., Hill, R.C., Rozar, G.E. 1989 Partial anomalous pulmonary venous connection to the right side of the heart. *J Thorac Cardiovasc Surg* 98, 861–8.

Najm, H.K., Williams, W.G., Chuaratanaphong, S., Watzka, S.B., Coales, J.G., Freedom, R.M. 1998 Primum atrial septal defect in children: early results, risk factors, and freedom from reoperation. *Ann Thorac Surg* 66, 829–35.

42

Atrioventricular septal defects

THOMAS L. SPRAY MD
Alice Langdon Warner Professor of Surgery, Department of Cardiothoracic Surgery, University of Pennsylvania School of Medicine; Division Chief of Cardiothoracic Surgery, The Children's Hospital of Philadelphia, Philadelphia, Pennsylvania, USA

HISTORY AND ANATOMY

Atrioventricular septal defects (AVSDs) include deficiencies in the inferior portion of the atrial septum, the inflow portion of the ventricular septum, and the tissue forming the left and right atrioventricular (AV) valves.

1a Anatomically, AVSDs have been divided into partial, incomplete, and complete subtypes. Partial AVSDs have an ostium primum–type atrial septal defect (ASD) above the AV valve with a cleft or commissure between the superior and inferior cleft AV valve leaflets, associated with varying degrees of AV valve insufficiency. In incomplete AVSD, the atrial ostium primum defect is present, and the junction between the left and right AV valves is separated from the crest of the ventricular septum via a membrane of tissue. In these patients, the left and right AV valves have separate orifices but with abnormal structure, and the ventricular septal defect (VSD) component beneath the AV valve leaflets may be restrictive and filled in by chordal tissue. In complete AVSD, the common AV valve bridges over the VSD. The AV valve apparatus and AVSD has what can be considered as five leaflets in the complete form and six leaflets in the partial form. In complete AVSD, a superior and inferior bridging leaflet is always present with two additional right-sided lateral and anterosuperior leaflets and a left lateral or 'mural' leaflet.

The degree of bridging and chordal attachments of the common AV valve leaflets have been used to create the Rastelli classification of AVSDs.

1b In Rastelli type A defect, the superior bridging leaflet is split at the ventricular septum, and the left superior leaflet is over the left ventricle and the right superior leaflet over the right ventricle, with chordal attachments to the ventricular septum.

1c In Rastelli type C, the superior bridging leaflet floats freely over the ventricular septum without chordal attachments to the crest of the ventricular septum. The posterior bridging leaflet may be attached or free in either Rastelli type A or C classification. Rastelli type B is between the A and C extremes and is very rare.

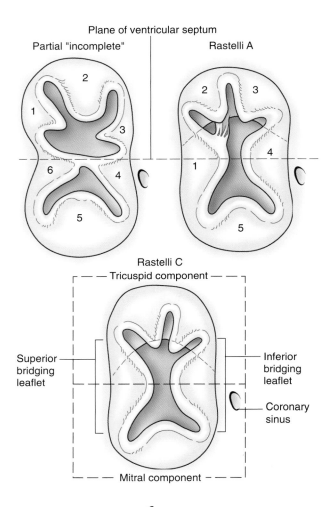

2 An additional consideration in AVSD repairs is the location of the AV conduction tissue, which is displaced posteriorly in AVSD toward the coronary sinus. The conduction tissue generally lies between the coronary sinus and the VSD. The ostium primum ASD distorts the coronary sinus orifice more posteriorly and inferiorly toward the left atrium, distorting the triangle of Koch. The bundle of His generally travels from the location near the coronary sinus along the crest of the VSD, under the inferior bridging leaflet on the rim of the VSD.

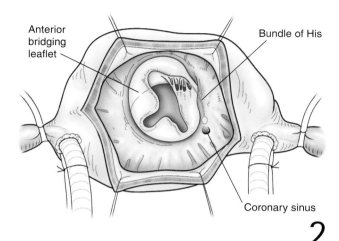

PRINCIPLES AND JUSTIFICATION

Patients with AVSDs have symptoms related to the magnitude of the associated left-to-right shunt and the magnitude of associated lesions such as AV valve insufficiency. Patients with partial AVSDs may have physiology similar to that of patients with secundum ASDs with no symptoms and a similar cardiac murmur, with right heart volume overload on echocardiography. When associated left AV valve insufficiency is present, cardiac failure and pulmonary congestion with dyspnea can occur. Because complete AVSD is associated with more significant left-to-right shunting, patients often have congestive heart failure, fatigue, and dyspnea with failure to thrive. Severe pulmonary hypertension eventually develops in the majority of patients, resulting in death in up to 65 per cent of infants with the complete form before 1 year of age without surgery. The majority of patients with complete AVSDs has Down syndrome, which may exacerbate the development of pulmonary hypertension. Echocardiography is the diagnostic procedure of choice in patients with AVSDs; valve anatomy and function can be accurately assessed.

Patients with partial AVSD usually undergo elective repair before school age, unless symptoms of heart failure are present. If significant AV valve insufficiency is present, then earlier operation is indicated. Patients with complete AVSDs generally require complete correction between 2 and 4 months of age. Operation at an early age may prevent the development of progressive pulmonary hypertension, which is a significant source of morbidity, and also may prevent early postoperative pulmonary hypertensive events that can increase postoperative morbidity and mortality. Patients who have significant congestive heart failure, failure to thrive, and poor weight gain can be operated on at any age, including the newborn period, although the requirement for operation in the neonatal period is rare and generally reserved to those patients with severe heart failure with associated significant AV valve insufficiency. Pulmonary artery banding is generally contraindicated, as complete anatomical repair can be performed at essentially any age in patients with AVSDs.

Contraindications to surgical intervention are based on the severity of pulmonary vascular resistance. Severely elevated pulmonary resistance above 10 Wood units may be a relative contraindication to repair, and significant unbalancing of the flow through the common AV valve to the left or right ventricle may be an indication for either delayed repair and preliminary pulmonary artery banding or consideration of a single ventricle surgical strategy.

PREOPERATIVE CARE

Patients with complete AVSDs often require the use of digitalis and diuretics to control congestive heart failure. If weight gain is sluggish or nonexistent, early operation is indicated. Prolonged attempts at feeding or placement of nasogastric tubes or gastrostomy tubes for continuous feeding in hopes of weight gain are generally ill-advised, as weight gain can continue to be poor, and progressive congestive heart failure may lead to more instability postoperatively.

If patients present late, after 4 months of age, and have signs of significant elevation of pulmonary vascular resistance, then cardiac catheterization should be considered for assessment of the pulmonary vascular bed under conditions of oxygen, nitric oxide, and prostacycline to assess reversibility of the pulmonary vascular disease before initiation of complete repair.

ANESTHESIA

Anesthetic management for patients with AVSDs is similar to that for other neonates or infants undergoing complex cardiac procedures. Narcotic anesthesia is generally used and, because of the potential for pulmonary vascular resistance elevation, hyperventilation early postoperatively is generally preferred. Nitric oxide can be used if pulmonary resistance is significantly elevated in the early postoperative period. This strategy decreases the risk of pulmonary hypertensive crises that were a cause of significant morbidity and early mortality in early series of AV canal defect repairs when operation was undertaken at over 6 months of age.

OPERATION

A standard median sternotomy is performed, and thymic tissue is removed if necessary. A portion of the anterior pericardium is excised and set aside for use as a patch in the atrium. The pericardium can be fixed in glutaraldehyde solution if desired. The aorta and vena cavae are cannulated, and a cardioplegia needle is inserted into the aortic root. It is generally advisable to mobilize the ligamentum arteriosum and ensure complete ductal closure by ligation, as echocardiography may occasionally miss the presence of a small patent ductus arteriosus with the excess turbulent flow out the pulmonary outflow tract from the large left-to-right shunt. After cardioplegic arrest is accomplished, the caval tapes are tightened, and a right atriotomy incision is made parallel to the AV groove and extending downward near the inferior vena caval cannula to gain maximum exposure of the atrium. Stay sutures may then be placed to allow adequate exposure of the common AV valve.

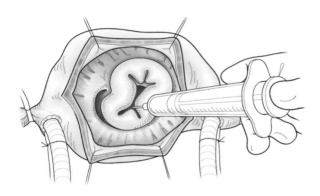

3a

3a–c The AV valve is exposed, and saline is injected into the ventricle to float the AV valves to assess the areas of coaptation. The area of coaptation between the left superior and left inferior bridging leaflet is then identified and secured with a suture (Figure 3b). Identification of this coapting area is important to prevent distortion of the AV valve during the repair and associated mitral regurgitation (Figure 3c). The size of the VSD is then examined, and a patch of Dacron material or Gore-Tex cut in a semicircular fashion suitable to the height of the defect from the right side of the ventricular septum to the bridging AV valves. The anterior posterior dimension is then measured. Inferiorly, a slightly larger length of the patch must be permitted to extend beyond the posterior aspect of the VSD underneath the inferior leaflet to protect the common bundle of His; superiorly, the patch is cut in a concave 'scooped out' fashion to accommodate the common AV valve attachment.

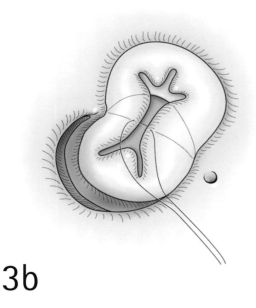

3b

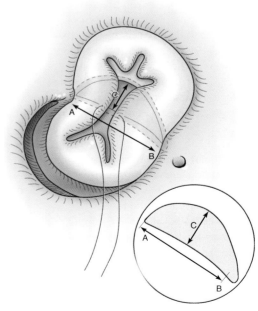

3c

4 The patch of Dacron material is then secured into the VSD starting at the midportion of the patch, inferiorly to the right of the crest of the ventricular septum. Using a running technique, the patch can then be anchored into place using traction on the suture to gain exposure superiorly and inferiorly near the hinge points of the bridging leaflets of the common AV valve. If chordal attachments of the inferior bridging leaflet obscure the margin of the septum, secondary chordae can be divided as the patch is inserted. Posteriorly, the suture is brought through the base of the bridging leaflet at the level of the annulus to avoid penetrating the bundle of His. Superiorly, the suture is brought through the annulus at the appropriate site of the superior bridging leaflet.

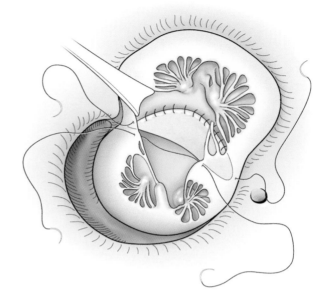

4

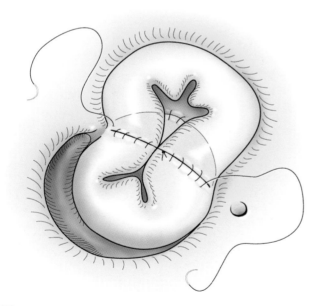

5

5 Next, the superior margin of the VSD patch is secured to the common AV valve leaflets using a running technique, incorporating the crest of the VSD patch below the AV valve tissue. A mattress technique may be necessary in some cases to avoid chordal attachments, and care must be taken to bring the coapting surfaces of the left superior and inferior bridging leaflets together at the initially marked point to ensure good coaptation of the left-sided component of the AV valve. After completion of the VSD patch implant, injection of saline into the left- and right-sided components of the common AV valve assess the degree of insufficiency.

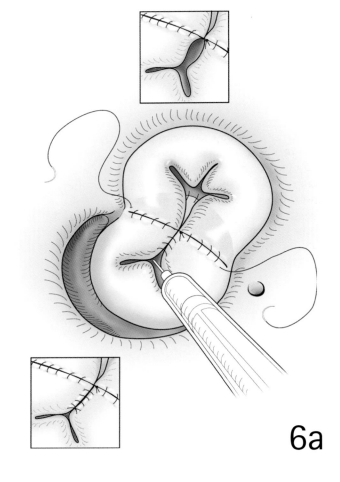

6a

6 a, b The commissure or cleft between the left superior and inferior bridging leaflet is then closed to the point of chordal attachments at the tip of the leaflet using a running suture, generally of 6/0 Gore-Tex material that does not cut through the delicate valve leaflet tissue. AV valve competence is then assessed again with saline injection and, if additional regurgitation at the coaptation areas is present, small pledgeted annuloplasty sutures may be required at the commissures.

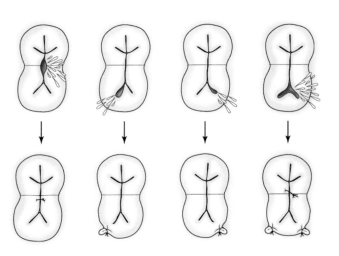

6b

7 After AV competence is assured, the ostium primum ASD component of the canal defect is closed with the homologous pericardial patch. The pericardium is cut to an appropriate size and shape, and then the suture line at the level of the common bridging AV valve leaflets is created using a running technique, reinforcing the VSD closure against the common AV valve with the suture to prevent valve dehiscence.

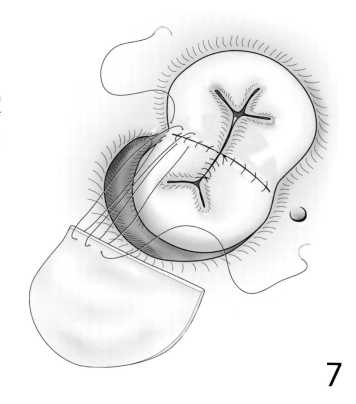

7

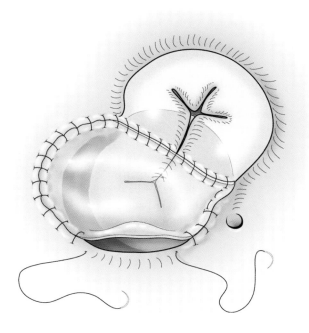

8

8 Posteriorly, the suture line is carried along the leaflet tissue at the annulus of the posterior bridging leaflet to allow the suture line to deviate away from the coronary sinus before connection to the atrial septum, to avoid the AV node and leave the coronary sinus in the right atrial aspect of the repair. The ASD closure is completed, and then the right atrium is closed with a running suture.

Primary closure of ventricular septal defect component

9 An alternative to two-patch repair of AVSD has been popularized by Nunn. In this repair, the VSD patch is omitted, and pledgeted mattress sutures are taken from the right-sided aspect of the VSD and then brought directly through the bridging leaflets of the AV valves and through the lower portion of the atrial septal patch. When the sutures are tied, the common AV valve leaflets are brought down to the crest of the ventricular septum. Although this technique would seem to potentially distort the AV valve leaflets and possibly create subaortic stenosis, experience to date has shown that good results can be obtained with this technique, with achievement of AV valve competence and no higher incidence of subaortic obstruction. Care, however, must be taken to place the sutures accurately to avoid distortion of the AV valve. The technique appears to be most suitable in patients with Rastelli type C anatomy, but it has been used in all types of AVSDs with good success.

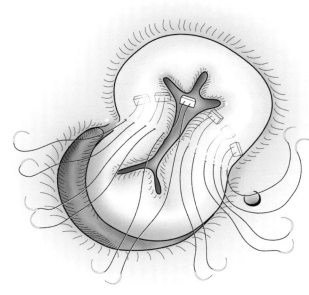

9

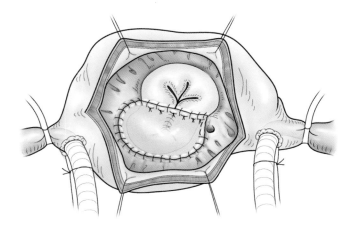

10

Repair of partial atrioventricular septal defect

10 The repair of partial AVSD involves the ASD patch as done in the complete form of AVSD. A pericardial patch is secured to the AV valve at the bridging tissue between the left and right valve orifices, and the cleft or commissure of the mitral valve between its left superior and inferior leaflets is closed with a running suture. After assessment of AV competence is performed, the ASD patch is completed, leaving the coronary sinus on the right atrial aspect of the repair.

POSTOPERATIVE CARE

Postoperative complications include pulmonary hypertensive events, left AV valve insufficiency, and complete heart block. Intraoperative transesophageal echocardiography is used routinely to assess the competence of the AV valves after the repair; and if significant regurgitation is present, then immediate reoperation with additional attempts to create AV valve tissue coaptation is important to prevent postoperative pulmonary hypertension and increased operative mortality. If patients are older at operation or have significant pulmonary hypertension preoperatively, generally such infants are kept sedated and paralyzed for 24 hours before emerging from anesthesia to decrease the risk of pulmonary hypertensive events. Nitric oxide is used, if necessary, to control the pulmonary vascular bed. Younger patients and those without significant pulmonary hypertension generally are allowed to awaken from anesthesia and are extubated within 24 hours of surgery.

Postoperative AV valve insufficiency is present in as many as 10–15 per cent of patients, but this problem is generally mild to moderate in degree. Patients are often managed with inotropic support consisting of milrinone to decrease afterload and improve right ventricular function and are converted to oral afterload-reducing agents before discharge from the hospital.

OUTCOME

The surgical results with repair of AVSDs have progressively improved. Partial AVSD repairs have a mortality rate similar to that of isolated secundum ASDs, with a mortality of 1 per cent or less. Nevertheless, these patients may have an incidence of reoperation for left AV valve insufficiency or stenosis, and reoperation may be associated with significant mortality and morbidity if there is deficiency of left AV valve tissue resulting in either significant mitral stenosis or progressive mitral insufficiency. These patients may, on occasion, come to valve replacement after repair attempts have failed.

The surgical results with complete ASD repairs have also progressively improved. Most major centers now have an operative mortality of 3 per cent or less for complete AV canal repair, with reoperation rates of 10–15 per cent. When competence of the common AV valves has been achieved, long-term valve function has been excellent, with rare reoperation on late follow-up. Mild to moderate degrees of AV valve regurgitation are generally well-tolerated, although reoperation may be required if regurgitation progresses and the patient shows signs of congestive heart failure or pulmonary hypertension. Reoperation for secondary repair of the left AV valve has been associated with good results, with only rare need for valve replacement in large series.

FURTHER READING

Canter, C.E., Spray, T.L., Huddleston, C.B., Mendeloff, E. 1997. Interoperative evaluation of atrioventricular septal defect repair by color flow mapping echocardiography. *Annals of Thoracic Surgery* 63, 592.

Elliott, M.J., Jacobs, J.P. 1997. Atrioventricular canal defects. In Kaiser, L.R., Kron, I.L., Spray, T.L. (eds), *Mastery of Cardiothoracic Surgery*. Philadelphia: Lippincott-Raven Publishers, 742–58.

Rastelli, G.C., Kirklin, J.W., Titus, J.L. 1966. Anatomic observations on complete form of persistent common atrioventricular canal with special reference to atrioventricular valves. *Mayo Clinic Proceedings* 41, 296.

Rastelli, G.C., Ongley, P.A., Kirklin, J.W., McGoon, D.C. 1968. Surgical repair of the complete form of persistent common atrioventricular canal. *Journal of Thoracic and Cardiovascular Surgery* 55, 299.

Thiene, G., Wenink, A., Anderson, R.H., *et al.* 1981. Surgical anatomy and pathology of the conduction tissues in atrioventricular septal defects. *Journal of Thoracic and Cardiovascular Surgery* 82, 928.

43

Fontan procedure for functionally single ventricle and double-inlet ventricle

GORDON A. COHEN MD, PHD
Senior Lecturer, Department of Cardiothoracic Surgery, University College London; Consultant Cardiothoracic Surgeon, Cardiothoracic Unit, Great Ormond Street Hospital for Children National Health Service Trust, London, UK

MARC R. DE LEVAL MD, FRCS
Professor of Cardiothoracic Surgery and Consultant Cardiothoracic Surgeon, Cardiothoracic Unit, Great Ormond Street Hospital for Children National Health Service Trust, London, UK

HISTORY

In 1971, Fontan and Baudet published their landmark paper describing a surgical correction whereby the pulmonary and systemic circulations were placed in series in a patient with tricuspid atresia. Since that time, the indications for this procedure have been extended to include all defects with a functionally univentricular heart. Despite the early success of this procedure, longevity and efficiency of this circulatory arrangement have been of constant concern, leading to numerous modifications of the original operation. Some of the early modifications dispensed with the inlet and outlet valves and ultimately led to the direct connection of the functional right atrium to the pulmonary circulation.

The usefulness of the right atrium in this connection has been questioned, and this concern led to the concept of lateral tunnel or total cavopulmonary connection (TCPC). In this operation, the superior and the inferior caval veins are connected to the pulmonary arteries. However, the superior vena cava undergoes a direct connection, whereas the inferior vena cava (IVC) is connected via a prosthetic conduit. The inferior connection takes the form of either an intra-atrial tunnel or an extracardiac conduit.

PRINCIPLES AND JUSTIFICATION

The basic principle of the original Fontan operation was to divert systemic venous return back to the pulmonary artery without the use of a functional ventricle. This arrangement then allowed the functional ventricle of the heart to be used

for providing systemic blood flow. Since it was originally described in 1971, the operation has undergone numerous modifications. Despite the evolution of the procedure, that central principle remains the basis of the various techniques that are used to perform the operation today.

A number of factors influence the approach to the repair of the patient with a functionally single ventricle. The main considerations include:

1 The use of the atrium as a contractile chamber and the use of valved conduits
2 Whether or not to perform a staged repair (bidirectional Glenn shunt followed by completion Fontan procedure)
3 The timing of the repair
4 The type of repair performed: lateral tunnel versus conduit, fenestrated versus completed.

The product of these considerations is a short list of surgical options for a functional single ventricle that includes systemic–pulmonary artery shunting, bidirectional Glenn shunt, and fenestrated Fontan and completed Fontan procedures. None of these options represents a complete repair; and in fact, all are palliative, with varying advantages and disadvantages. Unfortunately, the indications and timing for each of these procedures remain poorly defined. As a result, the application of these options varies from center to center.

The initial Fontan procedure and early modifications attempted to use a contractile atrial chamber as a pump to assist blood flow into the pulmonary arteries. However, the TCPC, which is the modification performed in contemporary times, does not depend on the contractile properties of the atrium. The TCPC directs, rather than pumps, systemic venous return into the pulmonary arteries. It is generally accepted that an atriopulmonary connection is an inefficient system. *In vitro* flow studies and hydrodynamic models that examine flow energetics have demonstrated this principle to be the case. Such a connection has flow disturbances at the inlet and the outlet of the atrial cavity and additional energy losses at the level of the atriopulmonary anastomosis. In addition, the pulsatile activity of the chamber exaggerates turbulence, which is inherently present in such a connection. Thus, the TCPC appears to be an appropriate alternative to the atriopulmonary connection for complex Fontan operations.

The traditional approach to the patient with a functional single ventricle had been a neonatal palliative procedure (shunt, pulmonary artery band, or complex reconstruction) followed by a completed Fontan procedure later in life. However, in 1990, surgeons from Children's Hospital in Boston advocated the bidirectional Glenn shunt (superior cavopulmonary anastomosis) as an intermediate step between a neonatal palliative procedure and a completion Fontan (TCPC). The staged repair was thought to reduce the morbidity and the mortality of the subsequent Fontan procedure. Consequently, the concept of performing a bidirectional Glenn shunt as an intermediate step has received relatively widespread acceptance.

The issue of timing for a Fontan procedure as definitive palliation is poorly defined. A review of the literature demonstrates published series with a broad spectrum of ages. Children younger than 1 year of age as well as adults in their mid-40s are among the patients who have undergone a successful Fontan procedure. However, the approximate average age of patients who undergo the operation in contemporary series is somewhere between 4 and 5 years. Despite the large number of patients who have undergone a Fontan procedure worldwide, no 'ideal' age or 'optimal' timing exists for the operation that has yet been identified. Moreover, the timing of a Fontan procedure may differ depending on the underlying diagnosis (i.e. hypoplastic left heart syndrome vs. tricuspid atresia, etc.).

Scientifically and clinically, patients who undergo a TCPC have been shown to have a better hemodynamic configuration as well as improved mortality and morbidity when compared with those who have an atriopulmonary connection. However, the clinical differences between the various modifications of the TCPC are unclear. The two most common modifications of the TCPC that are performed today are the lateral tunnel Fontan and the total extracardiac TCPC (extracardiac conduit). No good clinical series has been published to date that demonstrates one modification to be superior to the other. A comparison of series in the literature from centers that perform higher volumes of the TCPC show similar results for either operation.

Nonetheless, theoretical concerns may favor one procedure over the other. The extracardiac conduit has the benefit of being able to be performed on bypass at normothermia with a beating heart, with no need for aortic cross-clamping. Moreover, by its very nature of being extracardiac, no foreign material is placed within the systemic ventricle; and thus, a theoretical benefit exists in reducing the risk of thrombosis. In contrast, the lateral tunnel Fontan procedure requires systemic cooling and arresting of the heart; it also has foreign material within the systemic ventricle. The lateral tunnel has the benefit of being able to be performed on children of all ages because growth is not a significant issue since part of the tunnel consists of the native atrial wall. The extracardiac conduit, on the other hand, needs to be performed on larger children, in whom the conduit size is not a future issue; otherwise, conduit replacement may become necessary in the future.

In the early stages after a Fontan procedure, the extracardiac TCPC has the theoretical benefit of decreased atrial arrhythmias due to the absence of atrial suturing. However, no significant difference between the two groups has been demonstrated.

Anatomical issues can be important in determining which procedure to perform. The extracardiac conduit can be used to account for difficult pulmonary venous anatomy in cases in which obstruction of a pulmonary vein may occur with a lateral tunnel Fontan procedure. However, the lateral tunnel Fontan can account for difficult systemic venous anatomy when multiple systemic venous orifices drain into the right atrium. Despite these theoretical concerns, no significant differences in survival have been demonstrated between the two procedures. In one series in which large numbers of both procedures had been performed, survival for the two groups was equivalent, but the number of ventilator and ICU days was less in the group that underwent an extracardiac TCPC.

The placement of a fenestration between the systemic and pulmonary circulations at the atrial level as part of a TCPC results in decreased systemic venous pressures, decreased arterial oxygen saturations, and higher cardiac outputs. Fenestration carries with it the risk of potential paradoxical embolization because of the communication that exists between the pulmonary and systemic circulations.

A multi-variate analysis of a series of 500 consecutive patients at Children's Hospital in Boston demonstrated that fenestration was associated with a lower mortality. However, in the series from The Hospital for Sick Children in Toronto, fenestration was not associated with a lower mortality and also did not affect the duration of chest tube drainage. Thus, the issue of fenestration and its potential benefits still is not entirely defined.

PREOPERATIVE ASSESSMENT AND PREPARATION

Preoperative assessment of a patient for a Fontan procedure should include a thorough history, including patient age, physical examination, chest x-ray, and electrocardiogram. However, more sophisticated tests are necessary to determine the precise anatomy and physiology of the congenital cardiac defect. Transthoracic echocardiography is useful for identifying the cardiac morphology. Color flow Doppler echocardiography is useful in providing information about the competence of the atrioventricular valve(s) and data on left ventricular outflow tract obstruction, as well as other hemodynamic information. Cardiac catheterization is also useful for identifying cardiac morphology, and it provides a clear picture of great vessel anatomy. However, the greatest utility of cardiac catheterization is its ability to provide precise data on pulmonary vascular resistance as well as pressure measurements and oxygen saturations throughout the heart and great vessels. Cardiac catheterization also gives information as to the presence of the collateral circulation.

Historically, the focus was on the *selection* criteria for a TCPC. In fact, in 1977, Choussat *et al.* published the so-called 10 commandments, which were the strict selection criteria for performing a Fontan procedure. With time, those criteria became more extended to include patients with more complex congenital cardiac defects and patients who fulfilled fewer of Choussat *et al.*'s original criteria. However, the emphasis has now evolved away from selection and into *preparation* for a Fontan procedure. Infants are currently palliated and staged, with early removal of the volume load from the systemic ventricle. Correctable hemodynamic lesions are dealt with before a TCPC is performed. This shift in attitude has most likely contributed in large part to the improvements in mortality and morbidity that have been seen with the Fontan procedure in contemporary times.

ANESTHESIA

Critical issues in the anesthetic management of a patient who is undergoing a Fontan procedure begin immediately upon entry into the operating room. The decision as to the type and location of venous access is critical to the long-term success of the operation. Because of the risk of venous thrombosis that is associated with indwelling central venous catheters, many centers have a policy of avoiding central lines in the superior vena cava at any time. Femoral lines are considered to be more desirable for central venous access in a patient who is undergoing a TCPC.

After the surgical pathway has been constructed and the patient is weaned and separated from cardiopulmonary bypass, it is important to ensure that he or she has appropriate and adequate intravascular volume status. The goal is to optimize cardiac output at the lowest possible central venous pressure. To achieve this, it is necessary to minimize pulmonary vascular resistance. Measures to reduce the pulmonary vascular resistance include avoiding hypoxia and hypercarbia, correcting a metabolic acidosis, and rewarming of the patient. Patients should also be ventilated with the lowest possible airway pressure to reduce intrathoracic pressure.

Van Arsdell and coworkers have published their results on interventions that are associated with minimal Fontan mortality. They reported that the use of modified ultrafiltration after cardiopulmonary bypass was associated with a lower mortality and suggested that this was at least in part due to a reduction in pulmonary vascular resistance. In the same report, they also identified the institution of inotropic and vasodilator support at the time of separation from cardiopulmonary bypass to be associated with lower mortality. The authors suggested that this approach carried the potential benefit of avoiding a postoperative fall in cardiac output and the inherent delay in treatment that is associated with late recognition. They also noted that patients in their higher-mortality group arrived in the intensive care unit on lower doses of inotropic support but had reached equivalent doses to the lower-mortality group by 6 hours postoperatively.

Therapy in the postoperative period, at the time of separation from cardiopulmonary bypass and in the intensive care unit, can be aided by the intraoperative placement of a left atrial line. The ability to measure atrial pressure and to calculate transpulmonary gradient will guide in the pharmacological management of the patient. When the transpulmonary gradient is elevated, pulmonary vasodilators, such as inhaled nitric oxide, nitroglycerin, or phosphodiesterase inhibitors, can be used to reduce pulmonary vascular resistance. These key issues in the anesthetic management of the Fontan patient are also critical during the postoperative period in the intensive care unit.

OPERATION

As discussed earlier, the Fontan procedure has evolved and undergone a number of modifications. Numerous variations of the TCPC exist. For the purpose of this chapter, we describe the most common modifications.

Bidirectional cavopulmonary anastomosis

Staging of the Fontan procedure has become routine and is now an accepted standard in many institutions. Common to all modifications of the operation is a superior cavopulmonary anastomosis (bidirectional Glenn shunt). The superior cavopulmonary anastomosis is an end-to-side anastomosis of the superior vena cava to the right pulmonary artery (or, in the case of a left superior vena cava, to the left pulmonary artery).

The operation is performed via median sternotomy, with cardiopulmonary bypass and systemic cooling. The superior vena cava and the right pulmonary artery are fully mobilized. Extreme care is taken to avoid injury to the phrenic nerve. Once the patient is heparinized, the aorta is cannulated in a routine fashion. Venous return to the bypass circuit is through a cannula placed into the right atrial appendage, and a second small cannula is placed high up on the superior vena cava near the innominate vein. Cardiopulmonary bypass is initiated, and the patient is cooled to 28°C. Any systemic–pulmonary artery shunts that are present should be dissected and controlled. If a right shunt is present at the time of surgery, it should be disconnected from the pulmonary artery immedi-ately after the institution of cardiopulmonary bypass. The end of the shunt is then oversewn with a fine Prolene suture. When a shunt is present, the opening that is created in the right pulmonary artery by removing the shunt is extended centrally, and the anastomosis can later be performed to this area.

The operation itself is performed on a beating heart. A snare is passed around the superior vena cava and snugged down onto the venous cannula. If azygos continuation of the IVC is not present, the azygos vein is ligated. Some surgeons choose to divide the azygous vein if further mobilization of the superior vena cava is necessary to create a tension-free anastomosis.

A vascular clamp is then applied to the superior vena cava, just above the cavoatrial junction, taking care not to injure the sinus node. The superior vena cava is then divided above the clamp, and the atrial end of the superior vena cava is over-sewn with a running 6/0 Prolene suture. Once this step has been accomplished, the clamp is released. The right pul-monary artery is then fully mobilized all the way out to the first divisions. If the decision has been made to maintain for-ward flow in the patient, the main pulmonary artery is mobi-lized but not divided. However, if this is not to be the case, the main pulmonary artery is divided. The proximal pulmonary artery is then oversewn in two layers using a 4/0 Prolene suture, making sure to catch the valve leaflets with each stitch so that no dead space is left behind that could become a site of later emboli. This closure is reinforced with two strips of Teflon felt. The distal end of the divided main pulmonary artery can then either be directly closed or patched with a small piece of bovine pericardium or Gore-tex.

1 To perform the actual superior cavopulmonary anastomosis, a side-biting vascular clamp is applied along the superior surface of the right pulmonary artery start-ing at the point of its bifurcation from the main pulmonary artery. A long incision is then made on the superior aspect of the right pulmonary artery nearly the entire distance from its origin to its branching.

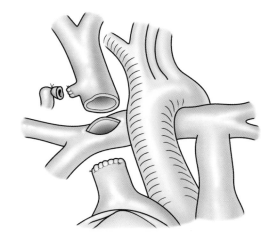

1

2 The cavopulmonary anastomosis is then carried out with a running 6/0 Prolene suture, which is interrupted in two areas to avoid a purse-string effect at the suture line and to maintain a widely patent anastomosis. The patient is then fully rewarmed, and the bypass is discontinued.

In the case of bilateral superior venae cavae, a bilateral, bidirectional, superior cavopulmonary anastomosis is necessary. In this instance, the cavae must be cannulated separately; and thus, three venous cannulae are required to perform this operation. Alternatively, two venous cannulae can be used, and the superior cannula is repositioned during the operation to the side on which the anastomosis is being performed. In this situation, the hemiazygos vein is ligated and divided, unless there is hemiazygos continuation of the IVC.

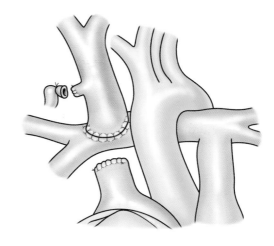

2

Lateral tunnel cavopulmonary anastomosis

Lateral tunnel cavopulmonary anastomosis is a modification of the Fontan operation that uses the placement of an intra-atrial Gore-tex baffle to route blood from the IVC along the lateral wall of the right atrium through the previously oversewn orifice of the superior vena cava up into the right pulmonary artery. This operation is performed following bidirectional cavopulmonary anastomosis and, as discussed earlier, usually occurs in a staged manner.

This operation is carried out by reopening the chest via the median sternotomy that was previously performed for the con-struction of the superior cavopulmonary anastomosis. Once the patient is fully heparinized, aortic cannulation is done in a routine fashion. Bicaval cannulation is performed by placing a venous cannula directly into the superior vena cava, and an additional cannula is placed in the IVC just above the diaphragmatic surface. Cardiopulmonary bypass is initiated, and the patient is then cooled to 25°C. Next, the aorta is cross-clamped, the cavae are snared, a right atriotomy parallel to the crista terminalis is performed, and cardioplegia is adminis-tered.

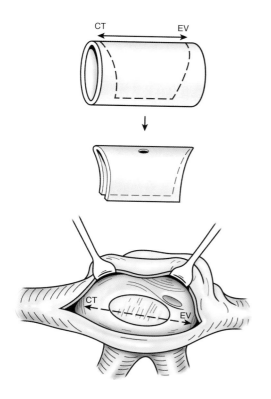

3 The intra-atrial baffle is then cut from a segment of Gore-tex tube and is fashioned so that a smooth, tubular intra-atrial tunnel can be created. Before the creation of the intra-atrial tunnel, the portion of the atrial septum within the confines of the oval fossa is excised. Before the Gore-tex baffle is sewn into place, a 4-mm fenestration is made using either a scalpel or an aortic punch. The superior cavoatrial junction, which had been previously oversewn at the time of the superior cavopulmonary shunt, is now opened.

3

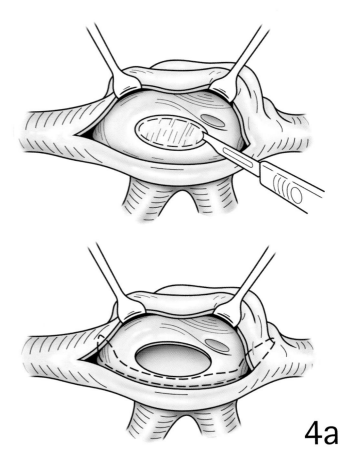

4a, b Once this step is complete, the baffle is sewn into position, starting at the orifice of the inferior cavoatrial junction, running the suture line posteriorly up to the superior cavoatrial junction. The suture line is then constructed around the entrance of the IVC into the atrium. It is important to note that the coronary sinus should be left on the pulmonary venous atrial side of the baffle so as to avoid injury to the conduction system. When the suture line reaches the inferior cavoatrial junction at its lateral aspect, the Gore-tex baffle can be trimmed to optimize the fit.

4a

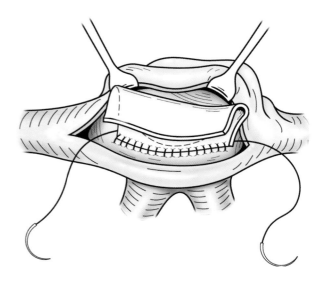

4b

5 The suture line is then carried around so that the remainder of the baffle is sutured to the lateral wall of the atrium. The suture line to the lateral wall of the atrium can be incorporated into the closure of the right atriotomy. The right atriotomy is then closed in two layers. It is important to avoid placing sutures into the crista terminalis, as this is thought to contribute to the later development of atrial arrhythmias. Once this is complete, the previously transected and now open superior cavoatrial junction can be anastomosed to the undersurface of the right pulmonary artery or to the site of the divided main pulmonary artery. This anastomosis is performed in a manner similar to that which was used to perform the superior cavopulmonary shunt. However, because the aorta is currently cross-clamped, it is not necessary to place an additional vascular clamp across the right pulmonary artery. The right pulmonary artery should be well mobilized before the creation of this anastomosis.

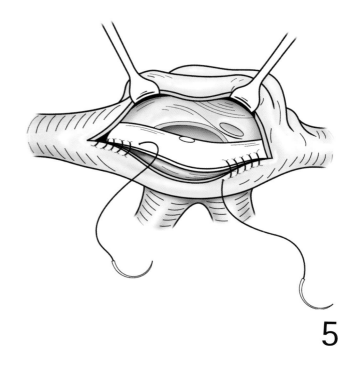

5

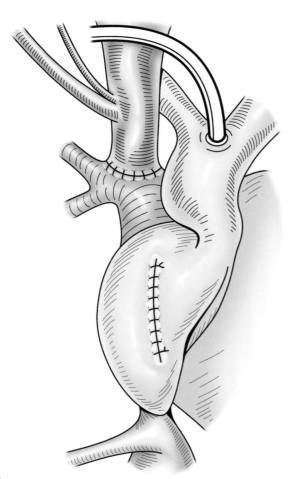

6

6 The completed lateral tunnel TCPC is demonstrated. Once this step is complete, the heart is deaired, the aorta unclamped, and the patient fully rewarmed.

Extracardiac conduit

The extracardiac conduit is an anatomical option that allows the creation of an extra-atrial pathway from the IVC to the pulmonary artery. This operation is performed using a Gore-tex tube as the conduit to divert the blood from the IVC to the right pulmonary artery. In general, this technique should be reserved for somewhat older patients so that growth and the long-term adequacy of the conduit size do not become an issue.

This technique is also performed using cardiopulmonary bypass. As described earlier, the chest is re-entered through the previous median sternotomy. Again, the right pulmonary artery is fully mobilized. The aorta is cannulated in a routine fashion. Venous return to the pump is via bicaval cannulation, with a small cannula placed in the superior vena cava and an additional cannula positioned in the IVC just above the diaphragmatic surface. Once cardiopulmonary bypass is initiated, the patient is cooled to 28°C. One of the benefits of this technique is that it does not require cross-clamping of the aorta.

The IVC is snared down to the venous cannula. A vascular clamp is placed at the inferior cavoatrial junction, taking care not to injure the coronary sinus. The IVC is divided just below the vascular clamp. The atrial end of the IVC is then oversewn in two layers with a running 5/0 Prolene suture, and the clamp is released. Next, a Gore-tex tube is sized to run from the cut end of the IVC up to the undersurface of the right pulmonary artery. The Gore-tex tube should be sized so that a gentle curve is formed just lateral to the heart. The IVC is then anastomosed to the Gore-tex tube using a running 5/0 or 4/0 Prolene suture. Once this step is completed, a snare is placed around the superior vena cava, which is snared down onto the venous cannula. Alternatively, a vascular clamp can be placed below the superior vena cava cannula. If the main pulmonary artery is still intact, it is divided and oversewn as described previously. However, the opening on the pulmonary arterial side is left open, and this opening is used for the anastomosis. If the main pulmonary artery had previously been divided, an arteriotomy is then performed on the undersurface of the fully mobilized right pulmonary artery. A small sump-suction can be placed in the pulmonary arteriotomy to facilitate visualization of the anastomosis.

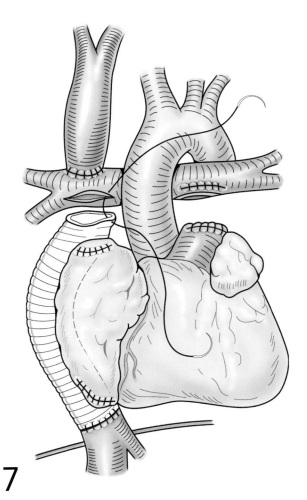

7 The end of the Gore-tex tube is then spatulated, and an anastomosis is created between the Gore-tex tube and the undersurface of the right pulmonary artery using a running 6/0 Prolene suture. Once the connection is completed, the snare and ligatures are released, followed by removal of the vascular clamp. The patient is then fully rewarmed and can be weaned from cardiopulmonary bypass.

If a fenestration is desired, this goal can be accomplished with a side-to-side anastomosis between the Gore-tex conduit and the atrial wall. This anastomosis can be performed either by using a side-biting vascular clamp on the atrial wall or a very short period of aortic cross-clamping, if necessary.

7

8a–c To create the anastomosis, a fenestration is made in the conduit adjacent to the atrium. A small opening is then made in the right atrium, which is next anastomosed circumferentially around the fenestration in the conduit 3–4 mm outside the perimeter of the fenestration. A 5/0 Prolene or Gore-tex suture can be used, taking full-thickness bites through the edge of the atriotomy and partial-thickness bites in the wall of the Gore-tex conduit.

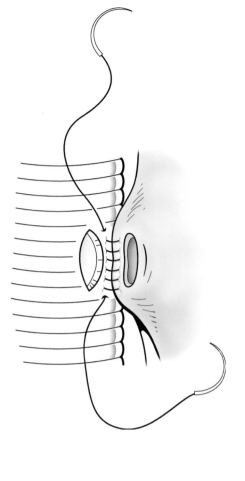

8b

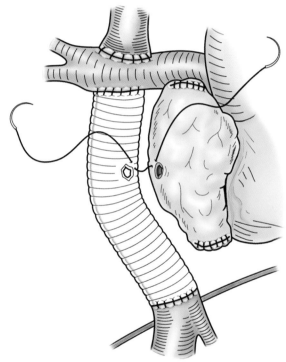

8a

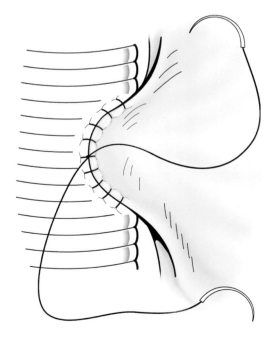

8c

Intra–extra cardiac conduit

An intra–extra cardiac conduit is an alternate technique that is particularly useful in patients with multiple hepatic venous orifices that drain into the right atrial chamber. As with the other techniques, this approach is undertaken via a median sternotomy. After full heparinization, the aorta is routinely cannulated. Venous drainage is via bicaval cannulation, with the inferior cannula placed low down in the IVC just above the diaphragmatic surface. The patient is placed on cardiopulmonary bypass and cooled to 22°C to allow for reduction in flow. The cavae are snared, and the aorta is cross-clamped. Cold cardioplegia solution is administered to arrest the heart. A right atriotomy is performed toward the inferior cavoatrial junction. Flow is reduced, and the inferior caval cannula is clamped, removed, and replaced with a small sump sucker.

9a The orifice to the IVC (or multiple orifices from hepatic veins and IVC) should be clearly visible. An appropriate-sized Gore-tex tube is then spatulated to provide the inflow into the conduit. This tube is sewn into place around the IVC and/or hepatic vein orifices. This step is most easily accomplished by starting at the most medial edge of the IVC orifice. Once the inferior caval end of the Gore-tex is anastomosed, the conduit is brought outside the heart through the right atriotomy. An appropriate spot is picked for a fenestration inside the right atrium so that flow can occur easily into the atrial chamber. A 4-mm fenestration is created with either a scalpel blade or an aortic punch.

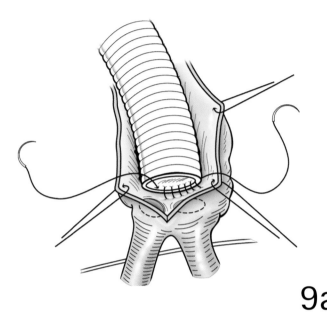

9a

9b Once this opening is made, the edges of the atriotomy are sewn to the outer surface of the Gore-tex tube using a running 5/0 or 6/0 Prolene suture. The length of the conduit is then assessed so that it fits neatly to the undersurface of the right pulmonary artery. Once this distance has been estimated, the end of the conduit is cut in a spatulated fashion. The undersurface of the right pulmonary artery is then opened, and the incision is extended from just beyond the origin of the right pulmonary artery all the way out to the branching of the right pulmonary artery (depending on the anatomy, the divided main pulmonary artery can alternatively be used).

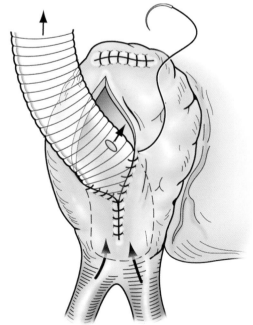

9b

9c An anastomosis is then created using a running 6/0 Prolene suture. Once this anastomosis is complete, the sump sucker is removed from the purse-string in the IVC, and the venous cannula is replaced into this location. At this point the aorta is filled with blood and deaired, the patient is fully rewarmed, and the aorta is unclamped.

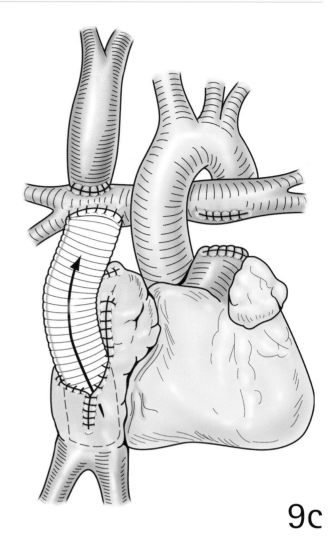

9c

POSTOPERATIVE CARE

The primary goal in the postoperative management of a patient having a Fontan procedure is to achieve the optimal cardiac output at the lowest possible central venous pressure. On arriving in the cardiac intensive care unit from the operating theater, the patient is most likely still intubated and on ventilatory support. Early weaning from the ventilator and extubation is often necessary to achieve the optimal hemodynamics. Positive pressure ventilation increases mean airway pressures, and positive expiratory pressure can increase pulmonary vascular resistance and intrathoracic pressure, leading to decreased ventricular filling. Hence, a suboptimal cardiac output state may be improved simply by returning the patient to spontaneous ventilation. However, if a patient is in a relatively severe low cardiac output state, he or she should remain ventilated, as spontaneous breathing can make the situation worse.

The patient may have a relative degree of cyanosis due to right-to-left shunting through a fenestration secondary to increased pulmonary vascular resistance and high central venous pressures. Patients who cannot be weaned from ventilatory support should be evaluated early for diaphragmatic activity, as the phrenic nerve is at risk. Injury to the phrenic nerve may have more dire consequences in patients with a Fontan circulation than in those with other types of cardiac repair. Other potential causes for failure to wean from ventilatory support should also be investigated, including pleural effusions, lung consolidation, pneumothorax, and an unsatisfactory repair. Arrhythmias following the Fontan procedure can be significantly problematic in this group of patients. As a result, it is imperative to place atrial and ventricular temporary pacing wires at the time of surgery. Loss of atrioventricular synchrony may result in a low cardiac output state as the result of an increased dependence on the so-called 'atrial kick' in patients with this anatomical arrangement. Tachycardias are also poorly tolerated and may result in severe hemodynamic deterioration. Ultimately, tachycardias result in a low cardiac output state due to an attenuated stroke volume secondary to reduced ventricular filling times. Because of the severe consequences of postoperative arrhythmias in patients who have undergone a Fontan procedure, atrial and ventricular pacing wires must both be placed so that they are available to help optimize a patient's hemodynamics should an arrhythmia occur.

As stated earlier, the primary objective in the early postoperative management of a Fontan procedure is achieving the optimal cardiac output at the lowest possible central venous pressure. Thus, a strategy of aggressive evaluation of low cardiac output states must be used. Factors such as mechanical ventilation and arrhythmias are obvious causes of a low cardiac output state. However, other factors, such as inadequate volume status (i.e., low preload due to hypovolemia), elevated pulmonary vascular resistance, ventricular failure, and an anatomical obstruction in the surgical pathway, are all additional causes of a low cardiac output state. To assist with postoperative management and the potential need to evaluate a low cardiac output state, intraoperative placement of a central venous catheter and a common atrial line is imperative, as they are invaluable tools in the management of a postoperative Fontan patient. Postoperative echocardiography should also be used as an additional diagnostic tool in the management of these patients, as this, too, can provide invaluable information as to ventricular function and possible anatomical obstructions in the systemic venous pathway. Echocardiography can also provide information about atrioventricular valve regurgitation, ventricular outflow obstruction, and tamponade, which can all be additional causes of low cardiac output states. In some cases, early cardiac catheterization may be necessary to evaluate the quality of the surgical repair. Aggressive therapy to correct any or all of the factors that may contribute to a low cardiac output state is mandatory in this group of patients, as the early postoperative period is a critical time in the successful outcome of this operation.

In terms of the late postoperative issues in patients who have undergone a Fontan procedure, pleural and pericardial effusion is one of the more frequent causes of a prolonged hospitalization. The use of modified ultrafiltration and fenestrations has reduced the incidence and severity of pleural and pericardial effusions but has not eliminated them altogether. Thus, chest drains should be placed in the mediastinum as well as both pleural spaces intraoperatively and should not be removed until the drainage has dropped off completely. In patients in whom ongoing drainage to the chest tubes continues to occur, problems with protein losses, fluid losses, and electrolytes need to be addressed in an attentive manner. Often, ongoing pleural drainage can be managed with the use of medium-chain triglyceride enteral feeds, or, in the more extreme cases, total parenteral nutrition may be necessary. In patients who experience prolonged drainage, early cardiac catheterization is often necessary to look for surgically correctable causes of the persistent fluid losses.

Anticoagulation regimens to prevent thromboembolic complications in patients who have undergone a Fontan procedure are not uniform and often seem to be instituted as a matter of physician preference. After the Fontan procedure, patients can certainly be at increased risk of venous thrombosis. Low cardiac output, a foreign body in the circulation, and increased blood viscosity all contribute to the risk of thrombosis. Thus, anticoagulation therapy with warfarin or antiplatelet therapy with aspirin is often used in Fontan patients. However, no strict or uniform guidelines exist to date. A multicenter, prospective randomized trial is just beginning on an international basis to better address this issue.

Finally, a late complication of the Fontan procedure is the development of protein-losing enteropathy. This problem can be severe and debilitating. The condition itself is poorly understood in this group of patients but can be so exaggerated that it is an indication for cardiac transplantation. Other late complications of the Fontan procedure include atrial arrhythmias, cyanosis due to the formation of arteriovenous fistulae, and late cardiac failure.

OUTCOME

Follow-up data from Children's Hospital in Boston on 196 of 220 patients who underwent a lateral tunnel Fontan procedure over a 4-year period (1987–1991) provided some insight into 10-year outcomes of this particular modification of the operation. Kaplan-Meier estimated survival in their series was 93 per cent at 5 years and 91 per cent at 10 years. Freedom from failure was 90 per cent at 5 years and 87 per cent at 10 years. Freedom from new supraventricular tachyarrhythmia was 96 per cent at 5 years and 91 per cent at 10 years; freedom from bradyarrhythmia was 88 per cent at 5 years and 79 per cent at 10 years.

In 1998, Hagler published data from the Pediatric Cardiac Care Consortium. These data represented a total of 1 124 patients who had undergone the Fontan procedure between

Table 43.1 *Summary data of patients undergoing a Fontan procedure (as reported to the Pediatric Cardiac Care Consortium 1984–1993)*

Total no. of patients	1124
Previous palliative operation	925 (82.3%)
Systemic–pulmonary shunt	589
Pulmonary artery banding	238
Glenn procedure	179
Mortality	
Overall 30-day	14.4%
Without previous operation	12%
With previous operation	14.9%
Infants (<1 yr of age)	36.3%
Children aged 1–5 yr	15.5%
Children aged 5–10 yr	10.5%
Children aged 10–21 yr	12.2%
Adults aged 21.1–44.4 yr	15.4%
Adults >35 yr	50.0%
Children 5–10 kg	32.1%

1984 and 1993. This group represents patients of all ages and accounted for 3.8 per cent of all operations reported to the Pediatric Cardiac Care Consortium. The results are summarized in Table 43.1 above.

These mortality data are consistent with and in the same general range as those of other series that have been reported over the past two decades. In the data reported by the Pediatric Cardiac Care Consortium as well as most other series, patients who have a primary diagnosis of tricuspid atresia and undergo a Fontan procedure seem to have an overall lower mortality. In addition, these patients appear to have better long-term survival.

ACKNOWLEDGMENTS

The authors thank Ms. Faith Hanstater and Dr. Marco Ricci (Great Ormond Street Hospital, United Kingdom) and Mr. Phillip Weinstein (Sony Pictures, United States) for their assistance in the preparation of this chapter.

FURTHER READING

Choussat, A., Fontan, F., Besse, P., *et al.* 1977. Selection criteria for Fontan's procedure. In Anderon, R.H., Shinebourne, E.A. (eds), *Paediatric cardiology*. Edinburgh: Churchill Livingstone, 559–66.

de Leval, M.R., Kilner, P., Gewillig, M., Bull, C. 1988. Total cavopulmonary connection: a logical alternative to atriopulmonary connection for complex Fontan operations. *Journal of Thoracic and Cardiovascular Surgery* 96, 682–95.

Fontan, F., Baudet, E. 1971. Surgical repair of tricuspid atresia. *Thorax* 26, 240–48.

Gentles, T.L., Mayer, J.E., Gauvreau, K., *et al.* 1997. Fontan operation in five hundred consecutive patients: factors influencing early and late outcome. *Journal of Thoracic and Cardiovascular Surgery* 114, 376–91.

Hagler, D.J. 1998. Fontan. In Moller, J.H. (ed.), *Perspectives in pediatric cardiology.* Surgery of Congenital Heart Disease: Pediatric Cardiac Care Consortium 1984–1995. Vol. 6. Armonk, NY: Futura Publishing Co., 345–52.

Jonas, R. 1994. Indications and timing for the bi-directional Glenn shunt versus the fenestrated Fontan circulation. *Journal of Thoracic and Cardiovascular Surgery* 108, 522–4.

Stamm, C., Friehs, I., Mayer, J.E., *et al.* 2001. Long-term results of the lateral tunnel Fontan operation. *Journal of Thoracic and Cardiovascular Surgery* 121(1), 28–41.

Van Arsdell, G.S., McCrindle, B.W., Einarson, K.D., *et al.* 2000. Interventions associated with minimal Fontan mortality. *Annals of Thoracic Surgery* 70, 568–74.

44

Bidirectional Glenn and hemi-Fontan procedures

J. MARK REDMOND MD, FRCS

Consultant Pediatric Cardiac Surgeon, Our Lady's Hospital for Sick Children, Crumlin, Dublin, Ireland

The construction of an anastomosis between the superior vena cava (SVC) and the pulmonary artery (PA) is now well established in the management of the functional single ventricle either as a preliminary procedure in staged Fontan palliation or as an alternative procedure to the Fontan, occasionally as part of a one-and-a-half ventricle reconstruction.

HISTORY

Although Carlon in Italy first reported an experimental method for creating an anastomosis between the SVC and the right PA in 1951, the shunt bears the name of Glenn, whose pioneering research in right heart bypass in dogs paved the way for widespread clinical application of a direct end-to-end SVC to right atrium connection. In the Soviet Union, Meshalkin reported the first successful clinical use of the shunt in 24 children with 21 survivors in 1956. Glenn first performed the shunt on a 7-year-old boy with right ventricular hypoplasia and pulmonary stenosis in 1958.

As more complex intracardiac repairs became feasible and the safety of the shunt in infants was questioned, its popularity waned during the 1960s, only to be embraced once more in the 1970s as the logical first stage toward complete Fontan right heart bypass. In 1966, Haller and coworkers experimented with an end-to-side cavopulmonary shunt, without ligation of the right PA, in a canine model. Glenn had recognized that the normally occurring minute precapillary arteriovenous connections in the lung in patients with end-to-end SVC-to-PA shunts could enlarge, resulting in arterial desaturation. Because of Glenn's experience with the value of axillary arteriovenous fistulae, it was believed that the introduction of pulsatile flow into the pulmonary circuit could prevent the development of such fistulae. The end-to-side SVC-to-right PA modification was therefore adopted and became known as the bidirectional Glenn shunt (BDG).

To simplify the completion Fontan operation in patients with hypoplastic left heart syndrome, further modification of the shunt was popularized by Norwood as the hemi-Fontan procedure.

PRINCIPLES AND JUSTIFICATION

The BDG is currently defined as an anastomosis that diverts systemic venous return from the SVC (or cavae) to both lungs. The value of the operation is as an intermediate stage to render the patient with single physiology as ideal a candidate as possible for later Fontan completion. The BDG removes the obligatory volume overload imposed on the ventricle by a systemic-to-PA shunt, allowing resolution of excessive ventricular hypertrophy and dilatation with concomitant increase in diastolic compliance before the completion Fontan procedure. Improvement in tricuspid regurgitation in some patients may also be achieved. Because augmentation of the PAs is occasionally required, particularly in patients with hypoplastic heart syndrome who have successfully undergone the first palliative stage, the hemi-Fontan operation, which also involves homograft patch enlargement of the PAs, is preferred by some surgeons. Although this latter procedure is more complex, involving placement of a dam between the right atrium and the PA, it facilitates the Fontan completion if performed using the intracardiac lateral tunnel technique. As intermediate procedures, the BDG or hemi-Fontan have been associated with improved ventricular function and decreased incidence of pleural effusions at the completion operation.

The BDG can be combined with intracardiac correction to incorporate a smaller tripartite pulmonary ventricle, and thereby create pulsatile pulmonary blood flow as the one-and-a-half ventricle repair. Direct visceral venous return containing the 'hepatic factor' is preserved, which, together with preservation of pulsatile pulmonary blood flow, may prevent development of pulmonary arteriovenous fistulae.

Finally, the BDG may be used as definitive palliation in the management of complex cyanotic heart disease in patients not considered ideal candidates for Fontan physiology because of common atrioventricular valve insufficiency or congenital or iatrogenic abnormalities of PAs. Substantial improvement in systemic oxygen saturations can be achieved with reduction in cardiac workload.

PREOPERATIVE ASSESSMENT AND PREPARATION

Before performing the BDG or hemi-Fontan, it is critically important to identify physiological or anatomical problems that may have developed after the first-stage neonatal palliative procedure for single ventricle, whether it be a shunt, PA band, or more complex procedure such as a stage I Norwood operation for hypoplastic left heart syndrome. Evaluation for congestive heart failure due to ventricular dysfunction and dilatation associated with progressive atrioventricular valve regurgitation in the presence of a systemic-to-PA shunt should be performed. Narrowing or distortion of the PAs should be ruled out, especially in patients who have undergone stage I palliation for hypoplastic left syndrome, in whom progressive cyanosis may also be a manifestation of shunt narrowing or restriction of the atrial septal defect. Aortic arch obstruction in this latter group can cause pulmonary overcirculation and elevation of pulmonary vascular resistance. Early intervention for these problems may stabilize patients and lower the morbidity of the BDG or hemi-Fontan procedures. Although echocardiography is a valuable test for screening, cardiac catheterization is strongly recommended not only as a diagnostic test, but also for intervention when indicated. Residual arch obstruction can be dilated, while aortopulmonary collateral vessels, if present, can be addressed. PA abnormalities can be delineated before surgery. Such an aggressive approach is of paramount importance to ensure that patients remain 'ideal' Fontan candidates.

ANESTHESIA

Patients are intubated using the nasotracheal or orotracheal route. They are ventilated using low mean airway pressures with long expiratory times and minimal positive end-expiratory pressure. A radial arterial line is preferable. Monitoring of cavopulmonary pressures can be achieved using a percutaneous internal jugular line, although we have found it convenient to place transthoracic 3-Fr lines in the common atrium and at the cavopulmonary connection through the appropriate suture lines intraoperatively.

OPERATION

Bidirectional Glenn shunt

The BDG anastomosis is performed using aortobicaval, normothermic cardiopulmonary bypass with a beating, decompressed heart. Cannulation of the SVC may be avoided by placing a pump sucker in the proximal orifice of the transected SVC. PA isolation and patch augmentation of the branch PAs can be performed if required at this stage. Moderate hypothermia (28°C), aortic cross-clamping, and cold blood cardioplegia are used if concomitant atrial septectomy or atrioventricular valve repair are necessary.

1a After median sternotomy, the aorta, PAs, and inferior vena cava (IVC) are dissected. The SVC is dissected and fully mobilized superiorly to the innominate and subclavian vein tributaries. The azygous vein is doubly ligated and divided. The medial and lateral aspects of the SVC are marked with 7/0 monofilament suture (Polypropylene, Ethicon, Somerville, NJ) to ensure correct orientation for the BDG anastomosis. Similar marking sutures can be placed to delineate the location and extent of the incision on the superior aspect of the right PA. Control of a systemic-to-PA shunt, if present, is obtained. The aorta is cannulated using a single aortic purse-string. Cannulation of the IVC (DLP, Grand Rapids, MI or RMI Research Medical, Midvale, UT) is followed by high SVC cannulation at the innominate vein junction using a right-angled cannula (DLP or RMI). Cardiopulmonary bypass is established, and the systemic-to-PA shunt is ligated and divided. The PA branches may be opened and patch augmentation performed at this point. Depending on the anatomy, the pulmonary trunk may need to be clamped during this maneuver to prevent air entry into the beating heart.

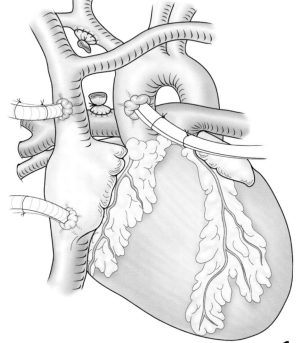

1a

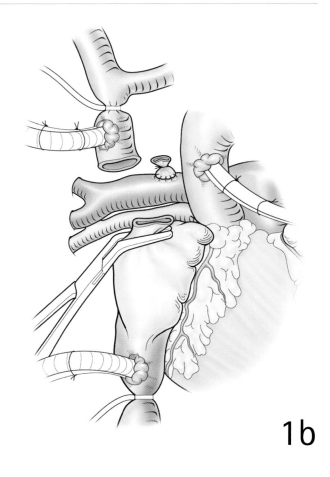

1b

1b, c
The tourniquet on the SVC is secured, and a clamp is positioned across the SVC–right atrial junction. The SVC is then transected. If the SVC has not been cannulated, the SVC is transected and a pump sucker carefully positioned in the cephalic end of the SVC to maintain adequate exposure during cardiopulmonary bypass. If an intracardiac procedure is required, the aorta is cross-clamped and cardioplegia administered. Then the IVC tourniquet can be secured and the right atrial incision made.

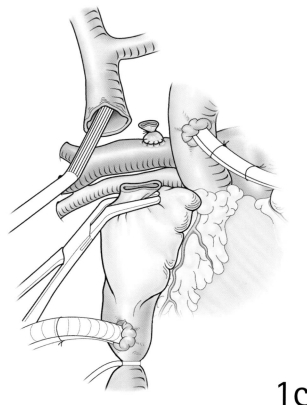

1c

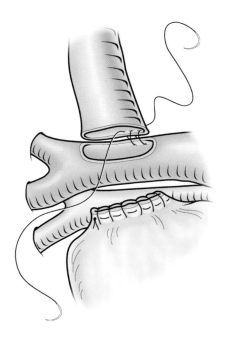

1d

1d, e With the vascular clamp on the SVC–right atrial junction, the cardiac end of the transected SVC is closed in two layers, using a running horizontal mattress suture of 5/0 polypropylene, followed by a running suture line after removal of the clamp. The PA is incised and the back wall of the SVC-to-right PA anastomosis begun at the medial end using a running 6/0 absorbable monofilament suture (Polydioxanone, Ethicon). The suture line is intermittently locked to prevent purse-stringing of the anastomosis. The anterior aspect of the anastomosis is completed with a similar suture line or with interrupted sutures if desired. Although rarely required, patch augmentation of the anterior aspect of the SVC-to-right PA anastomosis may be necessary to achieve a tension-free, large cavopulmonary connection. The tourniquet on the SVC is released, the heart allowed to fill and eject, and the patient separated from cardiopulmonary bypass. If an intracardiac procedure has been performed, deairing of the heart before removal of the cross-clamp and during rewarming is required.

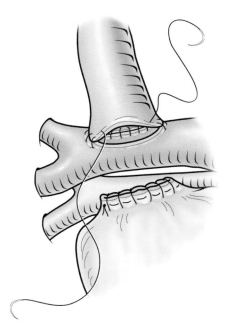

1e

Bilateral bidirectional Glenn shunt

2a Patients with a functional single ventricle, particularly those with heterotaxia, have anomalies of systemic and pulmonary venous return associated with splenic abnormalities. A high incidence of bilateral SVCs occurs in this group who, as suitable candidates for Fontan palliation, will require bilateral BDG shunts. If pulmonary atresia is present, a systemic-to-PA shunt is required in the neonatal period. If pulmonary stenosis is present, adequate pulmonary blood flow may be present initially, so that a bilateral BDG procedure may be the first intervention required, as in the example shown. Such anatomy occasionally affords the surgeon an opportunity to perform the BDG shunts sequentially, obviating the need for cardiopulmonary bypass.

After median sternotomy and subtotal thymectomy, the pericardium is opened and suspended with stay sutures. The great vessels are dissected and mobilized fully.

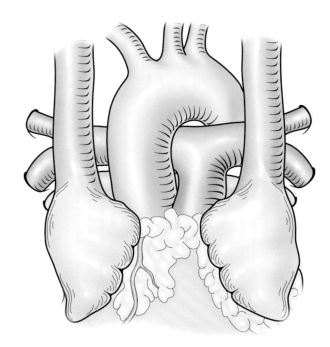

2a

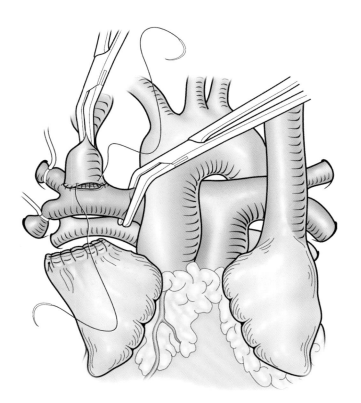

2b

2b Starting with the right SVC, marking sutures of 7/0 polypropylene are placed on the medial and lateral aspects. The right upper and lower PA branches in the hilum are encircled and tourniquets applied. The right PA is clamped medially, being careful to avoid distortion of the main and left PAs, and the tourniquets are secured laterally. Once oxygen saturations are stable, the SVC and cavoatrial junction are clamped, and the SVC is transected. The cardiac end of the transected SVC is closed in two layers, using a running horizontal mattress suture of 5/0 polypropylene, followed by a running suture line after removal of the clamp. The right PA is opened on its superior aspect, and an end-to-side cavopulmonary anastomosis is created using 6/0 polydioxanone suture as described previously. All clamps and tourniquets are removed.

2c After encircling the left upper and lower PAs in the left hilum, tourniquets are applied. The left SVC and the left-sided cavoatrial junction are clamped and the left SVC transected. Again, the cardiac end of the SVC is closed in two layers. The left PA is clamped medially, and the tourniquets are secured laterally. The left pulmonary is opened on its superior aspect, and once more, an end-to-side cavopulmonary anastomosis is created with 6/0 polydioxanone suture. The clamps and tourniquets are removed.

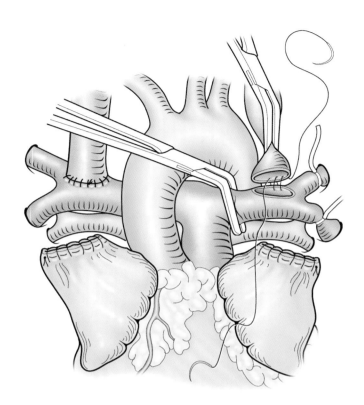

2c

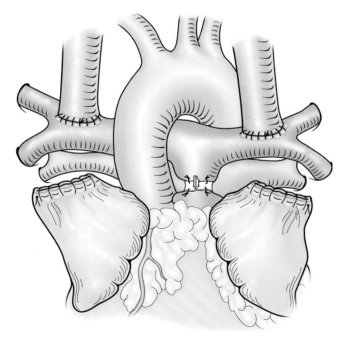

2d A PA band is applied to reduce the blood flow through the stenotic main PA. Transesophageal echocardiography and direct pressure measurements in the branch PAs can be used to guide tightening of the band.

2d

Hemi-Fontan I

3a The great vessels and relevant cardiac structures are dissected. The neoaorta and right atrium are cannulated. The right modified Blalock-Taussig shunt is encircled with a braided polyester ligature. The pulmonary bifurcation is mobilized as completely as possible before initiation of cardiopulmonary bypass. The shunt is ligated once bypass is established, and the PA dissection is completed, as the patient is cooled to a nasopharyngeal temperature of 18°C. When cooling is complete, circulatory arrest is established, the neoaorta is cross-clamped, and cardioplegia is administered. The venous cannula is removed from the right atrium. The SVC is opened at the cavoatrial junction. The incision spirals cephalad around the medial border of the SVC and ends posteriorly, adjacent to the PA. Caudally, it extends across the cavoatrial junction toward the sinus nodal artery, transection of which can occasionally be avoided. The PA is opened on its anterior aspect from a point immediately posterior to the SVC to the branch point of the left PA.

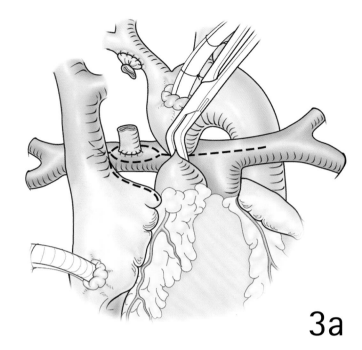

3a

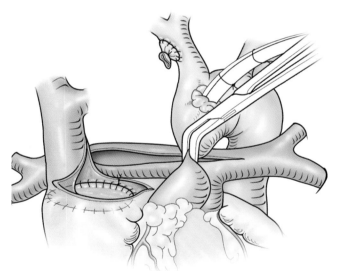

3b

3b A patch of Gore-Tex (Gore, Flagstaff, AZ, USA), appropriately tailored, is sewn into the right atrium immediately below the cavoatrial junction, through the incision, using 5/0 polypropylene suture. This patch serves to separate the right atrium from the cavopulmonary anastomosis and is excised during the subsequent Fontan completion procedure.

3c The posterior border of the cavoatrial opening is then sutured to the inferior edge of the pulmonary arteriotomy using a running 6/0 polypropylene suture.

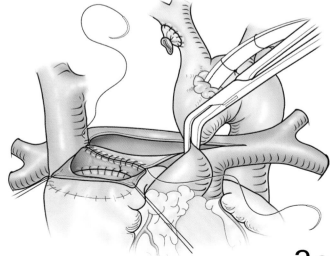

3c

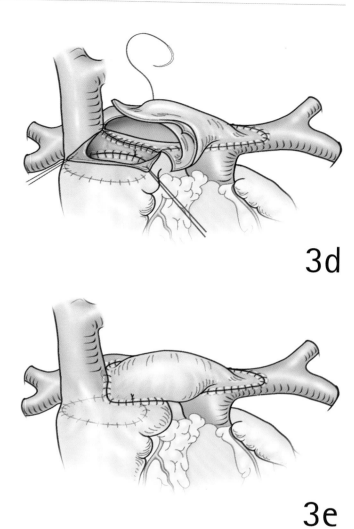

3d, e A generous triangular-shaped patch of cryopreserved pulmonary homograft is cut to the appropriate size. Using 6/0 polypropylene suture, the patch is sewn to the remaining margins of the pulmonary arteriotomy, starting at its leftward extent. The suture line is carried onto the cavoatrial junction, where it is completed. The right atrial cannula is replaced, and after deairing the heart, cardiopulmonary bypass is re-established and rewarming begun.

3d

3e

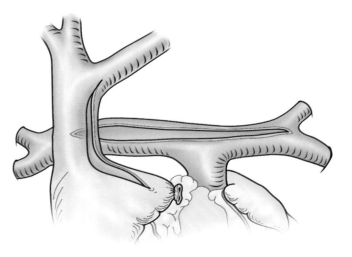

4a

Hemi-Fontan II

4a After dissection of the great vessels and relevant cardiac structures, the neoaorta and right atrium are cannulated. Cardiopulmonary bypass is initiated, and ligation of the right modified Blalock-Taussig shunt is performed. The dissection of the pulmonary bifurcation is completed; and after neoaortic cross-clamping, cardioplegia is administered. Circulatory arrest is begun. An incision is made in the PA from hilum to hilum. An incision is also made on the medial aspect of the SVC extending from just below the innominate vein junction, across the cavoatrial junction, onto the right atrial appendage.

4b The posterior margin of the SVC–right atrial incision is then sewn to the rightward end of the pulmonary arteriotomy using a running 6/0 polypropylene suture. This maneuver ensures a wide opening between the SVC and PA.

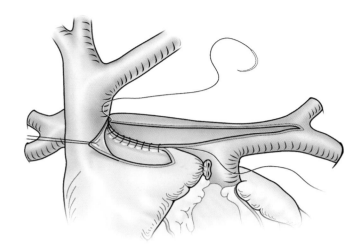

4b

4c, d A large triangular-shaped patch of cryo-preserved pulmonary homograft is tailored for augmentation of the pulmonary bifurcation. Beginning at the left hilum, the patch is sewn to the margins of the pulmonary arteriotomy using a running 6/0 polypropylene suture. The suture line connecting the patch and the inferior margin of the pulmonary arteriotomy is carried onto the cavoatrial junction along the margin of the incision in the right atrial appendage. The pulmonary homograft patch is then folded down, creating a dam at the level of the cavoatrial junction between the right atrium and the cavopulmonary anastomosis. This point is secured circumferentially with a 5/0 polypropylene suture. Careful incorporation of the double flap of pulmonary homograft is important to prevent any baffle leaks entering the right atrium. The cannula is replaced in the right atrium, the heart is deaired, and cardiopulmonary bypass is re-established.

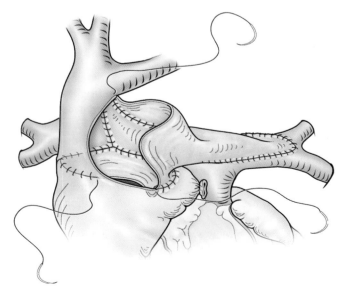

4c

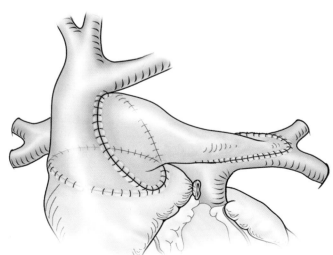

4d

POSTOPERATIVE CARE

After the procedure, patients are allowed to awaken and are extubated as early as possible. Expeditious removal from positive pressure ventilation improves hemodynamics across the pulmonary vascular bed. Head elevation and inhaled nitric oxide are used in the early postoperative phase if 'Glenn' pressures are temporarily increased. Pressure monitoring lines are removed as soon as hemodynamics have stabilized. Oxygen saturations in the mid–80 per cent range are typical after the procedure. Failure to wean rapidly from mechanical ventilation should initiate evaluation for phrenic nerve paralysis. Pleural effusions requiring intervention are unusual but should be ruled out. Although early sinus node dysfunction is not uncommon, normal sinus rhythm returns within 2 or 3 days of the procedure, and patients are generally ready for discharge by the fourth or fifth postoperative day.

OUTCOME

When used as an intermediate procedure in the staged palliation for hypoplastic left heart syndrome, perioperative mortality for the BDG and hemi-Fontan procedures is 1–2 per cent. With the use of modified ultrafiltration or aggressive postoperative diuresis, the incidence of pleural effusions requiring intervention is 5 per cent. PA thrombosis and heart block occur in less than 5 per cent of patients.

Our preference has been to perform the BDG rather than the hemi-Fontan. Some advantages of the BDG include the potentially lower incidence of dysrhythmias by avoiding incisions that interfere with sinus node function or blood supply. Hypothermic circulatory arrest and aortic cross-clamping can generally be avoided. If the surgeon's preference is to ultimately perform an extracardiac Fontan, then the BDG may be preferable, especially if fenestration is not considered routinely necessary. The improved energy conservation and hemodynamics obtained by offset of SVC and IVC flow are more readily accomplished when the BDG is used.

The hemi-Fontan, however, has several features that render it particularly suitable for patients with hypoplastic left heart syndrome. PA distortion or hypoplasia is common in these patients, a problem readily addressed by use of a generous patch of pulmonary homograft across the pulmonary bifurcation or the insertion site of the modified Blalock-Taussig shunt in the hemi-Fontan procedure. In addition, when the surgeon's preference is to perform an intracardiac lateral tunnel completion, which facilitates more reliable fenestration, then the hemi-Fontan may be more desirable. In the latter procedure, a dam is created at SVC–right atrial junction either as part of the pulmonary bifurcation patch, as described by Jacobs and Norwood, or as a separate patch, as

described by Bove. This patch is be easily resected at the time of the Fontan completion, rendering this procedure very straightforward.

A disadvantage of the hemi-Fontan is that the cavoatrial incision often transects the sinus nodal artery, with the potential for adverse consequences on sinus node function and for the development of late atrial dysrhythmias. The procedure requires hypothermic circulatory arrest with its attendant risk of neurological injury, although it does obviate the need for cannulation of the SVC.

When used as part of a one-and-a-half ventricle repair, the BDG has yielded favorable results, as long as the small or dysfunctional pulmonary ventricle is tripartite. Overall, survival of 90 per cent at 5 years has been reported, with the majority of patients experiencing a good clinical outcome. When the pulmonary ventricle is nontripartite, results have been unsatisfactory.

The commonest problem after the BDG procedure has been progressive cyanosis. This situation may be due to the development of systemic venous collaterals, which decompress the superior caval system into the inferior caval system. These collaterals usually can be treated by coil embolization. More difficult to deal with are the pulmonary arteriovenous collateral vessels arising from the brachiocephalic, bronchial, or intercostal arteries. Such left-to-right shunting can also place a hemodynamic burden on the systemic ventricle. Whereas discrete collaterals can be embolized, diffuse arteriovenous shunting is often not readily amenable to coil embolization. Presence of a BDG rather a completion Fontan procedure and older age are risk factors for these collaterals. Earlier Fontan completion may be indicated in such patients.

FURTHER READING

Douglas, W.I., Goldberg, C.S., Mosca, R.S., Law, I.H., Bove, E.L. 1999. Hemi-Fontan procedure for hypoplastic left heart syndrome: outcome and suitability for Fontan. *Annals of Thoracic Surgery* **68**, 1361–8.

Jacobs, M.L., Norwood, W.I. 1994. Fontan operation: Influence of modifications on morbidity and mortality. *Annals of Thoracic Surgery* **58**, 945–52.

Koutlas, T.C., Gaynor, J.W., Nicolson, S.C., et al. 1997. Modified ultrafiltration reduces postoperative morbidity after cavopulmonary connection. *Annals of Thoracic Surgery* **64**, 137–43.

Kreutzer, C., de Mayorquim, R., Kreutzer, G.O.A., et al. 1999. Experience with one and a half ventricle repair. *Journal of Thoracic and Cardiovascular Surgery* **117**, 662–8.

Seliem, M.A., Baffa, J.M., Vetter, J.M., et al. 1993. Changes in right ventricular geometry and heart rate early after hemi-Fontan procedure. *Annals of Thoracic Surgery* **55**, 1508–12.

45

Double-outlet ventricles

YVES LECOMPTE MD
Head Surgeon, Department of Pediatric Cardiology, Institut Jacques Cartier, Massy, France

PASCAL R. VOUHÉ MD
Professor of Cardiac Surgery, Paris V University; Consultant Cardiac Surgeon, Department of Pediatric Cardiac Surgery, Necker Hospital Group for Sick Children, Paris, France

Double-outlet ventricles represent a wide spectrum of pathophysiological malformations and include all anomalies of ventriculoarterial connection ranging from normal ventriculoarterial connection to complete transposition of the great arteries. In this chapter we discuss all types of anomalous ventriculoarterial connection in the presence of two adequate ventricles allowing biventricular repair, thus excluding patients with severe hypoplasia of one ventricle, one or more ventricular septal defects (VSDs), two atrioventricular valves, and normal atrioventricular concordance, thus excluding patients with discordant atrioventricular connection.

PREOPERATIVE ASSESSMENT

Choice of the type of repair

To classify malformations with double-outlet ventricles, it is usual to describe the ventriculoarterial alignment, the relationship between the great arteries, and the position of the VSD. Identification of hearts with double-outlet right ventricle, double-outlet left ventricle, or transposition of the great arteries with VSD is then possible. Although of value from a morphological point of view, this classification is of little help from a surgical standpoint.

The choice of the surgical procedure that provides anatomical repair (i.e. connecting the left ventricle with the aorta and the right ventricle with the pulmonary artery) depends on the following two anatomical determinants.

1   The distance between the tricuspid valve and the pulmonary valve: When this distance is sufficient, an unrestricted left ventricle–to–aortic valve tunnel can be constructed and the pulmonary orifice can be left as the natural outflow for the right ventricle.

2   The presence of pulmonary outflow tract obstruction (subvalvar and/or valvar).

Using these two anatomical determinants, the choice can be made between three types of anatomical repair:

1   Intraventricular repair (i.e. entirely within the right ventricle) when the distance between the tricuspid valve and the pulmonary valve is long enough (i.e. at least equal to the aortic valve diameter). A baffle is constructed that creates an unobstructed pathway from the left ventricle to the aortic orifice, and the natural right ventricular outflow tract passes around the left ventricular baffle but remains within the right ventricle. In the presence of concomitant pulmonary outflow tract obstruction, the right ventricular outflow tract may be enlarged using a prosthetic infundibular or transannular patch.

2   Arterial switch operation when the tricuspid to pulmonary distance is too short (i.e. significantly less than the aortic valve diameter) and in the absence of pulmonary outflow tract obstruction. A tunnel is constructed to connect the left ventricle with the pulmonary orifice, and an arterial switch operation is performed.

3   Réparation à l'étage ventriculaire (REV) when the tricuspid to pulmonary distance is too short and in the presence of pulmonary outflow tract obstruction. A left ventricle–to–aortic orifice tunnel is created including the pulmonary orifice; the main pulmonary artery is divided and translocated anteriorly onto the right ventricle.

Whatever the type of anatomical repair, an intracardiac tunnel must be constructed to connect the left ventricle with one of the arterial orifices (aortic orifice in intraventricular repair and REV procedure, pulmonary orifice in arterial switch operation). To create an unobstructed tunnel, enlargement of the VSD is often necessary. Enlarging the VSD is indicated in two circumstances:

1   When a portion of the interventricular septum (usually the infundibular septum) interposes between the VSD and the arterial orifice to which the left ventricle must be connected. To create a tunnel that is as short and straight as possible, this portion of the interventricular septum must be resected, even if the VSD is large.
2   When the VSD itself is small and may be a potential cause of postoperative subaortic stenosis. Depending on the intracardiac anatomy, septal enlargement may then involve either the infundibular septum or the muscular septum forming the anterior margin of the VSD.

Preoperative evaluation

The type of symptoms and the age at which they appear are very variable, although in most cases the presence of congenital heart anomaly becomes evident very early in life. The information that is necessary to choose the type of repair and to plan the surgical procedure can almost always be provided by echocardiographic evaluation alone. Invasive cardiac investigation remains, however, necessary in selected cases.

The optimal age for anatomical correction depends on the type of repair and, particularly, on the anticipated length of the intracardiac tunnel (i.e. the distance between the VSD and the arterial orifice to which the left ventricle is con-

nected). Primary repair is possible during the neonatal period or during early infancy when the length of the tunnel is short. On the other hand, if the anticipated length of the intracardiac baffle is more important, early palliative surgery (aortopulmonary shunt or pulmonary artery banding) is indicated, and anatomical repair is performed a few months later.

OPERATION

A median sternotomy is performed. Before initiating cardiopulmonary bypass, the great arteries are dissected and if an arterial switch operation or REV procedure is indicated, the pulmonary bifurcation and the pulmonary branches are freed from their pericardial attachments, including division of the ligamentum arteriosum.

Cardiopulmonary bypass is instituted using two caval cannulas and an ascending aortic cannula. A vent is placed directly into the left atrium. Moderate hypothermia is induced (profound hypothermia and circulatory arrest are not used), and intraoperative myocardial preservation is achieved using multi-dose blood cardioplegia. Myocardial hypothermia is maintained using an intrapericardial cooling blanket. After aortic cross-clamping and during the administration of the initial dose of cardioplegic solution, the right atrium is opened, and an atrial septal defect, if present, is closed.

Cardiac incision

In some patients (i.e. those with near normal ventriculoarterial connection), intracardiac repair may be carried out through a right atrial approach. However, in most cases, a right ventricular approach is warranted.

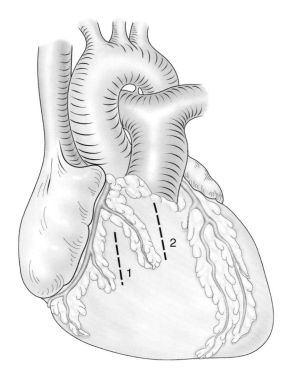

1   The right ventricle is opened either below the aortic orifice (incision 1) or below the pulmonary orifice (incision 2) when pulmonary outflow tract enlargement is anticipated. Great care is taken to preserve as many coronary arteries as possible; a long conal coronary artery is often present and should be avoided. The incision is begun at its caudal end and extended upward, taking care to preserve the aortic leaflets. In all cases, the incision must be planned and performed to provide excellent exposure of the aortic orifice and perfect assessment of the intracardiac anatomy.

As previously explained, the intracardiac step of the surgical procedure is essentially the same, regardless of the arterial orifice to which the left ventricle has to be connected (aortic orifice in intraventricular repair or REV procedure, pulmonary orifice in arterial switch operation). The procedure is described for the construction of a left ventricle–to–aortic orifice tunnel.

Septal resection: indications

The next step is to decide whether septal resection is indicated.

2a When the distance between the tricuspid valve and the aortic valve is equal or greater than the tricuspid valve–to–pulmonary valve distance, the infundibular septum usually interposes between the VSD and the aortic orifice and, therefore, interferes with the intracardiac left ventricle–to–aorta tunnel. The infundibular septum must be resected, even if the VSD itself is large.

2b In the other cases, the infundibular septum lies anterior to the anticipated intracardiac tunnel. The septum does not need to be resected and actually can be used to construct the anterior wall of the tunnel.

2c However, in some patients, the anterior margin of the VSD may bulge inside the anterior aspect of the left ventricle–to–aortic valve tunnel. Options then include either resection or incision of the anterior margin of the VSD to prevent postrepair subaortic stenosis. This type of septal resection is particularly hazardous, as this portion of the interventricular septum may contain important coronary arteries.

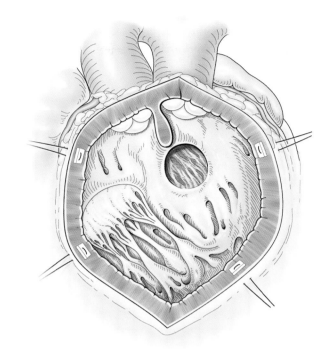

2a

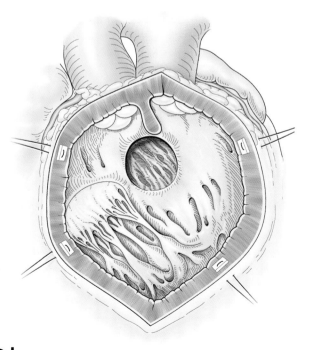

2b

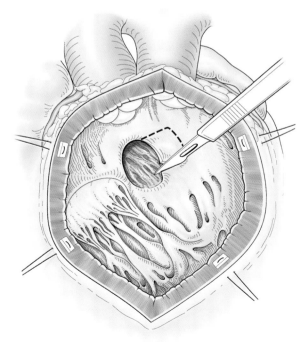

2c

Septal resection: technique

When resection of the infundibular septum is performed, it must be complete. Adequate alignment of the aortic orifice with the newly created left ventricular outflow tract depends on the extensiveness of the septal resection. This step is facil- itated by the introduction of a Hegar dilator through the pul- monary orifice and into the left ventricular cavity. This maneuver greatly improves the exposure of the infundibular septum and protects the mitral valve apparatus.

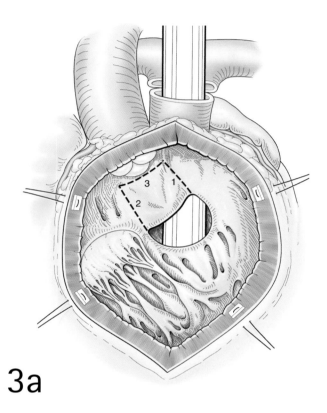

3a

3a Three incisions are then made: two anteriorly and posteriorly from the upper margin of the VSD up to the aortic annulus (incisions 1 and 2), and one parallel to the aortic annulus (incision 3). The infundibular septum is resected, the upper incision being carried out obliquely to avoid injury to the pulmonary valve.

3b When abnormal attachments of the tricuspid valve onto the infundibular septum are present, the sep- tum cannot be excised. Only incisions 1 and 3 are made. The infundibular septum is then mobilized and pulled back later- ally, allowing the construction of the left ventricle–to–aorta tunnel on the left ventricular side of the mobilized septum. After construction of the tunnel, the infundibular septum can be reattached on the prosthetic patch, if needed.

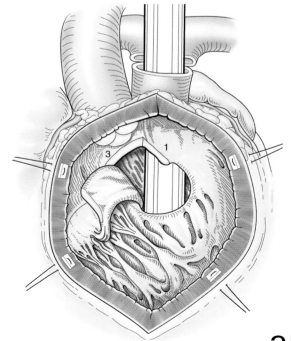

3b

Construction of the intracardiac tunnel

The intracardiac tunnel is created using a prosthetic patch (made of either heterologous pericardium or Dacron velvet lined with pericardium on the left side). The important technical point is the perfect tailoring of the patch. To prevent the development of subaortic stenosis, oversizing the patch is sometimes recommended. However, this technique is ineffective and may be harmful. In most cases, an obligatory angulation between the lower part of the tunnel close to the tricuspid valve and the upper part close to the aortic valve is present. If the patch is oversized, the summit of this angulation may protrude to the left side and cause subaortic obstruction. Extensive resection of the infundibular septum and perfect tailoring are the best ways to avoid subaortic obstruction, not oversizing of the patch.

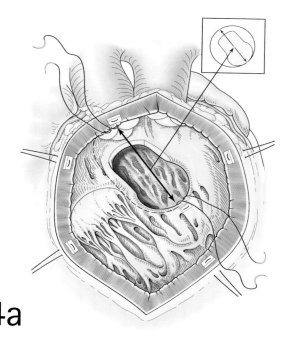

4a The distance between the inferior margin of the VSD and the anterior margin of the aortic annulus is measured precisely. The prosthetic patch is tailored as a circle having this distance as its diameter.

4b The prosthetic patch is secured first to the inferior margin of the VSD using interrupted horizontal mattress sutures. According to the anatomy, the sutures are either passed through the base of the septal leaflet of the tricuspid valve or anchored to the muscular rim that lies between the VSD and the tricuspid valve.

The suture line then goes up to join the right portion of the aortic annulus and goes around the annulus to reach the upper point of the intracardiac tunnel. For this portion of the suture, a continuous suture is used, reinforced with interrupted pledgetted stitches.

At this point, the patch must be precisely tailored. This step is done by trimming the anterior margin of the patch such that it reaches the anterior limit of the tunnel without tension, but also without bulging. As previously stated, at this point two different options exist, however, the rule to adequately tailor the patch remains valid. Only the anterior limit of the tunnel, in respect to the pulmonary orifice, may vary.

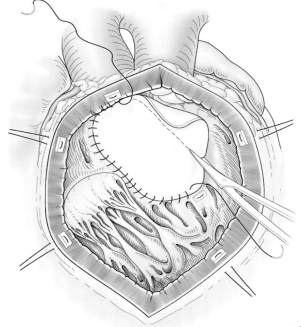

4c When the tricuspid-to-pulmonary valve distance is sufficient (at least equal to the aortic valve diameter), the anterior limit of the tunnel runs posteriorly to the pulmonary orifice, and intraventricular repair is performed. After completion of the intracardiac tunnel, the right ventricular incision is closed, primarily in the absence of pulmonary outflow tract obstruction. In the presence of pulmonary outflow tract obstruction, the pulmonary pathway is enlarged using either an infundibular patch or a transannular patch, just as for repair of tetralogy of Fallot.

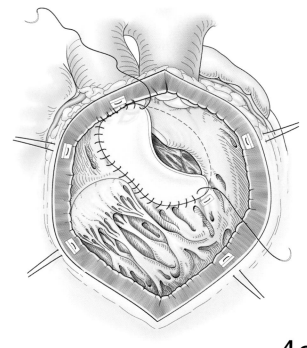

4c

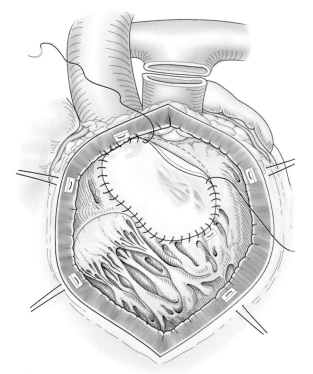

4d

4d When the tricuspid-to-pulmonary valve distance is too short to allow intraventricular repair, the anterior limit of the intracardiac tunnel runs anteriorly to the pulmonary orifice, and the pulmonary artery must be translocated onto the right ventricle (REV procedure).

Intracardiac tunnel in case of arterial switch operation

When an arterial switch operation is indicated (short tricuspid-to-pulmonary distance without pulmonary outflow tract obstruction), the intracardiac tunnel has to be constructed between the left ventricle and the pulmonary orifice.

Nonetheless, the surgical principles regarding septal resection, as well as tailoring and anchoring of the patch, are very similar to those described for the construction of a left ventricle-to-aortic orifice baffle.

5a In most cases, the infundibular septum is located anterior and to the right of the tunnel and can be used for the construction of the tunnel.

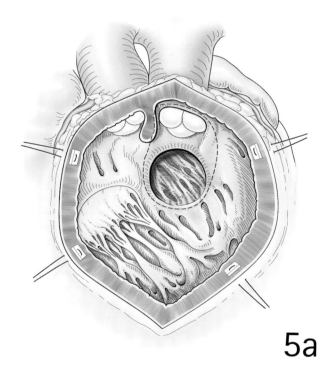

5a

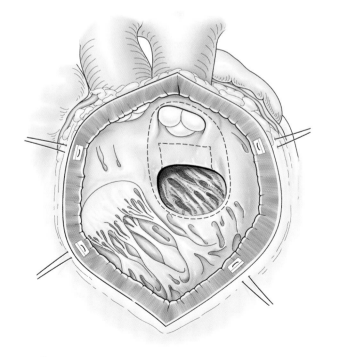

5b

5b However, the infundibular septum may also interpose between the VSD and the pulmonary orifice and must then be extensively resected.

Pulmonary outflow tract obstruction, (REV) procedure

When the REV (réparation à l'étage ventriculaire) procedure is indicated (short tricuspid-to-pulmonary valve distance with pulmonary outflow tract obstruction), the main pulmonary artery must be divided and reimplanted onto the right ventricle.

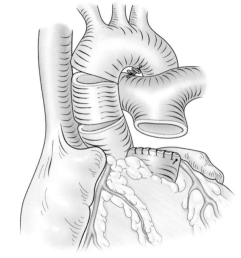

6a

6a The relationship between the great arteries is variable. In most cases (approximatively 75 per cent), the relationship is more or less anteroposterior. In this situation the pulmonary bifurcation should be translocated anterior to the ascending aorta, exactly as it is done for the arterial switch operation. The ascending aorta is divided. The pulmonary branches are extensively mobilized beyond the pericardial reflection, and the pulmonary bifurcation is translocated anterior to the ascending aorta. The ascending aorta is reconstructed by end-to-end anastomosis after a generous resection of the ascending aorta to facilitate the direct reimplantation of the pulmonary trunk onto the right ventricle. When the great arteries are side by side, this maneuver is usually unnecessary and leaving the pulmonary trunk either on the left or on the right side of the undivided ascending aorta is usually better.

In all cases, the cardiac end of the pulmonary trunk is closed primarily, great care being taken not to distort the coronary arteries, which often run very close to the pulmonary annulus.

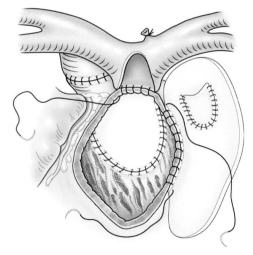

6b The posterior half of the circumference of the distal pulmonary trunk is directly anastomosed to the upper part of the right ventricular incision. The anterior wall of the pulmonary trunk is incised vertically up to the bifurcation. A prosthetic patch, calibrated according to the patient's body surface area, is inserted to reconstruct the pulmonary pathway. A monocuspid pericardial valve is inserted in the upper part of this patch.

6b

6c Unlike the intraventricular patch, the extracardiac patch, which reconstructs the pulmonary outflow tract, must be generous, particularly in its longitudinal axis. An obligatory angulation exists between the intracardiac portion of the right ventricular outflow tract and the extracardiac portion. If the prosthetic anterior patch is too flat (dotted line), this situation may create an obstruction at the level of the summit of this angulation.

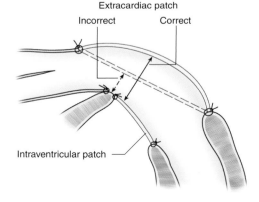

6c

OUTCOME

Postoperative Management

Patients undergoing surgical repair of double outlet right ventricle should be evaluated with intraoperative transesophageal echocardiography following separation from cardiopulmonary bypass. Specifically, the intraventricular tunnel directing left ventricular blood flow to either the aorta or pulmonary artery may be restrictive from either inadequate enlargement of a restrictive VSD or from distortion of the tunnel patch. Left to right shunting through a residual VSD may result in excessive pulmonary blood flow and compromise the hemodynamic status. The right ventricular outflow tract should also be evaluated and right ventricular outflow tract obstruction can occur from inadequate relief of existing pulmonary stenosis, inadequate muscle resection, or from bulging of the intraventricular tunnel patch into the RV outflow tract. Residual defects should be corrected prior to leaving the operating room. Repair of double outlet right ventricle frequently requires a prolonged period of myocardial ischemia and myocardial dysfunction can occur. Thus, the children should be sedated with a continuous narcotic infusion and receive neuromuscular blockade. In some children, allowing a residual right to left shunt through an atrial communication may be useful to maintain systemic cardiac output at the expense of some arterial desaturation. If the hemodynamics are marginal, delayed sternal closure may also be necessary. In children who have had unrestricted pulmonary blood flow prior to repair, pulmonary hypertension can occur in the postoperative period and should be managed with sedation, paralysis, hyperventilation, and treatment with a pulmonary vasodilator, such as inhaled nitric oxide.

FURTHER READING

Lecompte, Y., Batisse, A., Di Carlo, D. 1993. Double outlet right ventricle: a surgical synthesis. In Karp, R., Laks, H., Wechsler, A. (eds), *Advances in Cardiac Surgery*, vol. 4. Chicago: Mosby–Year Book, 109–36.

46

Ebstein's anomaly

ROLAND HETZER MD, PHD
Professor of Surgery, Humboldt University of Berlin; Chairman, Deutsches Herzzentrum, Berlin; Head, Department of Cardiothoracic and Vascular Surgery, Berlin, Germany

MIRALEM PASIC MD, PHD
Professor of Cardiac Surgery, Humboldt University Berlin, Deutsches Herzzentrum, Berlin, Germany

HISTORY

Ebstein's anomaly is a rare, complex, congenital malformation of the tricuspid valve and the right ventricle with variable pathological anatomy. This anomaly is named after Dr. Wilhelm Ebstein, the German pathologist who originally described this malformation in 1866. This congenital heart anomaly occurs in approximately 0.3 per cent of all congenital heart defects and accounts for approximately 0.8–1.2 per cent of all cardiosurgical procedures for congenital heart disease seen in a large heart center.

Operative treatment of Ebstein's anomaly, particularly for tricuspid incompetence, its most prominent sequela, has long been controversial with regard to indication, suitable operative technique (valve replacement or repair), the appropriate type of repair, and the optimal timing for surgery. Repair of the tricuspid valve had not been generally accepted, first, because of the immense variety of pathological features of the anomaly that makes the evolution of a standardized repair concept difficult; second, because few surgeons have had the opportunity to gain sufficient experience due to the rarity of the defect. Many surgeons have favored replacement of the tricuspid valve, as the most straightforward procedure, after the first successful replacement reported in 1963 by Barnard and Schrire. Hunter and Lillehei described the original concept of valve repair in 1958. This technique was clinically used by Hardy and was further modified by Danielson, who has been credited for popularization of valve repair in a large series of patients, which now numbers more than 400. In addition to repair of the tricuspid valve, the techniques include the transverse plication of the so-called atrialized chamber. Later, Carpentier introduced a technique of valve repair with longitudinal (instead of transverse) plication of the atrialized chamber. This technique was further modified by Quaegebeur. In contrast to these techniques, Hetzer introduced a concept of tricuspid valve repair in which the atrialized chamber remained untouched. Unlike the results of surgery achieved in older children and adults, all surgical attempts in infants, including palliative shunt procedures, were generally unsuccessful until Starnes used a procedure that included closure of the tricuspid orifice, enlargement of an interatrial communication, and a central shunt, which was later followed by a Fontan-type operation.

Anatomy of Ebstein's anomaly

The main characteristic of Ebstein's anomaly is that the septal and/or posterior leaflets of the tricuspid valve are variably deformed, predominantly dysplastic, and displaced downwards into the right ventricular cavity without normal attachment to the true tricuspid valve annulus. The anterior leaflet is usually enlarged and sail-like, but it is attached to the annulus at the normal position. This leaflet may have multiple chordal attachments to the ventricular wall. The displace-ment of the valve towards the apex of the right ventricular cavity divides the right ventricle into a portion that lies supravalvular on the atrial side of the tricuspid valve (i.e. the so-called atrialized chamber) and a subvalvular, small, residual right ventricular portion (i.e. the so-called true right ventricle). The annulus of the tricuspid valve and the right atrium are almost always dilated, and the tricuspid valve itself is usually incompetent.

Carpentier's classification of Ebstein's anomaly

1a–d Taking into account the main variables of the defect, Carpentier in 1988 proposed a classification, which is valuable for making surgical decisions as to the most appropriate procedure and for estimating individual surgical risk. In type A (minimal disease), the septal and posterior leaflet origins are only moderately displaced downwards into the right ventricle, the atrialized chamber is small, and a relatively large trabecularized right ventricular cavity is preserved. The anterior leaflet is large and mobile. The volume of the true right ventricle is adequate (Figure 1a). In type B (intermediate disease), the relationship between the volume of the atrialized chamber and the true right ventricle is reversed: a large atrialized chamber and a smaller contracting ventricle both are present. The anterior leaflet is also large and mobile (Figure 1b). In type C (severe disease), the anterior leaflet is restricted in motion by adherence to the anterior right ventricular wall by fibrous bands or abnormal chordae tendineae. This restriction may cause significant obstruction of the right ventricular outflow tract (Figure 1c). In type D (tricuspid sac lesion), the entire right ventricle is lined by broadly adherent fibrous leaflet tissue and almost completely atrialized with the exception of a small infundibular portion. Thus, the entire right ventricle forms a so-called tricuspid sac (Figure 1d).

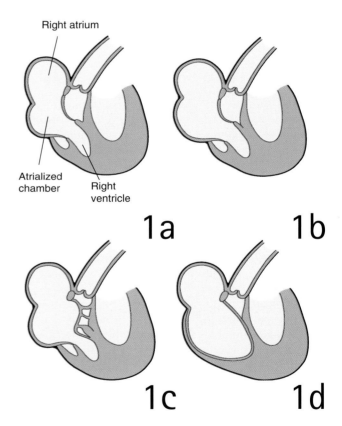

Right atrium

Atrialized chamber

Right ventricle

1a   1b

1c   1d

Associated anomalies

An interatrial communication, commonly in the form of a patent foramen ovale or an atrial septal defect, is a very frequent finding (occurring in approximately 90 per cent of patients) that is accompanied by a right-to-left shunt and systemic arterial desaturation and cyanosis. A Wolff-Parkinson-White type of accessory pathway is present in approximately 10–15 per cent of patients. Other rare anomalies are ventricular septal defect, atrioventricular (AV) septal defect (AV-canal malformations), tetralogy of Fallot, transposition of the great arteries, valvular and subvalvular pulmonary stenosis, pulmonary atresia, and malformation of the mitral valve.

PRINCIPLES AND JUSTIFICATION

Indications for medical or surgical treatment

The management of patients with Ebstein's anomaly is aimed at preventing and treating the complications. In general, medical management is recommended for those patients with only mild symptoms. This approach concentrates on medications for heart failure, arrhythmias, and anticoagulation. The classic indication for operative treatment is the presence of severe, chronic heart failure with symptoms of functional New York Heart Association (NYHA) class III or IV. Based on the favorable results of surgical treatment, indications for operation have been extended, and currently, most patients can be surgically treated with good results. The extended indications for operative treatment include the following:

- Less symptomatic patients with functional NYHA class II and progression of symptoms
- Increasing cyanosis
- Deterioration of exercise tolerance
- Retardation of growth curve in children
- Paradoxical embolization
- Brain abscess
- Rhythm disturbances with atrial tachyarrhythmias or ventricular arrhythmias
- Progressive increase in cardiac size
- Worsening of the echocardiographic findings, such as an increase of tricuspid valve regurgitation, enlargement of the right atrium and right ventricle, and deterioration of right ventricular function.

Contraindications

No specific contraindications exist for surgical treatment relative to the anomaly *per se*. The contraindications include the general surgical contraindications for open heart surgery, for example, the inability to improve the patient's quality of life or life expectancy (e.g. malignancy, neurological damage).

Types of operative treatment

TRICUSPID VALVE REPAIR

Tricuspid valve repair is preferred to valve replacement to avoid the problems of valve dysfunction, anticoagulation, and the need for repeat valve replacement in childhood due to growth. The excellent functional results enable an extension of the scope of repair, even for cases that hitherto were predominantly reserved for primary valve replacement. According to the different institutional policies, tricuspid valvuloplasty is feasible in 40–98 per cent of patients, with a reoperation rate of 3–15 per cent. Numerous surgical techniques and modifications have been proposed. Five main valve repair techniques exist: Hardy, Danielson, Carpentier, Quaegebeur, and Hetzer. According to the mode of plication of the atrialized chamber, the techniques can be divided into three types: transverse plication techniques (Hardy and Danielson), longitudinal plication techniques (Carpentier and Quaegebeur), and no plication technique (Hetzer).

TRICUSPID VALVE REPAIR WITH TRANSVERSE PLICATION (TECHNIQUES OF HARDY AND DANIELSON)

This technique consists of the reconstruction of the tricuspid valve by the use of the mobile anterior leaflet as a closing mechanism of the valve. The procedure is performed by transposing the displaced septal and posterior leaflets to the normal level of the tricuspid valve. Thus, the atrialized chamber is plicated and obliterated in a transverse plane (parallel to the true tricuspid annulus). This technique brings the body of the anterior leaflet towards the true tricuspid annulus and allows anterior leaflet coaptation with the atrialized septum. Danielson modified this technique by additional posterior annuloplasty to reduce the diameter of the tricuspid annulus.

TRICUSPID VALVE REPAIR WITH LONGITUDINAL PLICATION (TECHNIQUES OF CARPENTIER AND QUAEGEBEUR)

Carpentier's repair technique includes the detachment of the anterior and/or posterior leaflets at their origin at the annulus, transection of fibrous bands between leaflets and the right ventricular wall, longitudinal plication of the atrialized chamber, and the reinsertion of the detached leaflets to the true annulus above the plicated chamber. Also, the leaflets are moved clockwise towards the posterior part of the septal annulus. To reduce tension of this new leaflet attachment line, transection and reattachment of the papillary muscles of the anterior leaflet may be necessary, particularly those of its anterior part. Stabilization of this new valve annulus with a prosthetic ring is strongly recommended. Quaegebeur modified the Carpentier technique in two ways: first, instead of insertion of a ring to hold the annulus in a certain shape and at a reduced size, he introduced a suture annuloplasty along the posterior leaflet annulus, which further reduced the size of the annulus. Subsequently, the second modification was no need for transection and reimplantation of papillary muscles of the anterior leaflet.

TRICUSPID VALVE REPAIR WITHOUT PLICATION (TECHNIQUE OF HETZER)

This technique restructures the valve mechanism at the level of the true tricuspid annulus by the use of the most mobile leaflet for valve closure, but without plication of the atrialized chamber. The Hetzer repair permits sufficient repair of the tricuspid valve so that even in cases in which only the posterior leaflet or part of the anterior leaflet can be remodeled, they can act as a valve-closing structure.

TRICUSPID VALVE REPLACEMENT

Tricuspid valve replacement is indicated only if the tricuspid valve is not amenable to reconstruction. According to different institutional experiences, its frequency differs widely, from 2 to 50 per cent of patients. The clear indications for tricuspid valve replacement are lack of valvular tissue and the presence of the Carpentier's type D lesion ('tricuspid sack lesion'). A prosthesis can be implanted in the standard manner with insertion of the prosthetic sewing ring in the true tricuspid annulus, or by the use of a slightly modified technique as recommended by Barnard and Schrire. In their classic report, they described the placement of a prosthetic valve on the atrial side of the coronary sinus to minimize the risk of complete heart block. Thus, the coronary sinus is left to drain into the right ventricle. However, heart block cannot be avoided in every case, and some patients require the insertion of a pacemaker. The standard prosthetic replacement of the tricuspid valve can be performed either with or without concomitant plication of the atrialized chamber. If the atrialized chamber is excessively dilated and the volume of the functional ('true') right ventricle is normal, the plication of the atrialized chamber may then be included with valve replacement. No uniform opinion exists as to which type of prosthesis (mechanical or biological) should be used. The decision is made in agreement with the patient, who is fully informed about the advantages and disadvantages of both types of prostheses.

SURGICAL OPTIONS FOR VERY SEVERE ANOMALIES (TYPES C AND D ACCORDING TO CARPENTIER'S CLASSIFICATION)

In severely sick patients with severe anomalies, any one of the various repair techniques carries a high operative risk. In such patients, a combination of tricuspid valve repair and a cavopulmonary anastomosis (Glenn shunt) may be applied, or alternatively, primarily orthotopic heart transplantation may be considered.

Importance of the atrialized chamber

The crucial questions that have to be raised refer to the importance of the atrialized chamber. Hardy, Danielson, Carpentier, and Quaegebeur consider it important to obliterate or, at least, to reduce this chamber for various reasons. On one hand, this chamber, when exposed to right ventricular pressure, might have a similarly negative effect on ventricular energy economics as a left ventricular aneurysm on the left ventricle. Also, stasis within the non-contractile sac could promote clot formation. Thus, plication of the atrialized chamber might enhance right ventricular function and might obviate the characteristic rhythm disturbances. On the other hand, transverse plication, at least in the more pronounced cases of types B and C (according to the classification of Carpentier), may cause high tension on both the plication sutures and the tissue, with unknown effects on the already abnormal septum and the left ventricle. In contrast, longitudinal plication does not cause ventricular distortion and preserves the apex-to-base distance of the right ventricle. However, most of the proponents of tricuspid valve replacement leave the atrialized chamber untouched, and no negative sequelae have been reported. Similarly, the Hetzer repair technique makes no attempt to obliterate or to reduce this chamber and results in neither further enlargement of the right ventricle nor any other undesirable effects. Furthermore, the incorporation of the atrialized chamber into the contracting right ventricle may be beneficial in allowing sufficient right ventricular filling during diastole, which could stimulate the remaining musculature in the atrialized chamber wall towards hypertrophy and even contribute to right ventricular contraction. However, this field is open for further investigation.

PREOPERATIVE ASSESSMENT AND PREPARATION

Clinical manifestations

Patients with Ebstein's anomaly become symptomatic according to the severity of the anomaly. Neonates, who are highly symptomatic, have massive cardiac enlargement, severe cyanosis, and metabolic acidosis, and they require urgent surgery. In these patients, physiological pulmonary atresia is present due to the inability of the right ventricle to produce sufficient pressure to open the pulmonary valve. This situation causes a right-to-left shunt through an inter-atrial communication with systemic arterial desaturation and cyanosis. Some patients may have symptoms of chronic heart insufficiency with progressive cyanosis, paradoxical embolization, brain abscess, and rhythm disturbances such as atrial or ventricular arrhythmias. Paroxysmal atrial tachycardias may cause progressive cardiac failure or worsening of cyanosis, and may even cause syncope. Some patients with a mild form of the anomaly may be oligosymptomatic or even asymptomatic up to adulthood. In these patients, the diagnosis is usually made by echocardiographic examination after the finding of cardiac enlargement.

Preoperative examination

CHEST X-RAY

2 The chest x-ray is characterized by massive enlargement of the right atrium, which gives the heart a triangular shape with a broad, symmetrical base on the diaphragm. The pulmonary arteries and the aorta are usually small, and the pulmonary vasculature is diminished.

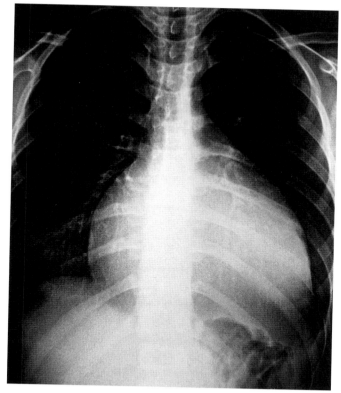

2

ECHOCARDIOGRAPHY

The most important diagnostic procedure nowadays is echocardiography with Doppler evaluation of regurgitant tricuspid flow, the interatrial shunt, and the characteristic anatomy of the anomaly. Echocardiographic analysis focuses on the degree of tricuspid incompetence and on the size of the right atrium, the atrialized chamber, and the 'true' right ventricle, the last being the most decisive for the assessment of risk and the outcome of surgical repair. Also of great importance are the size and the mobility of the predominant tricuspid leaflet, which is the anterior leaflet in most cases. Furthermore, determination of the shape, size, and function of the usually distorted left ventricle is important, because these attributes may be further impaired by the repair techniques with plication of the atrialized chamber. The location and the size of the interatrial communication and the degree of shunt can be well determined by echocardiography Doppler techniques.

HEART CATHETERIZATION

With modern echocardiographic technology, cardiac catheterization has lost gravitas, but may be desirable to detect further cardiac anomalies and disease, such as coronary artery disease, which is extremely rare in the age group operated on hitherto. Preoperative pressure recordings, especially in the right atrium, may be helpful for postoperative comparison. Oximetric quantification of the shunt may be required to underline the Doppler echocardiographic findings.

ELECTROPHYSIOLOGICAL EVALUATION

Preoperative electrophysiological evaluation is warranted in patients with arrhythmias. Electrophysiological mapping is necessary for the localization and ablation of the accessory conduction pathway.

ANESTHESIA

The principles of anesthesia follow those for standard open heart procedures. No specific anesthetic requirements exist for perioperative management relative to the anomaly. At our institution, the standard anesthesia protocol includes induction with etomidate and fentanyl, pancuronium for muscle relaxation, and propofol infusion for maintenance of anesthesia.

OPERATION

General procedures before valve repair

SURGICAL APPROACH AND INSPECTION OF THE HEART

The operation is carried out via standard full-length or partial median sternotomy. After opening the pericardium, a piece of it is harvested for a patch, which can be optionally fixed in glutaraldehyde. Then, the intraoperative situs is inspected. Typically, the right atrium is enormously enlarged, and the right ventricle appears to be dilated. This situation encompasses both the atrialized chamber and the remaining portion of the right ventricle. The atrialized chamber can be well defined from outside at the acute margin and along the inferior aspect of the heart. The left ventricle is displaced towards the left side and winds around the right ventricle like a curved cucumber.

CARDIOPULMONARY BYPASS

Cardiopulmonary bypass is established using aortic and separate caval cannulation, total cardiopulmonary bypass, and mild systemic hypothermia of 30°C. The aorta is cross-clamped, and cardioplegic arrest is induced.

MYOCARDIAL PROTECTION

Myocardial protection is performed according to institutional and surgical preferences. At our institution, cardioplegic arrest is initially afforded by aortic root infusion of crystalloid arrest solution (Cardioplegin). Myocardial protection is maintained by repeated infusions of cold hydroxyethylene starch solution.

3 **Opening of the right atrium**   The right atrium can be opened in one of three alternative ways: an angulated oblique incision (A), an oblique incision from the right atrial appendage towards the inferior vena cava (B), or a straight incision parallel to the AV groove (C).

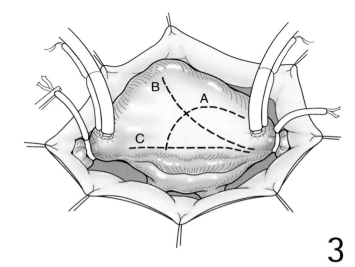

3

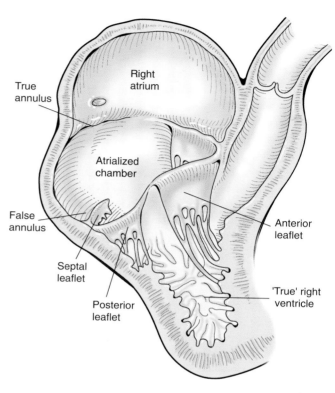

4a

4a, b
Intracardiac inspection For this complex defect, the intracardiac pathological anatomy is typically widely varied in all patients, and no case equals another in every respect. However, the characteristic features of Ebstein's anomaly are easily found in every patient. The anatomical annulus of the tricuspid valve is grossly distended, and the septal leaflet is displaced in its origin towards the right ventricular cavity. The posterior and the anterior leaflets show marked variety. The annular attachment of the posterior leaflet is also displaced and gives rise to the formation of a so-called 'atrialized chamber' of greatly differing size (see the section 'Carpentier's classification of Ebstein's anomaly'). The anterior leaflet is the largest leaflet in most cases. This leaflet can be fully mobile or can be partially or completely attached to the adjacent right ventricular free wall by a varying number of fibrous bands that restrict leaflet mobility. In some patients, the posterior leaflet is quite substantial and mobile and is almost the same size as the anterior leaflet, or it may be even larger. The anterior leaflet may show clefts or deep fenestrations. Rarely, a fourth, smaller, accessory leaflet exists with its origin in the anteroseptal commissure.

DECOMPRESSION OF THE LEFT SIDE OF THE HEART

Decompression of the left atrium and left ventricle is achieved by placing a sucker or a vent catheter across the patent foramen ovale or atrial septal defect. Alternatively, a left ventricular vent catheter can be inserted through the right upper pulmonary vein.

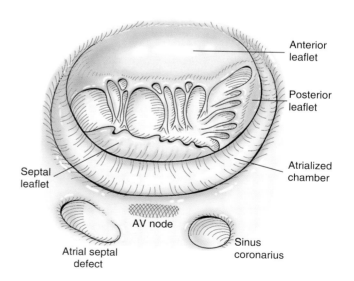

4b

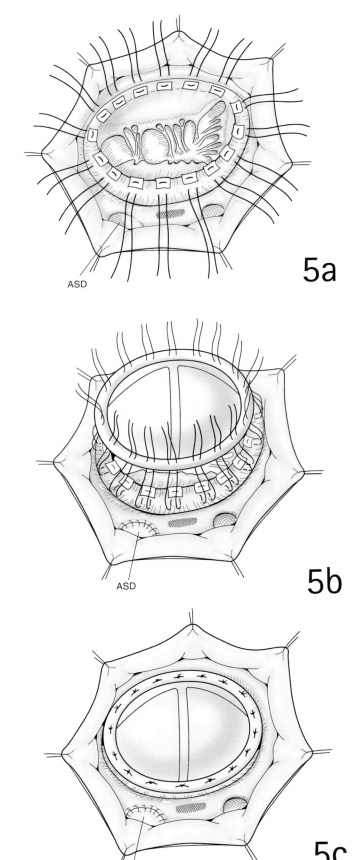

Specific valve procedures

Tricuspid valve replacement

5a–c Standard implantation technique without plication of the atrialized chamber The leaflets and the chordal attachments are left in place to preserve right ventricular function. Where obstruction of the right ventricular outflow tract by leaflet tissue occurs, commissurotomy-like radial incisions are made in the tissue of the leaflets to open up the right ventricular outflow tract. Interrupted mattress sutures buttressed with Teflon pledgets are placed through the true tricuspid annulus tissue and then through the prosthetic sewing ring. Care must be taken to avoid the area of the bundle of His by placing the sutures on the septum below the natural annulus (at least in the anteroseptal area) and also to avoid suturing between the coronary sinus and the tricuspid annulus. A prosthesis, usually with a diameter of 31–33 mm, is positioned into the annulus of the tricuspid valve. When the sutures are tied, the sewing ring of the prosthesis lies on the anatomical tricuspid annulus. The atrialized chamber is not plicated and remains below the prosthesis.

6 Standard implantation technique with plication of the atrialized chamber If the atrialized chamber is excessively dilated and the volume of the functional ('true') right ventricle is normal, plication of the atrialized chamber may be undertaken in addition to valve replacement. Interrupted mattress sutures with Teflon pledgets are placed close together on the false annulus at the attachments of the posterior and septal leaflets, again through the true annulus, and then through the prosthetic sewing ring. When tying the sutures, the atrialized chamber is obliterated. The tricuspid valve leaflets are not excised, as described previously.

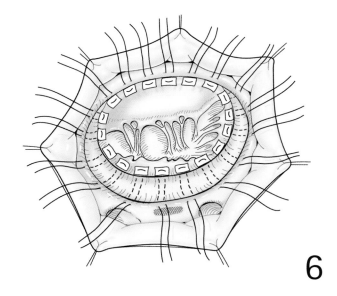

6

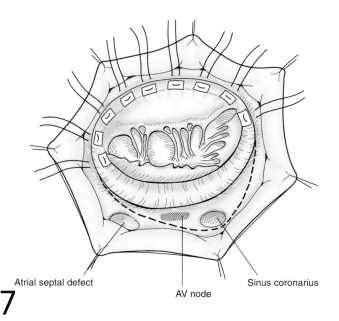

Atrial septal defect

AV node

Sinus coronarius

7

7 Modified technique The suture line is placed posterior to the AV node and around the coronary sinus to avoid injury to the conduction system. Thus, the prosthetic valve lies on the atrial side of the coronary sinus, which leaves the coronary sinus to drain into the ventricle. The atrialized chamber is not plicated. However, if plication of the atrialized chamber is added to this modification, this step has to be performed with a separate suture line to avoid obstruction of the coronary sinus.

TRICUSPID VALVE REPAIR

Valve repair with transverse plication of the atrialized chamber (Danielson technique)

8a **Placement of transverse ventricular plication sutures** Interrupted mattress sutures with Teflon pledgets are placed along the ventricular rim of the atrialized chamber and again on the true tricuspid annulus.

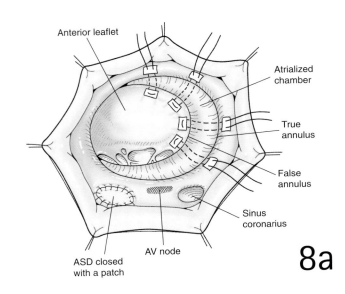

8a

8b **Transverse plication of the atrialized chamber** The plication sutures are tied, which pull the posterior and septal leaflets towards the true tricuspid annulus; thus, the atrialized chamber is plicated and obliterated in a transverse plane that lies parallel to the true tricuspid annulus.

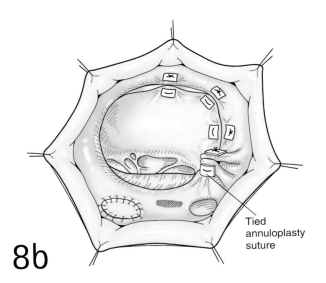

8b

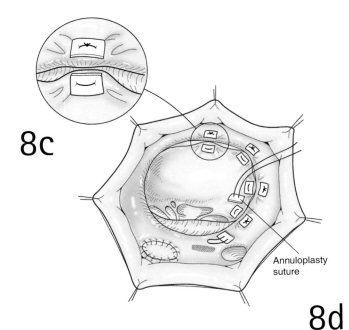

8c

8d

8c, d **Posterior annuloplasty of the tricuspid annulus** The diameter of the tricuspid annulus is reduced by a posterior annuloplasty by the use of polypropylene 3/0 mattress suture with Teflon pledgets. The posterior annuloplasty suture is placed at the level of the coronary sinus to avoid injury to the conduction bundle.

The tricuspid valve is tested for competence by the instillation of saline solution into the right ventricle. After repair, the tricuspid valve functions as a monocusp valve.

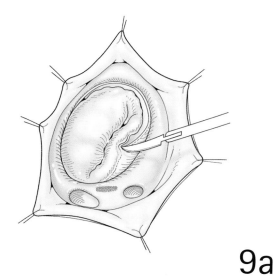

9a

Valve repair with longitudinal plication of the atrialized chamber (techniques of Carpentier and Quaegebeur)

Carpentier technique

9a, b Mobilization of the anterior and posterior leaflet   The anterior leaflet and the adjacent portion of the posterior leaflet of the tricuspid valve are detached from their hinge along the annulus. The incision starts at the anteroseptal commissure, but the attachment of the anterior leaflet at the level of the anteroseptal commissure should be left untouched. The detached leaflets are further mobilized by cutting accessory trabeculae, fibrous bands, and adhesions to the ventricular wall. Interchordal spaces are fenestrated if obliterated. The corresponding papillary muscle is also fully mobilized by cutting the muscular bands that are inserted on the lateral wall of the right ventricle. An inadequate mobilization of the muscle may cause unsatisfactory leaflet coaptation due to excessive traction on the leaflets.

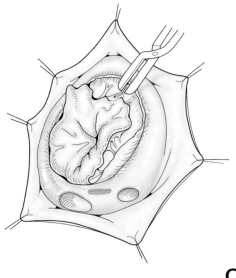

9b

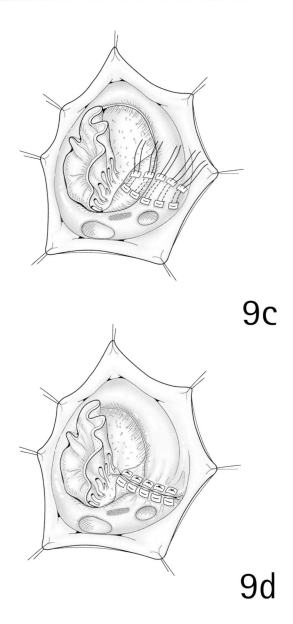

9c

9d

9c, d Longitudinal plication of the atrialized chamber

The atrialized chamber is obliterated by placing the sutures perpendicular to the true tricuspid annulus. Plication is performed by the use of either single mattress sutures with Teflon pledgets or a running suture reinforced with a number of interrupted stitches. Care should be taken not to perforate the myocardial wall or to injure the coronary arteries. Plication of the atrialized chamber reduces the diameter of the tricuspid annulus.

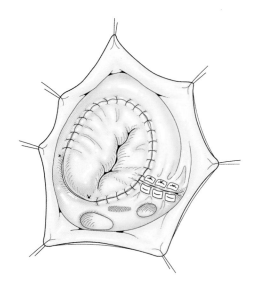

9e

9e Rotation and reattachment of the mobilized leaflets

The anterior and posterior leaflets are rotated in a clockwise direction and then reattached to the new, smaller annulus by the use of continuous 5/0 polypropylene suture. The needle stitches should pass through the tissue away from the AV node to prevent heart block. The dangerous zone is the septal portion of the annulus next to the orifice of the coronary sinus; and therefore, the suture should stop at the level of the coronary sinus. After suturing the mobilized anterior leaflet to the annulus, the leaflet functions as a monocusp valve and covers the whole valve orifice area. Thus, the tricuspid annulus is reduced by the amount of atrialized chamber plication, and the anterior leaflet is swung clockwise to cover the entire length of the annular portion of the anterior and posterior leaflet.

The tricuspid valve is tested for competence by the instillation of saline solution into the right ventricle. After repair, the tricuspid valve functions as a monocusp valve with the anterior leaflet. If the leaflet coaptation is insufficient because of inadequate papillary muscle mobilization, the muscle can be translocated from the lateral ventricular wall and reimplanted at a higher position on the ventricular septum.

9f **Reinforcement of the tricuspid annulus** For stabilization of the annulus, an annuloplasty ring is implanted. The ring further decreases the diameter of the dilated tricuspid annulus, and thereby improves leaflet coaptation and the competence of the valve. The ring should be omitted in children and may not be necessary in patients with type A lesions (according to Carpentier's classification).

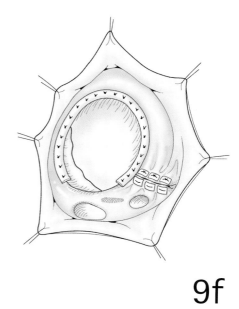

9f

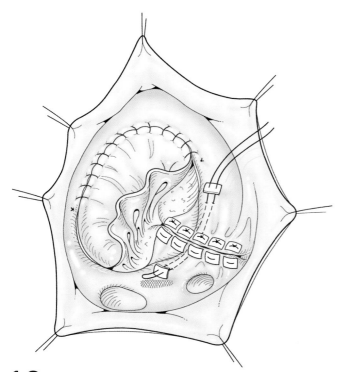

Quaegebeur technique

10 **Posterior annuloplasty of the tricuspid annulus** In this modification of the Carpentier technique, no prosthetic ring is used to reinforce the annulus. The diameter of the tricuspid annulus is reduced by posterior annuloplasty by the use of polypropylene 3/0 mattress suture with Teflon pledgets. Thus, in contrast to Carpentier's technique, the newly reinserted leaflets do not come under excessive tension; and therefore, transection and translocation of the papillary muscle become necessary. The posterior annuloplasty suture is placed next to the coronary sinus to avoid injury to the conduction bundle.

10

Valve repair without plication of the atrialized chamber (technique of Hetzer)

Anterior leaflet is large and intact

11a–c
Mobilization of the leaflet and suture placement   The anterior leaflet is examined for mobility. The fibrous bands between the leaflet and the right ventricular wall, if present, are dissected to enhance leaflet mobility. The original orifice of the tricuspid valve is reduced by obliteration of the posterior part of the tricuspid ostium with 4–6 interrupted mattress sutures of 3/0 polypropylene supported by pledgets of autologous pericardium or Teflon felt. The new tricuspid valve orifice should measure at least 2.5 cm in diameter. To ensure this orifice size, the first suture is placed as a test suture. This suture runs through the true annulus in the region of the anterior leaflet and then through the opposite point on the septum. The suture divides the original orifice of the tricuspid valve into two parts: the anterior one that will become a new orifice, and the posterior part that will be obliterated. The valve is tested by instillation of saline into the right ventricular cavity to prove that the anterior leaflet can effectively close the new orifice. The remaining sutures are placed consecutively to obliterate the posterior part of the tricuspid ostium. The suture line is placed at the level of the true annulus, except in the region of the septum. In this area, to avoid injury of the AV node, the sutures lie in the muscular region of the atrialized chamber just below the true annulus. The atrialized chamber is left intact without plication.

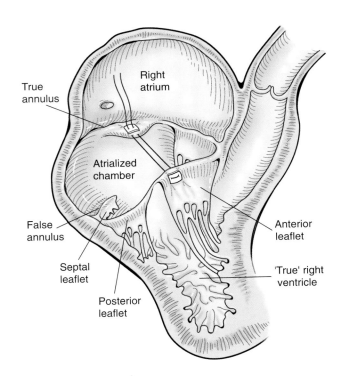

11a

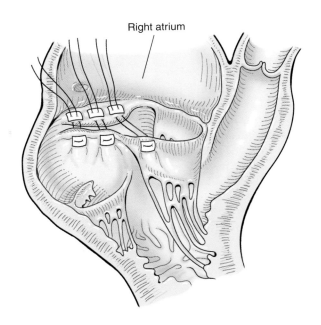

11b

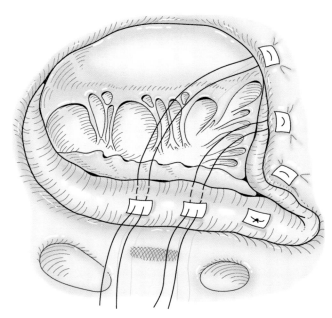

11c

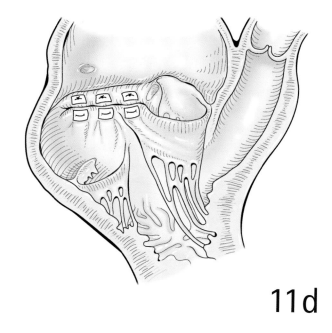

11d

11d, e
Obliteration of the posterior part of the annulus The sutures are tied, which results in the obliteration of the posterior part of the original tricuspid orifice. Thus, the anterior annulus is approximated to the septum.

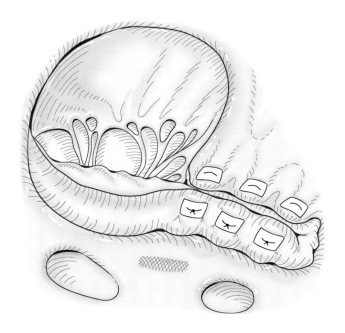

11e

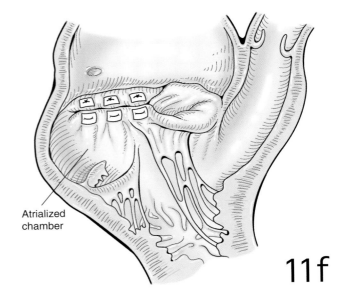

Atrialized
chamber

11f

11f, g **Proof of valvular competence** Valve
competence is tested by filling the right
ventricular cavity with saline solution, and the anterior part
of the anterior leaflet coapts with the atrialized septum. The
atrialized chamber is incorporated into the contracting right
ventricular cavity.

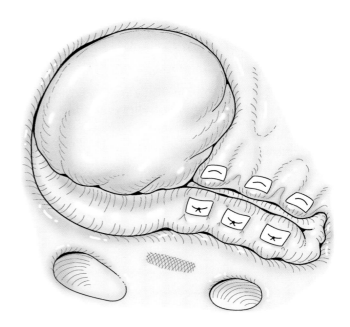

11g

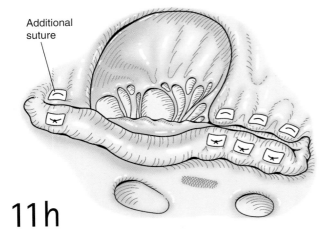

Additional
suture

11h

11h Rarely, the tricuspid ostium is additionally
narrowed at the anteroseptal commissure to correct some residual valve regurgitation.

Anterior leaflet is divided by a cleft or several fissures

12a Inspection and mobilization of the anterior leaflet The anterior leaflet is split by a cleft and deep fissures. Some chordal adhesions of the leaflet to the right ventricular wall are present and are dissected.

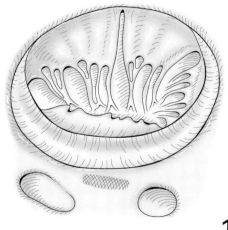

12a

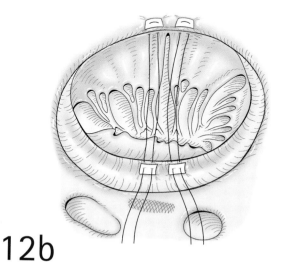

12b

12b Suture placement Two 3/0 polypropylene mattress sutures, supported with autologous pericardium or with Teflon felt, are passed through the middle portion of the anterior annulus in the region of the cleft and the opposite atrialized septum, just below the true septal annulus.

12c Creation of a valve The sutures are tied, and the anterior annulus is approximated to the septum, dividing the valve into two orifices. The two separate anterior leaflet parts coapt with the opposing septum.

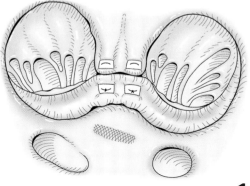

12c

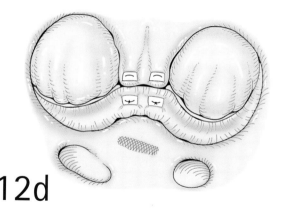

12d

12d Proof of valvular competence Valve competence is tested by filling the right ventricular cavity with saline solution. The 'double orifice' valve is closed with two parts of the anterior leaflet. The atrialized chamber is then incorporated into the contracting right ventricular cavity.

General procedures after valve repair

CLOSURE OF AN INTERATRIAL COMMUNICATION

A patent foramen ovale is closed directly by a running suture. Larger atrial septal defects should be closed with a patch of impermeable material such as autologous pericardium or polytetrafluoroethylene.

CORRECTION OF ADDITIONAL CONGENITAL DEFECTS

Other associated anomalies (such as ventricular septal defect, AV-canal defect, mitral valve pathology, and valvular and subvalvular pulmonary stenosis) are corrected in the standard fashion either before tricuspid valve repair or thereafter, as is appropriate.

TREATMENT OF ATRIAL ARRHYTHMIAS

Intraoperative ablation of AV node re-entry tachycardia or intraoperative ablation of an accessory conduction pathway in patients with Wolff-Parkinson-White syndrome can be performed as a part of the operative treatment. The Cox-Maze procedure (i.e. standard biatrial maze procedure, isolated left atrial or right atrial technique) can be performed concomitantly with valve repair to control chronic or paroxysmal atrial fibrillation or flutter. The maze procedure is done either surgically as a 'cut and sew technique' or by the use of a radiofrequency catheter technique.

RIGHT REDUCTION ATRIOPLASTY AND CLOSURE OF THE RIGHT ATRIUM

The closure of the right atrial incision is preceded by a significant reduction of the giant right atrium. A substantial part of the dilated and redundant atrial wall may be excised or wrapped by the closing suture line. The right atrium is closed with a continuous 4/0 polypropylene suture.

DEAIRING OF THE HEART

Deairing is performed in the institutional standard manner. To avoid air embolization, carbon dioxide can be insufflated into the pericardium during surgery.

INTRAOPERATIVE ECHOCARDIOGRAPHIC ASSESSMENT

Once the heart is closed and beating, intraoperative transesophageal echocardiography is carried out to assess tricuspid valve competence and orifice area, to exclude a residual shunt and to observe left and right ventricular function.

PERIOPERATIVE MONITORING AND WEANING FROM CARDIOPULMONARY BYPASS

Atrial and ventricular epicardial wires are placed for postoperative pacemaker stimulation, left and right atrial pressures are monitored, and the patient is weaned from cardiopulmonary bypass.

PERIOPERATIVE AND POSTOPERATIVE CARE

Taking the patient off extracorporeal circulation may require inotropic support and, in rare cases, even mechanical circulatory support, such as intra-aortic balloon counterpulsation. The addition of nitrous oxide to respirator ventilation air to reduce pulmonary vascular resistance may be liberally applied to support right ventricular function. The institution's standard management of patients after open-heart surgery is applied.

Repair as a single ventricle in infants

When severe symptoms arise as early as in infancy, the degree of malformation is extensive and the valve tissue immature, which precludes conventional repair. These children have functional pulmonary atresia, which results from increased pulmonary vascular resistance of the neonate and severe tricuspid regurgitation. No antegrade blood flow occurs from the right ventricle to the pulmonary artery, and these infants remain dependent on ductal patency. They may present in a state of advanced cardiorespiratory failure, with cyanosis and metabolic acidosis. A palliative surgical procedure is required to enable the patient to survive for either future surgical correction or heart transplantation. Palliation is achieved either by central or peripheral systemic-to-pulmonary artery shunt (e.g. Blalock-Taussig shunt), or by a bidirectional cavopulmonary anastomosis (Glenn shunt). These palliative procedures increase pulmonary blood flow and thereby decrease cyanosis. Although better oxygenation can be provided in this way, results have been unfavorable due to persistent tricuspid valve regurgitation and subsequent cardiac enlargement, which may maintain or even aggravate circulatory failure. More recently, a procedure to create a 'true' tricuspid atresia was introduced by Starnes, which provided better results. With this procedure, not only is a systemic to pulmonary shunt installed, but also the tricuspid valve orifice is closed, and the atrial septal defect is enlarged. Infants may then survive and grow, and the decision for further surgical correction (bidirectional cavopulmonary anastomosis and intra-atrial or extracardiac Fontan-tunnel procedure in one or two sessions) then follows according to the established principles for correction of tricuspid atresia, or the child may be listed for heart transplantation.

STARNES TECHNIQUE

13a **Cardiopulmonary bypass and opening of the right atrium** After median sternotomy, pericardium is harvested for patch material, which can optionally be fixed in glutaraldehyde. Cardiopulmonary bypass is established by the use of standard aortic and bicaval cannulation. Systemic cooling is started, aiming at a deep hypothermia of 20°C. After cross-clamping of the aorta and administration of cardioplegic solution, the right atrium is opened obliquely from the right appendage to the inferior vena cava. Inspection of the heart shows the characteristic findings of Ebstein's anomaly.

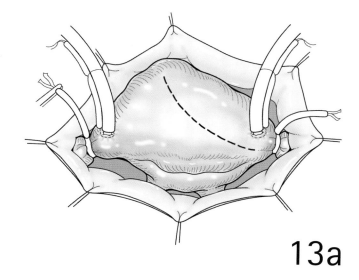

13a

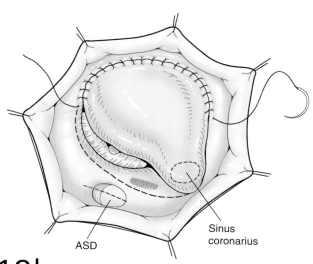

ASD

Sinus
coronarius

13b

13b **Closure of the tricuspid valve** The tricuspid valve is closed with an autologous pericardial patch using a continuous 6/0 polypropylene suture. The suture line begins at the level of the anteroseptal commissure and runs clockwise along the true annulus. The suture passes through the pericardial patch and then through the true tricuspid annulus, except in the area of the coronary sinus. At the level of the annulus that corresponds to the posterior leaflet, the suture line leaves the true annulus and surrounds the coronary sinus to reduce heart block (dashed line). Note that the coronary sinus is left beneath the patch.

13c **Enlargement of the atrial septal defect and reduction atrioplasty** An atrial septal defect or patent foramen ovale is enlarged (or created if it does not exist) to ensure unrestricted mixing of the blood at the atrial level. The incision is made downward, to the lower rim of the fossa ovalis, and a few millimeters upward, through the atrial septal muscles toward the entrance of the vena cava superiorly. A right atrial reduction plasty is performed by excision of a part of the enlarged anterior free wall of the right atrium. The right atrium is closed with a running suture of 6/0 polypropylene, and the patient is rewarmed.

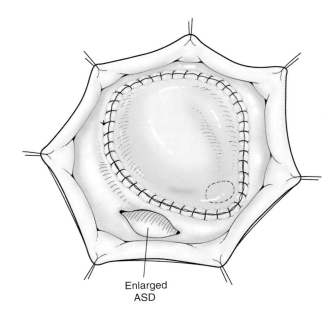

Enlarged
ASD

13c

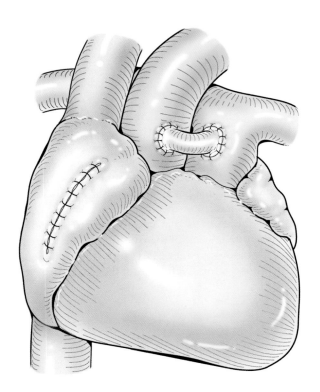

13d

13d **Insertion of a central shunt** During the rewarming phase, a central shunt is inserted between the ascending aorta and the main pulmonary artery by the use of a 4-mm-diameter polytetrafluoroethylene prosthesis. The patient is weaned from cardiopulmonary bypass with necessary support (e.g. dopamine, epinephrine, infusion of prostaglandin E$_1$, nitric oxide insufflation, hyperventilation).

OUTCOME

The early mortality rate varies from 2.9 to 8 per cent in different series of patients. The late results are excellent, with a survival rate of approximately 90 per cent at one year and 80 per cent at two years. Nearly all patients show a substantial improvement of their preoperative status, and most patients are in NYHA class I or II with a significant improvement of oxygen saturation. Usually, patients have a postoperative reduction in heart size and fewer arrhythmias.

Specific complications of surgery

Specific perioperative and postoperative complications include complete heart block, injury to the right coronary artery, low cardiac output syndrome, myocardial insufficiency that necessitates mechanical circulatory support, persistent atrial arrhythmias, ventricular arrhythmias, residual tricuspid insufficiency or tricuspid stenosis after valve repair, and prosthetic dysfunction after valve replacement.

Postoperative surveillance

All patients should be followed on a regular basis, with outpatient visits at least once a year. This follow-up should include clinical and echocardiographic examinations, electrocardiography, and Holter monitoring.

FURTHER READING

Carpentier, A., Chauvaud, S., Macé, L., *et al.* 1988. A new reconstructive operation for Ebstein's anomaly of the tricuspid valve. *Journal of Thoracic and Cardiovascular Surgery* 96, 92–101.

Danielson, G.K., Maloney, J.D., Devloo, R.A.E. 1979. Surgical repair of Ebstein's anomaly. *Mayo Clinic Proceedings* 54, 185–92.

Ebstein, W. 1866. Ueber einen sehr seltenen Fall von Insufficienz der Valvula tricuspidalis, bedingt durch eine angeborene hochgradige Missbildung derselben. *Arch F Anat Physiol Wissensch Med Leipz*, 238–55.

Hetzer, R., Nagdyman, N., Weng, Y.G., *et al.* 1998. A modified repair technique for tricuspid incompetence in Ebstein's anomaly. *Journal of Thoracic and Cardiovascular Surgery* 115, 857–68.

Quaegebeur, J.M., Sreeram, N., Fraser, A.G, *et al.* 1991. Surgery for Ebstein's anomaly: the clinical and echocardiographic evaluation of a new technique. *Journal of the American College of Cardiology* 17, 722–8.

Starnes, V.A., Pitlick, P.T., Berstein, D., Griffith, M.I., Choy, M., Shumway, N.E. 1991. Ebstein's anomaly appearing in the neonate: a new surgical approach. *Journal of Thoracic and Cardiovascular Surgery* 101, 1082–7.

47

Ventricular septal defect

CARL LEWIS BACKER MD
A. C. Buehler Professor of Surgery, Division of Cardiovascular-Thoracic Surgery, Children's Memorial Hospital, Professor of Surgery, Northwestern University Feinberg School of Medicine, Chicago, Illinois, USA

If a single operation 'defines' congenital heart surgery, it is probably closure of a ventricular septal defect (VSD). This procedure is not only one of the most common congenital heart operations performed, but it is an integral part of many other complex procedures (e.g. tetralogy of Fallot, truncus arteriosus, Rastelli procedure). Hence, understanding the anatomy and pathophysiology of VSDs along with the techniques of VSD closure is an integral and essential part of any congenital heart surgeon's repertoire.

HISTORY

The pathological finding of a VSD was first described by Roger in 1879. Eisenmenger in 1897 described the autopsy findings of a 32-year-old cyanotic patient with a large VSD and overriding aorta. The first surgical intervention for VSD occurred in 1952, when Muller and Dammann performed a pulmonary artery band to limit the pulmonary artery blood flow in a patient with a large VSD. The first intracardiac repair of a VSD was performed in 1954 by C. Walton Lillehei. Lillehei used controlled cross circulation, with the child's parent acting as the pump oxygenator. John Kirklin and associates reported successful transventricular repair of a VSD using a mechanical pump oxygenator in 1956. In 1961, Kirklin reported successful repair of a VSD in infancy, thereby eliminating the need for a pulmonary artery band.

ANATOMY AND NOMENCLATURE

A VSD is defined as an opening or hole in the interventricular septum. Isolated VSDs occur in approximately 2 of every 1 000 live births and constitute over 20 per cent of all congenital heart defects. Because isolated VSD is one of the most commonly recognized forms of congenital heart disease, numerous nomenclature schemes have been used to describe and classify this lesion. This text attempts to unify the concept of VSD anatomy using the classification scheme advocated by

Robert Anderson. This classification divides VSDs into three main types: perimembranous defects that are bordered directly by the fibrous continuity between the atrioventricular (AV) valves and an arterial valve, muscular defects that are completely embedded in the septal musculature, and doubly committed juxta-arterial defects that are bordered directly by the fibrous continuity of the leaflets of the aortic and pulmonary valves (Table 47.1).

Table 47.1 *Anatomy and nomenclature of ventricular septal defect*

Doubly committed juxta-arterial (subarterial, supra-cristal, conal)
Perimembranous (paramembranous, conoventricular)
    Outlet
    Trabecular
    Inlet
Muscular
    Outlet
    Trabecular
    Inlet

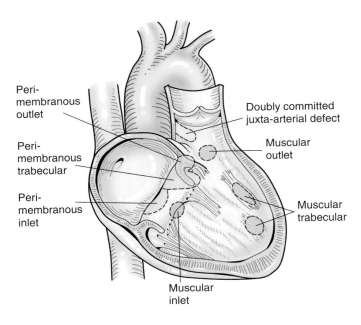

1

1 Perimembranous and muscular defects have been subdivided into three subgroups based on whether they open mainly into the inlet, trabecular, or outlet portion of the right ventricle. The anatomy of the VSD is quite important, as the indications for VSD closure vary significantly depending on the anatomical location of the VSD.

Perimembranous defects are the most common and account for 80 per cent of all defects. Muscular and doubly committed juxta-arterial defects are equally split in most surgical series at 10 per cent each.

INDICATIONS FOR VENTRICULAR SEPTAL DEFECT CLOSURE

With steadily improving results of VSD closure secondary to improvements in cardiopulmonary bypass techniques, myocardial protection, and postoperative intensive care unit management, the indications for VSD closure have been expanded, and the age of the patients at the time of correction has steadily decreased. In general, the indications for VSD closure are based on a comparison between the natural history of VSD and the results of surgical intervention. For the individual patient, the four main considerations are: the anatomy of the defect, the child's age and symptoms, the pulmonary vascular resistance, and associated intracardiac anomalies. Our general indications for VSD closure are shown in Table 47.2. Infants with a large VSD present with a loud systolic murmur and symptoms of congestive heart fail-

Table 47.2 *Indications for ventricular septal defect closure*

Nonrestrictive ventricular septal defect with congestive heart failure and pulmonary hypertension
Restrictive ventricular septal defect with Qp/Qs >1.5:1.0
Aortic valve prolapse or aortic valve insufficiency
All doubly committed juxta-arterial defects
Prior episode of bacterial endocarditis

ure. These symptoms include sweating with feeds, failure to thrive, and frequent upper respiratory tract infections. Older children with a smaller VSD usually present with a harsh pansystolic murmur. They may be otherwise asymptomatic. The diagnostic evaluation of a child with a VSD includes chest x-ray, electrocardiogram, two-dimensional color Doppler echocardiogram, and, in select cases, cardiac catheterization.

Chest x-ray helps to reveal the size of the cardiac silhouette. Patients with large VSDs have cardiomegaly and evidence of increased pulmonary blood flow. The electrocardiogram shows right and left ventricular hypertrophy if there is a large VSD. The two-dimensional color Doppler echocardiogram is diagnostic in most cases. The echocardiogram demonstrates the location of the VSD, the size of the VSD, and, by Doppler evaluation of tricuspid valve regurgitation, gives an assessment of right ventricular pressure. Cardiac catheterization was historically performed for all patients with a VSD, but in the past 10 years it has become less frequently used due to the increasing diagnostic accuracy of echocardiography. However, cardiac catheterization remains the only way to determine the precise degree of left-to-right shunt (Qp/Qs) and the exact pulmonary artery pressures in borderline cases. Cineangiography at the time of cardiac catheterization gives an anatomical 'picture' of the defect.

The size of the VSD and the pulmonary vascular resistance determine the magnitude of intracardiac left-to-right shunting. At birth, the pulmonary vascular resistance is predictably high and blunts the potential left-to-right shunt. Within weeks to months after birth, the pulmonary vascular resistance falls, resulting in increasing left-to-right shunt that results in progressive manifestations of congestive heart failure as described previously. If the patient has a large nonrestrictive VSD, defined as a VSD the same size or larger than the aortic valve annulus, right ventricular and pulmonary artery pressures may be systemic. In these patients, the VSD should be closed at 3–6 months of age to prevent the development of pulmonary vascular obstructive disease. Patients with this unrestricted pulmonary blood flow may develop irreversible pulmonary vascular obstructive disease by 1–2 years of age. This is referred to as *Eisenmenger's syndrome*. These patients have a progressive elevation of pulmonary vascular resistance that eventually leads to the shunt changing from a left-to-right shunt to a right-to-left shunt, with resultant cyanosis and eventual right ventricular failure. Closure of a VSD when the pulmonary vascular resistance has progressed to a point at which it is not reversible results in right ventricular failure and death after VSD closure.

A restrictive VSD is one that is smaller than the aortic valve annulus. In these patients, right ventricular and pulmonary artery pressures are less than systemic. These patients may be managed medically in infancy unless they meet other surgical criteria. Spontaneous closure is observed in nearly 80 per cent of all small muscular and perimembranous VSDs. The mechanisms of spontaneous closure include fibrosis of the defect margins, muscle bundle hypertrophy, and tricuspid valve pouch adherence to the defect. The incidence of spontaneous closure is highest in the first year of life and continues to a lesser degree until approximately 5 years of age, after which spontaneous closure is rare. For patients with a restrictive VSD not affecting the aortic valve, closure should be performed after 4 years of age if they continue to have a harsh IV/VI murmur, or if the Qp/Qs by cardiac catheterization is greater than 1.5:1.0.

Patients with perimembranous and doubly committed juxta-arterial VSDs may develop aortic valve prolapse as the cusps of the aortic valve sag into the VSD. Left unrepaired, aortic valve prolapse may lead to progressive valve insufficiency. If the VSD is closed when the patient has only aortic valve prolapse or mild aortic insufficiency, the aortic valve disease does not progress. If the aortic insufficiency is mild to moderate at the time of VSD closure, consideration should be given to resuspending the aortic valve at the time of VSD closure. All patients with aortic valve prolapse or aortic valve insufficiency associated with the VSD should undergo VSD closure. Doubly committed juxta-arterial VSDs are located in the conal septum and are immediately beneath the aortic and pulmonary valves. These patients have a very high incidence of aortic valve prolapse leading to aortic valve insufficiency. These VSDs should be closed, even if they are very small, because of the high incidence of aortic valve prolapse leading to aortic valve regurgitation.

For children with a VSD, the incidence of bacterial endocarditis is 14.5 per 10 000 patient years. This incidence is 35 times the normal population–base rate for bacterial endocarditis. Surgical closure reduces the risk of subacute bacterial endocarditis (SBE) by over 50 per cent. Prevention of SBE is a consideration for VSD closure in borderline cases. All patients with a VSD who have had a prior episode of SBE should have surgical closure of their VSD.

OPERATION

The operative approach to VSDs has evolved considerably over the past several decades. The current technique of VSD closure emphasizes an approach that is either transatrial or transpulmonary, hence avoiding a ventriculotomy in nearly all cases. Several general principles of VSD closure which apply to nearly all VSDs will be covered first. Each individual anatomical subtype of VSD has technical points related specifically to that diagnosis and each will be covered separately.

General principles

The general principles of surgical VSD closure are summarized in Table 47.3. VSD closure is performed using cardiopulmonary bypass and hypothermia. Most VSDs can be successfully closed without the use of circulatory arrest, although this technique has been useful for some subgroups, such as VSD with interrupted aortic arch and small premature babies less than 2 or 3 kg in size. Bicaval venous cannulation allows cardiopulmonary bypass to continue during VSD closure and avoids the possible complications of circulatory arrest. Aortic cross-clamp with cold blood cardioplegia administration allows VSD closure to be performed in a quiet field. A vent in the right superior pulmonary vein makes for a bloodless field by suctioning blood from the left atrium and left ventricle. The operative approach varies according to the type of VSD. Perimembranous VSDs are usually repaired through a right atrial approach. Doubly committed juxta-arterial defects are approached through the pulmonary artery. Muscular VSDs are usually approached through the right atrium, although they may also be approached through the pulmonary artery or through a limited right or left ventriculotomy. Some perimembranous and subarterial VSDs, particularly those with significant associated aortic valve insufficiency, may be best approached through the aorta and the aortic valve. These different approaches are illustrated in Table 47.4.

Table 47.3 *General principles of ventricular septal defect closure*

Aortic and bicaval venous cannulation
Cardiopulmonary bypass
Hypothermia (28°–32°C)
Vent
Right superior pulmonary vein or left atrial appendage
Aortic cross-clamp
Cardioplegia

Table 47.4 *Approaches for ventricular septal defect closure*

Type of defect	Approach
Perimembranous	Right atrium
Doubly committed juxta-arterial	Pulmonary artery, aorta, right ventricle
Muscular	Right atrium, right ventricle, left ventricle
Inlet	Right atrium

Specific technique based on anatomy of ventricular septal defect

PERIMEMBRANOUS

Essentially all perimembranous VSDs are approached through the right atrium.

2a, b A 'medial' atriotomy provides the optimal exposure of the tricuspid valve orifice, especially for closure of VSDs that extend into the outlet septum. This atriotomy begins at the base of the right atrial appendage and extends parallel to the right coronary artery, staying at least 1 cm away from the right coronary artery. The incision extends between the right coronary artery and the inferior vena cava cannula and concludes adjacent to the coronary sinus. Stay sutures placed on the edges of the atriotomy are used to hold open the right atrium and expose the tricuspid valve orifice.

The perimembranous VSD is identified by retracting the septal and anterior leaflets of the tricuspid valve. One clue to the location of the VSD is a portion of the tricuspid valve that is pulled into the defect by the suction of the vent. Another clue to the location of the VSD is fibrotic hemodynamic changes in the right ventricular muscle adjacent to the VSD orifice.

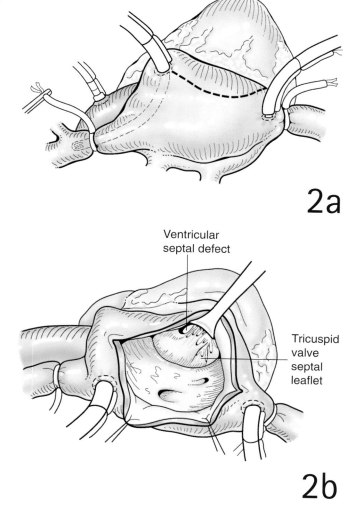

2a

Ventricular septal defect

Tricuspid valve septal leaflet

2b

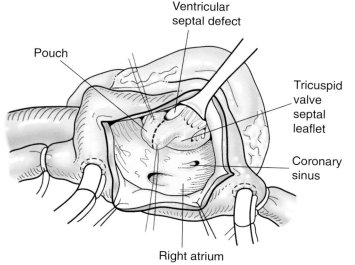

Pouch

Ventricular septal defect

Tricuspid valve septal leaflet

Coronary sinus

Right atrium

3

3 In some instances, the VSD perimeter cannot be completely identified because of the overlying tricuspid valve tissue. This situation is called a *tricuspid valve pouch*.

4 In the case of a tricuspid valve pouch, opening the tricuspid valve in a radial fashion from the leading edge of the septal leaflet to the tricuspid valve annulus is advantageous. Doing so allows exposure of the entire perimeter of the VSD, although not necessarily all at one time – only a portion of the VSD perimeter needs to be visualized at any one time. Fine stay sutures placed at the leading edge of the tricuspid valve before opening the leaflet assist in precisely repairing the tricuspid valve after VSD closure. The next step is to inspect the VSD and, in particular, examine it for the location of the aortic valve leaflets. The aortic valve leaflets may prolapse into the defect and must be avoided during suture placement.

The technique of VSD closure that we have used at Children's Memorial Hospital for over 40 years is to encircle the perimeter of the VSD with multiple, interrupted, pledget-based Dacron sutures. The sutures are then sequentially placed through an appropriately sized patch, the patch is lowered into the defect, and the sutures are tied and cut. The suture placement for a perimembranous VSD must avoid the area of the AV node and the conducting system.

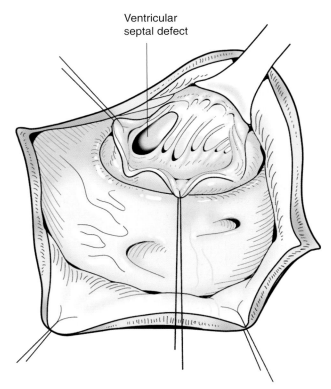

Ventricular septal defect

4

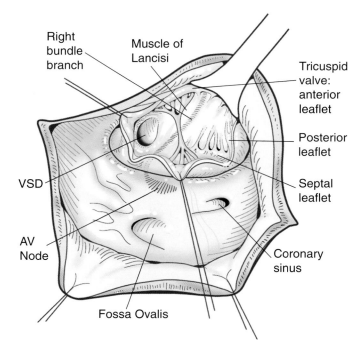

Right bundle branch

Muscle of Lancisi

Tricuspid valve: anterior leaflet

Posterior leaflet

VSD

Septal leaflet

AV Node

Coronary sinus

Fossa Ovalis

5

5 The location of the AV node is shown.
To avoid injury to the conducting system, the sutures should be placed superficially and carefully along the inferior and posterior margins of the defect and stay on the right ventricular side of the VSD. This closure begins from the area of the insertion of the muscle of Lancisi (medial papillary muscle of the conus) to the annulus of the tricuspid valve near the region of the apex of the triangle of Koch. The borders of the triangle of Koch are the tricuspid valve annulus, the orifice of the coronary sinus, and the tendon of Todaro. In some cases, the sutures are passed from the right atrial side of the tricuspid valve annulus, through the annulus itself, into the right ventricular side. Care must be taken when placing these sutures to avoid the aortic valve cusp, which is just on the other side of the tricuspid valve annulus. Once all of the pledgetted sutures have been placed around the perimeter of the VSD, a Dacron or Gore-Tex patch is cut to the appropriate size. The size of the patch is usually approximately 1.5 times the size of the actual hole in the septum. This size allows a space for the pledgetted sutures to be placed with a 2–3 mm rim of patch between the suture placement and the edge of the patch.

6 The sutures going through the patch are shown. After all of the sutures have been passed sequentially through the patch, the patch is lowered into the defect, and care is taken to make sure that all of the loops of the sutures are pulled up. Then, all of the sutures are tied.

The selection of Dacron versus Gore-Tex for the VSD patch is the individual surgeon's preference. The Dacron patch is somewhat more forgiving and elastic than the Gore-Tex patch. The Dacron patch is incorporated by the fibrous reaction of the body to the patch, and any small residual needle holes or small residual defects at the perimeter of the patch often close because of this fibrotic reaction. When the Dacron patch is looked at years after the patch placement, it is completely covered with endothelium. The Gore-Tex patch has the advantage that it may be cut more precisely, and needle holes may be placed closer to the edge without tearing through. However, Gore-Tex does not incite as much of a tissue reaction as does the Dacron patch. We commonly use Dacron for perimembranous defects and are more apt to use Gore-Tex for doubly committed juxta-arterial defects when aortic valve insufficiency might be striking the patch. An aortic insufficiency jet striking a Dacron patch may lead to unremitting hemolysis.

After the patch has been anchored by tying all the pledgeted sutures, the tricuspid valve is repaired. This repair is facilitated by the stay sutures placed at the leading edge of the tricuspid valve before dividing the tricuspid valve.

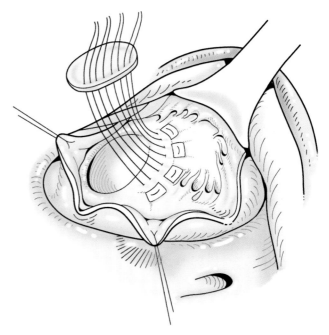

6

7 The repair of the tricuspid valve is accomplished with multiple interrupted fine sutures (usually 6/0 Prolene). When the tricuspid valve repair is completed, the right ventricle can be irrigated with a large bulb syringe filled with cold saline. This maneuver gives the surgeon an idea of whether significant tricuspid valve regurgitation has been caused by the tricuspid valve repair. This issue can then be addressed further as needed. The completion of the VSD closure is accomplished by closing the atrium. This step is accomplished with two layers of running Prolene suture, the first layer placed as a mattress suture. The heart is deaired by turning the sump off and allowing the bronchial collateral circulation to fill the left atrium with blood. Air is evacuated from the right side of the heart by temporarily occluding the inferior vena cava (IVC) cannula, releasing the IVC tourniquet, and evacuating air through the right atrial suture line. The cardioplegia needle, which is at the high point of the left side, is then aspirated with a syringe, evacuating air from the left side of the heart. Once the heart is fully deaired, then the aortic cross-clamp is removed. As soon as the cross-clamp is removed, the sump is restarted to aspirate any residual air that might come up from the pulmonary veins during the rewarming and ventilating process. In addition, the cardioplegia needle in the ascending aorta can be converted to a vent to the bypass circuit to capture any other air bubbles that might go out the aorta. The patient is rewarmed and typically will resume a spontaneous normal sinus rhythm. If not, the heart is defibrillated (1 J/kg). The patient is ventilated; and after being ventilated and having good cardiac action, the vent is removed. This step is done during a Valsalva maneuver to increase the pressure in the left atrium and prevent aspiration of air through the vent site. The patient is then weaned from cardiopulmonary bypass.

We have used intraoperative transesophageal echocardiography (TEE) for most VSD closures since 1992. TEE is used to confirm the preoperative diagnosis and to assure the integrity of the repair after the closure by evaluating for residual intracardiac left-to-right shunting. If residual shunting exists, TEE can give the surgeon an idea of where the residual VSD is located and of the magnitude of the residual shunting. TEE can also demonstrate significant postoperative tricuspid valve insufficiency if it is present. Transesophageal echocardiography is especially useful in those cases where aortic valve insufficiency is repaired, to assess the degree of aortic insufficiency pre- and postoperatively.

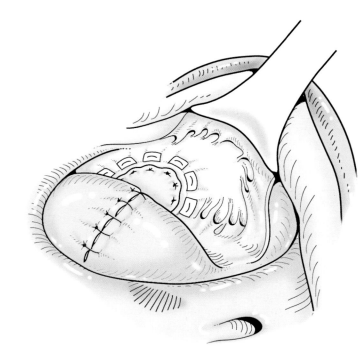

7

DOUBLY COMMITTED JUXTA-ARTERIAL (SUBARTERIAL, SUPRA-CRISTAL, CONAL) VENTRICULAR SEPTAL DEFECTS

Doubly committed juxta-arterial VSDs account for 5–10 per cent of all VSDs closed surgically in Western countries. In reviews from Asian countries, doubly committed juxta-arterial VSDs are more frequent, representing approximately 30 per cent of VSD closures. All patients with a doubly committed juxta-arterial VSD should undergo closure, because of the high risk of development of aortic valve prolapse followed by aortic valve insufficiency.

8 The approach to these defects is through the main pulmonary artery and then the pulmonary valve. Cardiopulmonary bypass maneuvers are the same as for perimembranous VSD. However, after cardioplegia has been administered, the exposure of the defect is accomplished through a vertical incision in the pulmonary artery. This incision typically extends from the main pulmonary artery into the sinus of the pulmonary valve, anteriorly and to the patient's right. Retraction of the pulmonary artery opening is accomplished with stay sutures. Small vein retractors are used to gently retract the pulmonary valve and demonstrate the doubly committed juxta-arterial VSD.

Pledgetted sutures are placed circumferentially around the perimeter of the VSD. A critical part of the closure involves placing sutures directly in the base of the pulmonary valve cusps as an anchoring point where no muscular septum separates the aortic and pulmonary valves. These steps are illustrated in Figures 9 and 10.

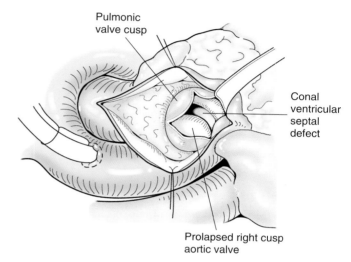

Pulmonic valve cusp

Conal ventricular septal defect

Prolapsed right cusp aortic valve

8

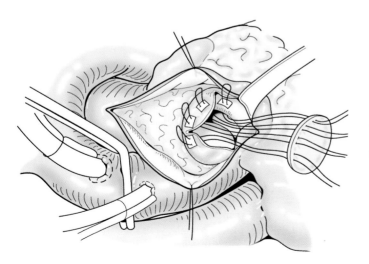

9 The location of the pledgeted sutures not only in the top of the muscular septum, but also in the base of the pulmonary valve cusp, is shown.

9

10 The lateral projection of the superior portion of the defect, showing pledgetted sutures passing through the base of the pulmonary valve cusp and the relationship to the aortic valve cusp, is shown.

These sutures must be very carefully placed to avoid injuring the aortic valve or the pulmonary valve. Once the sutures are placed around the perimeter of the ventricular septal defect, they are passed through the patch, which is then lowered into the defect and all of the sutures are tied.

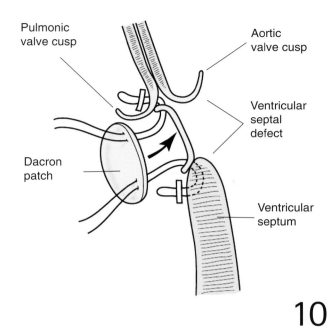

10

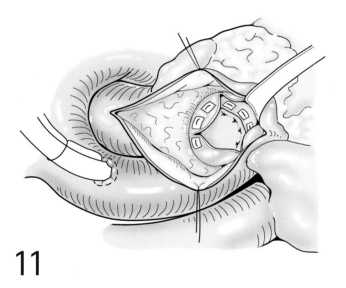

11

11 The completed patch closure is shown.

After the VSD is closed, the opening in the pulmonary artery is closed with a running Prolene suture. The left and right sides of the heart are deaired as for a perimembranous VSD before removing the aortic cross-clamp.

RIGHT VENTRICULAR APPROACH

An alternative approach for the patient with a doubly committed juxta-arterial VSD is through the infundibulum of the right ventricle. Of note, some of these patients have an associated right ventricular outflow tract stenosis that requires resection. Some surgeons have felt that the approach through the infundibulum facilitates the excision of infundibular stenosis and the exposure for the VSD closure. However, we have preferred to avoid a ventriculo-tomy and have not used it since the early 1980s. Two types of right ventriculotomy incisions are possible, transverse and vertical. The transverse incision may have the advantage of limiting injury to the circular muscular fibers. However, exposure through this approach may be restricted. This approach is also usually inadequate when enlargement of the infundibulum with a patch is required.

12 If a vertical incision is used, it should be limited to the infundibular area.

Examining the coronary artery distribution before beginning any ventriculotomy is important. If a left anterior descending coronary artery originates from the right coronary artery, ventriculotomy is dangerous and should be avoided because of the possible injury to the distribution of the left anterior descending coronary artery. Infrequently, these arteries, as they cross the infundibulum, are intramyocardial and may not be seen on the myocardial surface. The preoperative aortic angiogram location of the coronary arteries should be evaluated. Alternatively, an echocardiogram can also show the location of the coronary arteries.

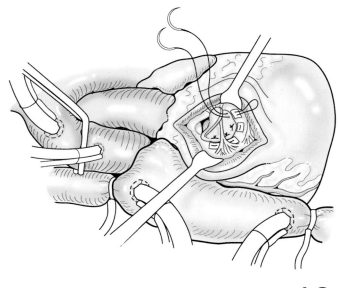

12

TRANSAORTIC APPROACH

If the patient has associated aortic valve insufficiency, he or she may require a simultaneous aortic valve suspension. Vertical suspension in patients such as these was initially described in great detail by Dr. George Trusler from Toronto. In our series of conal VSD patients, four patients required aortic valve suspension. In three of these patients, the VSD was closed through an aortotomy rather than through the pulmonary artery. This approach was because the primary indication for the procedure was the aortic valve insufficiency.

13 After cardioplegia, an obliquely curved incision is made, starting on the anterior aspect of the ascending aorta curving down into the noncoronary sinus. This incision may be extended as needed transversely toward the left. The aortic valve leaflets are retracted carefully to expose the defect. Often, a superior muscular or fibrous rim of the defect is absent, making suture placement somewhat difficult. In this situation, sutures may be passed through the aortic wall from the inside of the aortic valve sinus in a fashion analogous to the placement of suture through the base of the pulmonary valve cusp, as described previously. However, we do not always use pledgets on the aortic side to prevent adhesions at the base of the aortic valve cusp with resultant aortic insufficiency. The transaortic approach to a VSD is illustrated in this figure.

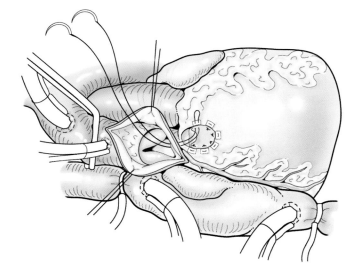

13

MUSCULAR VENTRICULAR SEPTAL DEFECTS

The operative approach to muscular VSDs is not as straight-forward as that for perimembranous and doubly committed juxta-arterial defects. Muscular defects are often multiple and are technically often difficult to reach. Historically, these lesions (especially when multiple) were managed by first placing a pulmonary artery band, and then later (in 6 months to 1 year) removing the band and closing the defects when the patient was older and larger. More recently, a distinct trend toward repairing muscular defects in infancy has evolved, even if they are multiple. In one series reviewing 130 patients with multiple VSDs operated on between 1980 and 1991, 32 per cent had a preliminary pulmonary artery band. The perimembranous septum was involved in 102 patients, the muscular septum in 121 patients, and the conal septum in 9 patients. Fifty patients had the 'Swiss cheese' form of lesion. In that same experience, right atriotomy was used in 82 patients (63 per cent), right ventriculotomy in 32 patients (24 per cent), and left ventriculotomy in 14 patients (10 per cent). Left ventriculotomy was only used in low apical muscular VSDs. That series used the same technique for closure that we have used at Children's Memorial Hospital – interrupted pledget-based mattress sutures and an elastic Dacron patch. The division of trabeculations within the body of the right ventricle facilitates the exposure and, hence, accurate closure of muscular VSDs. In particular, the moderator band can be divided in cases of midtrabecular muscular VSDs. However, doing so causes right bundle branch block. These trabeculations become hypertrophied with a pulmonary artery band and hence more and more surgeons are electing to repair these lesions in infancy rather than placing a pulmonary artery band first. An alternative approach to these defects (apical muscular) is the use of catheterization-delivered devices.

LEFT VENTRICULAR APPROACH

Use of this operative exposure is limited to certain muscular VSDs, particularly those with multiple apical perforations ('Swiss cheese'). These defects may be easier to patch on the left ventricular side because of the relatively smooth septum, lack of heavy trabeculations, and single orifice, as compared to multiple orifices on the right ventricular side.

14 The ventricular incision is usually a vertical one starting in a relatively avascular left ventricular apical area with limited extension. The coronary artery distribution must be carefully analyzed to minimize injury to the coronary arteries. Left ventricular incisions, however, may be associated with significant long-term ventricular dysfunction and should be avoided whenever possible, except for small apical incisions that are probably well tolerated.

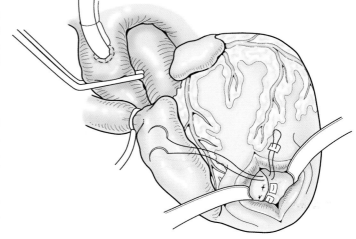

14

ALTERNATIVE TECHNIQUES

Although our experience at Children's Memorial Hospital has been using pledgeted interrupted sutures for the majority of VSDs, there are certain exceptions to this practice. For very tiny infants, (i.e. less than 3 kg), the VSD is often surrounded by relatively friable neonatal muscle. Placement of sutures with pledgets and then tying all of the sutures separately may actually increase the chances of the sutures pulling through the delicate neonatal myocardium. In this circumstance, we have used a running suture technique using 6/0 Prolene suture.

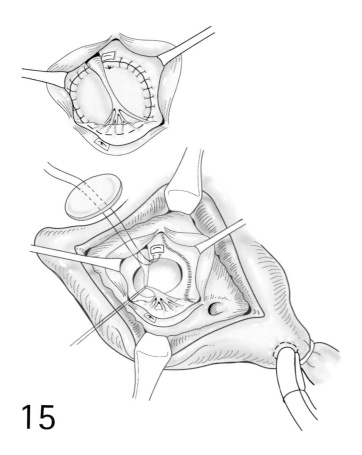

15 The suture is anchored with a pericardial pledget, and we then use a pericardial patch fixed in glutaraldehyde for the VSD closure. The pericardial pledget is passed through the portion of the VSD that is furthest away from the surgeon. The suture is passed through the tanned pericardium and then tied. The two remaining ends of the sutures are then used in a running fashion, one superiorly and one inferiorly, and the pericardial patch is sutured to the edge of the VSD. The suture is then completed on the tricuspid valve annulus, and the knot is tied outside of the tricuspid valve. Again, we have found this procedure most useful for neonates with friable myocardium.

Our reasoning for using the interrupted pledgeted technique has been to minimize the incidence of residual VSD. However, some centers use a running suture technique for essentially all VSDs. Some surgeons have recommended using a strip of pericardium as the pledget to reinforce a portion of the VSD repair.

15

POSTOPERATIVE CARE

The postoperative care of the patient with a VSD is dictated by the age of the patient and the size and morphology of the VSD. Infants with large VSDs have the potential to develop pulmonary hypertensive crisis and are treated differently than older children with VSDs, who are often extubated in the operating room. A wide spectrum of potential postoperative strategies exists between these two extremes. For the small infant with a large nonrestrictive VSD, we keep the patient paralyzed and ventilated for the first 12–24 hours postoperatively. These patients are also treated expectantly with pulmonary vasodilators, afterload reduction, and inotropic support. This treatment typically includes low doses of dopamine and dobutamine (2.5–5 mcg/kg/minute) and intravenous milrinone (0.5 mcg/kg/minute). These patients are also kept on Versed and morphine drips, along with a Pavulon drip for the first 12–24 hours. We then stop the Pavulon infusion; and if the child does not have pulmonary hypertensive crisis, we wean the sedation and the ventilation and extubate the child at 48–72 hours after the procedure. If the child shows evidence of pulmonary hypertensive crisis (arterial desaturation, hypotension), we reinstate his or her paralysis. If he or she has evidence of pulmonary hypertensive crisis despite paralysis and ventilation, then we add nitric oxide therapy (20 parts per million inhaled through the endotracheal tube). In the current era, in which most babies with large VSDs undergo a prompt operative repair within the first several months of life, pulmonary hypertensive crises are really quite rare. This problem was more common when children were allowed to go to an age of 1–2 years (or older) before closure of large VSDs. Most patients with a nonrestrictive VSD will have been on digoxin, Lasix, and captopril before the surgery. We discontinue their digoxin and captopril, but we do keep them on Lasix for several weeks after the procedure. Usually 4–6 weeks after the operation, they are off of all medications. For the older child with a restrictive VSD who is being repaired for indications of aortic valve prolapse or aortic valve insufficiency, he or she often is weaned off cardiopulmonary bypass without any inotropic support. These patients are frequently extubated in the operating room and are monitored in the intensive care unit for only 12–24 hours after the procedure. They then recover on the regular ward (1–2 days) and are usually discharged without any medications.

OUTCOME

At Children's Memorial Hospital between 1980 and 1992, 417 patients had closure of a VSD – perimembranous (327), doubly committed juxta-arterial (44), and muscular (46). Four deaths (0.9 per cent) occurred, three patients had heart block and required a pacemaker (0.7 per cent), five patients required reoperation while in the intensive care unit (1.2 per cent), and four patients had a significant residual VSD (1 per cent). The four deaths were all related to pulmonary hypertension and occurred in patients who were 1 month, 6 months, 8 months, and 11 years old, all with nonrestrictive VSDs and systemic pulmonary artery pressures preoperatively. Between 1980 and 1989, 36 children with a doubly committed juxta-arterial VSD underwent intracardiac repair at Children's Memorial Hospital. The mean age was 5 years. No mortality occurred, and no patient had heart block. In patients undergoing 'elective' VSD closure (i.e. patients over 1 year of age with a pulmonary-to-systemic flow ratio less than 2), almost no complications occurred. Between 1980 and 1991, 141 patients at Children's Memorial Hospital had closure of a restrictive VSD at an age of older than 1 year. The mean pulmonary artery pressure was 26 mm Hg, and the mean pulmonary-to-systemic flow ratio was 1.6:1.0. Aortic valve prolapse was present in 45 per cent of patients, aortic valve insufficiency in 18 per cent of the patients, and 3.5 per cent of the patients had prior bacterial endocarditis. No early or late deaths and no major morbidity occurred. No patient required a ventriculotomy to accomplish VSD closure. The mean intensive care unit stay was 1 day, and the mean hospital stay was 5 days. No instances of permanent complete AV dissociation occurred. No reoperations were performed for bleeding, and no patient developed postoperative wound infection. In addition, no reoperations were required for residual or recurrent VSDs. This review (published in 1993) led us to call for a re-evaluation of historical indications for VSD closure. The surgical risk of VSD closure (as defined by this experience), when compared with the known natural history studies, is less than the lifetime risks of developing bacterial endocarditis or progressive aortic valve prolapse leading to aortic valve insufficiency. VSD closure also removes the socioeconomic stigma associated with living with an uncorrected cardiac defect (which is not insignificant).

Special consideration: heart block

If in the operating room after full rewarming the patient is not in sinus rhythm, temporary wires should be placed on the surface of the right ventricle. These temporary wires can be used to pace the ventricle safely to wean the child from cardiopulmonary bypass. Many times, as the child recovers from the cardioplegia or is started on inotropic support, the heart block resolves. However, if the heart block does not resolve, we recommend using the temporary wires to pace the child and then recommend observing the child for a period of 7–10 days. We have not urgently reoperated to revise the patch. During the period of observation many children resume sinus rhythm. Should this situation occur, we then perform a 24-hour Holter monitor to establish the resolution of heart block and resumption of sinus rhythm before discharging the patient. However, after 7 days, the chances of the child resuming normal sinus rhythm become remote, and at this point (somewhere between 7 and 10 days), we recommend placement of a dual-chamber pacing system. Currently, we recommend placement of steroid-eluting epicardial leads and dual-chamber pacing. This placement is performed in an epicardial fashion for the majority of patients who have VSD closure, as these patients are usually less than 1–2 years of age. For the occasional older child who has heart block after VSD closure, we recommend placement of a dual-chamber transvenous pacing system.

Residual ventricular septal defect

If a residual VSD is suspected in the operating room either because of a thrill palpable on the anterior surface of the right ventricle or a color jet seen on the TEE, several considerations exist. The TEE can estimate the size of the color Doppler jet (i.e. tiny, mild residual, moderate residual, or severe residual). The surgeon should consider a re-exploration for moderate or severe residual defects. If TEE is not available, or in cases that are not easily classified, one can measure the intracardiac shunt in the operating room and use this information to decide whether to re-explore. Two separate syringes with fine needles are used to aspirate blood from the right atrium and the pulmonary artery. The oxygen saturation of the blood in the right atrium versus that in the pulmonary artery, along with the known aortic saturation (usually 100 per cent), can then be used to calculate the shunt (Qp/Qs), using the following formula:

$$\frac{AoSat - PASat}{AoSat - RASat} = \frac{Qp}{Qs}$$

where $AoSat$ = oxygen saturation in aorta, $PASat$ = oxygen saturation in pulmonary artery, and $RASat$ = oxygen saturation in right atrium.

Unless the residual shunt is more than 2 to 1, the residual defect will probably close over time.

SUMMARY

Anatomically, the three main types of VSD are perimembranous (80 per cent), doubly committed juxta-arterial (10 per cent) and muscular (10 per cent). Indications for VSD closure include congestive heart failure, Qp/Qs greater than 1.5:1.0, aortic valve prolapse, aortic valve insufficiency, all doubly committed juxta-arterial defects, and prior episode of SBE. The results of operative closure of VSDs in the current era are extremely good. The risk of death for all patients, including those with severe pulmonary hypertension, is less than 1 per cent. For elective patients over 1 year of age, the risk of death approaches zero. The risk of major morbidity, such as heart block, emergent reoperation, or significant residual VSD, is approximately 1 per cent each. For elective patients over 1 year of age, the risk of major morbidity approaches zero. The great majority of patients who have VSD closure have an excellent outcome, and the long-term prognosis for these patients is very close to that of a normal child.

FURTHER READING

Backer, C.L., Idriss, F.S., Zales, V.R, et al. 1991. Surgical management of the conal (supracristal) ventricular septal defect. *Journal of Thoracic and Cardiovascular Surgery* 102, 288–96.

Backer, C.L., Winters, R.C., Zales, V.R., et al. 1993. Restrictive ventricular septal defect: how small is too small to close? *Annals of Thoracic Surgery* 56, 1014–19.

Gersony, W.M., Hayes, C.J., Driscoll, D.J., et al. 1993. Bacterial endocarditis in patients with aortic stenosis, pulmonary stenosis, or ventricular septal defect. *Circulation* 87[Suppl I], I-121–6.

Jacobs, J.P., Burke, R.P., Quintessenza, J.A., Mavroudis, C. 2000. Congenital heart surgery nomenclature and database project: ventricular septal defect. *Annals of Thoracic Surgery* 69[Suppl I], S25–35.

Serraf, A., Lacour-Gayet, F., Bruniaux, J., et al. 1992. Surgical management of isolated multiple ventricular septal defects. *Journal of Thoracic and Cardiovascular Surgery* 103, 437–43.

Trusler, G.A., Williams, W.G., Smallhorn, J.F., Freedom, R.M. 1992. Late results with repair of aortic insufficiency associated with ventricular septal defect. *Journal of Thoracic and Cardiovascular Surgery* 103, 276–81.

48

Tetralogy of Fallot

TOM R. KARL MD, MS
Director of Cardiothoracic Surgery and Professor of Surgery, University of California, San Francisco, School of Medicine; Professor of Pediatric Cardiothoracic Surgery, UCSF Medical Center, San Francisco, California, USA

CHRISTIAN P.R. BRIZARD MD
Cardiac Surgical Unit, Royal Children's Hospital, Melbourne, Australia

HISTORY

Tetralogy of Fallot (TOF), one of the most frequently encountered surgical lessons, is an important entity for the cardiac surgeon. TOF was the first cyanotic lesson to be formally described, and some of the initial palliative and definitive operations for congenital heart disease were performed for treatment of TOF. Probably more is known about TOF than about any other complex cardiac abnormality, and consequently, this lesson has served as a model for the natural history of cyanotic congenital heart disease and our ability to alter that history with surgery. Our understanding of cardiac physiology, myocardial protection, cardiopulmonary bypass (CPB), molecular biology, and other areas has been enhanced by the study of TOF. Finally, TOF is a fatal lesson without treatment, but one that now has a quite favorable natural history after an appropriate surgical strategy.

The first operations for TOF were performed by Blalock and associates at Johns Hopkins Medical Center in 1948. The Blalock strategy was to divert blood from the systemic circulation to the pulmonary circulation to neutralize the effect of right-to-left shunting within the heart. A more direct approach to TOF was first used by Lillehei and associates at the University of Minnesota in 1954. Open correction of TOF was performed by this group using cross circulation between the child and a support patient, and later using a bubble oxygenator and CPB. Although numerous strategic and technical modifications have been introduced since these initial efforts, Lillehei's work set the standard for the modern surgical approach to TOF.

The anatomical features of TOF are described in detail in Chapter 38 in this book by Anderson, whose general approach to congenital heart disease and its nomenclature has improved our surgical understanding significantly. The basic features relevant to the surgical repair of tetralogy are shown in Figure 1.

1 **Anatomical features of tetralogy of Fallot**   Anterior and
cephalad displacement of the infundibular (muscular
outlet) septum results in malalignment ventricular septal
defect (VSD), right ventricular outflow tract obstruction
(RVOTO), and RV hypertrophy. The pulmonary arterial
(PA) tree may show any degree of hypoplasia.

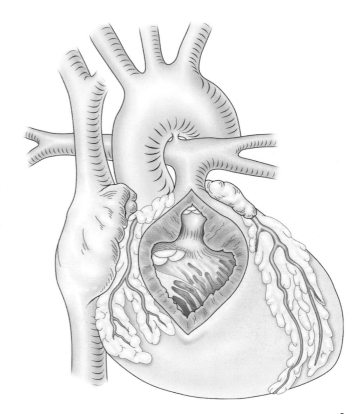

1

PRINCIPLES AND JUSTIFICATION

For most patients with TOF, the diagnosis can be established in the neonatal period. Depending on the anatomy of the RVOT and PAs, as well as the degree of collateral circulation and other factors, a plan for timing and strategy can be developed (Figure 2).

2a–d Imaging in tetralogy of Fallot (clockwise): 2-D echocardiograms demonstrating aortic override of the large VSD, RV hypertrophy, and malalignment of ventricular septal segments that generates the VSD and override of approximately 50 per cent; hypoplasia of PA tree with severe RVOTO demonstrated by right ventriculogram; cardiac gated T-1 weighted spin echo (magnetic resonance imaging) showing confluent branch PAs with a severe stenosis just proximal to the LPA bifurcation. Pulmonary stenosis and aortic enlargement are also shown.

Preoperative investigation is based primarily on 2-D echocardiography, which provides information about the RVOT, VSD, the central PA tree, and the proximal coronaries. In some cases, angiography may be required to delineate unusual features. The decision to perform a complete repair is predicated on the presence of an adequate PA tree (i.e. the ability of the pulmonary circulation to accept the full cardiac output after septation, with a subsystemic RV pressure). Many formulas have been proposed to assess this feature, but none is infallible.

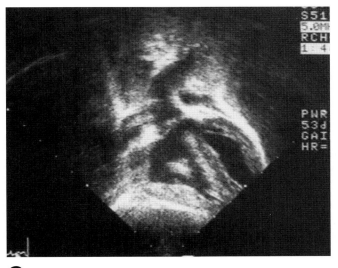

2a

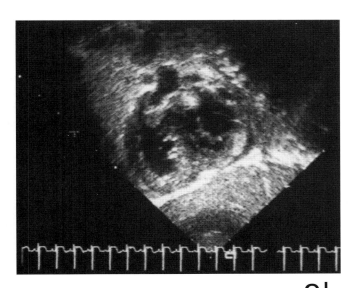

2b

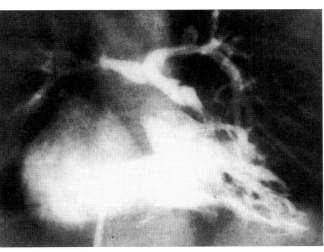

2c

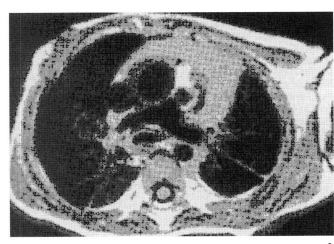

2d

3 Treatment strategy for tetralogy of Fallot In the current era, most cardiac surgical teams elect complete repair whenever possible for the symptomatic patient. Although the strategy of intracardiac repair in totally asymptomatic neonates has little to recommend it, the perceived best age for elective repair in stable patients varies from birth to 1 year of age. The trend worldwide over the past decade has been toward earlier (3–6 months of age) elective repair. Other factors that may influence timing of repair in a given cardiac center include the general medical condition of the baby, prematurity, very low birth weight, possible need for an extracardiac conduit, the presence of additional intracardiac problems, discontinuous PAs, etc. However, in various centers worldwide, good early results have been achieved with diverse timing strategies, involving both one- and two-staged approaches (i.e. complete repair; or modified Blalock-Taussig shunt followed by complete repair, followed by complete repair at an interval).

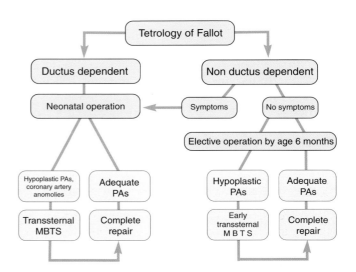

3

OPERATION

Modified Blalock–Taussig shunt

The indication for this procedure is cyanosis of unacceptable degree in a patient believed to be unsuitable for complete repair for one of a variety of reasons (see above). The best approach is via median sternotomy, which can be limited to the upper half of the sternum if desired. Use of the transsternal approach allows continued ventilation during the operation and a more stable hemodynamic situation. The thymus is resected, and the upper pericardium is opened longitudi-

nally. The preferred side for the shunt is the right in all cases, irrespective of arch anatomy (i.e. to right or left of trachea). Performing the shunt at this site facilitates closure at subsequent complete repair. The polytetrafluoroethylene (PTFE) shunt can be easily dissected medially to the superior caval vein, clipped and divided immediately after the commencement of CPB (see below).

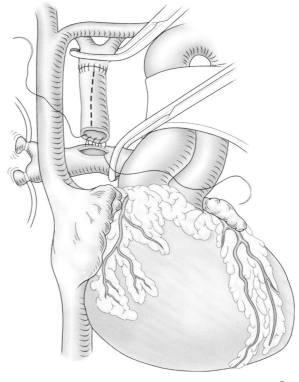

4a, b **Transsternal approach for modified Blalock shunt** The brachiocephalic artery and PA are dissected with electrocautery and isolated within Silastic loops. Heparin is administered systemically (1 mg/kg), and the RPA is controlled with a vascular clamp. A PTFE graft (3.5 or 4.0 mm, for infants under and over 3.5 kg, respectively) is cut on a bevel and anastomosed to the brachiocephalic artery with running polypropylene suture. The clamp is left in place while the distal end of the shunt is sutured to the RPA using either a second clamp or traction on the vessel loops. Excessive length of the shunt may result in a kink, which can lead to early occlusion. Clamps are removed, and the pericardium and sternum are closed over a Silastic drain. Common early postoperative problems include mild metabolic acidosis and unilateral hyperemia on chest x-ray, both usually transient. Chylous or serous effusions may also occur, but the incidence of either may be decreased by limiting the extent of mediastinal dissection and avoiding instrumentation of the shunt, respectively. Postoperatively, patients receive heparin (1 unit/kg/hour) until oral aspirin (5 mg/kg/day) can be started.

4a

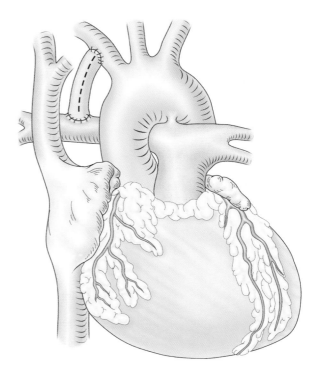

4b

Open correction of tetralogy of Fallot

The goals of complete repair are to provide adequate relief of RVOTO, to septate the heart completely, and to preserve the contractile, electrical, and valvular function as much as possible. The original techniques used for TOF repair were based on the use of a large right ventriculotomy for both VSD closure and relief of RVOTO. An approach using transatrial VSD closure and limited or no ventriculotomy was promoted by Hudspeth, Edmunds, and others. The best strategy available for most patients is the transatrial-transpulmonary repair, described in Figures 5a–e.

5a–e Transatrial-transpulmonary repair of tetralogy of Fallot The operative approach is via full median sternotomy, using a relatively short skin incision. The thymus is resected, and the pericardium is opened to the left of the midline. A suitable pericardial patch adequate for VSD closure and RVOT reconstruction is excised, immersed for 10 minutes in 0.1 per cent glutaraldehyde solution, and rinsed several times in saline. The patient is heparinized (3 mg/kg) and cannulated for CPB via the superior and inferior caval veins and the ascending aorta (at the base of the brachiocephalic artery). The modified Blalock-Taussig shunt, if present, is dissected, clipped, and divided as CPB is commenced. The patient is cooled systemically to 32°C. The arterial ligament (or duct) is dissected and ligated. The aorta is clamped, and crystalloid cardioplegia is delivered into the aortic root. The caval vein snares are tightened around the venous cannulas, and the right atrium (RA) and pulmonary trunk are opened longitudinally. A vent sucker is placed through the oval foramen, which may require enlargement with a scalpel. The pulmonary valve is inspected, and fused commissures are opened right back to the sinotubular junction (Figure 5a). A 3-mm 45° Hegar dilator is passed retrogradely into the RV to facilitate identification and inspection of the RVOT. Exposure is then changed to the transtricuspid valve aspect via the RA. With the anterior leaflet of the tricuspid valve (TV) retracted, the RVOT is exposed. The septoparietal trabeculations of the muscular outlet septum (parietal extension of the infundibular septum) are excised as completely as possible (Figure 5b), taking care to avoid the rim of the VSD and aortic valve leaflets. Additional obstructing muscle bands in the RVOT are mobilized and excised as well, and this exercise may be repeated working through the pulmonary valve. The goal of RVOT resection is to allow free passage of a Hegar dilator that is 2 mm larger than predicted for the normalized pulmonary valve diameter. In approximately 50–75 per cent of cases, a small, transannular extension of the PA incision (10–15 mm) will be required, and this extension should be made through the anterior commissure of the pulmonary valve, extending onto the free wall of the RV (Figure 5c). Care should be taken to avoid injuring coronary artery branches.

The VSD is then closed, working through the TV (Figure 5d). Polypropylene mattress sutures (5/0 or 6/0 with pledgets) are placed through the base of the septal tricuspid leaflet

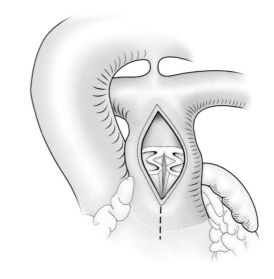

5a

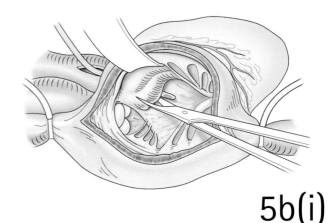

5b(i)

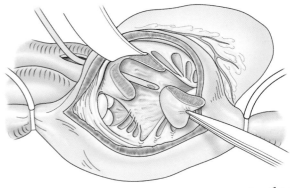

5b(ii)

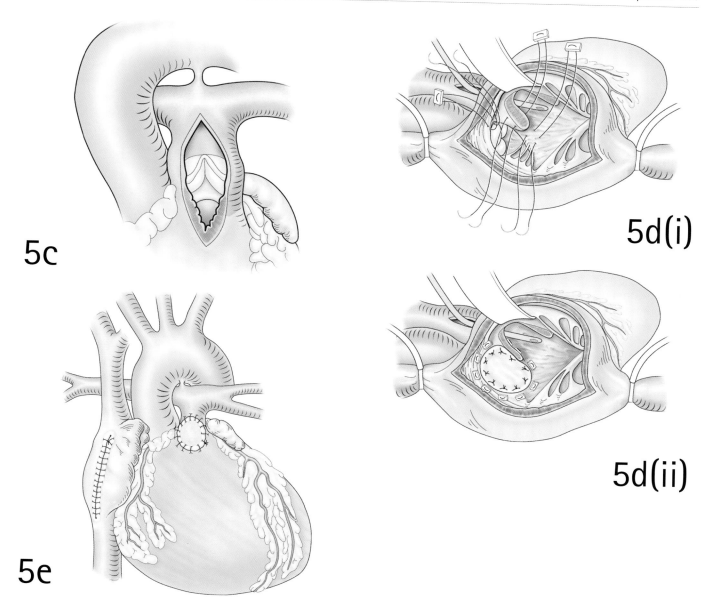

5c

5d(i)

5d(ii)

5e

and around the rim of the VSD. The aortic leaflets should again be identified through the VSD and protected, as should the area of the atrioventricular (AV) conduction tissue along the posterior rim. In the conduction area, a distance of 5 mm from the VSD rim is maintained (as in other perimembranous defects). The sutures are passed through a glutaraldehyde-treated pericardial (or woven Dacron) patch, which is tucked beneath the TV septal leaflet, and then tied and cut. The patch size approximates that of the aortic diameter at the junction with the left ventricle (LV). The oval foramen or atrial septal defect is closed with a polypropylene suture, and the heart is deaired via the aorta and the foramen, before tying the sutures. The aortic clamp is removed, and the

patient is warmed to 37°C. Proper apposition of the TV leaflets is checked and adjusted with a septal-anterior commissural suture as required.

The RA incision is closed with running polypropylene, and the caval vein tapes are removed. The incision in the PA (and RVOT) is either closed directly (if the caliber has been judged to be adequate) or repaired with a second small oval pericardial patch (Figure 5e). The width of the patch is based on the prior dilator measurements, and the patch is sutured to the epicardial and arteriotomy edges with running polypropylene. CPB is discontinued after application of atrial and ventricular pacing wires and, in some cases, after left atrium or RA line insertion.

Special considerations for tetralogy of Fallot repair

CORONARY ARTERY ANOMALIES

Coronary artery anatomy in TOF deviates from the expected pattern for normal hearts in 5–30 per cent of cases. Of concern to the surgeon are cases in which an abnormal coronary branch crosses the RVOT, imposing limitations on the safe extent of the ventriculotomy (should it be required).

6 Patterns of anomalous coronary arteries in 36 cases encountered in the Royal Children's Hospital (RCH) series (Melbourne). The most frequently appearing anomaly was an anterior descending branch from the right coronary artery. All patterns shown could preclude a classical transventricular approach to repair.

Coronary abnormalities can usually be imaged preoperatively with 2-D echocardiography, although aortography with steep caudocranial angulation may be more sensitive. A number of strategies have been proposed for dealing with anomalous coronaries at the time of TOF repair, including the use of extracardiac RV–PA conduits. Mobilization of the coronary to accommodate a patch beneath it is not recommended. In our experience, most cases can be handled with the transatrial-transpulmonary repair strategy described previously without compromising the adequacy of RV–PA reconstruction (see Outcome).

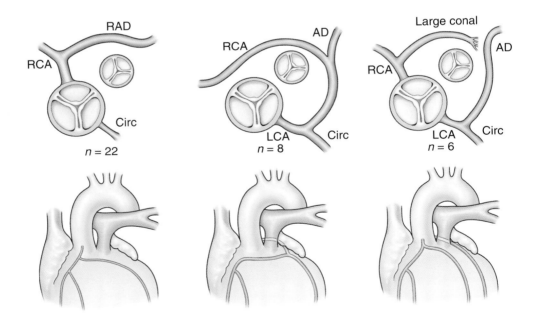

6

7 Transatrial-transpulmonary repair in the presence of an anomalous coronary (**anterior descending from right coronary**) The small transannular patch stops short of the coronary branch and can be deviated leftward. In patients with the anterior descending coronary artery arising from the right coronary artery, extension of a transannular patch laterally may be possible. In those with the right coronary artery arising from the left anterior descending, the patch must stop short of the transverse pathway of the coronary, and a more extensive muscle resection may be required. In a minority of patients, alternative strategies such as extracardiac conduits can be used with acceptable outcome.

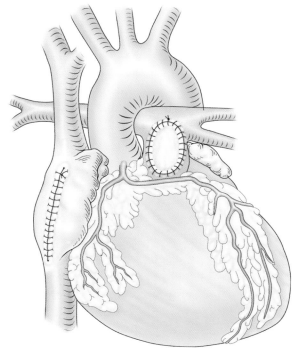

7

TETRALOGY OF FALLOT WITH ATRIOVENTRICULAR SEPTAL DEFECT

Atrioventricular septal defect (AVSD) complicates TOF in 1.0–6.5 per cent of cases. Conversely, TOF occurs in 2.7–10.0 per cent of cases of AVSD. The overall incidence of the 2 lesions together is less than 1 per cent, and a strong (greater than 75 per cent) association exists with Down's syndrome. Anatomical features of both AVSD and TOF are present, but there is a wide spectrum of AV valve and RVOT and PA anatomy. The VSD typically (but not invariably) extends under the inferior bridging AV valve leaflet, which makes the anatomy distinctly different from that of TOF. The superior bridging leaflet is freely floating (Rastelli type C).

The surgical procedure for TOF and AVSD is an extensive one. Complete repair is possible at any age, but in general, the results are not as good as those for either lesion in isolation. If possible, the operation should be performed at approximately 1 year of age, when the AV valve repair is more reliable and more surgical options are available. In practice, an earlier operation is often required due to severity of the RVOTO and/or AV valve insufficiency. The main operative considerations are maintenance of AV and pulmonary valve competence. The operative strategy for repair is a combination of those used for isolated AVSD and TOF. Initial steps of the operation are similar to those for isolated TOF, up to the point of VSD closure.

Repair of TOF with a VSD

8 For this part of the operation, a large comma-shaped patch is used. Pledgeted sutures are placed around the aortic valve and the inlet portion of the VSD and then through the patch, which is seated beneath the tricuspid chords. Sutures are placed through the crest of the VSD patch, through the AV valve leaflets, and through one edge of a second autologous pericardial patch, to partition the single large AV valve into two nonstenotic orifices. The LV is then filled with cold saline to assess AV valve competence. Sutures are placed in the accessory septal commissure (or AV valve cleft) as required (see Chapter 41 'Atrial septal defect'). Other valve repair techniques, such as commissuroplasty or semi-circular annuloplasty, may also be required. A similar exercise is used for the RV and tricuspid portion of the partitioned AV valve, with the PA temporarily occluded. The ostium primum is then closed with the autologous pericardial patch, leaving the coronary sinus in either the LV or RV, depending on the amount of fibrous tissue present in the area between the coronary sinus and AV valve tissue. The heart is deaired, and the aortic clamp is removed. RVOT reconstruction is then performed as for isolated TOF. Recently, we have used mono-cusp-bearing patches and, occasionally, complete homograft RV-to-PA conduits as *in situ* pulmonary valve replacements in patients who would otherwise have severe pulmonary incompetence due to lack of leaflet tissue or extent of right ventriculotomy. The hemodynamic burden of residual AV valve and pulmonary valve incompetence may result in an unstable postoperative course, and inotrope, ventilator, and vasodilator support may be required for several days.

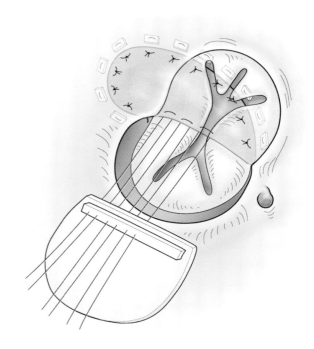

8

Absent pulmonary valve syndrome

Absent pulmonary valve syndrome (APVS) is a Fallot variant characterized by moderate pulmonary stenosis and severe incompetence, with variable (sometimes extreme) dilation of the main and branch PAs. The dilation usually extends to the main lobar branches in the lung hilum. The pulmonary valve is rudimentary, and the annulus is moderately hypoplastic. Intrinsic abnormalities of the PA wall and ventriculoarterial junction are also encountered. Some infants with APVS have tracheobronchomalacia and airway compression of the major lobar branches. Intrinsic airway and vascular abnormalities may extend to the level of the small bronchi. Repair may be required within the first few months of life if airway compression is severe. In less-symptomatic patients, the timing of surgery can be similar to that for TOF. The basic operative strategy consists of transatrial-transpulmonary repair, as outlined for TOF. In addition, the caliber of the enlarged branch PAs is reduced by resection of the main PA and the anterior (and/or posterior) wall of both primary PA branches. A short homograft valved conduit or monocusp-bearing patch is then used to reconstruct the RVOT, as continued pulmonary insufficiency may contribute to further aneurysmal dilation of the abnormal PAs (Figure 9a–d).

9a–e Repair of absent pulmonary valve syndrome

The main PA and an ellipse of branch PA anterior wall are excised. The lateral portion of the PA branches is closed directly, and a short incision is made in the RVOT. A cryopreserved aortic homograft is sutured to the annulus. The homograft anterior mitral leaflet is used to augment the RVOT. A homograft monocusp patch (inset) can also be used.

Some surgeons rely on PA aneurysm reduction alone, and in such cases, repair is performed with a direct valveless RVOT reconstruction. The main PA may be resected to bring the branches forward and possibly relieve the bronchial compression. An alternate approach, which we have favored in more recent years, is to divide the aorta just above the valve, fully mobilise the branch pulmonary arteries, and perform a Lecomple maneuver (anterior translocation of the pulmonary arteries). The aorta is then anastomosed, and central tracheobronial compression is largely eliminated (Figure 9e). With either approach, the postoperative course may be difficult in infants with APVS, with a requirement for prolonged ventilator support due to established tracheobronchomalacia.

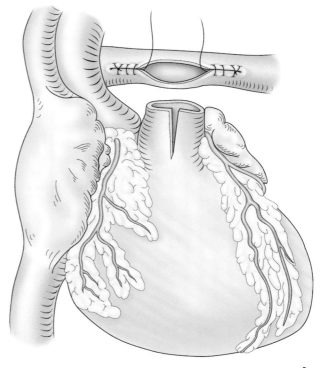

9b

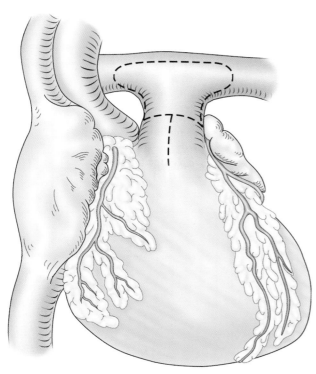

9a

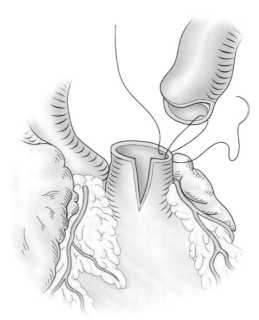

9c

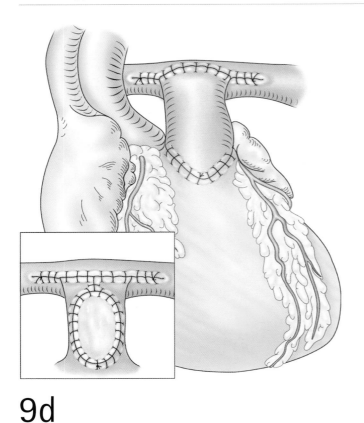

9d

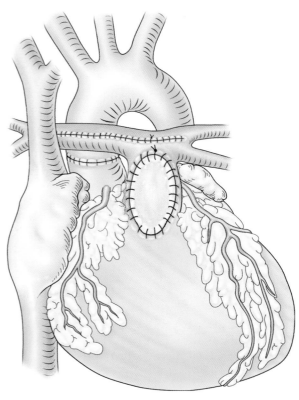

9e

Older patients with tetralogy of Fallot

In some less-developed parts of the world, cardiac surgical teams are sometimes faced with very late diagnosis or referral of patients with tetralogy of Fallot. Teams receiving overseas patients from such areas occasionally face the same problems. Such patients may present with four different clinical presentations and past histories:

Patients who have been previously satisfactorily palliated with an additional blood supply (e.g. a modified or classical Blalock-Taussig shunt or a Waterston shunt). The LV has been adequately preloaded, and the RV is hypertrophied and well developed. Repair can be undertaken at minimal risk. An aortogram may be indicated to eliminate aortopulmonary collaterals if the shunt seems minimally functional. One should be wary of left PA (previous Waterston) or right (previous Blalock-Taussig shunt) distortion.

Patients who have had no palliation but are minimally cyanotic. The anatomy is usually as expected, with predominantly valvar stenosis and well-developed PA branches. The repair is always very well tolerated, and the postoperative course is fairly simple. These patients can be quite old by tetralogy standards, even up into the fifth decade.

Patients who have had no palliation and are deeply cyanotic. SaO$_2$ is less than 70 per cent, and hematocrit is greater than 65 per cent (sometimes up to 85 per cent). The anatomy is usually favorable for a repair, with well-developed PA branches and predominantly severe infundibular stenosis. Despite the favorable PA anatomy, such patients should be treated carefully, and complete repair may be contraindicated in some cases. One should not embark on complete repair for these patients without a full awareness of the potentially very difficult postoperative physiology. Complete repair may generate a surgical risk significantly higher than that of patients with other clinical presentations. The threshold for temporary palliation depends on the culture of the unit, the past experience with such patients, and the possibilities for postoperative ventricular assist. The appearance of the LV and RV on investigations will guide the prognosis. Some aspects are very worrisome: the LV can be small relative to the right and, at times, very echogenic. This finding may apply to the whole thickness of the LV wall. Systolic function can be depressed. A very small heart on the chest x-ray is suggestive of very low Qp/Qs, with total flow distributed over two ventricles.

Almost certainly, the RV will not be adapted to receive a normal cardiac output postoperatively, with or without a transannular patch. The pathophysiology of the right or global ventricular failure after total repair in such cases is multifactorial. High LV preload may be required that cannot be matched by the failing RV, especially in the presence of a transannular patch. The failure of the RV can be systolic, diastolic, or both, even without a transannular patch. The PA pressure is usually initially low, but rapid elevation can be observed. Underdevelopment of the pulmonary lymphatic system in these patients may be the origin of severe pulmonary edema with moderately elevated left atrial pressure. The LV failure can be due to myocardial intrinsic properties or to the shift of the septum to the left, secondary to RV failure. The systemic resistances are extremely low preoperatively (as an adaptation to the high blood viscosity), and they remain extraordinarily low postoperatively. The role of an atrial septal defect placed initially or after the onset of the failure is not clear, and may not prevent all of the above problems.

CPB for patients with extremely high hematocrit is challenging. Rheology, hemostasis, and systemic resistance are the most obvious difficulties with which to deal. Conversely, all these risk factors can be corrected by a systemic–PA shunt or a percutaneous pulmonary valvotomy for a period of a few weeks to a few months, associated with a gentle exchange hemodilution. Isolated exchange hemodilution as a distant or immediate preparation to total repair is extremely dangerous. The association of decreased systemic resistances with decreased oxygen transport ability is usually not compensated by a modest increase in saturation.

Patients deeply cyanotic after a very recent history of deterioration. Bronchial infection, viral or bacterial pneumonitis, and endocarditis must be ruled out with certainty before total repair can be contemplated. In the presence of infection and persistent life-threatening cyanosis, urgent palliation is indicated, and total repair is contraindicated.

POSTOPERATIVE CARE

Basic principles of postoperative management for infants apply. Low-dose inotropic support (dopamine 3 µg/kg/minute) and a period of mechanical ventilation may be required, but early (in some cases, immediately postoperative) extubation may be preferable. The main problems encountered are moderately low cardiac output due to right heart failure and atrial arrhythmias. Both may be due to a combination of factors, including RV damage during resection, ventriculotomy, induced tricuspid insufficiency, and intrinsic myocardial abnormalities specific to TOF. RV pressure may be greater than 50 per cent of LV pressure transiently after transatrial-transpulmonary repair, due to high endogenous catecholamine levels. These problems are usually self-limited, and most infants can be supported with fluid restriction, diuretics, low-dose inotropes, and avoidance of excessive beta agonist stimulation. In all cases with persistent hemodynamic problems, an assiduous search should be made for a residual VSD and/or anatomical components of RVOTO, which may require early revision.

OUTCOME

The outcome of tetralogy surgery in the current era is excellent, considering the unfavorable natural history of the disease. At the Royal Children's Hospital (RCH), data has been analyzed for the first 611 cases (to December 1997). Median weight at the time of repair (1995–97) was 8.9 kg (5.5–54.0 kg). Transatrial-transpulmonary repair was possible in 599/611 cases. Operative mortality was 0.9 per cent (CL 0–2 per cent). The mean systolic RV-to-PA gradient at late follow-up (1–12 years) was 15 mm (+/– 24 mm). Late survival has been excellent, with a flat survival curve out to 10 years. A similarly low early mortality (0/100, CL = 0–4 per cent) has been achieved at Children's Hospital of Philadelphia for patients with tetralogy (1995–99) who had an *elective repair* within the first 6 months of life, at a median weight of 5.3 kg (range 2.7–9.6 kg). Of this subset, 59 per cent were operated with a transventricular approach, and the remainder had a transatrial-transpulmonary repair. Circulatory arrest was used in 47 cases, and 77 per cent had a transannular patch. The median hospital stay was 5 days.

The operative risk for 36 patients with anomalous coronaries (operated at the RCH) was 0 per cent (0–11 per cent), with a late RV-to-PA gradient of 19 +/– mm ($P = 1$, $P = 0.23$, respectively). The presence of an anomalous coronary was not a risk factor for poor outcome, either early or late after repair. The stratified risk of reoperation for all patients is presented in Figure 10.

For APVS, the outcome is related primarily to the degree of preexisting tracheobronchomalacia. In 19 infants with APVS and airway obstruction operated on at the RCH, hospital mortality was 16 per cent (CL 7–29 per cent). Reoperation has been required in 25 per cent for PA problems within 5 years of the initial procedure.

For the combination of TOF and AVSD, results have also been, in general, less favorable. At the RCH, 22 patients have been operated on for this lesion (4.9 per cent and 8.4 per cent of the total TOF and AVSD cases, respectively, during the same period). The operative risk was 3.7 per cent (CL = 0.9–19.0 per cent), but to date, 10 children have required reoperations, primarily for AV valve insufficiency. Two late deaths have also occurred.

For very long-term outcome after tetralogy repair, we can look to the experience of surgeons who have been performing the operation since the early days. Lillehei himself published results for 106 hospital survivors, six of whom were operated with cross circulation. The 30-year survival probability was 77 per cent, with a 91 per cent freedom from reoperation.

TOF repair results

10 Kaplan-Meier freedom from reoperation after repair of tetralogy of Fallot, for patients with and without anomalous coronary arteries ($P = 0.92$).

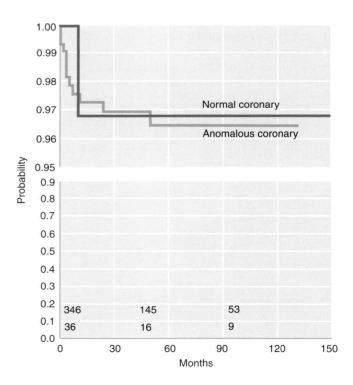

Nollert *et al* reported follow-up for 490 survivors of hospitalization, operated between 1958 and 1977. The 10-, 20-, 30-, and 36-year survival probabilities were 97 per cent, 94 per cent, 89 per cent, and 85 per cent, respectively The annualized risk of death increased from 0.0024 to 0.0094 during the follow-up period, primarily due to congestive heart failure or (presumed) arrhythmia. Mortality risk factors were operation before 1970, polycythemia, and the use of an RVOT patch ($P < 0.01$). For patients without these risk factors ($n = 164$), the 36-year actuarial survival probability was 96 per cent. Finally, Knott-Craig *et al* reported a 20-year postoperative survival probability of 98 per cent for 294 tetralogy patients. The freedom from reintervention at latest follow-up was 91 per cent in their series.

In conclusion, although some problems remain unsolved, surgical treatment has effectively altered the natural history for all Fallot variants. The most problematic patients are those with AVSD and APVS. The long-term outlook for less-complex cases is excellent.

FURTHER READING

Brizard, C.P.R., Sohn, Y.S., Mas, C., Cochrane, A.D., Karl, T.R. 1998. Transatrial trans-pulmonary repair of tetralogy of Fallot with anomalous coronary arteries. *Journal of Thoracic and Cardiovascular Surgery* 116, 770–9.

Karl, T.R. 1995. Tetralogy of Fallot. In Laks, H. (ed.), *Glenn's thoracic & cardiovascular surgery*, 6th edition, vol. 2. New York: Appleton-Century-Crofts, 1345–67.

Karl, T.R. 1997. Atrioventricular septal defect with tetralogy of Fallot or double outlet right ventricle: Surgical considerations. *Seminars in Thoracic and Cardiovascular Surgery* 9(1), 26–34.

Karl, T.R., Sano, S., Pornvilawan, S., Mee, R.B.B. 1992. Transatrial transpulmonary repair of tetralogy of Fallot: favourable outcome of non-neonatal repair. *Annals of Thoracic Surgery* 54, 903–7.

Lillehei, C.W., Varco, R.L., Cohen, M., *et al.* 1986. The first open heart corrections of tetralogy of Fallot. A 26–31 year follow-up of 106 patients. *Annals of Surgery* 204(4), 490–502.

Nollert, G., Fischlein, T., Bouterwek, S., Bohmer, C., Klinner, W., Reichart, B. 1997. Long term survival in patients with repair of tetralogy of Fallot: 36-year follow-up of 490 survivors of the first year after surgical repair. *Journal of the American College of Cardiology* 30(5), 1374–83.

49

Pulmonary atresia with ventricular septal defect

FRANK L. HANLEY MD
Professor of Cardiothoracic Surgery, Stanford University School of Medicine; Director, Pediatric Heart Center, Lucille Packard Children's Hospital, Stanford, California, USA

V. MOHAN REDDY MD
Assistant Professor, Children's Hospital, Indiana University, Indianapolis, Indiana, USA

MARK D. RODEFELD MD
Assistant Professor of Surgery, Section of Cardiothoracic Surgery, Indiana University School of Medicine, James Whitcomb Riley Hospital for Children, Indianapolis, Indiana, USA

HISTORY

Definition

Pulmonary atresia with ventricular septal defect (PA-VSD) is an uncommon complex congenital cardiac lesion in which no luminal continuity exists between the right ventricle (RV) and the pulmonary arteries. PA-VSD represents the most severe end of the spectrum of tetralogy of Fallot and is often referred to as 'tetralogy of Fallot with pulmonary atresia.' The intracardiac anatomy is consistent and similar to that of tetralogy of Fallot with an anteriorly malaligned VSD, a well-developed left ventricle (LV), and a variable degree of RV infundibular hypoplasia. The extracardiac pulmonary blood supply, however, has great morphological variability as a hallmark characteristic.

Collaterals

Blood flow to the lungs is supplied from the systemic arterial circulation via a patent ductus arteriosus (PDA) or aortopulmonary collaterals. This feature represents the greatest challenge to surgical reconstruction. If a PDA is present, normally sized and arborizing confluent pulmonary arteries are typically found. Surgical repair is relatively straightforward, with closure of the VSD, ligation of the PDA, and creation of unobstructed continuity between the RV and central pulmonary arterial system. When the ductus arteriosus is absent, major aortopulmonary collateral arteries (MAPCAs) provide systemic blood flow to the lungs. Great variation in the number, origin, size, course, and destination of these MAPCAs exists. MAPCAs frequently have intrinsic stenoses. Additionally, MAPCAs may be the exclusive source of blood flow to both lungs, one or more lobes of each lung, or particular lung segments, or they may be part of a dual supply along with the true pulmonary arteries. The morphology of the true pulmonary arteries themselves varies widely, ranging from complete absence to normal caliber, although typically they are markedly hypoplastic and centrally confluent, exhibiting distinct arborization abnormalities. The morphological and physiological details of the true pulmonary arteries and MAPCAs are of critical importance in designing the reconstructive operation.

Because of the morphological and physiological complexity of the pulmonary blood supply in PA-VSD/MAPCAs, attempts at surgical repair have been undertaken only relatively recently. Before the 1980s, this entity was considered inoperable. In the 1980s, several groups began to approach the lesion using multiple-staged palliative procedures. In 1995, a systematic approach for one-stage complete repair, including reconstruction of the pulmonary blood supply and intracardiac repair, was described.

PRINCIPLES AND JUSTIFICATION

The natural history of PA-VSD hinges on the adequacy of pulmonary blood flow. Based on this principle, patients can be loosely categorized into three anatomical subgroups. Patients with well-developed confluent pulmonary arteries and a large PDA represent 50 per cent of those with PA-VSD.

With the ductus arteriosus as the sole or dominant source of pulmonary blood flow, these infants typically present soon after birth with profound cyanosis as the ductus closes. Due to the ductal dependent source of the pulmonary blood flow, 90 per cent die within the first year of life if untreated. The second category, representing 25 per cent of patients, have moderately developed pulmonary arteries with a moderate number of MAPCAs. Clinical presentation may be later in life compared to that of the first group, but the majority become symptomatic within the first year. Untreated, mortality approaches 90 per cent by the tenth year of life. The third category, representing 25 per cent, are those patients with extremely hypoplastic or absent central pulmonary arteries and extensive systemic collaterals to the lungs. Presentation may be delayed beyond early infancy. Patients in this anatomical subgroup also typically present within the first year of life with cyanosis. However, these patients generally have a longer life expectancy if untreated, with mortality near 90 per cent by the third decade of life. Conversely, in a small number of cases with large aortopulmonary collaterals and few stenoses, the clinical presentation may be with heart failure rather than cyanosis, which develops at 4–6 weeks of life as pulmonary vascular resistance falls. However, many patients with MAPCAs do not fall easily within specific categories, but rather the morphological variability of the pulmonary arteries and MAPCAs describes a spectrum.

The size of the central pulmonary arteries may vary from complete absence to normal size. This situation depends on the degree of communication between the MAPCAs and the pulmonary arteries. Nonconfluent right and left pulmonary arteries are found in approximately 30 per cent of cases. A particular segment of the lung may receive blood flow solely by either the true pulmonary arteries or the aortopulmonary collaterals, or dually by both. Connections between the two systems may be located at central or peripheral points and at single or multiple sites. Although collaterals originate most commonly from the anterior aspect of the descending thoracic aorta, they may also arise from the ascending aorta, transverse aortic arch, subclavian arteries, abdominal aorta or one of its branches, or, rarely, the intercostal or coronary arteries.

MAPCA stenoses commonly follow a course of progression to severe stenosis or occlusion. Stenoses may play an early protective role in preventing overcirculation and development of hypertensive pulmonary vascular disease, but, untreated, they often result in distal arterial hypoplasia and underdevelopment of its supplied lung segment. When stenoses are absent or mild, unrestricted systemic pulmonary blood flow at systemic pressures can promote pulmonary vascular disease in those patients surviving beyond infancy.

Surgical goals

The ultimate surgical goal in repair of PA-VSD is to establish completely separated, in-series pulmonary and systemic circulations, with the lowest possible pressure in the RV.

Achieving these goals is based on four objectives. First, the true pulmonary arteries and MAPCAs must be 'unifocalized,' with a goal of achieving the maximal possible cross-sectional 'neopulmonary' artery area to supply the total pulmonary capillary bed. Second, reconstruction of the central pulmonary arteries may be required, depending on the extent of central pulmonary hypoplasia. Third, RV-to-pulmonary artery continuity must be established via right ventriculotomy and placement of a valved conduit. Fourth, the VSD is closed to separate the systemic and pulmonary circulations.

The actual repair performed is tailored to the individual patient based on the morphological severity of the defect. The most important physiological factor signifying a favorable outcome after complete repair is the postrepair peak RV pressure, which should be as low as possible. This factor is dependent on the number of lung segments unifocalized, the status of the pulmonary microvasculature in those segments, and the absence of obstruction in the pathway from the RV to the lung microvasculature.

Staged approach

The traditional surgical approach to the management of PA-VSD has generally been based on the concept of staged unifocalization of the pulmonary blood supply, followed by central pulmonary artery reconstruction and VSD closure, thus requiring multiple operations before complete repair is achieved. Although associated with excellent long-term results in selected patients, this approach has a number of theoretical and practical disadvantages. First, multiple procedures are required to achieve complete repair, including thoracotomy to access the lung hilum for peripheral pulmonary arterial reconstruction. Second, staged repair results in delay in achieving normal circulatory physiology. Third, iatrogenic loss of lung segments often occurs by occlusion using a staged approach. Fourth, some lung segments may be exposed for long periods to high-pressure MAPCAs. Fifth, peripheral conduits have no growth potential and tend to calcify, leading to difficulty in centralizing these grafts when reconstructing the RV outflow tract from a midline approach at a subsequent operation.

Rationale for one-stage repair

The longer a given lung segment is exposed to MAPCA physiology, the higher the likelihood that it will develop either hypertensive pulmonary vascular obstructive disease or will atrophy. Because stenoses with MAPCAs progress over time, even a vessel with the perfect degree of stenosis at birth will not remain that way. The pulmonary vascular bed is healthiest at birth and declines thereafter. Thus, the earlier that the repair can be made, the greater the chance of incorporating the largest number of healthy lung segments into the unifocalized pulmonary circuit. The number of lung segments recruited into the pulmonary arterial system correlates strongly with low postrepair pulmonary arterial pressures and calculated pulmonary vascular resistance.

Based on this argument, we have adopted a strategy of early complete unifocalization of the pulmonary blood flow with intracardiac repair and an RV-to-pulmonary artery conduit in a single stage as the procedure of choice for repair of PA-VSD. Prosthetic material in the lung periphery is eliminated with a single-stage approach. Native tissue-to-tissue apposition provides better theoretical growth potential and is given priority in planning reconstruction. Establishment of RV-to-pulmonary artery continuity at the time of the first operation allows for subsequent catheter access for percutaneous interventions, such as balloon angioplasty, if needed. The ideal age of repair of this lesion is unknown. If the patient is well balanced physiologically, we prefer to perform this procedure at 3–4 months of age. However, if the patient is severely cyanotic or is overshunted and in heart failure, repair is feasible as early as the first week of life.

The morphological variability of the lesion, the timing of referral, and prior interventions sometimes preclude adoption of a single-stage approach. In patients whose collaterals are not adequate to allow one cardiac output because of distal stenosis, either naturally occurring or secondary to shunt procedures, we prefer to completely unifocalize the collaterals but not close the VSD. In the small subgroup of patients with small true pulmonary arteries and a paucity of MAPCAs, we have performed an aortopulmonary window as a palliative step to promote growth of the pulmonary arteries and facilitate later repair. In approximately 5 per cent of cases with severe stenoses that are not surgically amenable or are difficult technically to repair, unifocalization is performed electively in stages via thoracotomy.

PREOPERATIVE ASSESSMENT AND PREPARATION

Investigation and decision making

Echocardiography provides the initial diagnosis and identifies any additional associated cardiac malformations. The echocardiographic appearance of PA-VSD is similar to that of tetralogy of Fallot but differs in lack of continuity between the RV and pulmonary artery. Difficulty may exist in delineating the presence and extent of the true pulmonary arteries or the sources of systemic arterial supply with echocardiography. Because of this deficiency, detailed angiography is essential in all cases to clearly assess the anatomical and hemodynamic characteristics of the true pulmonary arteries and MAPCAs

and to plan the optimal surgical management of patients. Angiography provides critical information regarding MAPCA numbers, size, location, presence and location of stenoses, and sites of communication with the true pulmonary arteries (see Figure 1). Each MAPCA is selectively injected to demonstrate whether it connects with a true pulmonary artery or enters the lung parenchyma as a sole supply to a particular lung segment. Identification of stenoses and pressure measurements is important. Pulmonary vein wedge angiography may be useful to visualize the central pulmonary arteries. In selected cases with well-developed confluent central pulmonary arteries and a large PDA, angiography may not be required. However, one should be certain that no evidence of significant collateral vessels is seen by echocardiography.

Angiography is performed at diagnosis in the neonatal period to define the anatomy of the pulmonary arteries and MAPCAs and to identify ductal tissue. If ductal tissue is present with MAPCAs, the ductus typically provides flow to the left pulmonary artery. In these cases, neonatal repair is undertaken, as the entire left lung is in jeopardy of being lost if surgery is delayed. If surgery is electively scheduled at 3–4 months of age, then repeat angiography is mandatory, because new stenoses may develop.

Preparation

Thorough preoperative planning of MAPCA reconstruction is a necessity. One must have a 'mental image' of MAPCA numbers, origins, and courses before surgery, as well as an idea of how they may be best unifocalized. Selected angiographic images or cineangiograms may be helpful to have available for review during the reconstruction. The total cross-sectional area of the neopulmonary arterial unifocalization is the most important determinant of the postrepair RV/LV pressure ratio (pRV/pLV); however, flawless technical execution of the unifocalization procedure is also necessary, as poorly constructed anastomoses and/or kinking of unifocalized MAPCAs can add critical amounts of resistance to the pulmonary vascular circuit.

If the patient is ductal dependent, infusion of prostaglandin E_1 maintains stability before surgery. Ductal closure results in hypoxemia and cyanosis and necessitates emergent repair if adequate systemic collateral vessels are absent. In contrast, in the few cases with a large PDA or collateral shunt, patients may manifest clinical features of congestive heart failure. To optimize the preoperative pulmonary status, diuresis, inotropic support, and mechanical ventilation may be needed.

OPERATION

1 Case that illustrates the importance of careful angiography in a characteristically complex and heterogeneous anomaly   This patient has multiple unusual collaterals to the right lung and a single collateral to the left lung. No true central pulmonary arteries are present. The left lung is supplied by a single collateral (1) originating from the lower aspect of the aortic arch. This collateral arborizes into a near-normal pulmonary arterial pattern to supply all segments of the left lung. This supply was originally thought to be of ductal origin, but intraoperative findings failed to demonstrate the presence of the recurrent laryngeal nerve below its origin, thus confirming that this vessel is an embryological collateral rather than ductal tissue. The right lung is supplied by four collaterals without any segmental stenoses. A collateral of pericardiophrenic artery origin (2) arising from the internal mammary artery pedicle supplies three medial segments of the right lower lobe. A collateral originating from the thyro-cervical trunk (3) supplies most middle and upper lobe segments. A small collateral from the descending aorta (4) supplies several medial lung segments. A dominant and large intercostal artery (5) originates from the descending aorta and travels to its lateral-most extent before penetrating the lung and branching to supply the majority of the right lower lobe. The collateral supply to the right lung in this case is similar to that seen in pulmonary sequestration. This patient underwent one-stage complete repair as a neonate.

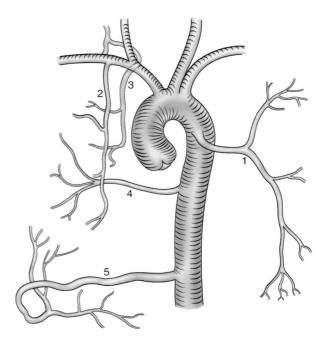

1

Incision and exposure

2a **Extended midline incision and sternotomy, subtotal thymectomy** Wide exposure is obtained by extended midline incision and median sternotomy. Combined with generous sternal retraction, this approach improves exposure of both lungs. A subtotal thymectomy is performed, and both pleural spaces are opened widely. Care is taken to avoid the phrenic nerves, particularly where they are located more anteriorly in the upper mediastinum.

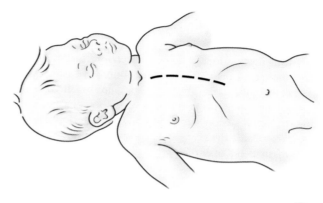

2a

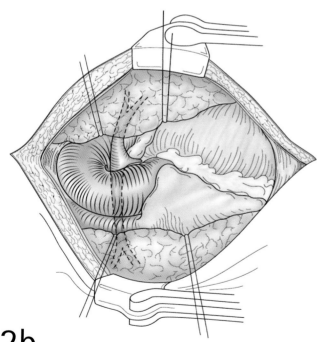

2b

2b **Wide harvest of pericardial patch, pericardial edges suspended** A large anterior patch of pericardium is harvested, and the pericardial edges are suspended with stay sutures. These sutures can then be moved and pinned appropriately to greatly improve exposure and facilitate hilar dissection in both lungs.

Mediastinal dissection

3a **Mediastinal dissection of true pulmonary arteries and major aortopulmonary collateral artery origins** The aorta and central pulmonary arteries are widely dissected. Extensive dissection is performed in the posterior mediastinal space superior to the left atrium (asterisk). This critical maneuver provides space for mobility during relocation of collateral vessels. This area is best approached through the space between the aorta and superior vena cava. The transverse sinus is widely opened, and the posterior mediastinal soft tissues are dissected. The central collaterals are identified and dissected over their entire course, extending toward their aortic origins. The descending aorta itself is dissected as needed in the posterior mediastinal space to expose MAPCA origins. Any further collaterals in the subcarinal space from the proximal descending aorta, transverse aortic arch, and ascending aorta are identified and dissected.

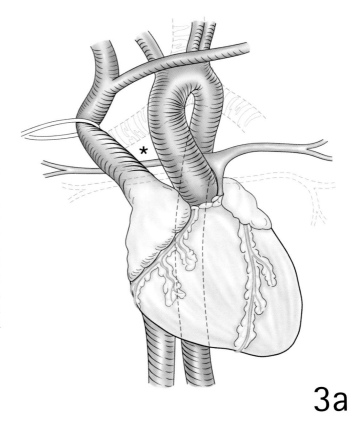

3a

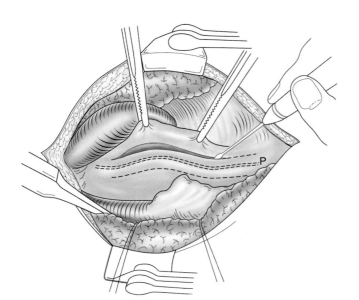

3b

3b **Pericardium and parietal pleura on both sides incised longitudinally above and below the phrenic nerve** To facilitate hilar dissection, as well as isolation, rerouting, and unifocalization of collaterals, the pericardium and pleura are incised above and below the phrenic nerves bilaterally, leaving a strip of pericardium as a vascularized and physically supporting pedicle to the phrenic nerve. Care is taken to avoid phrenic nerve injury by stretching or cautery.

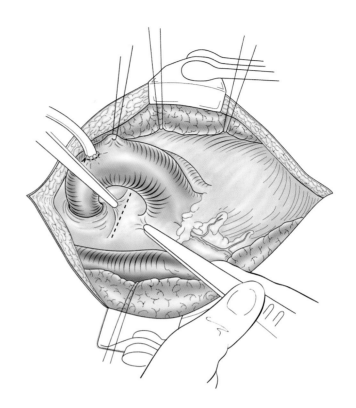

4a

Right hilar dissection The right lung is left *in situ*, and the right pulmonary artery is dissected as peripherally into the hilum as possible. This dissection usually extends into the lung parenchyma to the first- or second-level bifurcation of the true pulmonary artery.

4a

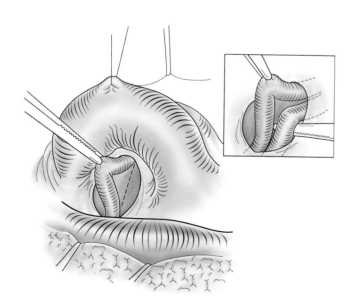

4b

4b Right collaterals are identified and mobilized into the hilum. This step is often achieved as a natural progression of the central mediastinal dissection. Often, however, the right lung is retracted anteriorly out of the right chest cavity, and the collateral is dissected along its posterior route into the right hilum.

5a **Left hilar dissection** The left lung is left *in situ,* and the left pulmonary artery is dissected as peripherally into the hilum as possible, similar to right lung dissection.

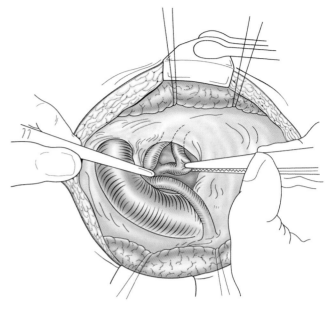

5a

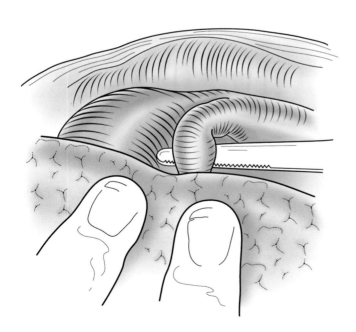

5b

5b Left collaterals are identified and mobilized into the hilum.

Institution of cardiopulmonary bypass and control of collaterals

6 All collaterals are identified, dissected completely, and controlled with vessel loops before initiation of cardiopulmonary bypass. This approach prevents damaging pump flow run-off into the lungs and maximizes systemic perfusion. The patient is systemically heparinized and prepared for aortic and bicaval cannulation. Before initiating cardiopulmonary bypass, as many collaterals as possible are permanently ligated at their origin, mobilized, and unifocalized to minimize pump time. When oxygen saturations approach a compromising level, the remaining MAPCAs are snared or occluded, the patient is cannulated, and cardiopulmonary bypass is initiated. The remainder of the collaterals are then unifocalized at mild to moderate hypothermia with the heart beating.

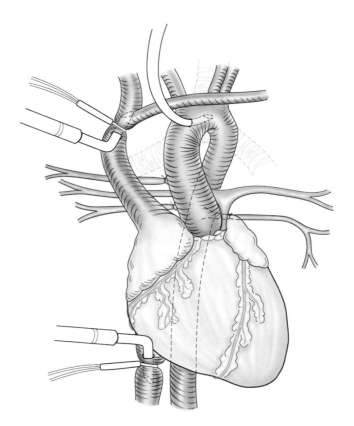

6

Peripheral unifocalization

7a **Anastomotic techniques to maximize neopulmonary artery cross-sectional area** Achieving the best reconstruction depends on advanced planning, flexibility in reconstruction, aggressive mobilization, and creative rerouting of MAPCAs. Reconstruction of the pulmonary arteries is performed with the highest priority given to maximally using the length of the MAPCAs in the anastomoses, preservation of autologous tissue apposition, and avoidance or minimizing use of synthetic conduits or allograft tissue in the periphery. Absorbable fine (7/0 or 8/0) monofilament suture is used for anastomoses (Maxon). Mobilized collaterals are typically routed through the transverse sinus and delivered to the true pulmonary arteries for subsequent unifocalization; however, occasionally they are best routed above the hilum. Even collaterals that are part of a dual supply to a lung segment also supplied by a native pulmonary artery are often unifocalized to maximize the cross-sectional area of the reconstructed neopulmonary arteries. Techniques that generally maximize the neopulmonary artery area include the following:

1 Side-to-side anastomosis of collaterals to central pulmonary artery (augments the hypoplastic central pulmonary artery)
2 Side-to-side anastomosis of collateral to collateral
3 End-to-side collateral to peripheral native pulmonary artery
4 End-to-side collateral to collateral
5 End-to-end or end-to-side of collateral to central allograft conduit
6 Allograft patch augmentation of collateral stenosis
7 Button of aorta giving rise to multiple unobstructed collaterals to native pulmonary arteries
8 Reconstruction of neocentral pulmonary arteries with allograft tissue patch

The use of allograft tissue patch material is common; however, a patch is used noncircumferentially to augment the central pulmonary arteries out to the level of the hilum on both sides so that the growth potential of the native tissue is maintained. Rarely, the central pulmonary arteries are of adequate size, and patch augmentation is unnecessary.

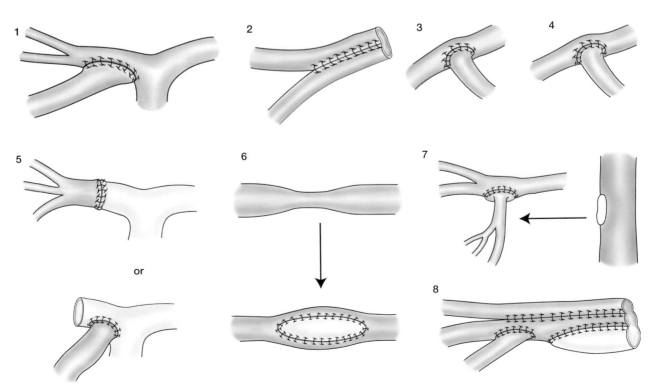

7a

7b Completed unifocalization of case illustrated in Figure 1 Collateral 2 was taken from its origin and transposed across the central mediastinum to create central continuity with the left lung collateral (1). The remaining right-sided collaterals were carefully anastomosed to collateral 2 to create a unifocalized right-lung vascular supply. A central pulmonary arterial augmentation was created with homograft patch material.

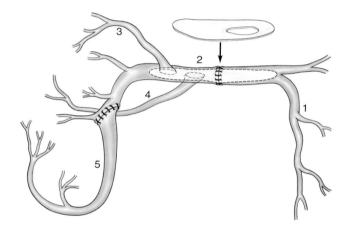

7b

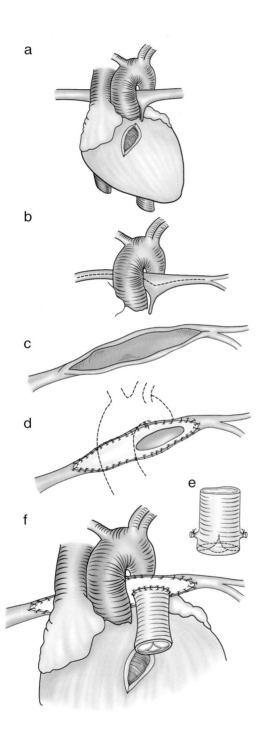

8 **Right ventriculotomy and distal RV-to-pulmonary artery anastomosis** After peripheral unifocalization, the aorta is cross-clamped, and cardioplegia is administered. A longitudinal ventriculotomy is made in the RV infundibulum. The anatomy of the infundibulum is inspected, and any obstructive tissue and/or hypertrophic muscle bundles are resected. An appropriate-sized allograft valved conduit is then selected to connect the RV to the unifocalized neopulmonary arterial system. Because of the possibility of somewhat elevated right-sided pressures, an aortic allograft is preferred. The distal end is typically anastomosed end-to-side to the centrally augmented, reconstructed neopulmonary arteries. Rarely, a second non-valved conduit is needed to reconstruct the central left and right pulmonary arteries, usually in older patients with completely absent true pulmonary arteries and inadequate collateral tissue. Circumferential allograft conduits are always limited to the pericardial cavity due to concerns over growth potential.

8

9 **Intraoperative flow study** At this point, a decision must be made regarding VSD closure. In patients who are completely unifocalized, the total resistance of the neopulmonary artery vascular bed is estimated by an intraoperative flow study. After complete unifocalization and distal conduit anastomosis, while the patient is still supported by bypass, a pulmonary artery pressure catheter and a perfusion cannula are placed through the allograft conduit. The left atrium is vigorously vented. Incremental volumes of gradually increasing blood flow up to at least one cardiac index (2.5 L/minute/m²) are pumped through the unifocalized pulmonary arteries with the use of a standard roller pump. Mean pulmonary artery pressures are recorded at each steady state. If the pulmonary arterial pressure is less than or equal to 25 mm Hg at a flow equivalent to one cardiac output, a decision is made to close the VSD.

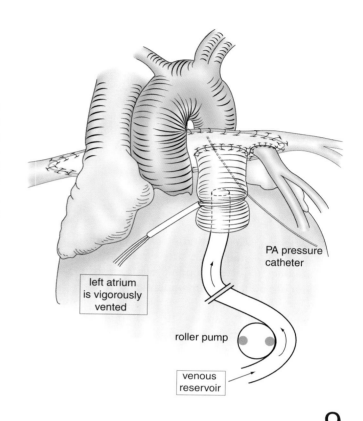

9

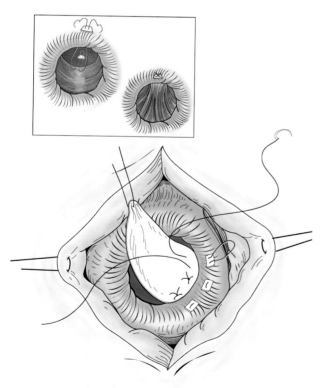

10 **Closure of VSD** The VSD is closed through the ventriculotomy with a Dacron or glutaraldehyde-treated autologous pericardial patch using pledgetted, braided, polyester interrupted mattress sutures or running nonabsorbable monofilament sutures, as preferred. The right atrium is opened to inspect the atrial septum. If an atrial septal defect or patent foramen ovale is present, it is partially closed in a fashion to leave a small, one-way, interatrial communication as a pop-off valve in the event of RV dysfunction (inset). In some cases with intact atrial septum, a small unidirectional interatrial communication may be intentionally created. After right atrial closure, the cross-clamp is removed, and rewarming is started.

10

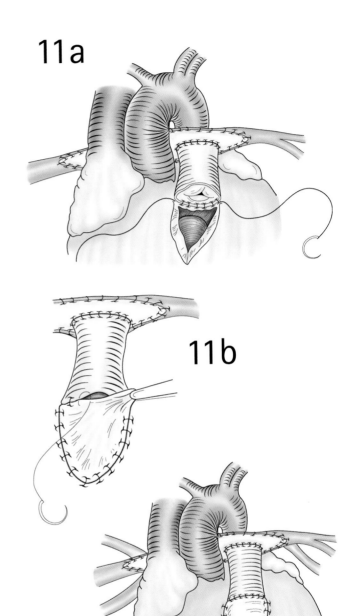

11a–c Completion of proximal RV-to-pulmonary artery conduit

The proximal RV-to-pulmonary artery conduit anastomosis is completed with running nonabsorbable monofilament suture. A pericardial or allograft tissue hood is fashioned to complete the infundibulotomy closure. A pressure-monitoring line is placed through the right atrial free wall, across the tricuspid valve, to monitor the RV pressure.

After separation from cardiopulmonary bypass, the aortic, RV, and left and right atrial pressures are monitored continuously. Intraoperative transesophageal echocardiography is routinely performed. Bilateral pleural and mediastinal drains are placed, and the sternum is closed. If bleeding or ventilation is an issue, the sternum is electively covered with a silicone rubber patch (Silastic). Secondary closure is then performed on the 2nd or 3rd postoperative day.

POSTOPERATIVE CARE

RV-pressure monitoring, as well as right- and left atrial-pressure monitoring, is routinely performed. Maneuvers to minimize the RV afterload and optimize pulmonary function include maintenance of a mild respiratory alkalosis and relatively high arterial oxygen concentrations, as pulmonary hypertension or high peak RV pressures are often an issue in the early postoperative period. Sedation and paralysis are maintained during the critical phase of the patient's recovery. Inotropic support is used routinely in the early postoperative period. Our typical regimen includes low-dose epinephrine, moderate-dose dopamine, and moderate-dose amrinone or milrinone.

Postoperative bleeding is managed similarly to that in other instances in which prolonged and extensive operations have been performed, with aggressive correction of coagulation abnormalities. Fresh frozen plasma, platelet, and packed red blood cell transfusions may be required. Antifibrinolytic medications are not used because of concerns over thrombosis in the neopulmonary arterial circuit, which has many fresh suture lines.

Minor lung hemorrhage is common and is managed expectantly. Catastrophic bleeding is rare. Fiberoptic bronchoscopy is sometimes performed if evidence of tracheobronchial obstruction exists before the operation. Postoperative bronchoscopy is sometimes performed for pulmonary toilet or to rule out tracheobronchomalacia. Lung reperfusion injury is seen commonly and is almost always self-limiting. Injury has been limited to segments that are severely underperfused before unifocalization. Recovery is evident within the first few postoperative days.

Phrenic nerve injury often is not apparent until attempting to wean the patient from the ventilator. Phrenic nerve praxia is typically temporary, and the incidence has markedly diminished as we have gained experience with the operation. In an occasional patient, pulmonary vasoreactivity is of concern, and inhaled nitric oxide may be used. This problem is sometimes an issue in older patients with an unprotected pulmonary vascular bed or large shunts. Monitoring of serum electrolytes, glucose, and hepatic enzymes in the perioperative period is strongly recommended, especially in the younger age groups. Splanchnic end-organ injury, manifested by acute hepatic insufficiency and, rarely, bowel necrosis, has been encountered on occasion in our experience.

OUTCOME

Predischarge echocardiography and perfusion lung scanning is routinely performed in all patients and is repeated at 6-month intervals thereafter. If the tricuspid regurgitation jet suggests elevated RV pressure and/or the lung scan shows maldistribution of flow, cardiac catheterization is performed promptly. Completely repaired patients are followed clinically and scheduled for cardiac catheterization approximately 1 year after surgery, or earlier if symptoms develop. Patients who do not undergo closure of the VSD at the time of the unifocalization are catheterized electively at 3 months postoperatively to assess the feasibility of complete repair. If the Qp/Qs ratio is greater than 2:1, the VSD is closed. If the Qp/Qs ratio is less than 2:1, the patient is assessed for further reconstruction. This goal may be achieved by percutaneous balloon dilatation and/or stenting, or by unilateral or bilateral patch augmentation of the pulmonary artery system.

To date, our series includes 130 patients operated on from 1992 to 2000. The mean age at surgery is 4 months, with a range from 5 days to 39 years. The number of MAPCAs unifocalized in a given operation ranges from two to nine, with a median of four. One-stage complete unifocalization has been achieved in 90 per cent of patients, with the remaining 10 per cent being completely unifocalized after two or three total operations. Sixty per cent of patients have had the VSD closed in a single stage; however, eventually, 95 per cent of all patients have had VSD closure with acceptable RV pressures (i.e. less than 50 per cent of the RV/LV ratio). Early postoperative reactive airway problems resolve over several weeks. Lung function is otherwise normal in all patients.

The most commonly observed postoperative events in our series have included phrenic nerve palsy, pulmonary parenchymal reperfusion injury, pulmonary hemorrhage, and bronchospastic hyperreactivity. Bleeding requiring re-exploration has been minimized due to the use of delayed sternal closure and mediastinal packing in selected cases (rate less than 5 per cent). Phrenic nerve praxia has been seen in approximately 5 per cent of cases; however, the incidence has declined as experience has been gained. Diaphragmatic plication has been required in a few patients. The rate of reintervention for pulmonary arterial stenoses, either percutaneous or surgical, is approximately 20 per cent. Aneurysm of the RV outflow tract has been seen in two patients. RV-PA conduit obstruction occurs at the same rate as that for other procedures requiring RV outflow tract conduit reconstruction.

The early mortality rate is 6 per cent, and late mortality is 5 per cent. Late mortality has been due to sudden hemoptysis in 2 patients, infection in 2 patients with immune compromise, and cardiac death in 3 patients.

FURTHER READING

Haworth, S.G. 1980. Collateral arteries in pulmonary atresia with ventricular septal defect. A precarious blood supply. *British Heart Journal* **44**, 5–13.

Iyer, K.S., Mee, R.B.B. 1991. Staged repair of pulmonary atresia with ventricular septal defect and major systemic to pulmonary artery collaterals. *Annals of Thoracic Surgery* **51**, 65–72.

Puga, F.J., Leoni, F.E., Julsrud, P.R., Mair, D.D. 1989. Complete repair of pulmonary atresia, ventricular defect, and severe peripheral arborization abnormalities of the central pulmonary arteries. *Journal of Thoracic and Cardiovascular Surgery* **98**, 1018–29.

Reddy, V.M., Liddicoat, J.R., Hanley, F.L. 1995. Midline one stage complete unifocalization and repair of pulmonary atresia with ventricular septal defect and major aortopulmonary collaterals. *Journal of Thoracic and Cardiovascular Surgery* **109**, 832–45.

Reddy, V.M., Petrossian, E., McElhinney, D.B., Moore, P., Teitel, D.F., Hanley, F.L. 1997. One-stage complete unifocalization in infants: when should the ventricular septal defect be closed? *Journal of Thoracic and Cardiovascular Surgery* **113**, 858–68.

50

Right ventricular outflow tract obstruction with intact ventricular septum

HILLEL LAKS MD
Professor and Chief of Cardiothoracic Surgery and Director of Heart and Heart-Lung Institute, UCLA School of Medicine, Los Angeles, California, USA

MARK D. PLUNKETT MD
Assistant Professor of Surgery, Division of Cardiothoracic Surgery, University of California, Los Angeles, UCLA School of Medicine; Pediatric Cardiac Surgeon, Division of Cardiothoracic Surgery, UCLA Medical Center, Los Angeles, California, USA

HISTORY OF PULMONARY STENOSIS

Although obstructive lesions of the right ventricular outflow tract are found in 25–30 per cent of children with congenital heart disease, isolated pulmonary stenosis at the valvar level with an intact ventricular septum accounts for approximately 8–10 per cent of all congenital heart defects. The etiology is undetermined and most likely multifactorial. An increased incidence of 2–4 per cent has been reported in siblings of patients with this defect. The initial pathological description of pulmonary stenosis is credited to Morgagni in 1761. The first attempt at surgical treatment of this lesion was by Doyen in 1913. The report describes a transventricular valvotomy using a tenotomy knife with an unsuccessful outcome. Subsequent reports followed in 1948 by Sellors and Brock describing successful blunt valve dilatation using a transventricular approach. Several successful reports of open pulmonary valvotomy using systemic hypothermia and ventricular fibrillation also followed. In 1953, with the advent of cardiopulmonary bypass, open pulmonary valvotomy was introduced as a successful approach to this lesion. Open valvotomy remained the primary therapy for patients with pulmonary stenosis until the technique of balloon valvotomy was introduced by Semb and associates in 1979. Currently, balloon valvotomy is used as the initial therapy in most patients with pulmonary stenosis.

PRINCIPLES AND JUSTIFICATION

In patients with valvar pulmonary stenosis, the pulmonary valve is typically dome-shaped with fusion of the leaflets at the commissures and a small central orifice. The pulmonary annulus may be normal in size or smaller than predicted. The right ventricle is normal in size and morphology, but secondary hypertrophy of the infundibulum develops early in life. Neonates with critical pulmonary stenosis who present in the newborn period develop severe cyanosis and congestive heart failure. The clinical findings are directly related to the severity of the stenosis as well as the degree of shunting across the atrial septum. Although severe pulmonary stenosis may present in the newborn period, most of these lesions do not manifest significant clinical findings until later in childhood. The timing of intervention is usually determined by the severity of clinical findings or a documented gradient of 50 mm Hg or greater across the right ventricular outflow tract. The results of treatment are directly related to the size of the right ventricle and the age of the patient at presentation.

According to recent reports, both balloon valvotomy and surgical valvotomy are associated with low morbidity and mortality rates and excellent long-term survival (see outcome sections). Each procedure has a significant incidence of recurrent stenosis requiring additional early or late interventions. There is a also a significant incidence of pulmonary valve insufficiency after surgical valvotomy (80 per cent) and balloon valvotomy (20 per cent). This pulmonary insufficiency also occurs and is tolerated remarkably well in most patients, and its long-term clinical importance is a topic of controversy. Although late mortality is not reportedly changed in patients with significant pulmonary insufficiency, the development of right ventricular enlargement, right ventricular dysrhythmias, and abnormal right ventricular response to exercise have been well documented. Operative intervention for surgical pulmonary valvotomy may be performed as an open technique using cardiopulmonary bypass or off-pump through a closed transventricular approach. Most off-pump procedures are performed with a cardiopulmonary bypass pump immediately available. Although an off-pump valvotomy may be performed using an inflow occlusion technique, this approach is rarely indicated.

PREOPERATIVE ASSESSMENT AND PREPARATION

On physical examination, most children with pulmonary stenosis present with a harsh holosystolic ejection murmur, an ejection click, and a palpable thrill over the pulmonic valve region. An electrocardiogram reveals right axis deviation, prominent P waves, and right ventricular hypertrophy. A chest radiograph often reveals prominent pulmonary artery shadows secondary to poststenotic dilatation. The cardiac shadow is normal except in severe cases associated with congestive heart failure. An echocardiogram establishes the severity of the stenosis and identifies any associated anomalies. Cardiac catheterization is performed for additional diagnostic information and intervention using balloon valvotomy.

ANESTHESIA

The anesthetic management of these patients is similar to that for any neonate or child with a right ventricular outflow tract obstruction. In the neonate, the ductus must be kept patent and pulmonary vascular resistance reduced to ensure adequate pulmonary blood flow. Systemic hypotension is avoided, as it may result in reduced ductal flow and subsequent hypoxemia. These patients may also have dynamic obstruction in the infundibular region secondary to right ventricular myocardial hypertrophy. Inotropes must be used with caution as increased contractility may cause increased functional obstruction across the pulmonary outflow tract and further compromise pulmonary blood flow.

OPERATIONS

Open pulmonary valvotomy using cardiopulmonary bypass

1 Open pulmonary valvotomy is performed through a median sternotomy using cardiopulmonary bypass and bicaval cannulation. The patent ductus arteriosus is ligated or snared before the initiation of cardiopulmonary bypass. An aortic cross-clamp is applied, and antegrade cardioplegia is administered through the aortic root to achieve myocardial arrest. The patent foramen ovale or atrial septal defect is closed directly through a right atriotomy incision using a primary or pericardial patch technique. A vertical arteriotomy is then performed on the anterior wall of the main pulmonary artery and extended down to the level of the pulmonary valve.

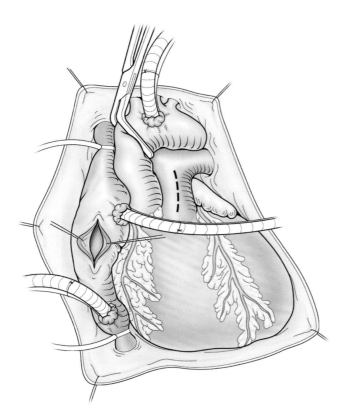

1

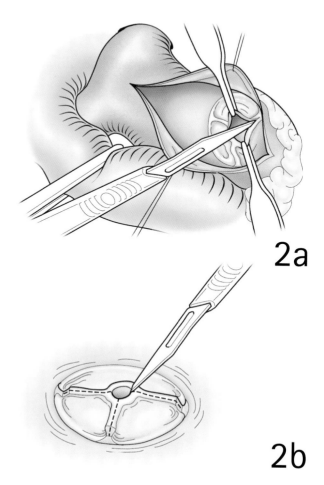

2a

2a–c
The stenotic valve is inspected, and the fused commissures are carefully incised with a No. 11 scalpel blade or fine vascular scissors. The incisions in the valve should extend to the annulus. Any valvular adhesions to the pulmonary arterial wall are sharply incised. A partial valvectomy may be necessary to remove thickened valve tissue or dense fibrous scarring on dysplastic leaflets. The infundibulum is then inspected through the valve for any subvalvular stenosis. Sharp infundibular resection may be performed if necessary. The arteriotomy is closed using a running polypropylene suture.

2b

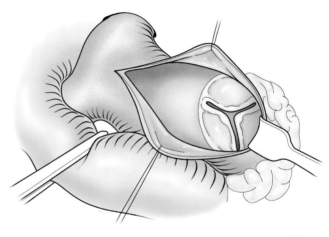

2c

Off-Pump transventricular pulmonary valvotomy

3 If no atrial septal defect is present, a pulmonary valvotomy may be performed through a median sternotomy using an off-pump transventricular technique. A pursestring suture is placed in the anterior wall of the right ventricle. An angiocatheter connected to a pressure transducer is first introduced through the pursestring in the right ventricle and into the pulmonary artery. Using the same technique, progressively larger metal dilators are then introduced across the valve membrane. If the valve tissue does not dilate easily, a long vascular clamp can be used to initially disrupt the valve tissue. After adequate dilation is achieved, the pursestring is tied and reinforced.

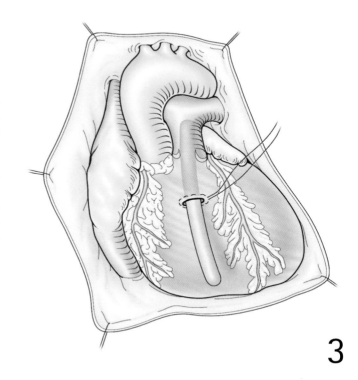

3

POSTOPERATIVE CARE

Most patients with pulmonary stenosis are operated on electively and require routine preoperative and postoperative care. In neonates, the management of acidosis, electrolyte derangements, and congestive heart failure should begin preoperatively and continue postoperatively. A residual gradient often exists across the right ventricular outflow tract. Inotropic support should be used judiciously to avoid exacerbation of any residual infundibular obstruction. Transesophageal echocardiography may be performed to assess any residual gradient. Mild and moderate residual gradients often resolve with increasing age and growth of the patient.

OUTCOME

A multi-institutional study by Hanley and associates reported a postoperative survival of 94 per cent, a 30-day survival of 89 per cent, and a 4-year survival of 81 per cent for all modes of intervention in neonates with critical pulmonary stenosis. Unfortunately, 26 per cent of these patients required re-intervention within 2 years for residual stenosis (defined as a gradient greater than or equal to 30 mm Hg). After successful pulmonary valvotomy (either after initial intervention or re-intervention), right ventricular size approaches normal in more than 90 per cent of these neonates. Furthermore, surgical intervention in older children is associated with minimal morbidity and mortality and excellent short- and long-term outcomes.

HISTORY OF PULMONARY ATRESIA WITH INTACT VENTRICULAR SEPTUM

In contrast to other forms of right ventricular outflow tract obstruction, pulmonary atresia with intact ventricular septum (PA/IVS) is an uncommon congenital cardiac malformation representing between 1–3 per cent of all congenital heart defects. Historically, surgical treatment of this defect was associated with a very high morbidity and mortality. The low incidence of this defect, combined with its extreme morphologic variability, delayed the development of a standardized approach to surgical therapy. The original Greenwold classification of PA/IVS described this defect by two types of right ventricles: type I with a hypoplastic right ventricle and type II with a normal or dilated right ventricle. More recently, some surgical approaches to PA/IVS have been based primarily on a quantitative Z-score assessment of the tricuspid valve diameter. This Z-score is determined by comparing the estimated diameter of the tricuspid valve (as measured by echocardiography) to the expected 'normal' size and calculating the difference in standard deviations. In 1989, Billingsley and associates from the University of California, Los Angeles (UCLA) School of Medicine introduced a surgically-oriented classification of mild, moderate, and severe hypoplasia of the right ventricle as described in the section. With a more systematic approach to this defect, increasing surgical experience, and improved diagnostic modalities, outcomes from the surgical treatment of PA/IVS have steadily improved.

PRINCIPLES AND JUSTIFICATION

Without early surgical intervention, children with PA/IVS have an extremely high mortality rate. The natural history is a 50 per cent mortality rate at 2 weeks and approximately 85 per cent mortality at 6 months. Death occurs secondary to severe hypoxemia and progressive metabolic acidosis secondary to closure of the ductus arteriosus. In general, most children with PA/IVS require multiple surgical interventions. Previous surgical experience has indicated that the surgical management of patients with PA/IVS should be based primarily on an anatomic classification system that specifically defines the degree of right ventricular hypoplasia. Using this approach, neonates with PA/IVS are initially separated into three groups of *mild*, *moderate*, and *severe right ventricular hypoplasia*. In patients with *mild right ventricular hypoplasia*, the tricuspid valve and right ventricular cavity are approximately two-thirds or greater of calculated normal size, and the right ventricular outflow tract is well developed. This situation correlates with a Z-score for the tricuspid valve of 0 to −2. In patients with *moderate right ventricular hypoplasia*, the tricuspid valve and the right ventricular cavity are approximately one-half of calculated normal size (with a range of one-third to two-thirds of normal), and the pulmonary outflow tract is usually developed enough to perform an effective pulmonary valvotomy. This situation correlates with a Z-score for the tricuspid valve of −2 to −4. In patients with *severe right ventricular hypoplasia*, the tricuspid valve and right ventricular cavity are one-third or less of calculated normal size, and the pulmonary outflow tract is not amenable to an effective pulmonary valvotomy. This situation correlates with a Z-score for the tricuspid valve of −4 to −6. This approach is not based on any single anatomic component, but instead assesses the overall right ventricular morphology and the degree of both tricuspid valve and right ventricular hypoplasia.

PREOPERATIVE ASSESSMENT AND PREPARATION

Although prenatal diagnosis is increasing for many congenital heart defects, most neonates with PA/IVS are diagnosed shortly after birth. Echocardiography remains the initial diagnostic study to identify the anatomic abnormalities and to assess the right ventricular morphology. Because of the complexity and variability of PA/IVS, the anatomy and morphology must be defined by echocardiography and right and left heart cardiac catheterization. Selective coronary injections and an injection into the right ventricle are also required for a complete evaluation. Classification is determined from these studies, and an appropriate operative procedure is selected based on the right ventricular morphology, tricuspid valve size, the right ventricular outflow tract, and the coronary circulation.

During the initial evaluation of patients with PA/IVS, special attention must be directed towards the anatomy of the coronary circulation. Right ventricle-to-coronary artery fistulae are present in 45 per cent of cases and are more common in those patients with a severely hypoplastic right ventricle and a small competent tricuspid valve. These connections are frequently accompanied by the development of fibrous intimal hyperplasia, resulting in stenosis or complete obstruction of the native coronary circulation. The presence of obstructive lesions in the proximal coronaries may produce a 'right ventricle-dependent coronary circulation' (RVDCC). Such patients are at high risk for myocardial ischemia, as desaturated blood from the right ventricle perfuses a significant portion of the myocardium. A greater risk of myocardial ischemia is incurred by reduced diastolic aortic pressure resulting from the creation of a systemic-to-pulmonary artery shunt. In such patients, decompression of the right ventricle by an outflow tract patch, pulmonary valvotomy, or tricuspid valvotomy is poorly tolerated and may lead to acute myocardial infarction.

In addition, an Ebstein's malformation of the tricuspid valve is present in 10 per cent of patients with PA/IVS. This group of neonates should be considered separately. Most of these patients have severe tricuspid valve insufficiency and a normal-sized or enlarged right ventricle. Massive dilatation of the right atrium also exists. The left ventricle is often compromised in these infants because of the dilated dysfunctional right ventricle. Although an aorta-to-pulmonary artery shunt may establish adequate pulmonary blood flow, left ventricular output remains compromised by the dilated right ventricle. Surgical intervention in these patients is associated with a greater than 50 per cent mortality. Orthotopic heart transplantation may be the only viable therapeutic option.

Selection of operations in neonates

Initial surgical management of most neonates with PA/IVS involves the establishment of a reliable and adequate source of pulmonary blood flow and optimizing the potential growth and development of the right ventricle and tricuspid valve. The selection of appropriate operations in these neonates is based primarily on the degree of right ventricular hypoplasia.

Neonates with PA/IVS and mild right ventricular

hypoplasia are best treated with a pulmonary valvotomy, insertion of an aorta-to-pulmonary artery shunt, and ligation of the ductus arteriosus. Occasionally, patients exist in whom a pulmonary valvotomy alone restores adequate pulmonary blood flow. Experience has shown that initial valvotomy alone often fails to produce effective palliation despite favorable anatomy. In most instances, performance of a small central shunt to ensure adequate pulmonary blood flow and promote subsequent growth of the branch pulmonary arteries is preferable.

Neonates with PA/IVS and moderate right ventricular hypoplasia are best treated with a pulmonary valvotomy, augmentation of the pulmonary outflow tract, insertion of an aorta-to-pulmonary artery shunt, and ligation of the ductus arteriosus. Pulmonary valvotomy and augmentation of the pulmonary outflow tract relieves right ventricular hypertension, reduces tricuspid regurgitation, and potentiates the growth of the tricuspid annulus and the right ventricular cavity. This approach may allow for a subsequent biventricular repair as the definitive procedure. A transannular pericardial patch may be necessary to augment the right ventricular outflow tract. This procedure can be performed off-pump without using cardiopulmonary bypass, which is preferred in neonates in whom a mixed circulation persists postoperatively.

Neonates with PA/IVS and severe right ventricular hypoplasia are more difficult to manage surgically. Balloon atrial septostomy is recommended at the time of cardiac catheterization. Pulmonary valvotomy is usually not effective in relieving right ventricular hypertension. These neonates are best treated with an aorta-to-pulmonary artery shunt or a subclavian artery-to-pulmonary artery (modified Blalock-Taussig) shunt. If no right ventricular sinusoids exist or if sinusoids are tortuous and narrow without broad coronary artery fistulae, the right ventricle is decompressed by incising the tricuspid valve. This step can be performed using a closed technique without cardiopulmonary bypass. In most cases, decompression of the right ventricle results in regression of the narrow tortuous type of sinusoids and does not result in myocardial ischemia (if the native coronary circulation is intact). Frequently broad fistulae from the coronary arteries to the right ventricle can be identified on the epicardial surface of the heart and directly ligated.

Selection of operations for older children

Infants with PA/IVS are followed closely after their initial palliative procedures. With improving results, an increasing number of patients are presenting for later interventions. A cardiac catheterization is performed at 3–6 months of age, depending on the infants initial morphology and the subsequent echocardiographic findings. In patients with severe right ventricular hypoplasia, repeat catheterization at 2–3 months is recommended, as a high mortality may occur in this group while awaiting repair. The selection of operative procedures is once again based primarily on right ventricular morphology and an assessment of the tricuspid valve and right ventricular growth since the previous intervention. Whereas in neonates the size of the tricuspid valve and the right ventricle usually correlate, in older children a significant discrepancy may exist between these two structures.

In patients with mild right ventricular hypoplasia, later surgical intervention includes closure of the atrial septal defect with an adjustable snare, enlargement of the right ventricular cavity and outflow tract by myocardial resection, and patch augmentation of the right ventricular outflow tract. To achieve a competent pulmonary valve, either a pericardial monocusp valve or a bioprosthetic tissue valve is inserted in the right ventricular outflow tract. A successful biventricular repair is achieved in the majority of these patients.

The use of an adjustable snare to close the atrial septal defect permits right-to-left shunting at the atrial level in children in whom right ventricular volume and compliance may limit forward outflow to the pulmonary arteries. The ability to adjust the size of the atrial septal defect allows for postoperative control of right-to-left shunting and allows the adjustment of forward flow through the right ventricle. This approach can be helpful in optimizing cardiac output and avoiding excessive cyanosis.

In patients with moderate right ventricular hypoplasia, later intervention is dictated by the previous growth of the right ventricle and the tricuspid valve. If the right ventricle is one-half to two-thirds normal size, then repair includes closure of the atrial septal defect with an adjustable snare, enlargement of the right ventricular cavity by myocardial resection, and a valved connection between the right ventricle and pulmonary artery. If the right ventricular volume and the tricuspid valve diameter are marginal (one-third to one-half normal) for a two-ventricle repair, a bidirectional cavopulmonary shunt (Glenn shunt) is performed. This shunt allows the channeling of one-third of the systemic venous return from the superior vena cava directly to the pulmonary arteries while the inferior vena cava (two-thirds of the systemic venous return) continues to pass through the tricuspid valve and right ventricle. This approach has been termed the *one and one-half ventricle* or *partial biventricular* repair. This plan limits the volume load on the right ventricle and provides obligatory pulmonary blood flow directly to the pulmonary arteries. A two-ventricle repair (with takedown of the Glenn shunt) or a completion Fontan reconstruction may follow based on the subsequent growth of the right ventricle and the tricuspid valve. The atrial septal defect is adjustable to control forward flow through the right ventricle. This approach enhances the growth and development of the right ventricle and the tricuspid valve and increases the likelihood of a two-ventricle repair.

In patients with PA/IVS and severe right ventricular hypoplasia, a biventricular repair is usually not possible. Most of these patients have a systemic-to-pulmonary artery shunt in the neonatal period with or without tricuspid valvotomy. The bidirectional cavopulmonary shunt is performed in the first 3–6 months of life with a plan for a Fontan procedure within the first 3–4 years. A fenestration of the Fontan is used as an atrial septal defect with an adjustable snare. The Fontan may be performed as a lateral tunnel or as an extracardiac conduit.

Selection of operations in children with right ventricle-dependent coronary circulation

In infants with RVDCC, systemic right ventricular pressure must be maintained to ensure adequate coronary perfusion to the myocardium. Decompression of the right ventricle in these patients by augmentation of the outflow tract or tricuspid valvotomy may lead to severe myocardial ischemia and acute cardiac failure. If an RVDCC is identified, a single ventricle surgical strategy is pursued. If epicardial connections between the right ventricle and the coronary circulation are identified and these coronary arteries do not have proximal obstruction which make them dependent on right ventricular pressure for adequate perfusion, surgical ligation of the epicardial fistulae may be performed safely.

If signs of myocardial ischemia exist, either preoperatively or intraoperatively, the patient with an RVDCC can be improved by creating an aorta-to-right ventricle shunt at the time of the cavopulmonary shunt or the Fontan procedure. This shunt theoretically reduces the right ventricular systolic pressure to equal the systemic pressure while elevating the diastolic pressure perfusing the coronary circulation. Flow through such a shunt appears to be bidirectional and biphasic. If myocardial ischemia results from decompression of an undiagnosed RVDCC, coronary artery bypass grafting using the internal mammary artery may be attempted. The use of coronary artery bypass grafting in these patients is limited by technical difficulties, conduit options, and the limited long-term patency of the grafts. Finally, in patients with RVDCC and severe right ventricular dysfunction, early shunt placement may be followed by orthotopic heart transplantation.

ANESTHESIA

The management of neonates with PA/IVS is similar to that described for neonates with severe pulmonary stenosis. Because no blood flow is pumped from the right ventricle to the pulmonary arteries, these patients are completely ductal dependent. Careful modulation of the pulmonary vascular resistance is essential to ensure adequate oxygenation. Patients with RVDCC must be carefully monitored for evidence of myocardial ischemia. Older children undergoing biventricular repairs should be managed to optimize antegrade pulmonary blood flow. Patients undergoing one and one-half and staged single ventricle repairs often require higher inotropic support. They also need reduction of their pulmonary artery pressures to maintain adequate flow in the Glenn and Fontan shunts.

OPERATIONS IN NEONATES

Shunts

Principles and techniques of systemic-to-pulmonary artery shunts are discussed in Chapter 39.

Off-pump insertion of a pulmonary transannular patch

4 A median sternotomy is performed, and a primed cardiopulmonary bypass pump is made available. A pediatric cross-clamp is placed immediately beneath the bifurcation of the main pulmonary artery. The ductus is kept patent to provide pulmonary blood flow. A vertical incision is made in the anterior aspect of the main pulmonary artery and extended down to the junction of the right ventricle. A partial thickness incision is continued down to the area over the right ventricular cavity. Epicardial muscle is resected to a depth of 2–3 mm to thin out the superficial wall of the right ventricle.

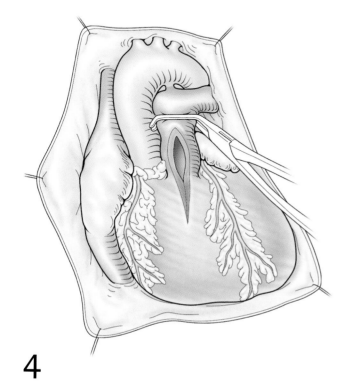

4

5 A pericardial patch is now sutured to the edges of the pulmonary artery and to the edges of the right ventricular incision. The sutures are left loose inferiorly, and a scalpel is used to incise the valve membrane and the remaining myocardium over the right ventricular cavity.

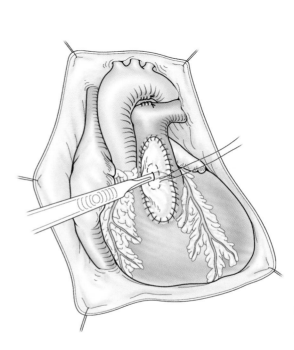

5

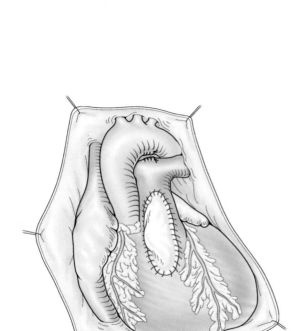

6

6 The sutures are pulled up to control the bleeding, and the cross-clamp is removed. Flow is re-established through the right ventricular outflow tract. The ductus arteriosus is ligated.

7 If the right ventricular pressure is not adequately reduced to one-third of systemic pressure, a rhizotomy knife is introduced through a pursestring in the pericardial patch, and the right ventricular muscle and pulmonary membrane are further incised.

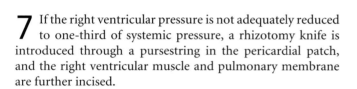

7

Off-pump transarterial pulmonary valvotomy

8 An open pulmonary valvotomy can be performed through a left thoracotomy without the use of cardiopulmonary bypass. The approach is through the fourth intercostal space, and the main pulmonary artery is cross-clamped immediately below the bifurcation. Pulmonary perfusion is maintained through the ductus arteriosus. A pursestring suture is placed in the anterior wall of the main pulmonary artery. The main pulmonary artery is incised vertically within the pursestring and retracted to expose the valve.

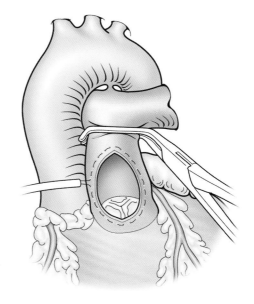

8

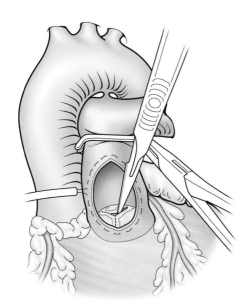

9

9 The fused commissures are identified and incised sharply with a No. 11 scalpel to the level of the annulus.

10 The pursestring is tightened, and a thin-bladed vascular C-clamp is quickly applied to the incision. The cross-clamp on the pulmonary artery is removed.

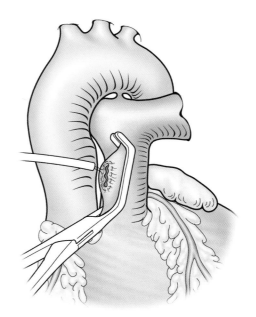

10

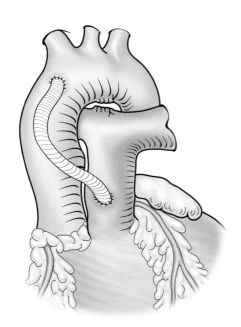

11

11 A Gore-Tex graft is sutured to the incision in the main pulmonary artery and to the left subclavian artery (LSA) to establish adequate pulmonary blood flow. After completion of the shunt, the ductus arteriosus is ligated.

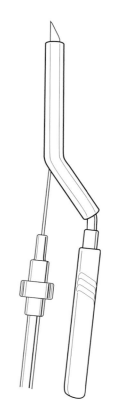

12a

Closed tricuspid valvotomy

12a, b Closed tricuspid valvotomy can be performed through a median sternotomy or a right thoracotomy without the use of cardiopulmonary bypass. An instrument is made using a rhizotomy knife with a small curved blade passed through a segment of red rubber tubing. A needle connected to a pressure transducer is placed into the tubing. The knife may be advanced or withdrawn in the rubber tubing, avoiding damage to structures on insertion or withdrawal.

The pericardium is incised, and a pursestring suture is placed in the right atrial appendage. The tubing is introduced into the right atrium and across the tricuspid valve. Once the pressure transducer confirms placement in the right ventricle, the knife blade is advanced and the tricuspid valve is incised anteriorly. Care is taken to avoid incising the area of the conduction system along the septal leaflet. When the right ventricular pressure has fallen to one-half of systemic or less, the knife is retracted into the tubing and the pursestring suture is tied to achieve hemostasis.

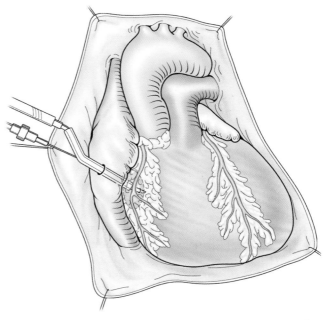

12b

OPERATIONS IN OLDER CHILDREN

Enlargement of right ventricular cavity and outflow tract

Enlargement of the right ventricular cavity is performed through a median sternotomy using cardiopulmonary bypass with bicaval cannulation. The heart is arrested with antegrade and retrograde delivery of cardioplegic solution. The right atrium is incised and opened. A second incision is made vertically from the main pulmonary artery, through the pulmonary annulus, and across the infundibulum to the main right ventricular cavity. The cavity is enlarged by extensive sharp resection of trabecular right ventricular myocardium through both incisions. A right angle clamp is used to avoid injury to underlying myocardium and the papillary muscles of the tricuspid valve. A glutaraldehyde-treated pericardial transannular patch is then sutured to the right ventricle and pulmonary artery. The atriotomy is closed using a running polypropylene suture in a two-layered technique.

Adjustable atrial septal defect

13 Creation of an adjustable atrial septal defect is performed through a median sternotomy using cardiopulmonary bypass and bicaval cannulation. If the atrial septal defect is small with firm edges, it may be closed with an adjustable snare. The snare is created by placing a No. 1 polypropylene suture as a pursestring around the tissue edges of the existing defect. Pericardial pledgets may be used for reinforcement. The No. 1 polypropylene suture is secured in its position with one or more interrupted polypropylene sutures around the edges of the defect. Both ends of the No. 1 polypropylene suture are then brought out through the interatrial groove. An 8-Fr polyethylene tube is cut to a length which reaches the linea alba from the atria and is passed over the ends of the suture to construct the snare. The proximal end of the tubing is sutured to the atrial wall with a single chromic suture. The snare is adjusted by tightening or loosening the ends of the suture at the distal end of the tubing. The length of the suture is fixed with medium vascular clips. The end of the snare is left under the subxiphoid linea alba where it can be retrieved (under local anesthesia) postoperatively for adjustment. An atrial pressure of approximately 12–15 mm Hg with an oxygen saturation of 88 per cent or more on 100 per cent fraction of inspired oxygen is considered optimal.

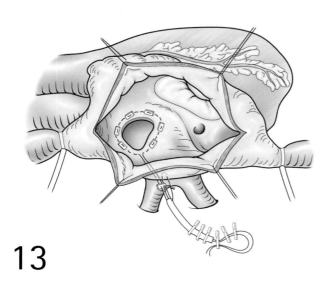

13

14 A similar technique can be used to create an adjustable atrial septal defect in a Gore-Tex patch. The defect in the suture line is left on the right side of the patch between the Gore-Tex and the posterior atrial wall. A pursestring No. 1 polypropylene suture snare is placed around the defect as described above. The atrial septal defect is left open until the patient is weaned from cardiopulmonary bypass. The defect is then slowly closed using the snare while the right atrial pressure and the arterial oxygen saturations are monitored.

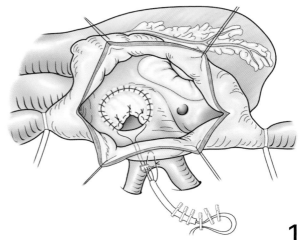

14

Transannular patch with over-sized porcine valve insertion

15a–c Insertion of a bioprosthetic valve and transannular patch is performed through a median sternotomy using cardiopulmonary bypass with bicaval cannulation. Myocardial arrest with cardioplegia is often used but may not be necessary. A transannular incision is made vertically across the pulmonary outflow tract and extended distally on to the left pulmonary artery and proximally down into the right ventricle. Any residual membrane in the region of the pulmonary annulus is resected. An over-sized (relative to the normal valve size of the child) porcine bioprosthetic valve is placed under a pericardial or Gore-Tex patch within the right ventricular outflow tract. If pericardium is used, it is treated with glutaraldehyde for 5 minutes and rinsed with saline. The sewing ring of the porcine bioprosthetic valve is seated below the level of the true pulmonary annulus. This approach allows a larger valve to be implanted and reduces the amount of compression that may result from sternal closure. A running polypropylene suture is used to anchor the porcine valve sewing ring to the right ventricular outflow tract posteriorly. The transannular patch is sewn to the edges of the pulmonary artery, and the porcine valve is anchored to the patch anteriorly. Implantation of the patch is completed by suturing the proximal edges to the remaining myocardial defect in the right ventricular outflow tract.

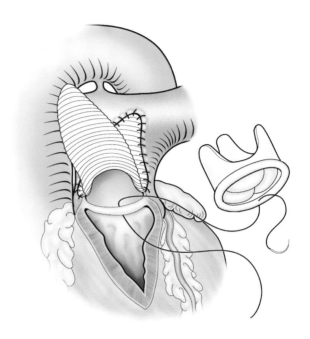

15b

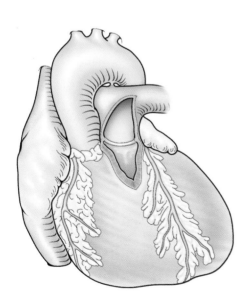

15a

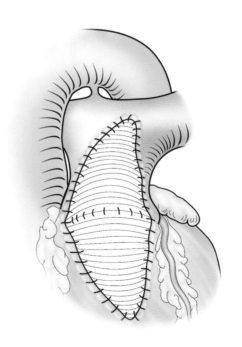

15c

Transannular patch with pericardial monocusp valve insertion

16a–c Insertion of a transannular patch with a monocusp valve is performed through median sternotomy using cardiopulmonary bypass and bicaval cannulation. After harvesting, the pericardium is treated with glutaraldehyde for 5 minutes and then rinsed in saline. The transannular patch and the monocusp valve leaflet are marked on the harvested pericardium using a sterile marking pen. Sizing of the monocusp valve is made using a metal dilator that approximates the expected 'normal' diameter of the pulmonary annulus. The width of the monocusp leaflet at its base should be approximately one-half of the circumference of the dilator. This width should also correspond with the width and shape of the proximal end of the transannular patch. The superior edge of the monocusp valve leaflet should be attached to the edges of the incised pulmonary artery several millimeters distal to the area of the true valve annulus. The monocusp valve is attached to the edges of the pulmonary artery and the right ventricle using the same suture that attaches the edges of the transannular patch.

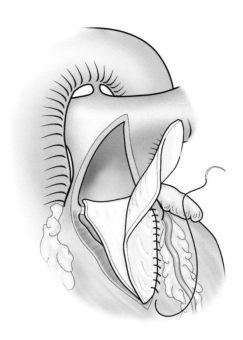

16b

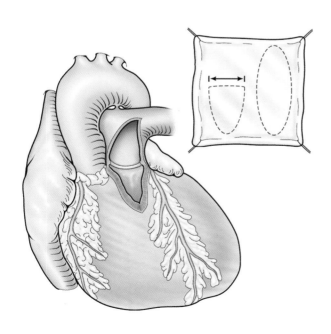

16a

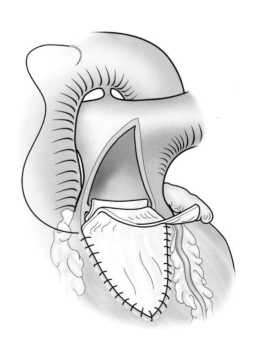

16c

Homograft valve insertion

17 The insertion of an aortic or pulmonary homograft is performed through a median sternotomy using cardiopulmonary bypass and bicaval cannulation. Cardioplegic arrest of the heart may or may not be necessary. An appropriately sized aortic or pulmonary homograft is selected, thawed, and trimmed to the correct length. The pulmonary artery is opened, and a running polypropylene suture is used for the distal anastomosis of the homograft to the pulmonary artery bifurcation.

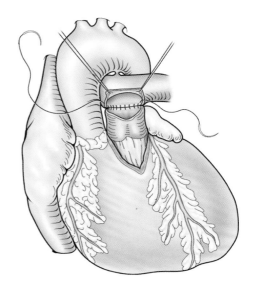

17

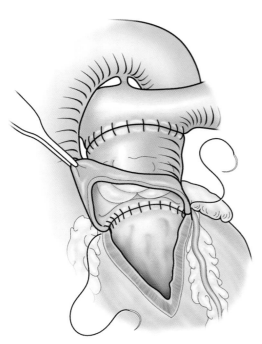

18

18 Proximally, the posterior edge of the homograft is sutured to the right ventricular outflow tract just below the pulmonary valve annulus using a running polypropylene suture. If the myocardium is friable, a reinforcing strip of glutaraldehyde-treated pericardium is used for this anastomosis.

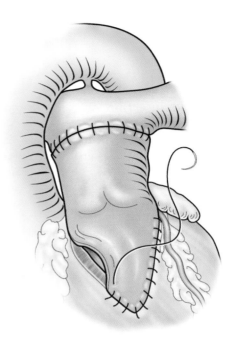

19a

19a, b The remaining anastomosis of the anterior edge of the homograft to the right ventriculotomy can be performed using the anterior leaflet of the mitral valve of an aortic homograft. Alternatively, this anastomosis may require a rectangular hood of Gore-Tex or pericardium. This hood enlarges the right ventricular outflow tract and avoids residual obstruction at the junction of the homograft.

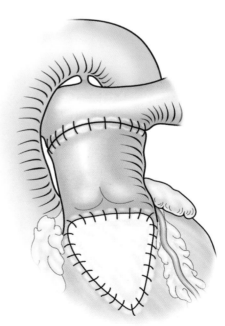

19b

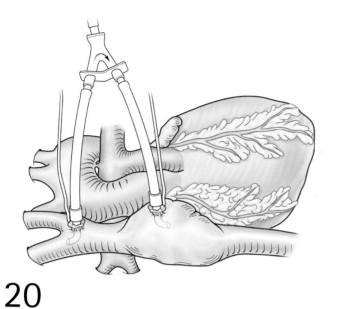

20

Off-pump bidirectional cavopulmonary shunt (Glenn shunt)

20 An off-pump bidirectional cavopulmonary shunt is usually performed through a median sternotomy. The azygous vein is identified and divided between ligatures. A pursestring suture is placed in the superior vena cava at the junction of the innominate vein. A second pursestring is placed in the right atrial appendage. The patient is heparinized, and a temporary bypass shunt is created using two modified aortic cannulae and a Y connector with a chapeau attachment.

21a–c The superior vena cava is then clamped at its junction to the right atrium and at its junction to the innominate vein. The superior vena cava is divided at the atrial junction. The open end of the superior vena cava is enlarged by an incision in the posterior wall of the vessel. This enlargement assures a widely patent anastomosis. The right pulmonary artery is clamped with a vascular C-clamp and a V-shaped incision is made on its superior aspect with the apex of the incision pointing anteriorly. The anastomosis is performed between the superior vena cava and the pulmonary artery. The anterior anastomosis may be enlarged with a patch of pericardium to assure patency and avoid tension. Any previously placed systemic-to-pulmonary artery shunt is now reduced in size to give an estimated ratio of pulmonary-to-systemic circulation of 1.3:1.0 or less.

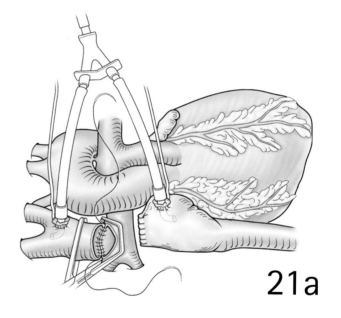

21a

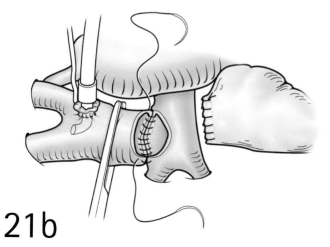

21b

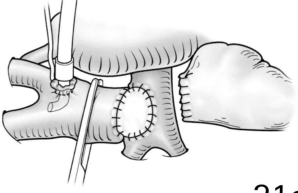

21c

Lateral tunnel Fontan with adjustable atrial septal defect

22 The lateral tunnel Fontan procedure is usually performed as the second-stage operation after a bi-directional cavopulmonary shunt. The procedure is performed through a median sternotomy using cardiopulmonary bypass with bicaval cannulation. After myocardial arrest with antegrade cardioplegia, a right atriotomy is performed just anterior to the linea terminalis. The coronary sinus is identified and cannulated with a retrograde cardioplegia catheter. A pursestring suture is used to secure the catheter in the coronary sinus. Cold cardioplegic solution is delivered intermittently both antegrade and retrograde to maintain myocardial arrest. The remaining atrial septum is completely excised. The superior vena cava orifice is identified from within the right atrium. The right pulmonary artery is incised adjacent to the opening in the stump of the superior vena cava. The posterior wall of the adjacent pulmonary artery and right atrium are sutured together. Anteriorly, the connection is bridged with a pericardial patch.

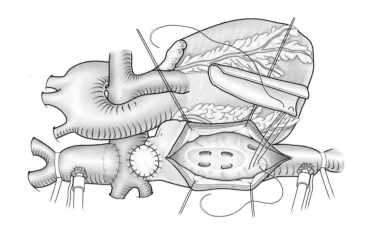

22

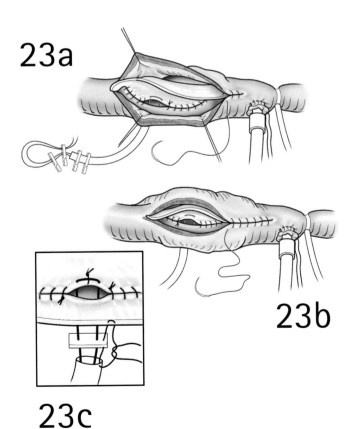

23a

23b

23c

23a–c Construction of the lateral tunnel is achieved using a rectangular Gore-Tex patch cut from a 0.8-mm Gore-Tex patch material. The length is carefully measured from the orifice of the inferior vena cave to the orifice of the superior vena cava. A running polypropylene suture is used for the posterior suture line starting inferiorly near the inferior vena cava and proceeding superiorly to the chosen site of the adjustable atrial septal defect. This site for the adjustable atrial septal defect between the common atrium and the Fontan tunnel is chosen where a natural recess exists close to the right superior pulmonary vein. A second suture line is begun at the superior end of the adjustable defect and extended around the superior vena cava orifice. The atrial septal defect is sized according to the age of the patient. As a general rule, the defect size is 4 mm for 2-year olds, 6 mm for 4-year olds, and 8 mm for 6-year olds and older. Before completing the anterior suture line, a snare is placed for the adjustable atrial septal defect (as previously described in operations in older children, Figures 13 and 14). The patch is now trimmed and the anterior part of the suture line is completed using full-thickness sutures through the atrial wall. The atrial septal defect snare is adjusted to achieve arterial saturations of 80–85 per cent while attempting to maintain the pressure in the lateral tunnel at 12–15 mm Hg.

Extracardiac Fontan with adjustable atrial septal defect

24 The extracardiac Fontan is performed through a median sternotomy using cardiopulmonary bypass and bicaval cannulation. A distinct advantage of this procedure is the ability to complete it in most patients without the need for cardioplegic arrest of the heart. A clamp is placed on the inferior vena cava near its junction to the right atrium. The inferior vena cava (IVC) is then divided between the snared venous cannula and the clamp. The atrium is repaired, and the clamp is removed.

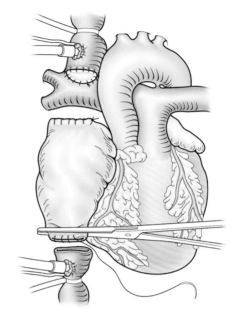

24

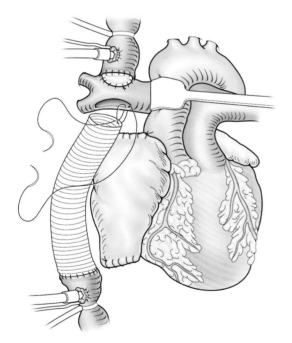

25 The open end of the inferior vena cava is anastomosed end-to-end to a Gore-Tex conduit (16–20 mm diameter) using a running Gore-Tex suture. The proximal anastomosis is performed end-to-side between the Gore-Tex conduit and the inferior aspect of the right pulmonary artery. The clamps are released, and flow is established between the inferior vena cava and the pulmonary arteries.

25

26a, b To create the adjustable atrial septal defect, a partial occluding vascular C-clamp is placed on the Gore-Tex graft. An 8.0-mm Gore-Tex graft is anastomosed end-to-side to the middle of the larger conduit. A similar technique is used to create an opening in the right atrium, and the other end of the 8.0-mm graft is anastomosed to this site. A snare may be placed to encircle the graft or, preferably, inserted on the atrial side (as previously described in Figures 13 and 14) to control the opening and closing of this 'atrial septal defect.' A distinct drawback to the extra cardiac Fontan is the need for anticoagulation with warfarin postoperatively for up to a year, with subsequent conversion to aspirin therapy.

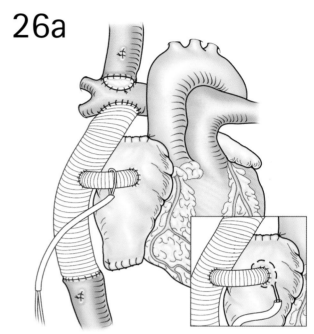

26a

26b

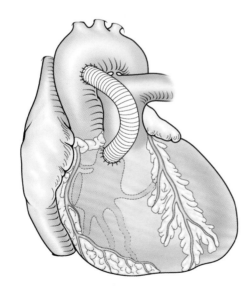

27

Aorta-to-right ventricle shunt

27 The aorta-to-right ventricle shunt is performed through a median sternotomy using cardiopulmonary bypass and bicaval cannulation. Cardioplegic arrest of the heart may or may not be necessary. The shunt is created using a 5.0-mm Gore-Tex graft. A partial occluding clamp is placed on the anterior wall of the ascending aorta. An aortotomy is created and an end-to-side anastomosis is performed between the graft and the ascending aorta using a running polypropylene suture. A ventriculotomy is made in the infundibular portion of the right ventricle and the distal end of the graft is anastomosed to this site using a running polypropylene suture.

POSTOPERATIVE CARE

Neonates

Neonates may be critically ill in the early postoperative period after operative intervention for PA/IVS. The presence of low cardiac output may require substantial inotropic support. In the presence of an aorta-to-pulmonary artery shunt, balanced pulmonary and systemic blood flow must be achieved. The management of pulmonary and systemic vascular resistance is critical to maintaining adequate oxygenation and cardiac output. Episodes of pulmonary hypertension must be managed quickly and may require the use of inhaled nitric oxide. An excessively large shunt may lead to pulmonary over-circulation and require adjustment or replacement of the shunt. Postoperative ischemia can develop due to unrecognized RVDCC and may be associated with electrocardiogram changes, ventricular dysrhythmias, and segmental wall dyskinesis on echocardiography. In patients with persistent hypoxemia despite adequate medical management, residual right ventricular outflow tract obstruction or severe tricuspid hypoplasia should be excluded.

Older children

Early management after the Fontan procedures should focus on optimizing cardiac output and reducing systemic venous pressure. Inotropes are routinely used, starting with dopamine and dobutamine. If additional inotropic support is needed, milrinone may be added. If systemic vascular resistance is low and additional inotropic support is needed, the use of epinephrine may be indicated. The adjustable atrial septal defect is useful because it allows as much as one-third of the systemic venous return to traverse the defect to the atrium, thus lowering the systemic venous pressure while increasing left ventricular preload and the cardiac output. With an estimated ratio of pulmonary-to-systemic circulation of 1.5:1.0, the arterial oxygen saturation should be approximately 85 per cent. A systemic venous pressure of 12–15 mm Hg is optimal. Of note, the presence of a patent right-to-left shunt increases the risk for paradoxical emboli from thrombus that may develop in the right atrium or the hepatic veins. Therefore, complete closure of the adjustable atrial septal defect should be performed when it is hemodynamically tolerated.

If the pulmonary vascular resistance is elevated postoperatively after a Glenn or Fontan procedure, an infusion of nitroglycerin and prostaglandin E_2 may be employed. These medications are more effective in lowering pulmonary vascular resistance if delivered directly into a catheter in the Glenn or Fontan tunnel. If these medications are not sufficient, nitric oxide is administered through the ventilator. Unlike the intravenous medications, nitric oxide does not result in the lowering of systemic vascular resistance. Extubation within the first 24 hours is generally attempted for Glenn and Fontan procedures. The development of pleural and pericardial effusions is anticipated, and mediastinal and pleural chest tubes are left for several days postoperatively until drainage is minimal.

OUTCOME

At the UCLA School of Medicine, the surgical approach to patients with PA/IVS has been based on classification of the degree of right ventricular hypoplasia. Between 1982 and 1997, a total of 111 patients with a diagnosis of PA/IVS underwent surgical intervention at our institution. Six patients had Ebstein's anomaly of the tricuspid valve and were excluded from analysis.

A total of 63 patients with PA/IVS underwent palliative procedures at UCLA as neonates. Twenty patients were classified as having severe right ventricular hypoplasia or demonstrated severe coronary abnormalities with RVDCC, or both. Three early deaths occurred in this group. Forty-three patients were classified as having mild to moderate right ventricular hypoplasia without significant right ventricle sinusoids or fistulae. These patients all underwent procedures to open the right ventricular outflow tract with or without a shunt. Three early deaths and two late deaths occurred in this group. Early survival in this total group is 90 per cent and late survival is 87 per cent.

A total of 80 patients surviving palliative procedures from UCLA and referring institutions underwent later interventions at UCLA based on our classification system. Nineteen of these patients underwent partial biventricular repair with a bidirectional cavopulmonary shunt. Three deaths occured in this group. Twenty-two of these patients underwent Fontan operations as a later intervention. Two early deaths and one late death occurred after discharge. Actuarial survival in this total group is 96 per cent at 1 year, 89 per cent at 5 years, and 83 per cent at 10 years. Our clinical experience with the aorta-to-right ventricle shunt is limited (eight patients), and the long-term patency and function of these grafts remains to be determined.

PA/IVS remains a formidable congenital heart defect that requires surgical intervention early in life. In the neonate with PA/IVS, we have found that surgical classification of right ventricular hypoplasia into mild (greater than two-thirds of normal) moderate (one-third to two-thirds of normal) and severe (less than one-third of normal) is useful in selecting a surgical approach. In older children, a similar classification is used, and patients are stratified into those who will benefit from an attempt to achieve a biventricular repair and those who are best suited to a Fontan procedure. By using this approach, the surgical mortality and morbidity has been markedly reduced, and long-term survival has been excellent.

FURTHER READING

Pulmonary stenosis

Hanley, F.L., Sade, R.M., Blackstone, E.H., *et al.* 1993. Outcomes in neonatal pulmonary atresia with intact ventricular septum: a multiinstitutional study. *Journal of Thoracic and Cardiovascular Surgery* **105**, 406.

Kan, J.S., White, R.I., Mitchell, S.E., Gardner, T.J. 1982. Percutaneous balloon valvuloplasty: a new method for treating congenital pulmonary stenosis. *New England Journal of Medicine* **307**, 540.

Polansky, D.B., Clark, E.B., Doty, D.B. 1985. Pulmonary stenosis in infants and young children. *Annals of Thoracic Surgery* **39**, 159.

Pulmonary atresia with intact ventricular septum

Laks, H., Gates, R.N., Grant, P.W., *et al.* 1995. Aortic to right ventricular shunt for pulmonary atresia and intact ventricular septum. *Annals of Thoracic Surgery* **59**, 342.

Laks, H., Pearl, J.M., Drinkwater, D.C., *et al.* 1992. Partial biventricular repair of pulmonary atresia with intact ventricular septum. Use of an adjustable atrial septal defect. *Circulation* **86(suppl II)**, 159.

Laks, H., Plunkett, M.D. 1998. Pulmonary stenosis and pulmonary atresia with intact septum. In Kaiser, L.R., Kron, I.L., Spray, T.L. (eds), *Mastery of cardiothoracic surgery*. Philadelphia: Lippincott-Raven Publishers, 805–18.

51

Left ventricular outflow tract obstruction

ROSS M. UNGERLEIDER MD
Professor of Surgery, Chief, Pediatric Cardiac Surgery, Section of Pediatric Cardiac Surgery, Doernbecher Children's Hospital, Oregon Health Sciences University, Portland, Oregon, USA

IRVING SHEN MD
Assistant Professor of Surgery, Section of Pediatric Cardiac Surgery, Doernbecher Children's Hospital, Oregon Health Sciences University, Portland, Oregon, USA

Left ventricular outflow tract obstruction (LVOTO) can be caused by a spectrum of lesions that obstruct the flow of blood from the left ventricle into the aorta. The site of obstruction is often classified anatomically as valvular, subvalvular, or supravalvular. Although these lesions usually occur separately, patients can present with combinations of the anatomic varieties. In this chapter, common presentations of LVOTO are considered, and the surgical management is discussed.

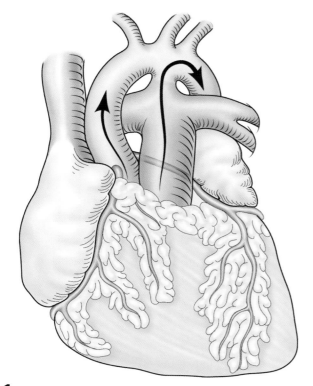

CRITICAL AORTIC STENOSIS OF THE NEONATE

1 Aortic stenosis in the newborn is a very serious defect. In contrast to aortic stenosis in adults, which can be followed for years as it progresses toward the need for intervention, aortic stenosis in neonates presents as an acute, life-threatening problem. The anatomy of the aortic valve leaflets can be very abnormal, ranging from bicuspid, with fusion of the commissures, to unicuspid, with an eccentrically located orifice and no obvious discernible commissural fusion. The valve annulus is usually small and produces a significant component of the stenosis. Because left ventricular outflow is restricted, systemic perfusion is impaired. In severe cases, perfusion to the body requires right-to-left shunting across a patent ductus arteriosus; thus, critical aortic stenosis of the newborn can be considered a 'ductal dependent' lesion.

Ductal dependent systemic perfusion explains why some infants may present *in extremis* shortly after birth when the ductus arteriosus closes. Left heart failure and poor cardiac output result in decreased systemic perfusion, delayed capillary refill, and severe metabolic acidosis. When they present, these infants are usually tachypneic to compensate for their metabolic acidosis. All their peripheral pulses are thready, in contrast to infants with aortic coarctation where the pulses are usually strong in the right arm. These critically ill infants appear ashen 'grey' and need immediate intensive resuscitation and simultaneous diagnostic workup. Infants with less severe LVOTO may present in the first few weeks of life with less acute left heart failure, irritability, and failure to thrive.

DIAGNOSIS OF AORTIC STENOSIS

Echocardiography is the single most useful diagnostic modality to establish the diagnosis. A parasternal long-axis view demonstrates a small aortic valve annulus (usually 4–6 mm) with abnormal or thickened valve leaflets. A minor axis view may help define the anatomy of the valve leaflets as being bicuspid or unicuspid. The left ventricle usually is dilated and has decreased contractile function. Echocardiography is also useful in estimating left ventricular size and whether other commonly associated cardiac anomalies are present. Hypoplasia of the left ventricle, where the echocardiographic measured cross-sectional area of the left ventricle is less than 2 cm^2, is associated with increased operative mortality after aortic valvotomy. Other associated anomalies include mitral stenosis (mitral valve annulus diameter less than 9 mm in a normal size infant), endocardial fibroelastosis of the left ventricle (signifying severe subendocardial ischemia with fibrosis of the left ventricular endocardium), aortic coarctation, and atrial or ventricular septal defect. The combination of many of these left-sided outflow obstructions defines Shone's Complex. A ductus arteriosus may be present; and if the patient has been started on prostaglandin E$_1$, knowing whether the ductus is patent is helpful.

Cardiac catheterization to gain additional anatomic information is seldom necessary. Measurement of the gradient across the valve is not useful, because in severely ill patients, the greatly reduced cardiac output may not generate a gradient commensurate with the severity of the LVOTO. However, when the left ventricle appears small on echocardiography, cardiac catheterization can provide a measurement of left ventricular volume. A left ventricular end-diastolic volume of less than 20 mL/m^2 is associated with increased risk of mortality after surgical aortic valvotomy.

PREOPERATIVE MANAGEMENT OF AORTIC STENOSIS

Management requires simultaneous resuscitative measures to stabilize these very ill patients and diagnostic efforts to define the anatomic abnormalities. Resuscitation requires management in the intensive care unit with central venous and arterial access, endotracheal intubation and mechanical ventilation to reduce the concomitant pulmonary hypertension, initiation of prostaglandin E$_1$ infusion to open or maintain ductal patency, and inotropic support. The patient should be sedated to minimize overall body oxygen consumption. Arterial blood gases should be monitored, and acidosis or hypoxia should be corrected to ensure adequate tissue oxygen delivery.

Indications for surgery for aortic stenosis

Neonates with critical aortic stenosis should be treated with urgency. Once they are stabilized and anatomic diagnosis has been established, therapeutic options are considered to formulate a treatment plan. Treatment should be initiated without delay. Neonates with critical aortic stenosis and adequate left ventricular volume (echocardiographic measured left ventricular cross-sectional area greater than 2 cm^2 or calculated left ventricular end-diastolic volume greater than 20 mL/m^2 based on cineangiographic measurements) should proceed with balloon or surgical valvotomy. If the left ventricular volume is inadequate or if the aortic stenosis is part of the hypoplastic left heart syndrome, these patients eventually may need to be staged to a Fontan procedure. Patients with less severe aortic stenosis, who present weeks to months after birth, can be treated more electively depending on the degree of LVOTO and whether they have important associated defects.

OPERATION

Valvular aortic stenosis

If the infant has 'isolated' valvular aortic stenosis without a significant associated defect, the treatment is to enlarge the aortic valve opening. This goal can be achieved either by catheter-based balloon valvotomy or by surgical open valvotomy. Results with balloon valvotomy have improved in recent years, and nonoperative dilation is becoming the preferred technique at many institutions. Surgical open valvotomy is rarely performed on infants with critical aortic stenosis.

A few approaches are available for open aortic valvotomy. Some centers prefer to employ inflow occlusion with open valvotomy without the use of cardiopulmonary bypass. This is performed by occluding the superior and inferior cavae with snares for a few cardiac cycles to allow the heart to empty. The aorta is then cross-clamped, a longitudinal aortotomy is made, and the appropriate valvotomy is performed. The aortotomy is then secured with a side-biting clamp, and the aortic cross-clamp and caval snares are removed. This technique allows the heart to reperfuse while the aortotomy is being repaired. Because this procedure requires speed and experience and subjects a compromised heart to added stress, we do not routinely employ this technique for open valvotomy.

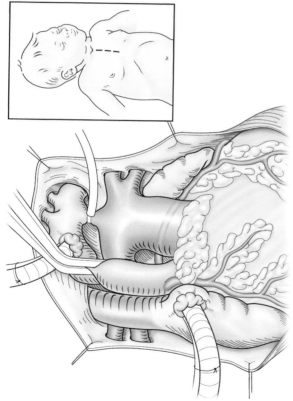

2 Our technique of open valvotomy employs cardiopulmonary bypass. The heart is approached through a median sternotomy. After systemic heparinization, the patient is cannulated for cardiopulmonary bypass with an arterial cannula in the distal ascending aorta and a single venous cannula in the right atrium. Shortly after inception of cardiopulmonary bypass, the patent ductus arteriosus, if one is present, should be temporarily occluded with a snare. Mild hypothermia (32° to 34°C) is employed. The aorta is cross-clamped, and the heart is arrested with antegrade cold blood cardioplegia. A transverse aortotomy is made to gain access to the aortic valve. Rewarming on bypass can begin immediately after the aorta is cross-clamped.

2

3–6 The stenotic aortic valve is inspected carefully, and the areas of commissural fusion are identified. In some patients, inserting a small cardiotomy sucker through the valve orifice can facilitate inspection of the stenotic aortic valve. The fused commissures are divided with a No. 11 scalpel blade. The incision should extend toward, but not into, the annulus to minimize postvalvotomy aortic insufficiency. Moderate to severe aortic insufficiency is poorly tolerated and leads to early valve replacement more often than mild residual stenosis. After performing the valvotomy, the aortotomy is repaired with a single line of continuous suture, the aortic cross-clamp is removed, and the patient is weaned from cardiopulmonary bypass. The ductus arteriosus should be ligated if the patient is stable. However, if the left ventricular output is inadequate even on aggressive inotropic support, the ductus can be left open and maintained patent on a prostaglandin E$_1$ infusion during the early postoperative period. This maneuver allows additional systemic perfusion from the right ventricle through the ductus.

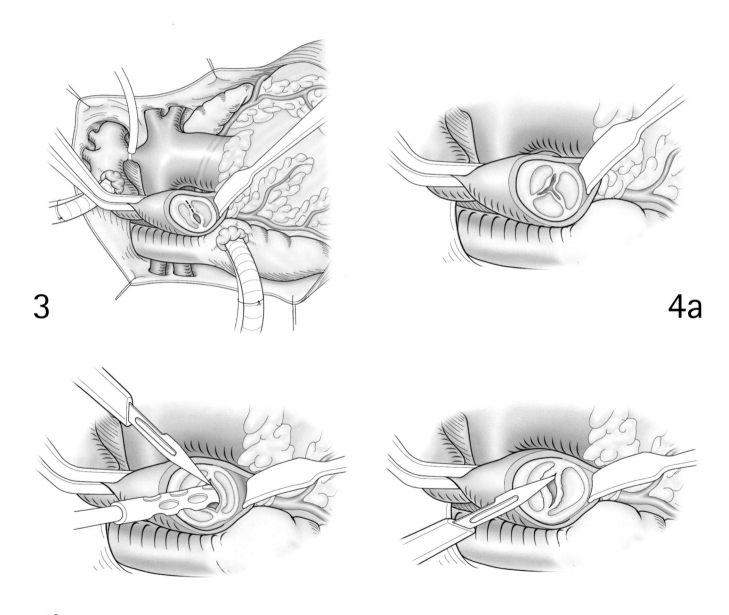

3

4a

4b

5

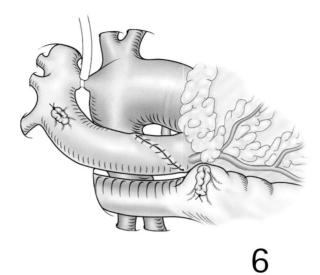

6

POSTOPERATIVE MANAGEMENT AFTER AORTIC VALVOTOMY

After surgical aortic valvotomy, infants may remain critically ill and require inotropic support for several days. The left ventricle may have significant diastolic dysfunction that leads to decreased ventricular filling and low cardiac output. This syndrome is manifested by tachycardia with marginal distal perfusion. Pulmonary hypertension can be managed by maintaining adequate oxygenation and respiratory alkalosis. In some extreme cases, the patient may require prostaglandin E_1 infusion to assist with distal perfusion.

Most infants with a properly performed aortic valvotomy and an adequate size left ventricle should improve over several days. The heart rate decreases as left ventricular compliance improves and allows an increase in stroke volume to maintain cardiac output. Prostaglandin can be stopped, and inotropes can be weaned. Ventilation can be normalized, and the patient can be removed from mechanical ventilatory support and allowed to begin oral feeding. Echocardiography demonstrates improved flow across the aortic valve, and there may actually be an increase in left ventricular outflow gradient compared to preoperatively as cardiac output across the aortic valve increases. A mild amount of aortic insufficiency is not uncommon if the valvotomy was adequate. The patient's clinical course is more important than these echocardiographic findings as long as the clinical course is one of continued improvement and progress. If the patient is not progressing through an expected course of convalescence, then further diagnostic tests must be performed to evaluate the importance of other associated defects. A large ventricular septal defect may require closure or pulmonary artery banding. Severe aortic coarctation may exist although it may not have been apparent when the ductus was maintained patent with prostaglandin E_1. If the valvotomy is inadequate, the patient needs repeat valvotomy or aortic valve replacement.

OUTCOME AFTER AORTIC VALVOTOMY

Complications of aortic valvotomy are few. Mild aortic insufficiency is common, but usually well tolerated. If the aortic annulus is small or if the valve is extremely dysplastic, the infant may have persistent severe LVOTO after the valvotomy. The infant can be treated by repeat valvotomy or by aortic valve replacement. Dissection of the aorta during advancement of balloon catheters has been encountered and may require surgical treatment. Local vascular complications at the insertion site of the balloon catheters can lead to pulse loss in the leg, but this problem can be treated with thrombolytic agents, often with good resolution.

The majority of infants with critical aortic stenosis benefit from open or balloon valvotomy and can be discharged from the hospital. However, aortic valvotomy is only palliative because the aortic valve remains anatomically abnormal in these patients. Eventually, all patients probably will require aortic valve replacement. For infants and children, the preferred choice for aortic valve replacement is the pulmonary autograft unless they have a contraindication for using their pulmonary valve.

OPERATION

Aortic valve replacement in infants

7, 8 Using the pulmonary autograft for pediatric aortic valve replacement (Ross procedure) is attractive because the valve has the potential to grow with the patient. The procedure is conducted through a median sternotomy and moderate hypothermic cardiopulmonary bypass. A single venous cannula can be used, although the authors prefer bicaval cannulation for venous drainage. A left ventricular vent is extremely helpful and administration of cardioplegia through the retrograde fashion protects the myocardium during the procedure. After cross-clamping the aorta, the aorta is transected at the level of the sinotubular junction. The aortic valve is inspected, and once a decision has been made that the valve is not repairable, the pulmonary valve is harvested to use for replacement. The main pulmonary artery is transected just proximal to the bifurcation of the right and left pulmonary artery. The pulmonary valve is inspected to ensure no abnormality exists. By pulling the main pulmonary artery anteriorly, the posterior investment of the valve is dissected free from the right ventricular muscle. A right-angle clamp is then placed across the pulmonary valve and used to identify the spot on the anterior right ventricular wall just inferior to the nadir of one of the sinuses. This opening is carefully extended in both directions around the base of the pulmonary valve in order not to damage the valve leaflets. A dissection plane usually develops along the posterior aspect of the valve where the region of previous posterior dissection is encountered; staying in this plane prevents deep incision into the interventricular septum and injury to the first septal perforating branch of the left descending coronary artery.

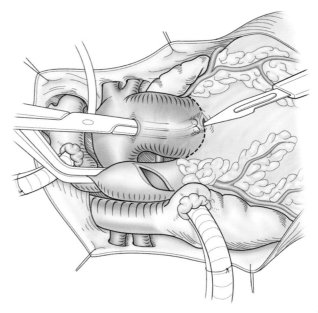

7

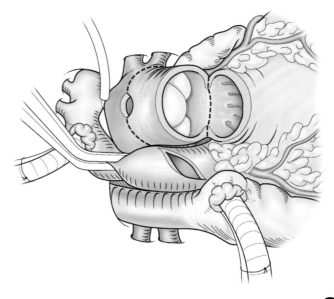

8

9–12

After harvesting the pulmonary valve, the coronary arteries are removed as buttons with a large amount of adjacent sinus wall. The aortic valve leaflets and the excess aortic wall tissue are removed. The pulmonary autograft is then sutured to the left ventricular outflow tract opening using continuous or interrupted sutures. Orientation of the autograft in such a way that the coronary buttons can be situated in the sinuses of the autograft without excessive tension or kinking is important. After the proximal suture line is completed, the left coronary artery is anastomosed to an appropriate portion on the posterior wall of the autograft. The autograft is then anastomosed to the distal aorta using a continuous suture. After completing the distal anastomosis, the neoaortic root can be distended with a dose of cardioplegia solution to allow determination of the most appropriate position for placement of the right coronary artery button. Marking the location of the commissures on the outside of the autograft is often helpful before completing the distal suture line to prevent inadvertent injury to the valve leaflet during implantation of the right coronary button.

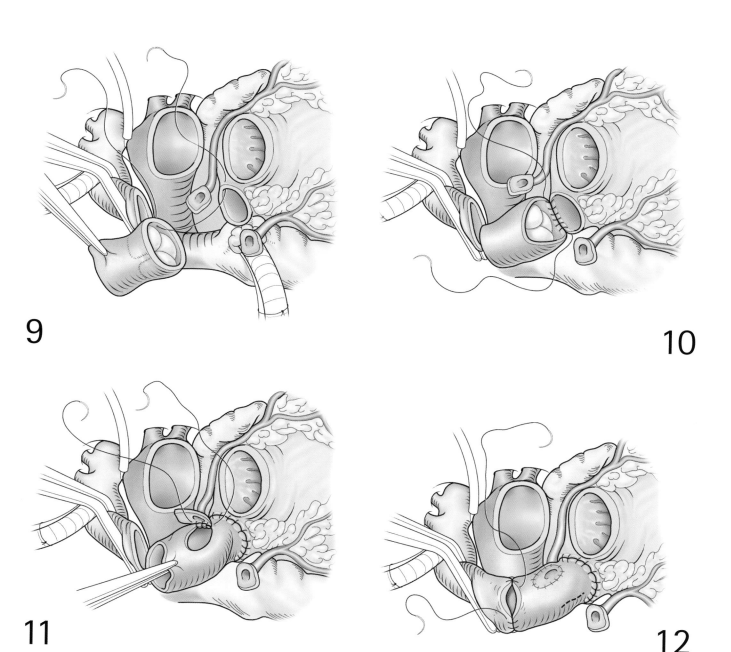

9

10

11

12

13 During the implantation of the autograft, an appropriate size cryopreserved pulmonary homograft is selected and thawed to use for reconstructing the right ventricular outflow. Performing the distal anastomosis first using a continuous suture is usually easiest. The proximal suture line is then performed, and air is evacuated from the right side of the heart before completing the suture line.

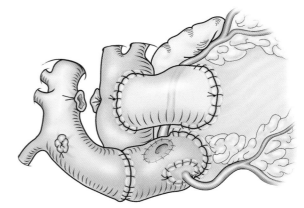

13

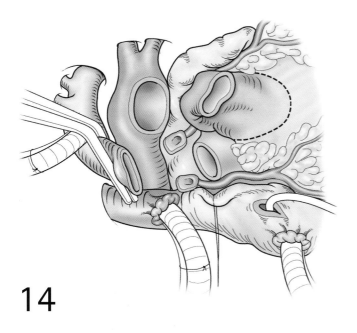

14

14 Occasions exist, especially in neonates, in which significant LVOTO is caused by annular or subannular narrowing. In these circumstances, an aortoventriculoplasty is performed to enlarge the left ventricular outflow tract in addition to valve replacement using a pulmonary autograft, an aortic homograft, or a mechanical valve. Currently, our preference is to incorporate the aortoventriculoplasty with the Ross procedure (Ross-Konno procedure). This procedure is performed using moderate hypothermic cardiopulmonary bypass through a median sternotomy. Protection of the myocardium using intermittent retrograde coronary sinus cardioplegia perfusion is extremely useful. After cross-clamping the aorta and arresting the heart, the ascending aorta is transected at the level of the sinotubular junction. After examining the aortic and pulmonary valves, the pulmonary autograft and the coronary artery buttons are harvested. For the Ross-Konno procedure, extra tissue is harvested from the anterior right ventricular free wall with the pulmonary autograft. This extra tissue is used to repair the ventricular septal defect resulting from performing the aortoventriculoplasty.

15–17 A perpendicular incision is then made from the transverse aortotomy down toward the commissure between the right and left coronary artery. This incision is carried into the interventricular septum creating a ventricular septal defect. The pulmonary autograft is then sutured to the base of the aortic annulus using a continuous suture. The pulmonary autograft is oriented in such a way so that the extra right ventricular free wall tissue is placed anteriorly to close over the ventricular septal defect. After reattaching the coronary artery buttons to the pulmonary autograft, the distal end is anastomosed to the transected aorta using a continuous suture. Finally, the right ventricular outflow tract is reconstructed with an appropriate size pulmonary homograft. A gusset using extra pulmonary artery tissue from the homograft or a Gore-Tex patch may be needed for the proximal anastomosis of the pulmonary homograft to the right ventricle, although this maneuver is frequently not necessary in neonates and infants.

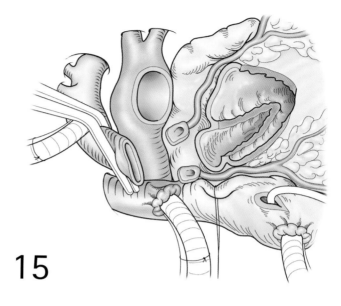

15

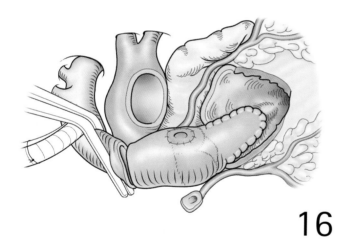

16

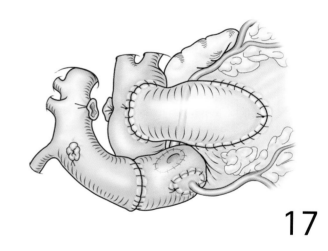

17

Success with the pulmonary autograft procedure has led many authorities to recommend aortic valve replacement for any child with critical aortic stenosis, and some use this procedure in lieu of aortic valvotomy. However, many infants with critical aortic stenosis not only survive a simple balloon valvotomy, but thrive and live for years before aortic valve replacement is necessary. Therefore, despite the attractiveness and success of the pulmonary autograft procedure, we recommend reserving aortic valve replacement for those patients in whom it is the only or distinctly the best option for survival. The pulmonary autograft procedure is contraindicated if the patient has collagen vascular disease, rheumatic heart disease, or abnormality of the pulmonary valve. We have also encountered a patient with an anomalous origin of the left descending coronary artery from the right coronary artery crossing the right ventricular outflow tract near the pulmonary valve annulus, in whom harvesting the pulmonary valve was not possible. Patients with conal septal ventricular septal defect and aortic insufficiency may not have adequate muscle under the pulmonary valve to allow for safe harvest of the pulmonary valve. In these cases, it may be more prudent to replace the aortic valve with a homograft than to attempt using an autograft.

As new 'tissue-engineered' valves become clinically available, some advantage may exist in using homografts, rather than autografts, for infant aortic valve replacement with the plan to replace these with adult-size tissue engineered valves at a subsequent setting. This strategy preserves the pulmonary valve. The use of mechanical valves in children has limited application owing to the long-term complications from anticoagulation and limitations in lifestyle.

OUTCOME AFTER AORTIC VALVE REPLACEMENT

Outcome after aortic valve replacement using pulmonary autograft is less than 2 per cent mortality with good long-term functional results. Greater than 90 per cent of patients should still have a functioning autograft 15 years after implantation. The need to replace the pulmonary homograft depends on the size inserted as much as the duration of follow-up, but the need for replacement should also be approximately 10 per cent at 15 years.

SUBVALVULAR AORTIC STENOSIS

The left ventricular outflow tract can also be obstructed by tissue inferior to the aortic valve. The most common form of this obstruction is by a discrete ridge of fibromuscular tissue or membrane located within a few millimeters below the aortic valve annulus. This shelf of tissue extends in a counter-clockwise direction from the membranous septum around the muscular septum to the region of the mitral valve below the commissure that separates the left and the non-coronary leaflet. Usually, the aortic valve itself is normal, although the turbulence created by the subvalvular stenosis may result in some degree of valvular insufficiency.

DIAGNOSIS OF SUBVALVULAR AORTIC STENOSIS

These patients usually present beyond the neonatal period and commonly after 2 years of age. They have decreased exercise capacity and a classic systolic crescendo-decrescendo murmur on physical examination. Echocardiography usually demonstrates the subvalvular ridge with turbulent flow beginning at the level inferior to the aortic valve. Doppler measurements of the LVOTO can quantify the gradient. Some of these patients also have mild to moderate degrees of aortic insufficiency. A cardiac catheterization is usually not necessary because echocardiography is diagnostic and displays the anatomy of the defect quite well.

INDICATIONS FOR SURGERY FOR SUBVALVULAR STENOSIS

Indications for surgery are controversial. The presence of subvalvular stenosis eventually leads to compromised aortic valve function, but this fact cannot be proven aside from individual patient experiences. Nevertheless, a discreet subvalvular stenosis should be resected if the gradient is greater than 30–40 mm Hg or if the patient develops new aortic insufficiency compared to previous echocardiograms.

OPERATION

Subvalvular aortic stenosis

18–21 Discrete subaortic stenosis is best treated by resection of the fibromuscular ridge through a median sternotomy on cardiopulmonary bypass and moderate hypothermia. A left ventricular vent placed through the right superior pulmonary vein is helpful during the procedure. The heart is arrested and protected with a dose of antegrade cardioplegic solution given after cross-clamping the distal ascending aorta. The aortic valve is exposed through a transverse or oblique aortotomy, and the aortic leaflets are retracted to expose the fibromuscular ridge. Extreme caution must be exercised so that the aortic valve leaflets are not damaged during the resection. This maneuver is particularly challenging in patients with bicuspid aortic valves. The fibromuscular ridge is excised sharply starting from the area near the membranous septum and working in a counter-clockwise fashion toward the region of the commissure that separates the left and the non-coronary leaflet. The location of the conduction tissue near the membranous septum should be identified, and deep incision in this region must be avoided. After excising the ridge, performing a septal myectomy by sharply excising a wedge of muscle from the interventricular septum below the right and left coronary leaflet is beneficial. Many surgeons believe that adding this septal myectomy improves outcome and reduces the likelihood for recurrence.

Complications of this procedure include creation of heart block, ventricular septal defect, and aortic insufficiency owing to injury to the aortic valve leaflet. Recurrence is reported in as many as 15–20 per cent of patients and may be reduced by adding a septal myectomy to the resection of the membrane. When a ventricular septal defect is created as a complication of the procedure, the VSD can be easily recognized on the postrepair intraoperative echocardiogram. Repair of such a ventricular septal defect has a high risk of concomitant complete heart block. In patients with significant aortic insufficiency and subvalvular stenosis, resection of the subaortic ridge can be performed as a part of the pulmonary autograft replacement of the aortic valve. If the major component of outflow obstruction is caused by subvalvular pathology, performing an aortoventriculoplasty and replacing the aortic valve with an autograft or an aortic homograft can enlarge the left ventricular outflow tract substantially.

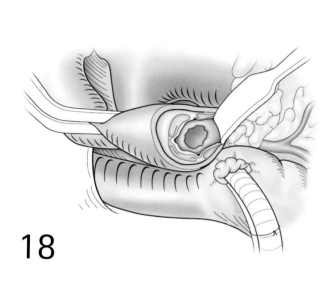

18

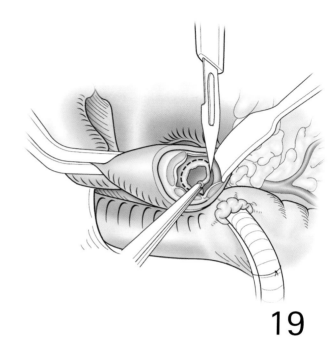

19

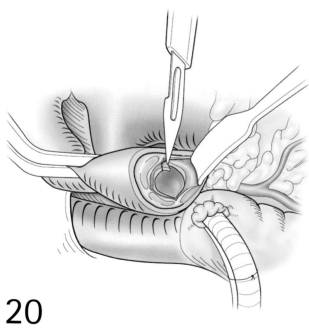

20

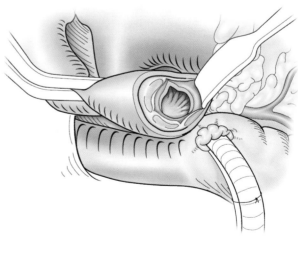

21

OUTCOMES FOR SUBVALVULAR AORTIC STENOSIS

Although operative mortality for resection of a subaortic membrane approaches zero per cent, the risk of recurrent subaortic stenosis can approach 20 per cent, especially when the resection is performed in patients under 3 years of age. Complete heart block requiring implantation of a permanent pacing system is a real risk of the procedure. Aortic valve pathology is also common with the presence of a bicuspid aortic valve or thickening of the leaflets, presumably from the turbulent subvalvular flow. For these reasons, many of these patients may eventually need aortic valve replacement later in life.

SUPRAVALVULAR AORTIC STENOSIS

LVOTO can be a result of a discreet or diffuse narrowing of the supravalvular aorta. This form of obstruction is uncommon and can be part of Williams Syndrome, which includes elfin features, mental retardation, and failure to thrive. Congenital discrete supravalvular narrowing usually occurs at the level of the sinotubular junction, and variable amounts of intimal thickening can create an internal shelf similar to aortic coarctation. The aortic valve leaflets are usually normal in this lesion, although mild thickening occasionally can occur. Discrete narrowing in other parts of the ascending aorta can be due to complication from previous cardiac surgery (at prior aortic cannulation site) or from intimal disruption after interventional catheterization. An isolated diffuse form of supravalvular aortic stenosis is less common, and can extend throughout the length of the ascending aorta and even into the aortic arch. Supravalvular aortic stenosis, whether in the discrete or the diffuse form, imposes an increased afterload to the left ventricle. This lesion most often presents later in childhood and is rarely seen in neonates and young infants.

Diagnosis of supravalvular aortic stenosis

Diagnosis might be suggested by echocardiography, but cardiac catheterization is usually necessary to fully delineate the features of the lesion. In the diffuse form, the entire ascending aorta, transverse arch, and descending aorta can be narrowed. In these patients, there is often narrowing of the branch pulmonary arteries. The discrete form usually presents with an intimal shelf at the sinotubular junction, although stenosis can be found in the distal ascending aorta if it is related to previous aortic cannulation or in the mid ascending aorta if it is related to intimal injury from catheterization. Whereas an angiogram can delineate the nature of the obstruction, pressure measurements can quantify its physiological significance.

INDICATIONS FOR SURGERY OF SUPRAVALVULAR AORTIC STENOSIS

The presence of discrete supravalvular stenosis with a pressure gradient greater than 30 mm Hg is probably an indication for surgery. Patients with lesser gradients, but who exhibit echocardiographic signs of left ventricular hypertrophy, can also be referred for surgical correction. In the diffuse form of the defect, surgical repair is more extensive, and good results are less likely. Therefore, the indications for repair of the diffuse form need to be individualized for each patient.

OPERATION

Supravalvular aortic stenosis

Surgical approach to the discrete form of supravalvular aortic stenosis requires cardiopulmonary bypass with aortic cannulation in the distal ascending aorta beyond the area of stenosis. If the area of stenosis is high in the ascending aorta, then it may be necessary to cannulate the iliac or femoral artery for cardiopulmonary bypass. If the patient is too small for groin cannulation, then the ascending aorta can be cannulated, and the repair is performed under a period of deep hypothermic circulatory arrest during which time the aortic cannula can be removed.

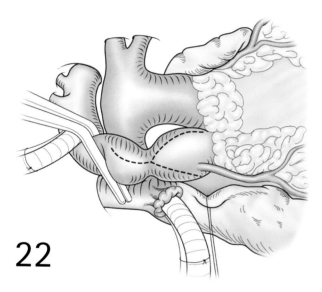

22

22–24 The heart is protected with hypothermic cardioplegic arrest after cross-clamping the distal ascending aorta. A longitudinal aortotomy is made across the area of stenosis and extends into the non-coronary sinus of Valsalva. Typically, another incision is made branching off from the initial aortotomy incision at the area of the tightest stenosis and extending into the right coronary sinus on the opposite side of the right coronary artery. We do not recommend routine excision of the intimal shelf because this procedure may weaken the integrity of the aortic wall and can lead to aneurysmal formation in the future. Most surgeons recommend placing either a generous piece of prosthetic or homograft patch on the ascending aorta to enlarge the narrowed area. In the typical situation in which the obstruction is at the sinotubular junction, the patch should be 'pantaloon' shaped and extends into the right and non-coronary sinuses. The diffuse form of supravalvular aortic stenosis is most commonly repaired by suturing a generous piece of homograft or polytetraflouroethylene (Gore-Tex) patch from the sinotubular junction all the way around the aortic arch using a period of deep hypothermic circulatory arrest. If the descending aorta needs to be enlarged, this procedure is more easily accomplished through a left thoracotomy with placement of an additional patch.

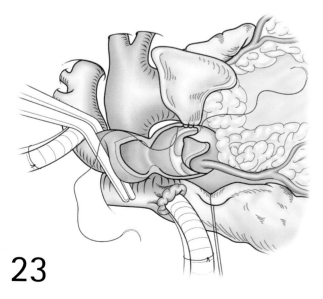

23

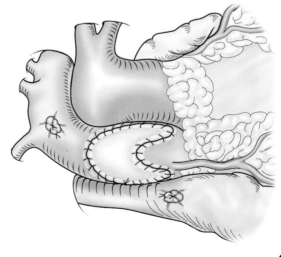

24

OUTCOME OF SUPRAVALVULAR AORTIC STENOSIS

Few complications occur after repair of the discrete form of supravalvular LVOTO. However, bleeding from the suture line in the aortic sinuses is a risk to which the surgeon should be aware of. As with any procedure on the ascending aorta, a risk of air or particulate embolism exists resulting in a stroke. The risks of repair for the diffuse form are similar, although probably at greater risk of bleeding due to the more extensive suture line and the longer period of hypothermic circulatory arrest.

FURTHER READING

Elkins, R.C., Knott-Craig, C.J., Ward, K.E., *et al.* 1994. Pulmonary autograft in children: realized growth potential. *Annals of Thoracic Surgery* 57, 1387–94.

Gaynor J.W., Bull C., Sullivan I.D., *et al.* 1995. Late outcome of survivors of intervention for neonatal aortic valve stenosis. *Annals of Thoracic Surgery* 60, 122–6.

Hawkins J.A., Minich L., Tani L.Y., *et al.* 1998. Late results and reintervention after aortic valvotomy for critical aortic stenosis in neonates and infants. *Annals of Thoracic Surgery* 65, 1758–62.

Rayburn S.T., Netherland D.E., Heath B.J. 1997. Discrete membranous subaortic stenosis: improved results after resection and myectomy. *Annals of Thoracic Surgery* 64, 105–9.

Reddy V.M., Rajasinghe H.A., Teitel D.F., *et al.* 1996. Aortoventriculoplasty with the pulmonary autograft: the 'Ross-Konno' procedure. *Journal of Thoracic and Cardiovascular Surgery* 111, 158–65.

Stamm C., Kreutzer C., Zurakowski J., *et al.* 1999. Forty-one years of surgical experience with congenital supravalvular aortic stenosis. *Journal of Thoracic and Cardiovascular Surgery* 118, 874–85.

52

Transposition of the great arteries with left-or-right ventricular outflow tract obstruction

CHRISTO I. TCHERVENKOV MD
Professor of Surgery, McGill University Faculty of Medicine; Director of Cardiovascular Surgery, The Montreal Children's Hospital, Montreal, Quebec, Canada

STEPHEN J. KORKOLA MD
Chief Resident, Cardiovascular Surgery, The Montreal Children's Hospital, McGill University Health Center, Montreal, Canada

HISTORY

Since successfully performed by Jatene in 1975, the arterial switch operation (ASO) has become the procedure of choice for d-transposition of the great arteries (TGA) with intact ventricular septum (IVS) and with ventricular septal defect (VSD). However, the presence of left ventricular (LV) or right ventricular (RV) outflow obstruction may complicate attempts at ASO or even preclude its use. The presence of significant fixed LV outflow tract obstruction (LVOTO) is usually a contraindication to ASO, as the subpulmonic area becomes the subaortic area after ASO. On the other hand, RV outflow tract obstruction (RVOTO) or subaortic obstruction (SAO) is frequently associated with aortic arch obstruction (AAO) in patients with TGA. After ASO, the aortic arch remains in the systemic circulation, whereas the subaortic area becomes the subpulmonary area. Therefore, residual AAO is a problem faced by the left heart, whereas preoperative SAO is a problem faced by the right heart and the pulmonary circulation after ASO. This chapter details surgical techniques that have been devised to achieve anatomical repair with these complex variants of TGA.

Left ventricular outflow tract obstruction

LVOTO can be dynamic or fixed and can be valvar, subvalvar, or both. Dynamic LVOTO is more common in patients with TGA-IVS and results from bowing of the interventricular septum into the left ventricular outflow tract (LVOT) of the low-pressure LV due to the systemic pressure in the RV. This obstruction may be exacerbated by abnormal systolic motion of the anterior leaflet of the mitral valve. This situation is still amenable to anatomical correction by the ASO in the absence of valvar pulmonary stenosis, as the dynamic obstruction corrects itself when the LV is connected to the systemic circulation. On the other hand, fixed forms of LVOTO, particularly in the presence of an abnormal pulmonary valve, may prohibit surgical correction by ASO. Fixed forms of LVOTO occur more commonly in TGA-VSD and may be subvalvar, valvar, or both. Posterior malalignment of the infundibular septum, fibromuscular bands or shelves, abnormal chordal insertions of the atrioventricular (AV) valves into the LVOT, and prolapsing of AV valve tissue through the VSD may all contribute, alone or in combination, to fixed LVOTO at the subvalvar level. In addition, valvar pulmonary stenosis or atresia may exist.

The Rastelli operation was designed to allow anatomical correction of patients with TGA-VSD and LVOTO by connecting the LV to the aorta. The procedure involves the creation of an intraventricular tunnel from the LV to the aorta through the VSD. The proximal main pulmonary artery (PA) and valve are oversewn, and RV-to-PA continuity is re-established with the use of a valved conduit, such as a pulmonary homograft. Because of concerns with the almost certain need for reoperation due to conduit obstruction in survivors of the Rastelli operation, Lecompte and associates modified the original procedure by connecting the RV to the PA without an extracardiac conduit. This so-called REV (réparation à l'étage ventriculaire) operation consists of the creation of a straight intraventricular tunnel from the VSD to the aorta, facilitated by the resection of the infundibular septum. After transection of the ascending aorta, the distal PA confluence is brought anterior to the aorta and sutured directly to the distal end of the ventriculotomy incision. The Rastelli operation and the subsequent Lecompte modification remain the procedures of choice for TGA-VSD and fixed LVOTO.

Patients with TGA-IVS and severe fixed LVOTO present a formidable surgical challenge in the absence of a VSD to allow for anatomical correction. We have successfully used the approach of creating a VSD in the subaortic area, followed by the Rastelli operation, which is then performed in the standard fashion. In cases in which the LVOTO is caused by accessory tissue, redundancy, or abnormal insertions of the mitral valve, mitral valve repair may be performed with an ASO. The shift in the interventricular septum towards the RV after the ASO further opens up the subaortic area.

Right ventricular outflow tract obstruction

RVOTO or SAO is rare in patients with TGA-IVS, but these problems may occur in 20–40 per cent of patients with TGA-VSD. These abnormalities are particularly common in patients with an anterior malalignment type of VSD. Whereas SAO is usually secondary to anterior malalignment of the infundibular septum itself, hypertrophied septoparietal trabeculations, prominent ventriculoinfundibular fold, and abnormal insertions of the AV valves into the right ventricular outflow tract (RVOT) may contribute as well. SAO may lead to preferential streaming of blood flow through the PA and patent ductus arteriosus during fetal life, leading to underdevelopment of the aortic arch such as tubular hypoplasia, coarctation of the aorta (CoA), or an interrupted aortic arch. Subaortic stenosis is usually still amenable to correction by the ASO, as this area becomes the subpulmonary area. Frequently, at the time of ASO, all that is required is direct resection of the obstructing muscle, followed by a pericardial patch augmentation of the RVOT incision after the VSD closure. In the presence of AAO, we advocate a single-stage ASO, VSD closure, and pulmonary homograft patch aortoplasty of the aortic arch. This approach results in anatomical repair and complete relief of any obstruction in the systemic circulation.

PRINCIPLES AND JUSTIFICATION

Rastelli operation

Current short- and long-term results with the ASO have been excellent, making it the procedure of choice in cases of TGA-VSD with LVOTO, when the obstruction is mild and amenable to primary resection. As mentioned, ASO is also the procedure of choice in dynamic forms of LVOTO that resolve when the LV is connected to the systemic circulation. However, when the LVOTO is fixed and diffuse and the pulmonary valve is stenotic, the Rastelli operation is the procedure of choice. Patients with TGA-VSD and LVOTO have traditionally been palliated with a systemic-PA shunt and balloon atrial septostomy. This strategy has allowed the child to grow to a size that would allow placement of a larger homograft at the time of the Rastelli operation. However, a palliative approach has certain disadvantages, such as persistent cyanosis and volume overload, that may lead to compromised ventricular function. Furthermore, the shunts may cause significant PA stenoses and/or distortions that subsequently complicate the intracardiac repair. Because of this possibility, we prefer to perform the Rastelli operation in early life as a primary procedure, even in the newborn period if required, consistent with the philosophy of early primary repair at our institution.

Arterial switch operation with aortic arch reconstruction

The surgical importance of AAO in association with TGA has only been appreciated recently. Diagnosing AAO in the form of CoA or interrupted aortic arch is relatively straightforward. However, recognizing the importance of tubular hypoplasia of the aortic arch has been less obvious. Whereas aortic arch hypoplasia is present in 62 per cent of cases of isolated CoA, this anomaly may be present in up to 93 per cent of cases of CoA associated with complex intracardiac defects. If left unrepaired, the residual obstruction in the aortic arch will be faced by a freshly repaired heart, with adverse consequences. Because of this danger, our procedure of choice for TGA-IVS or TGA-VSD with AAO is a single-stage ASO with concomitant aortic arch reconstruction.

Traditionally, these repairs were performed using a staged approach. The first stage involved CoA repair with pulmonary artery banding (PAB), usually performed through a left thoracotomy. This procedure was followed months to years later by debanding of the PA with ASO and intracardiac repair. Each stage, and the interval in-between, has been associated with significant morbidity and mortality. We have obtained superior results using a single-stage anatomical repair with ASO and aortic arch reconstruction in the neonatal period. We advocate the use of PA homograft patch aortoplasty for aortic arch reconstruction, as this procedure satisfies a number of important principles. The patch aortoplasty allows the arch repair to extend proximally and distally as needed to deal with obstruction at multiple levels, corrects the often-marked size discrepancy between the proximal neoaorta and the distal aorta, and allows for a single tension-free anastomosis. The single-stage approach to early repair of TGA with AAO has resulted in very low early and late mortality and recoarctation rate. In recent years, we have been able to perform all the aortic arch reconstructions without the use of deep hypothermic circulatory arrest.

Preoperative evaluation

Preoperative preparation requires a complete understanding of the intracardiac and great vessel anatomy to plan the optimal surgical repair. Although we plan our surgical repair based on the echocardiographic findings in the majority of cases, we insist on cardiac catheterization in some situations. Echocardiography can accurately define the morphology of the LVOTO, the size of the VSD, the location with respect to the great vessels, and the anatomy and size of the PAs. The echocardiogram is also useful to identify any factors that may alter the surgical approach, such as abnormal insertions of the AV valves into the LVOT or RVOT or around the edges of the VSD. Cardiac catheterization may be useful to rule out branch PA stenoses or distortions caused by palliative procedures.

A discussion must take place with the family regarding realistic expected outcomes and possible complications of the proposed surgical intervention. For the Rastelli procedure, early mortality is low in experienced centers, but late morbidity and mortality may be significant. The majority of patients undergoing the Rastelli operation requires reintervention in the future as a result of conduit obstruction. The ASO has enjoyed excellent short- and long-term results in recent years. Although the presence of AAO complicates the intracardiac repair, excellent results can still be anticipated using a single-stage anatomical correction in experienced centers.

ANESTHESIA

Standard principles of cardiovascular anesthesia are followed, but some specific points deserve mention. Neonates with AAO are fully resuscitated and stabilized as necessary in the pediatric intensive care unit (PICU) before coming to the operating room. This management involves the administration of prostaglandins to maintain ductal patency, correction of the metabolic acidosis, and reversal of acute renal failure, if present.

In the operating room, systemic steroids (methylprednisolone 30 mg/kg) are administered just after induction of anesthesia. In recent years, the acid–base management on cardiopulmonary bypass (CPB) has been to use a pH-stat strategy. After the repair and during rewarming, patients are hemoconcentrated to a hematocrit of 36 per cent. These measures have limited the degree of extracellular fluid accumulation associated with CPB.

OPERATIONS

Rastelli operation

1 After median sternotomy, the patient is prepared for cannulation for CPB. Patients are heparinized to achieve an activated clotting time greater than 400 seconds. In the case of a redo sternotomy, the administration of heparin is delayed until many of the adhesions in the pericardial cavity have been carefully taken down and any previously placed shunts have been exposed. In first-time operations, the pericardium is opened, and a piece of autologous pericardium is harvested for later use as a hood to augment the connection between the conduit and the RVOT. The distal ascending aorta is cannulated through a pursestring suture, snared in place, and connected to the arterial line after being deaired. Both vena cavae are cannulated with right angle cannulae and connected to the venous line with a Y-connector. CPB is instituted, followed immediately by ligation of the patent ductus arteriosus, if present, or clamping and division of any systemic-pulmonary shunts. The aorta is cross-clamped, and the vena cavae are then snared around their respective cannulae. Cold crystalloid or blood cardioplegia is administered into the aortic root to arrest the heart. The return from the coronary sinus is collected and discarded through a small right atriotomy incision. A cardiotomy sucker is also placed through this incision, into the left atrium, through an atrial septal defect or patent foramen ovale to decompress the left side of the heart. After a full dose of cardioplegia (30 mL/kg), a vertical incision is made in the RVOT, and a transverse incision is made in the proximal main PA just distal to the pulmonary valve annulus. The pulmonary valve is inspected to verify that it cannot be used as a systemic semilunar valve, thus necessitating a Rastelli operation.

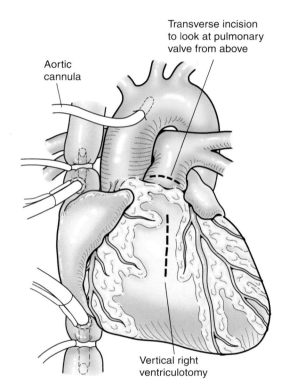

Aortic cannula

Transverse incision to look at pulmonary valve from above

Vertical right ventriculotomy

1

2 The ventriculotomy has been exaggerated for illustrative purposes. Pledgeted stay sutures are placed on the edges of the ventriculotomy to provide traction and aid in exposure. The intracardiac anatomy is then examined carefully. Particular attention is paid to the size and location of the VSD relative to the size and location of the aortic valve annulus. After examining the LVOTO and confirming that a Rastelli repair will be performed, an appropriately sized valved pulmonary homograft is thawed and prepared for later use. If the VSD is smaller than the diameter of the aortic valve annulus, it is enlarged at its leftward and anterior margin by resecting a wedge of the interventricular septum. The VSD can be further enlarged by resection of the infundibular septum.

Patients with IVS and fixed LVOTO may still be candidates for the Rastelli operation by creating a VSD in the subaortic area. An intraventricular tunnel can then be used to baffle the LV blood to the aorta. Similarly, in patients with a VSD remote from the aorta, baffling of LV to aorta is difficult. This VSD can be closed using standard techniques, and a new VSD can be created in a suitable location.

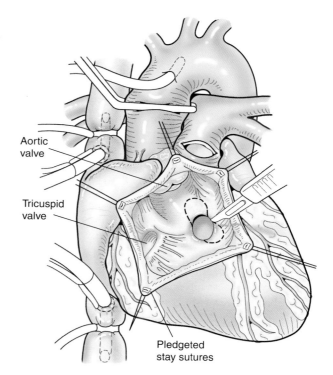

Aortic valve

Tricuspid valve

Pledgeted stay sutures

2

3a, b To create the intracardiac baffle, interrupted sutures of pledgeted 4/0 polyester are placed circumferentially to encompass the VSD and the aortic valve annulus. Superiorly great care is used to run the suture line close to the aortic valve annulus to avoid leaving trabeculations or myocardial crevices, which would result in a residual VSD. Inferiorly near the tricuspid valve, the suture line may need to be into tricuspid valve annulus in the absence of a muscle band. Occasionally, the sutures are placed through the right atrial aspect into the tricuspid valve annulus. Also, along the rightward inferior border of the VSD, the suture line is placed several millimeters away to avoid the conduction system. To decrease the myocardial ischemia time, we have in recent years used a running suturing technique using 4/0, 5/0, or 6/0 polypropylene, depending on the size and age of the patient, reinforcing the extensive suture line in several strategic places with interrupted pledgeted sutures. To create the intracardiac baffle, we prefer to use a 0.6-mm thick Gore-Tex patch (W. L. Gore and Associates, Flagstaff, Arizona, USA). To avoid obstruction through the baffle, the patch is cut with greater width to allow bowing into the RV. The final baffle takes on a semicircular orientation.

The main PA is then transected at the previous incision just above the pulmonary valve annulus, and the pulmonary valve and the PA stump are oversewn in two layers with a 4/0 polypropylene suture.

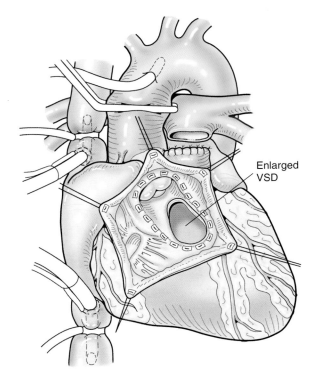

Enlarged VSD

3a

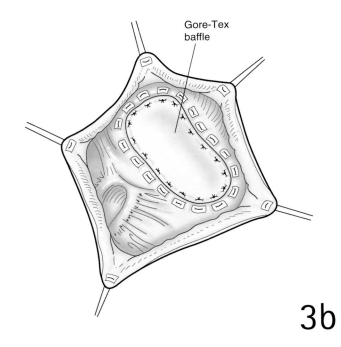

Gore-Tex baffle

3b

4 RV to distal PA continuity is then re-established with the pulmonary homograft, which has been trimmed to an appropriate length, leaving a small rim of muscle at the proximal end. The distal anastomosis is constructed with a running suture of 5/0 polypropylene. We prefer to construct these anastomoses with the heart arrested, believing that the slight increase in myocardial ischemia time is worth the increased accuracy of the anastomosis. Proximally, the pulmonary homograft is sutured to the distal end of the ventriculotomy incision with a running 5/0 polypropylene suture. The previously harvested autologous pericardium is used to augment the proximal anastomosis between the pulmonary homograft and the RV. The patient is rewarmed during insertion of the homograft. After the repair is complete, the cardiotomy sucker is removed from the left atrium, and any defect in the septum is closed after deairing by inflating the lungs. The patient is then placed in Trendelenburg position, and the aortic cross-clamp is removed, while the aortic root is vented. We continue to vent the aortic root with the patient's head down until the patient is weaned off CPB and the heart is ejecting to remove any residual intracardiac air. The patient is weaned from bypass at a rectal temperature of around 36°C, with infusions of inotropic agents as needed. Protamine is administered, and the heart is decannulated in the usual fashion once hemodynamic stability is achieved.

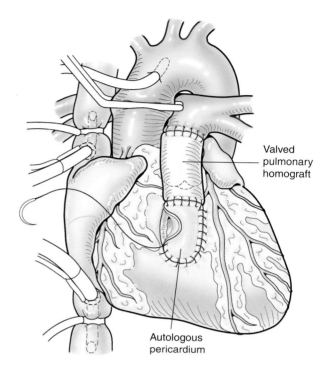

Valved
pulmonary
homograft

Autologous
pericardium

4

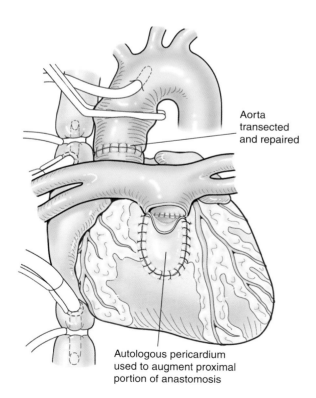

Aorta
transected
and repaired

Autologous pericardium
used to augment proximal
portion of anastomosis

5 The Lecompte modification avoids the use of an extracardiac conduit by anastomosing the PA directly to the right ventriculotomy. The aorta is transected, and the mobilized PA confluence is transferred anterior to the ascending aorta. The intracardiac repair involves extensive resection of the infundibular septum and the creation of an intraventricular baffle from the LV to the aorta, as with the Rastelli operation. The PA confluence is then anastomosed directly to the distal end of the right ventriculotomy incision. The anastomosis is augmented with a patch of autologous pericardium.

5

Arterial switch operation and aortic arch reconstruction

The details of the ASO are described by Dr. Lacour-Gayet in the chapter 'Anatomic repair of transposition of the great arteries.' CoA is the most common form of AAO occurring with TGA. However, as noted earlier, a high incidence of associated tubular hypoplasia of the aortic arch has been largely unrecognized until recently. We will perform a concomitant aortic arch augmentation if the diameter of the smallest part of the aortic arch is less than the baby's weight in kilograms ±1 mm. For example, in a 3-kg baby, if the aortic arch diameter is 4 mm or less, it will be enlarged.

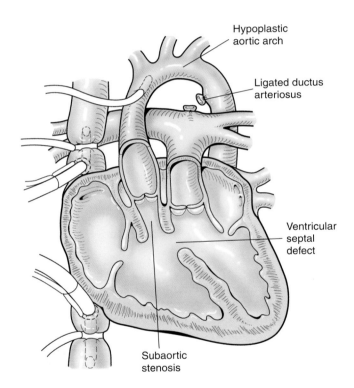

Hypoplastic aortic arch

Ligated ductus arteriosus

Ventricular septal defect

Subaortic stenosis

6 A sternotomy incision provides excellent exposure of the intracardiac anatomy and great vessels, as well as the entire aortic arch and proximal descending thoracic aorta. The pericardium is opened, and a piece is harvested if reconstruction of the RVOT is anticipated because of subaortic obstruction. The patient is heparinized to an activated clotting time of greater than 400 seconds. In recent years, all of our aortic arch reconstructions have been performed without the use of circulatory arrest. To facilitate this procedure, the right side of the distal ascending aorta is cannulated with a flexible 8-Fr arterial cannula (Bio-Medicus, Medtronic, Minneapolis, MN, USA), 5 mm proximal to the takeoff of the innominate artery. Standard bicaval cannulation is performed, and the patient is placed on CPB. The patent ductus arteriosus is ligated, and the patient is cooled to 18°C.

6

7a, b During cooling, the aorta is cross-clamped, and cold crystalloid or blood cardioplegia is administered into the aortic root. The vena cavae are snared, and the right atrium is opened to drain the cardioplegia from the coronary sinus. A cardiotomy sucker is placed into the left atrium through an atrial septal defect or patent foramen ovale to vent the left side of the heart.

If a VSD is present, the opening is first examined through the right atrial incision and closed with a 0.6-mm thick Gore-Tex patch by using a running suture of 5/0 or 6/0 propylene. If significant subaortic stenosis exists, a vertical right ventriculotomy is made to resect the obstruction and reconstruct the RVOT after closing the VSD. Occasionally, a difficult VSD is closed by running the suture line alternatively through the right atriotomy and ventriculotomy incisions. The suture line is reinforced in several places with interrupted pledgeted sutures to achieve a secure closure.

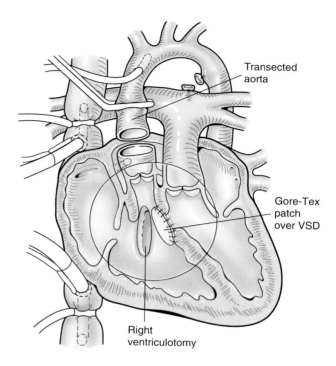

Transected aorta

Gore-Tex patch over VSD

Right ventriculotomy

7a

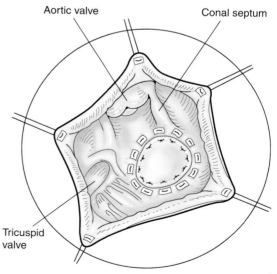

Aortic valve

Conal septum

Tricuspid valve

7b

8 After mobilizing the coronary buttons and transferring them to the neoaorta, a pantaloon-shaped autologous pericardial patch is used to reconstruct the sinuses of the proximal neopulmonary artery. At deep hypothermia, the aortic cannula is advanced into the innominate artery and snared in place. Pump flow is decreased to 0.5–1.0 L/minute/m^2, and continuous low-flow cerebral perfusion is maintained via the innominate artery. After the left common carotid and the left subclavian arteries are snared, the undersurface of the aortic arch is opened longitudinally. Ductal tissue is excised, and the incision is carried distally for 1 cm in the upper descending thoracic aorta. A clamp is placed on the descending thoracic aorta, distal to the incision, to limit backbleeding and improve exposure. Proximally, the incision is carried through the distal ascending aorta. The dotted line represents the proposed site to open the aortic arch.

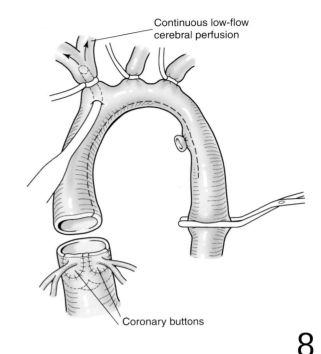

Continuous low-flow cerebral perfusion

Coronary buttons

8

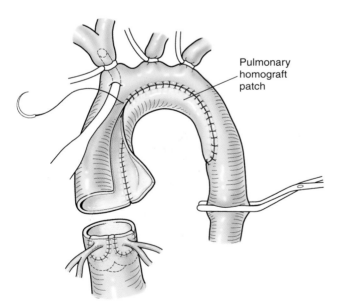

Pulmonary homograft patch

9

9 The aorta is opened on its undersurface from the proximal descending thoracic aorta to the site where the proximal ascending aorta had been transected. A patch of pulmonary homograft is used to enlarge the entire aortic arch and distal ascending aorta with a running 6/0 polypropylene suture. The clamp on the descending thoracic aorta is removed to allow the backbleeding to deair the aorta. The cross-clamp is then reapplied to the distal ascending aorta. The snares on the arch vessels are then removed, the arterial cannula is pulled back into the ascending aorta, and full flow is re-established.

10 This figure depicts the completed repair. Before completing the proximal aortic anastomosis to the neoaorta, the distal PA is brought in front of the aorta (Lecompte maneuver). The aortic anastomosis is completed with a continuous suture of 5/0 polypropylene, and the aorta is deaired while the patient is being rewarmed. The neopulmonary artery anastomosis is performed, connecting the main PA to the PA confluence with a running 5/0 polypropylene suture. After the ASO, the subaortic area becomes the subpulmonic area. To relieve the obstruction when present, a patch of autologous pericardium is used to augment the ventriculotomy incision. The aortic root is vented, and the patient is placed in Trendelenburg position before removing the aortic cross-clamp. We continue to vent the aortic root until the heart is ejecting, and the patient is weaned from bypass.

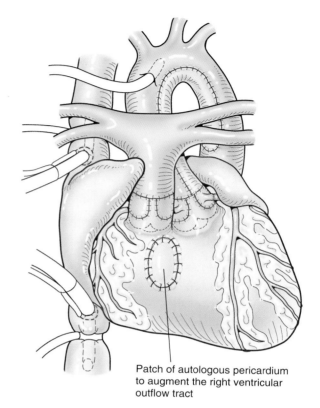

Patch of autologous pericardium to augment the right ventricular outflow tract

10

POSTOPERATIVE CARE

Before coming off bypass, we routinely place intracardiac lines in the left and right atrium. We have found these lines useful to guide fluid and inotrope administration when weaning off bypass. They have proved invaluable in the early postoperative care and in the PICU as well. Temporary atrial and ventricular pacemaker wires are also placed routinely, for therapeutic as well as diagnostic purposes, in the postoperative period. Multiple suture lines, especially in the case of ASO with aortic arch reconstruction, increase the risk of postoperative bleeding. After all surgical bleeding has been controlled, administration of platelets, fresh frozen plasma, and cryoprecipitate are given to correct any coagulopathy. Extra protamine may be required to reverse the effects of heparin, especially in those patients receiving heparinized pump blood that has been bagged for administration after the termination of CPB.

Patients should be kept warm with heating lamps and blankets while preparation is made for transfer to the PICU. On transfer, an accurate signover of the patient's pre- and intra-operative course is given to the PICU staff. Any anticipated problems should be outlined. Inotrope and fluid administration in the first 24–48 hours is guided by the arterial blood pressure, arterial blood gas, skin temperature, and urine output. We routinely use the phosphodiesterase inhibitor milrinone, especially in patients with anticipated RV dysfunction after ventriculotomy. Milrinone provides a degree of inotropic support, but more importantly, it decreases the afterload on the RV and LV by its vasodilator effect on the pulmonary and systemic vascular beds. In addition, the hematocrit is kept over 36 per cent to decrease any capillary leak that may be present with hemodilution.

The extensive mediastinal dissection, especially in patients undergoing aortic arch repair, may lead to lymphatic disruption and an increased risk of chylothorax. In these patients, feeding is introduced conservatively in the postoperative period. Patients are diuresed early and aggressively. The need for peritoneal dialysis is extremely rare, even in the sickest neonates undergoing the most complex repairs.

OUTCOME

Rastelli operation

Kreutzer and associates have published their results in 101 patients with TGA-VSD who underwent Rastelli operation at the Children's Hospital in Boston. The average age at the time of the Rastelli operation was 3.1 years of age, and 71 of the 101 patients had at least one prior palliative procedure. Seven early deaths (7 per cent) occurred, with no early deaths in the last 7 years of the study. Despite the excellent early results, late mortality, conduit obstruction, and arrhythmias were concerning long-term complications. Seventy-two reinterventions were performed for conduit stenosis, either operative (44 patients) or catheter-based (28 patients). Freedom from operation at 5, 10, and 15 years was 53 per cent, 24 per cent, and 21 per cent, respectively. A total of 17 late deaths occured, five of which were sudden.

Vouché and associates compared their surgical results in 62 patients with TGA-VSD and LVOTO using either the Rastelli operation or the Lecompte modification. Twenty-two patients had the Rastelli operation, whereas 40 patients underwent operation using the Lecompte modification. No difference existed between the two techniques with respect to early or late mortality. However, the likelihood of reoperation for PA outflow obstruction was significantly higher in the Rastelli group. They concluded that, although both operations provided satisfactory early and late results, the Lecompte modification might reduce the rate of reoperation by avoiding the use of an extracardiac conduit.

Arterial switch operation and aortic arch reconstruction

Since 1988 at the Montreal Children's Hospital, we have used a single-stage approach of ASO and concomitant aortic arch reconstruction for TGA complexes and AAO, with excellent short- and long-term results. Twenty-one of 22 such patients have undergone a single-stage repair, as described previously in this chapter. No early deaths and only one late death from a hepatoblastoma have occurred. One patient has required balloon dilatation for recoarctation, and no aneurysm formations have developed using the technique of pulmonary homograft patch aortoplasty to reconstruct the aortic arch. Since applying techniques to avoid circulatory arrest in recent years, no neurological morbidity has occurred.

FURTHER READING

Jatene, A.D., Fontes, V.F., Paulista, P.P., *et al.* 1975. Successful anatomic correction of transposition of the great vessels: A preliminary report. *Arquivos Brasileiros de Cardiologia* **28**, 461–4.

Kreutzer, C., De Vive, J., Oppido, G., *et al.* 2000. Twenty-five year experience with Rastelli repair for transposition of the great arteries. *Journal of Thoracic and Cardiovascular Surgery* **120**, 211–23.

Lecompte, Y., Neveux, J.Y., Leca, F., *et al.* 1982. Reconstruction of the pulmonary outflow tract without prosthetic conduit. *Journal of Thoracic and Cardiovascular Surgery* **84**, 727–33.

Rastelli, G.C., Wallace, R.B., Ongley, P.A. 1969. Complete repair of transposition of the great arteries with pulmonary stenosis. A review of a case corrected by using a new surgical technique. *Circulation* **39**, 83–95.

Tchervenkov, C.I., Tahta, S.A., Cecere, R., Béland, M.J. 1997. Single-stage arterial switch with aortic arch enlargement for transposition complexes with aortic arch obstruction. *Annals of Thoracic Surgery* **64**, 1776–81.

Vouché, P.R., Tamisier, D., Leca, F., Ouaknine, R., Vernant, F., Neveux, J.-Y. 1992. Transposition of the great arteries, ventricular septal defect, and pulmonary outflow tract obstruction. Rastelli or Lecompte procedure? *Journal of Thoracic and Cardiovascular Surgery* **103**, 428–36.

53

Anatomical repair of transposition of the great arteries

FRANÇOIS LACOUR-GAYET MD
Professor of Surgery, University of Colorado, Chairman Cardio-Thoracic Infant Department, The Children's Hospital, Denver, Colorado, USA

Anatomical repair, by restoring ventriculoarterial concordance, offers the optimal long-term survival to patients born with transposition of the great arteries. The arterial switch operation (ASO) has become, with time, a simplified operation. Almost all technical problems raised by an abnormal coronary artery anatomy and by associated cardiac lesions have found adapted solutions. The aim of this chapter is to describe the current surgical technique and some useful 'tricks' adopted during a 17-year experience at Marie Lannelongue, where the total number of ASOs performed by three surgeons reaches more than 1 300 cases.

This chapter focuses on coronary transfer and describes the anatomical classification of coronary arteries, cardiopulmonary bypass (CPB) and myocardial protection, preoperative management of transposition of the great arteries with intact ventricular septum (TGA-IVS), and the arterial switch technique.

HISTORY

The first successful arterial switch was achieved in patients with TGA-VSD by Abib Jatene in Sao Paolo in 1975. Arterial switch in TGA-IVS was first reported by Donald Ross in 1976 in a 20-month-old child with persistent ductus arteriosus. A two-stage arterial switch in TGA-IVS was reported by Yacoub et al. in 1976, whereas the first successful neonatal arterial switch attempted in a patient with TGA-IVS was reported by Aldo Castaneda in 1984. The description of the French maneuver by Yves Lecompte in 1981, avoiding the use of foreign material to reconstruct the pulmonary artery (PA), and our suggestion in 1985 to use a single posterior autologous pericardial patch, contributed to the wide success of the ASO.

MARIE LANNELONGUE ANATOMICAL CLASSIFICATION OF CORONARY ARTERIES

The Marie Lannelongue classification is based on the course of the coronary artery vessels and not on the origin. The main interest of this classification is that the coronary relocation technique is based on these different courses. In situs solitus, a left and a right coronary ostium are defined.

Four groups are recognized, according to the following coronary courses:

1 Normal course
2 Looping courses
3 Intramural course
4 Miscellaneous course associating intramural to looping courses.

Normal course (60 per cent)

1 The *normal course* of the coronary arteries is the most frequent and represents 60 per cent of cases. The left ostium gives the left anterior descending and the circumflex artery (CX), and the right ostium gives the right coronary artery (RCA). No vessel is crossing either in front of or behind the great vessels.

Looping courses (35 per cent)

The *looping courses*, those in which a coronary runs in front of and/or behind the great vessels, represent 35 per cent of cases. Three subgroups exist – the posterior looping course, the anterior looping course, and the double looping course.

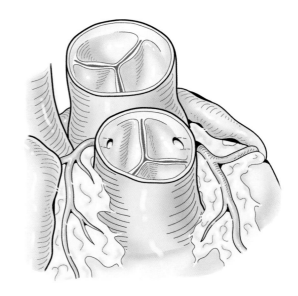

1

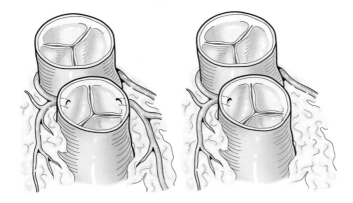

2

POSTERIOR LOOPING COURSE (20 PER CENT)

2 The *posterior looping course* is one in which a coronary runs posterior to the PA, and two subtypes exist. One is frequent, with the posterior looping coronary being the CX arising from the RCA, and the other is a single coronary ostium (1 per cent), with the common left trunk running behind the PA.

ANTERIOR LOOPING COURSE (1 PER CENT)

3 The *anterior looping course* is one in which a coronary runs anterior to the aorta, and three subtypes exist, including two single coronary forms. The pure anterior loop is very rare.

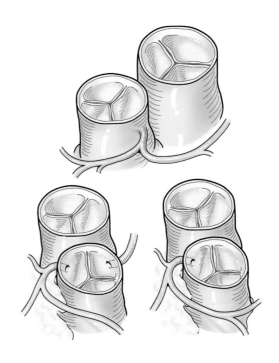

3

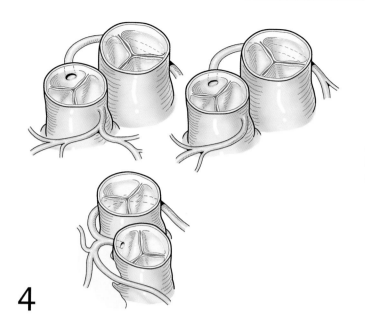

4

DOUBLE-LOOPING COURSE (14 PER CENT)

4 Two forms are frequent: one with a posterior loop, done by the common left trunk (8 per cent) (called *inverted coronary artery* by A. Castaneda) and one with a posterior loop done by the CX (5 per cent). One rare form is a single coronary (1 per cent).

Intramural course (5 per cent)

5 The intramural course is one in which, usually, the left coronary has an abnormal intramural course in the posterior aortic wall, crossing behind or above the posterior commissure from the right to the left sinus.

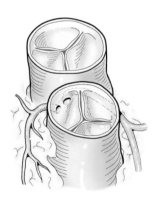

5

Miscellaneous course (0.1 per cent)

The *miscellaneous course*, associating intramural and looping courses, represents 0.1 per cent of cases.

CARDIOPULMONARY BYPASS AND MYOCARDIAL PROTECTION

Anesthesia follows the principles of neonatal cardiac surgery. The optimal CPB in neonates remains controversial. The principle uniformly followed is to limit as much as possible circulatory arrest and low flow. CPB is achieved using full flow at 100–150 cc/kg/minute with bicaval cannulation. The priming volume is currently 250 cc, using short tubing and miniaturized membrane oxygenators. The priming solution uses exclusively reconstituted blood, including fresh frozen plasma and red blood cells, to obtain a hematocrit of 30. The solution is buffered with calcium gluconate and sodium bicarbonate. The CPB is run at a temperature between 25°C and 30°C according to the complexity of the procedure.

Myocardial protection uses crystalloid or blood cardioplegia, injected antegradely at a dose of 30 mL/kg for the first injection, and repeated every 30 minutes at a dose of 10 mL/kg by direct injection in the coronary ostia, using a DLP cannula. The right ventricle is bathed with melting ice.

PREOPERATIVE MANAGEMENT OF TRANSPOSITION OF THE GREAT ARTERIES WITH INTACT VENTRICULAR SEPTUM

Antenatal diagnosis is obtained in 20 per cent of the patients and allows optimal management, with a delivery organized close to a pediatric cardiology unit. The protocol for patients with TGA-IVS routinely includes a Rashkind septostomy and prostaglandin E_1 infusion at a minimal dose to maintain patency at the ductus arteriosus. Preoperative angiography is not considered optimal to define the coronary anatomy; echocardiography is superior, particularly for the diagnosis of intramural coronary. The left ventricular (LV) myocardial mass is always calculated by echocardiography. A myocardial mass over 35 ± 5 g/m³ is required for safe anatomical repair. Operation is electively undertaken at the end of the first week of life.

OPERATION

Uniform arterial switch technique in normal coronary course

With time, the technique has been simplified and standardized. The technique described here is *applicable to all coronary anatomy* except the intramural pattern.

6 After median sternotomy, the thymus gland is partially resected, keeping a residual superior segment.

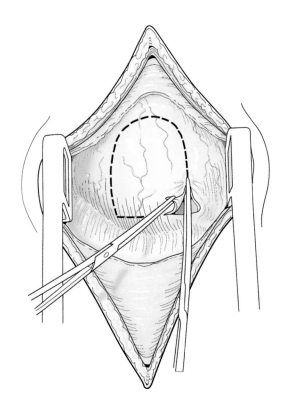

6

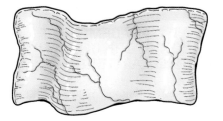

7

7 A large rectangular patch of anterior pericardium is harvested and kept in iced saline solution. The pericardium is used fresh.

INSPECTION

The pericardium is suspended, avoiding undue traction. Gentle retraction on the pursestring placed in the right atrial appendage helps to expose the great vessels. The anatomy is carefully analyzed, evaluating the following:

- Origin and the courses of the coronary arteries, recognizing the abnormal loopings. (Full evaluation of the coronary anatomy requires intra-aortic inspection.)

- The relationship of the great vessels, either anteroposterior or side by side. The relationship of the great vessels is either antero-posterior or side by side. It is most frequently a D Transposition with the aorta anterior and slightly to the right.

The technique is first described in the most frequent and simple condition, with a normal coronary artery course, an anteroposterior great vessel relationship, and no significant diameter size mismatch.

DISSECTION OF PULMONARY ARTERY BRANCHES AND DUCTUS ARTERIOSUS

8 All dissection is performed using electrocoagulation. The aorta and the right and left PAs are dissected and controlled by vessel loops. The ductus arteriosus wall is extremely fragile if prostaglandin has been continued, and its dissection is started below the right side of the aorta, on its right border. Traction on the left PA vessel loop helps to dissect the left border. The ductus is carefully controlled by a 3/0 suture, which will be tied when going on bypass. In case of torrential pulmonary flow by a large ductus arteriosus, occlusion of the right pulmonary branch with a tourniquet is helpful to increase the aortic diastolic pressure and improve the coronary blood flow.

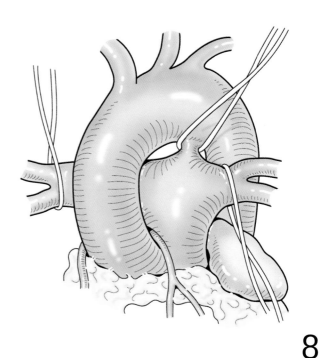

8

CANNULATION

9 Continuous bypass requires an accurate cannulation technique. The aorta must be cannulated very close to the brachiocephalic artery, using a small, straight, reinforced cannula. The superior vena cava venous cannula (straight, reinforced venous cannula, size 12 or 14) is introduced into the atrial appendage and placed in the right atrium. CPB is instituted with one venous cannula. After establishing bypass, the inferior vena cava venous cannula is introduced close to the inferior vena cava and snared. A left atrial (LA) venting cannula (Medtronic) is further introduced through the Sondergard sulcus, distant from the right pulmonary vein ostia. The superior venous cannula is then introduced into the superior vena cava and snared.

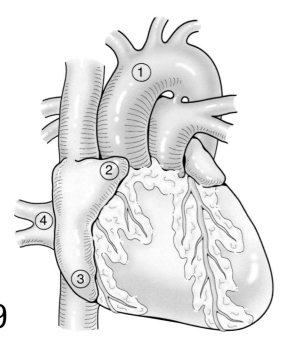

9

DUCTUS ARTERIOSUS DIVISION AND PROXIMAL AORTA DISSECTION

During cooling, the ductus arteriosus is divided. After prostaglandin infusion, the ductus walls are very fragile and should be managed carefully. The ductus is doubly ligated and then divided, with suturing of both ends. The aortic end can also be occluded by a vascular clip. Any tear or needle puncture of the ductal wall proximal to the ligation should be avoided, as a tear of the origin of the ductus arteriosus is difficult to control. Additional direct stitching usually worsens the hemorrhage, or it may create an isthmus stenosis. Serious hemorrhage at this stage is better controlled under circulatory arrest.

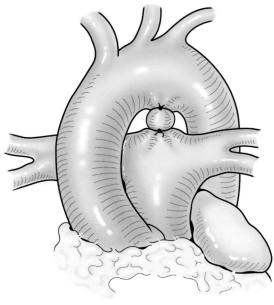

10

10 Patent ductus arteriosus ligation is shown.

11 Patent ductus arteriosus division is shown.

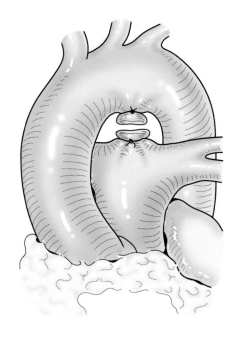

11

12 Patent ductus arteriosus suture – any tear or needle puncture of the ductal wall proximal to the ligation should be avoided.

The space between the aortic and pulmonary roots is carefully dissected. This dissection is performed more easily when the aorta is filled. This dissection runs close to the origin of the coronary trunks that are dissected, carefully using very low coagulation intensity. When the coronary trunks are not well seen, this dissection should not be done.

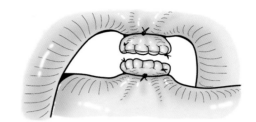

12

CROSS-CLAMPING, CARDIOPLEGIA, AND CLOSURE OF ATRIAL SEPTAL DEFECT

The aortic cross-clamp is placed very close to the aortic cannula. The cardioplegia is given through a needle placed at the level of the aortotomy. A short, longitudinal, right atriotomy allows good access to the atrial septal defect, which is closed using running suture. In case of a large atrial septal defect, patch closure is preferred to prevent potential arrhythmias.

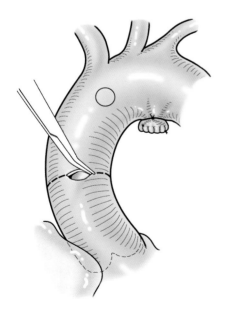

13

GREAT VESSEL TRANSECTION

13 This step is an important step, defining all landmarks of the arterial switch. The aorta is transected exactly at a middle point between the clamp and the aortic annulus. This incision should be high, to reduce the length of the reconstructed aorta that will lie behind the PA.

14 For the same purpose, the PA is transected in a low position, a few millimeters above the pulmonary commissures. This inferior incision leaves a good quantity of native tissue on the pulmonary bifurcation and also reduces the length of the future aortic root, allowing the Lecompte maneuver without compression.

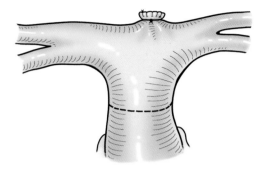

14

DISSECTION OF PULMONARY ARTERY BRANCHES

Helped by gentle traction on the vessel loops, the PA branches are fully dissected until the lobar branches are clearly seen. The pulmonary bifurcation is then pulled up in front of the ascending aorta. Using a second clamp or forceps, the aortic cross-clamp is mobilized and placed below the pulmonary bifurcation, closely in contact with the aortic cannula, to expose the maximum length of distal ascending aorta.

LECOMPTE MANEUVER

15 Notice that, after optimal transection of the great vessels, the future neoaorta is short, and the future neopulmonary artery long. The aortic clamp is blocked on the surgical field at twelve o'clock to stabilize the distal aorta.

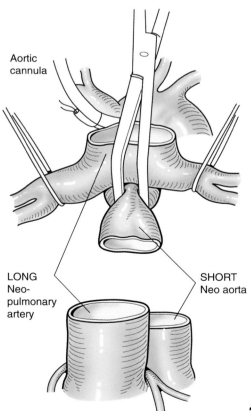

Aortic cannula

LONG Neo-pulmonary artery

SHORT Neo aorta

15

HARVESTING OF CORONARY BUTTONS

16 The harvesting of coronary buttons is crucial. The general principle is to take the largest possible button, removing almost all of the sinus of Valsalva, to perform safe anastomoses sufficiently distant from the coronary ostia. *These coronary buttons are in fact aortic buttons containing the coronary ostium.* Two traction sutures, one anterior and one posterior, help exposure. The locations of the ostia are carefully evaluated, particularly their proximity with the commissures and with the aortic annulus.

The left button is taken first. An anterior and vertical incision is made in the direction of the left lateral commissure, and the incision stays in close contact with the commissure until the bottom of the sinus. The second incision, which is posterior and vertical, similarly follows the posterior commissure. The last incision is horizontal and follows the aortic annulus. Depending on the location of the ostium, this incision is more or less in contact with the aortic annulus. In rare instances, when the ostium is very low, the aortic annulus itself should be resected. The origin of the left coronary trunk is dissected for 2–3 mm from the myocardium using coagulation until the button can be mobilized posteriorly without affecting the course of the left anterior descending and CX arteries. The right button is then harvested. Similarly, the incisions follow the commissures and the aortic annulus. The button is mobilized for a few millimeters using electrocoagulation to allow a posterior translation without distortion of the right coronary.

Three particular coronary anatomical conditions require appropriate management, as discussed below.

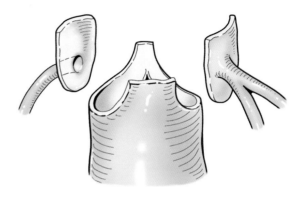

16

OSTIUM NEXT TO A COMMISSURE

In some instances, one ostium is located very close to or in contact with a commissure. Usually, the posterior commissure is involved, but rarely it can be the anterior commissure. In these cases deliberate detachment of the posterior commissure and harvesting a button that could include part of the annulus is crucial.

17 An ostium can be located very close to a commissure.

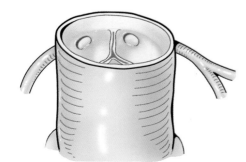

17

18 The commissure is to be taken down, to allow the harvesting of a large button.

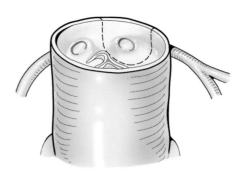

18

EARLY INFUNDIBULAR BRANCH

In other instances, an early branching of the infundibular artery arises from the left main trunk. This early branch blocks the posterior translation and can create a stenosis of the trunk. This branch should be dissected and mobilized. In most instances, this branch must be sacrificed and divided. More rarely, this early infundibular branching comes from the RCA but it should be managed the same way and sacrificed if necessary.

19a An early infundibular branch coming from the left main trunk can block the transfer and kink the left main trunk.

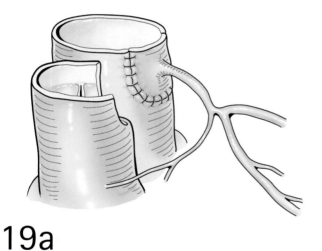

19a

19b An early branch of the infundibular artery can be dissected and mobilized when large. Otherwise, it should be sacrificed.

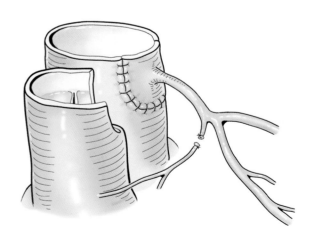

19b

20 Stabilization and exposure of the aorta. The aortic clamp is blocked at 12 H. The posterior part of the aortic anastomosis is started by three stitches to place the aorta in its final position.

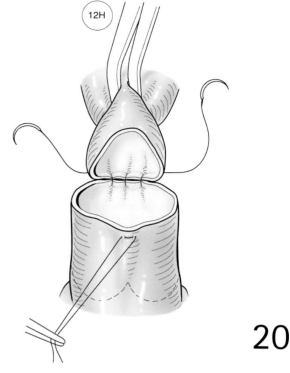

20

21 The aortic clamp is blocked at twelve o'clock. The posterior part of the aortic anastomosis is begun by four stitches to place the aorta in the final position.

CORONARY TRANSFER PRINCIPLES

Three points to consider are:

1   Always place the buttons laterally so that they are not compressed by the PA, which lies anteriorly.
2   Place the button on a curved aortic incision.
3   Place the left button in a low position and the right button in a high position, above the aortic anastomosis.

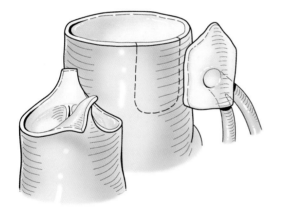

21

LEFT CORONARY BUTTON IMPLANTATION

22 The left button is transferred in a low left lateral position. The superior part of the button is tailored with an acute angle. To obtain a curved site for the button and also to reduce the neoaortic root that is always larger, a vertical, rectangular excision of the lateral left wall is performed. The inner excision line is defined by the left button's inner border and is usually 2–3 mm left of the anterior commissure. The depth of the excision should equal the button height and stops approximately 2 mm from the annulus.

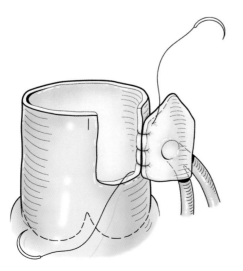

22

23 The anastomosis is performed using 7/0 or 8/0 suture and starts to close the base of the button. In the superior part of the anastomosis, the acute angle reduces the annulus.

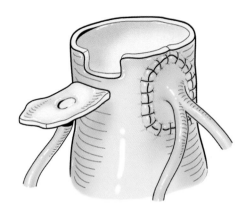

23

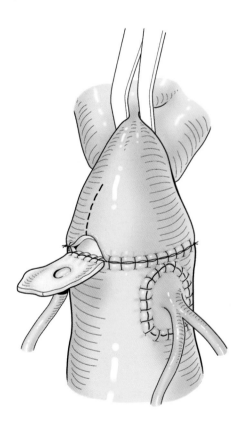

24

RIGHT CORONARY BUTTON IMPLANTATION

24 The right coronary button is transferred in high lateral right position across the aortic anastomosis. The superior part of the button is tailored with an acute angle. The lateral right free edge of the neoaorta is incised at a height from 2 to 8 mm according to the free movement of the coronary button. Mistakes occur from a button placed too low. The anastomosis is partially performed so as to place the inferior part of the button on the neoaortic root.

MALALIGNED COMMISSURES

Malaligned commissures is a very rare condition that never affects the right button transfer, which is located above the commissures. Impact is possible on the left button, which can be exactly located on the anterior commissure. The solution is to twist to the right proximal neoaorta so as to realign medially the anterior commissure. The proximal neoaorta is twisted 10°–40° to the right and fixed in position by starting the posterior anastomosis. After this twisting, the left button can be placed normally in the left lateral position.

AORTIC ANASTOMOSIS AND INCLUSION OF THE RIGHT BUTTON

25 The right button is included in the distal aorta by an incision directed vertically, close to the aortic clamp. This step is an important one because it will define the final position of the buttons. Some diameter mismatch always exists between the distal and the proximal segment. The aortic anastomosis starts on the right, using the initial stitch and meeting the posterior part of the right button. The left part of the anastomosis is then performed using the initial stitch. Keeping the stitch tight is crucial to prevent a loose suture. When reaching the anterolateral aorta, suturing in such a way that the left button remains located laterally on the left is important. When reaching the middle anterior line, the stay suture should be exactly at twelve o'clock. Crossing the line in the right anterior part, the suture becomes next to the right button. Almost always more tissue is present on the neoaortic root than on the distal aorta. The distal segment of the ascending aorta is then incised vertically towards the aortic clamp, on a length corresponding to the right button height. The last millimeters of midline anastomosis are performed, and the two stitches are tied together. The right button is then included in the distal aorta, starting on the posterior part reaching progressively the top and middle line.

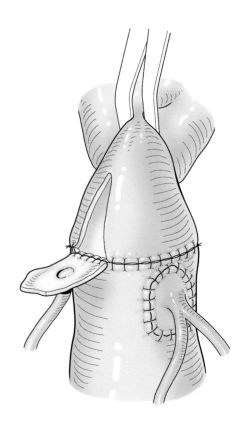

25

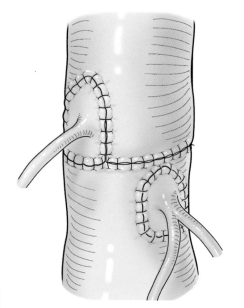

26 The technique shown controls the diameter mismatch and permits enlargement of the distal aorta and reconstruction of the sinotubular junction.

26

DEAIRATION AND CHECKING OF THE ANASTOMOSIS

Before finishing the anastomosis, the LA vent line is clamped, waiting for a good amount of blood to flush the LV. The stitches are then tied together, and the LA vent line is reopened.

To check the anastomoses, the two coronary trunks are very gently occluded using light forceps, and the aortic clamp is opened. Any source of bleeding should be stitched. When the anastomoses are perfectly dry, a very shallow layer of biological glue can be added on the suture lines.

27 After checking precisely the anastomoses, a light layer of glue is placed.

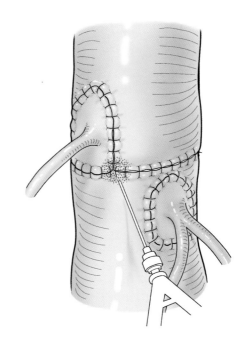

27

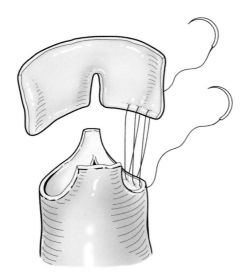

28

RECONSTRUCTION OF THE NEOPULMONARY ROOT

28 Reconstruction of the neopulmonary root is better done under aortic cross-clamping. In favorable cases, the aortic clamp can be removed and the coronary sinus blood flow suctioned with an additional suction line placed carefully through the tricuspid valve.

A large, rectangular, fresh patch of autologous pericardium is used. The patch is placed on the chest wall, and the anastomosis is performed distantly, starting on the left. When reaching the posterior commissure, the patch is incised vertically to place the posterior commissure in the posterior position. Excess tissue is resected.

When detached, the posterior commissure is reattached in the normal position.

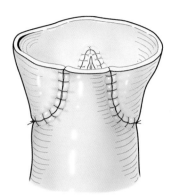

29 The final aspect of the reconstructed proximal PA is shown.

29

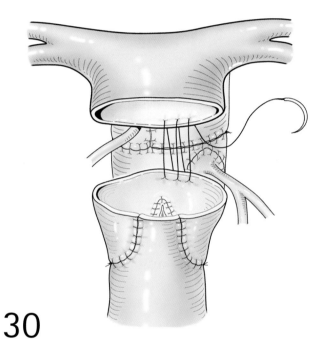

30

REMOVAL OF THE AORTIC CLAMP

The quality of the reperfusion is carefully evaluated, based on the coloration of the myocardium and on normal filling of the coronary arteries. The courses of the proximal coronary trunks are checked. When this evaluation is completed, the patient is rewarmed.

DISTAL PULMONARY ARTERY ANASTOMOSIS

30 The distal anastomosis is performed during rewarming.

31 Final results are shown.

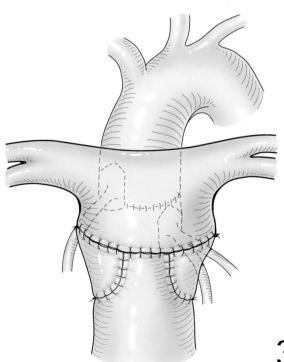

31

COMING OFF BYPASS

Before coming off bypass, the electrocardiogram, the coloration, and the contractions of all myocardial segments should be normal. Transesophageal echocardiography is useful in case myocardial ischemia is suspected. Bleeding should be minimal.

An LA line is routinely placed at the location of the LA suction line.

Atrial pacing is used to obtain a sinus rhythm of approximately 130–150 beats/minute. The need for inotropic support depends on the quality of LV function, varying from a small dose of dopamine to milrinone and epinephrine. Any suspicion of myocardial ischemia related to a kinking of a coronary trunk requires going back on bypass and redoing the anastomosis. LV dysfunction with normal coronary flow is usually related to poor LV mass and may require early extracorporeal membrane oxygenation.

Most frequently the sternum can be closed. But when any problem is expected, the sternum should be left open and the skin closed with polytetrafluoroethylene (Gore-Tex).

HEMOSTASIS

Hemostasis is a major complication of the ASO. With experience, major hemostatic problems are rare. When the bleeding cannot be easily controlled, going back on bypass and eventually taking down the distal pulmonary anastomosis to gain access to all bleeding points is preferable.

POSTOPERATIVE MANAGEMENT

In the simple forms, the postoperative course is unusually straightforward. Extubation should be undertaken only when the LV function is satisfactory.

The same coronary transfer technique is applied in looping courses

The technique described for a normal coronary course is applied to *all looping courses*. The risk of transfer follows the type of looping courses. *The posterior loop is associated with a risk of kinking and the anterior loop with a risk of stretching.*

The three points previously defined are applied:

1 Always place the buttons laterally so that they are not compressed by the PA, which lies anteriorly.
2 Place the button on a curved aortic incision.
3 The left button is to be placed in low position and the right button in high position, above the aortic anastomosis.

In addition, *extensive dissection of the coronary trunks* is necessary so that the translation does not induce a kinking or a stretching.

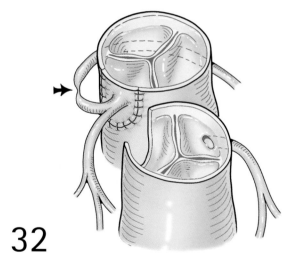

32 Anterior loop: stretching risk is shown.

33 Posterior loop: kinking risk is shown.

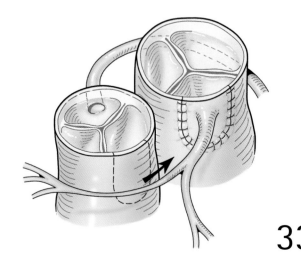

33

34 Posterior loop is shown. The circumflex comes from the RCA. The CX is dissected far away, behind the PA, to allow a safe mobilization.

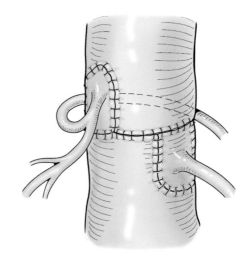

34

35

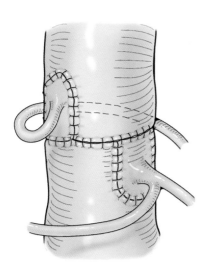

35 Double loop is shown. The posterior artery, here the CX, is extensively dissected. The anterior artery, here the RCA that crosses in front of the RV, is dissected for 20 mm and mobilized from the RV and the aorta.

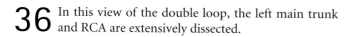

36 In this view of the double loop, the left main trunk and RCA are extensively dissected.

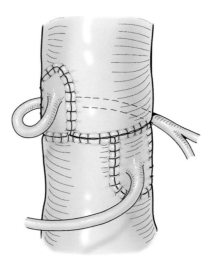

36

Single coronary ostium

Single coronary ostia are part of the looping course forms (4 per cent) (see Marie Lannelongue anatomical classification of coronary arteries), and their relocation follows the same principles. Notice that only one button is available for transfer. Extensive dissection of the coronary trunks is essential, either the posterior one (left trunk, CX) or the anterior one (RCA, left trunk, or left anterior descending). The risks are the same: stretching of the anterior vessel and kinking of the posterior

one. The right buttons are transferred in a high position and the left button in a low position.

Side-by-side vessels are frequent, and single left ostium, frequently found with side-by-side great vessels, requires a right translation of the PA bifurcation (see below in the next section). Three forms of single right coronary and one form of single left coronary exist. Miscellaneous forms with intramural coronary are, unfortunately, possible.

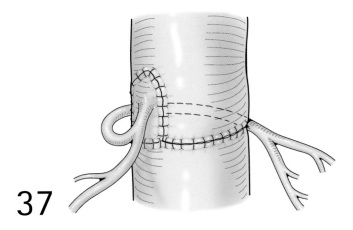

37

37 Single right coronary ostium: posterior looping from right button (1 per cent) is shown.

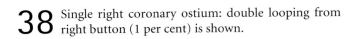

38 Single right coronary ostium: double looping from right button (1 per cent) is shown.

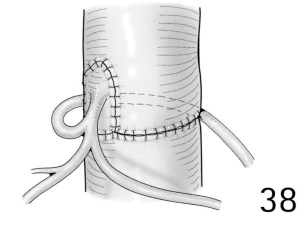

38

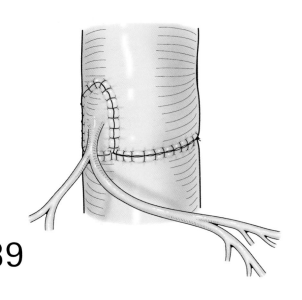

39

39 Single right coronary ostium: anterior looping from right button (1 per cent) is shown.

40 Single left coronary ostium: anterior looping from left button (1 per cent) is shown. The vessels are usually side by side, requiring a right transfer of the PA bifurcation (see below).

Side-by-side vessels

Side-by-side vessels are seen frequently in double loop (type E of Yacoub) and in Taussig-Bing hearts. After the Lecompte maneuver, the reconstruction of the pulmonary bifurcation can compress the left coronary button that includes an anterior looping coronary, which is always the RCA.

Mobilization of the pulmonary bifurcation to the right is necessary to prevent a compression of the RCA. The right PA is incised for 20 mm, and the reconstructed PA trunk is directly anastomosed to the right PA to mobilize the pulmonary trunk to the right. The left part of the PA trunk is then patched or directly closed to increase the left PA length.

The other option is not to do the Lecompte maneuver, which risks compression of the coronaries coming from the right button, namely, the RCA and the posterior looping vessels.

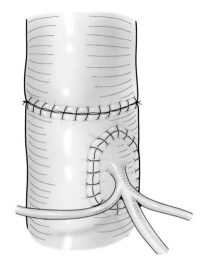

40

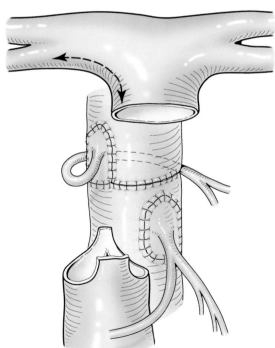

41 The patch reconstruction of the PA bifurcation can compress the left button, particularly the RCA that crosses in front of the previous aorta. The PA bifurcation is realigned on the right by an incision of the right PA for two-thirds of its length.

41

42 The pulmonary trunk has been transferred to the right to release the left coronary button. Direct anastomosis with the reconstructed PA root uses a large pericardial patch.

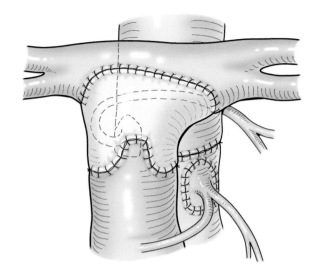

42

Intramural course

Coronary transfer with intramural course represents a major surgical difficulty. Preoperative echocardiogram is superior to angiocardiography for recognizing this rare pattern. The anomaly is confirmed after opening of the aorta. In many instances, this anomaly is discovered intraoperatively. Different techniques have been described. The technique described by Toshihide Azou and Roger Mee seems the safest one. The anomaly is, in almost all cases, related to an abnormal location of the left ostium on the right sinus in a high position, close to the posterior commissure. From this abnormal origin, the course of the left coronary is intramural. This intramural course can be very long and can cross the left sinus posteriorly. The right ostium also can have an abnormal location, moving superiorly and to the right, but it can occasionally be located in the left sinus. The two ostia are very close to each other, and sometimes only one ostium exists. In addition, the left ostium is frequently stenotic and hypoplastic.

The technique is to make two ostia. First, the posterior commissure is totally detached. The intramural course is evaluated using a coronary probe. The probe can be extremely long, measuring more than 20 mm. The left ostium is incised and 'unroofed' for a distance of 5 mm. After this opening, the two ostia are sufficiently distant to allow creation of two buttons. The harvesting of the left button should be very cautious, considering the very long intramural course, and aided by the use of a coronary probe. The final incision can, in fact, be made at the very end of the left sinus. The right sinus has quite a normal shape, but the left button is very abnormal and extremely long. The ostia are located very close to the edge of the button, which greatly increases the difficulty of the anastomosis. Use of 8/0 or 9/0 suture is mandatory to perform a precise anastomosis. The posterior commissure will be reattached on the pericardial pulmonary patch.

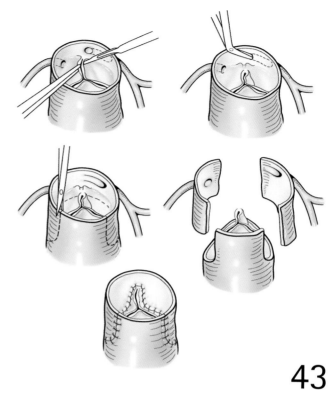

43 Two buttons are created in unroofing the left intramural course for a distance of 5 mm. The intramural course of the left button can be very long.

43

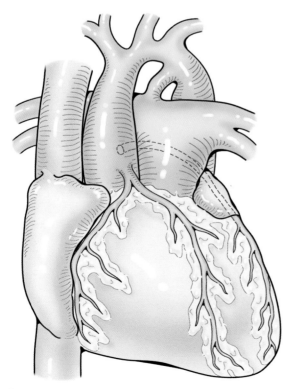

44

Major diameter mismatch between pulmonary artery and aorta

Major diameter discrepancy between the aorta and PA is seen in TGA-VSD and has an important impact on the coronary transfer. This feature is usually maximal in TGA-VSD with arch obstruction. The solution is to enlarge the distal aorta to correct the mismatch, which is done during the arch repair that is now performed under brain perfusion with the aortic cannula placed in the brachiocephalic artery.

44 Major PA-to-aorta diameter mismatch associated with side-by-side vessels and double-loop coronary course is shown here. This feature is seen in TGA-VSD coarctation or Taussig-Bing and coarctation.

45 The arch repair is performed using a brain perfusion; the aortic cannula is introduced in the brachiocephalic artery. The coarctation is resected and the transverse arch entirely incised.

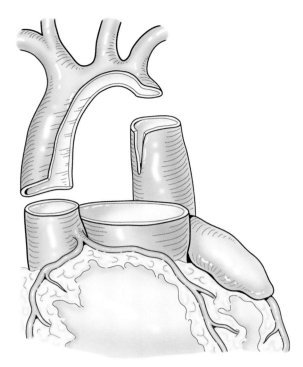

45

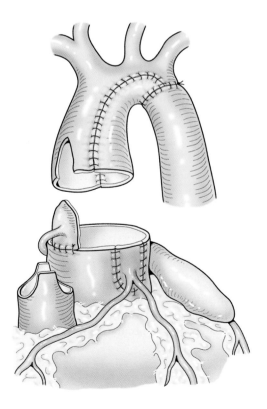

46

46 The distal ascending aorta and transverse arch are enlarged using a homograft patch. This step corrects the diameter mismatch. The right button is placed, as usual, in a high position.

OUTCOME

The arterial switch technique is now standardized, the coronary transfer being always the same. The relocation of the right button above the aortic anastomosis is helpful to reconstruct a harmonious aortic arch–sinotubular junction. The arterial switch is currently achieved with minimal mortality: from 0 per cent to 5 per cent in simple forms. Arterial switch performed in complex forms, including looping courses or intramural courses, is associated with an increased risk.

FURTHER READING

Asou T., Karl T.R., Pawade A., Mee R.B. 1994. Arterial switch: translocation of the intramural coronary artery. *Annals of Thoracic Surgery* 57, 461–5.

Castaneda, A., Norwood, I., Jonas, R., *et al.* 1984. TGA and IVS: Anatomical repair in the neonates. *Annals of Thoracic Surgery* 53, 438–43.

Lacour-Gayet, F., Piot, D., Zoghbi, J., *et al.* 2001. Surgical management and indication of left ventricular retaining in arterial switch for transposition of the great arteries with intact ventricular septum. *European Journal of Cardiothoracic Surgery* 20, 824–9.

Lacour-Gayet, F., Serraf, A., Galletti, L., *et al.* 1997. Biventricular repair of conotruncal anomalies associated with aortic arch obstruction: 103 patients. *Circulation* 96[Suppl II], 328–34.

Lecompte, Y., Zannini, L., Hazan, E., *et al.* 1981. Anatomic correction of TGA: New technique without use of a prosthetic conduit. *Journal of Thoracic and Cardiovascular Surgery* 82, 629–34

Planche, C., Lacour-Gayet, F., Bruniaux, J., *et al.* 1988. Switch operation for TGA in neonates. A study of 120 patients. *Journal of Thoracic and Cardiovascular Surgery* 96, 354–63.

Yacoub, M.H., Bernhard, A., Lange, P. 1980. Clinical and hemodynamical results of the two stage arterial switch for simple TGA. *Circulation* 62[Suppl I], 190–6.

54

Management of corrected transposition

PEDRO J. DEL NIDO MD
Professor of Surgery, Harvard Medical School; Senior Associate in Cardiac Surgery, Children's Hospital, Boston, Massachusetts, USA

HISTORY

The term *corrected transposition* was suggested by Rokitansky in 1875 when he first noted that, due to the position of the aorta and pulmonary arteries over the ventricular septum, the transposition was effectively 'corrected.' The term *congenitally corrected transposition* was added later to differentiate this anomaly from simple transposition that had undergone surgical repair. Lev described the abnormal position of the atrioventricular (AV) node in 1963, and Anderson and colleagues expanded on the anatomy of the conduction system in the 1970s. The first reports describing surgery for this cardiac anomaly came from the University of Minnesota in 1957. Initial reports describing physiological repair, leaving the morphological right ventricle as a systemic ventricle, were described in the 1970s and 1980s. Subsequently *anatomic correction* was described using the left ventricle as the systemic ventricle. Currently, the preferred method of repair is an anatomical approach in which the systemic venous return is diverted to the morphological right ventricle using an atrial baffle technique. Left ventricular-(LV) to-aortic flow is established either through a ventricular septal defect (VSD) baffle to the aorta or, in cases in which no LV outflow obstruction exists, an arterial switch procedure with coronary artery reimplantation.

PRINCIPLES AND JUSTIFICATION

Anatomy and physiology

The term *congenitally corrected transposition* is commonly applied to a spectrum of defects in which both AV and ventriculoarterial discordance exist, independent of situs. In this complex, the systemic veins are most often connected normally to a morphological right atrium, which connects to a morphological left ventricle. The LV outflow tract, if not atretic, connects to a semilunar valve leading to the pulmonary arteries. The pulmonary veins connect to a morphological left atrium, which is connected to a morphological right ventricle, which gives rise to the aorta. Typically, in situs solitus, the aorta is malposed to the left, and the pulmonary artery (PA) to the right of the aorta and slightly posterior.

The term *corrected* refers to the fact that the circulation is in series and systemic venous return first enters the pulmonary circulation via the native pulmonary arteries, and pulmonary venous return is ejected normally into the aorta. Thus, the term *congenitally corrected transposition of the great arteries* (CC-TGA) is frequently used. The Van Praagh convention, describing situs, ventricular looping, and relation of aorta to pulmonary artery, describes this lesion as either S,L,L (situs solitus, S; l-Loop, L; and left malposed aorta, L). In situs inversus, the defect is classified as I,D,D (situs inversus, I; d-loop, D; and right malposed aorta, D).

Of primary importance in this complex is the fact that the morphological right ventricle with its tricuspid valve is the systemic ventricle, receiving pulmonary venous return and connecting to the systemic circulation via the aorta. Associated defects are frequent and include ventricular septal defect, subpulmonary obstruction, and, more rarely, abnormalities of the tricuspid valve with Ebstein-like deformity. An additional important consideration includes the abnormal position of conduction tissue in situs solitus where the AV node and bundle of His are located anteriorly adjacent to the right AV valve orifice next to the orifice of the right atrial appendage. The elongated and tethered connection between the AV node and His bundle make these patients more susceptible to AV block.

Indications for surgery

In rare instances, corrected transposition exists as an isolated complex with no other associated defects. In these cases, the patients may remain asymptomatic, and reports exist of the diagnosis being made incidentally at the time of death from other causes. A VSD is present in the majority (approximately 70 per cent) of patients with CC-TGA. Symptoms of congestive heart failure, however, rarely are seen in infancy. LV outflow tract obstruction is seen in approximately 40 per cent, particularly in the presence of a VSD. In extreme cases, pulmonary atresia may exist. Tricuspid valve anomalies are frequent; however, the incidence of tricuspid valve regurgitation is low in younger children and increases with age, with as many as 40 per cent of adults developing at least moderate regurgitation. Ebstein-like deformity with short thick chordae tethering the valve can be seen but is uncommon.

The indications for surgical intervention are almost always dependent on the anatomical defects associated with CC-TGA. Operations in early infancy are indicated in cases in which severe subpulmonary stenosis or atresia are present resulting in severe cyanosis or ductal dependent pulmonary circulation. In such cases, palliative procedures to augment pulmonary blood flow such as subclavian-to-PA shunt are indicated, delaying corrective procedures to later in infancy. In rare cases, in the presence of a large VSD, congestive heart failure may be seen in early infancy, and usually PA banding to restrict pulmonary blood flow is performed in neonates. Tricuspid regurgitation is rarely an indication for surgery early in infancy and is usually due to tricuspid valve deformity. In such cases, anatomical repair is preferable because tricuspid valve repair is difficult and rarely completely successful, and replacement is associated with high intermediate mortality due to progressive right ventricular dysfunction. Most patients undergo repair within the first 1–2 years of life electively or because of progression of cyanosis or tricuspid regurgitation.

PREOPERATIVE ASSESSMENT AND PREPARATION

Anatomical features relevant to surgical repair of corrected transposition include situs, position of the apex of the ventricular mass, and the presence of associated defects, such as VSD and subpulmonary obstruction. Usually, children with CC-TGA present as older infants or children, and the symptoms are often subtle. Despite the frequent presence of a VSD, congestive heart failure is relatively uncommon in infancy due to the frequently associated presence of subpulmonary obstruction. The degree of subpulmonary obstruction also determines the degree of cyanosis, which is often the earliest presenting symptom. Bradycardia can also be the initial presenting symptom both in infancy and early childhood owing to the tenuous connection between the AV node and bundle of His. Spontaneous onset of complete AV block with slow ventricular rates can present as intermittent episodes of bradycardia. However, in most cases the presentation is that of sustained bradycardia that is permanent.

Diagnostic studies

The chest x-ray frequently indicates abnormalities of the ventricles due to the unusual position of the ventricular apex. Mesocardia or dextrocardia are not uncommon. The electrocardiogram may demonstrate the presence of AV block, varying from first degree to complete heart block.

The diagnosis of corrected CC-TGA is usually made by 2-dimensional echocardiography, demonstrating mitral valve morphology on the right-sided ventricle with two separate papillary muscles attaching to both valve leaflets. In S,L,L, the leftward ventricle has the typical morphology of a right ventricle with a trileaflet AV valve, direct septal attachments of the septal leaflet, and an infundibulum which gives rise to the leftward positioned aorta. Associated defects such as VSD, subpulmonary obstruction, and tricuspid valve abnormalities can also be detected by echocardiography. The degree of subpulmonary stenosis can be estimated by Doppler interrogation of the right-sided ventricular outflow tract. The competence of the AV valves can also be assessed.

Cardiac catheterization is usually reserved for assessment of the degree of subpulmonary obstruction and to directly measure PA pressures. Angiography is also helpful to assess PA branch size and potential distortion from previous surgical procedures such as systemic-to-pulmonary shunts.

ANESTHESIA

General anesthesia is used in all patients undergoing palliative or corrective procedures. The technique of anesthesia usually involves a combination of high-dose narcotics combined with muscle relaxants and inhalation agents and is not significantly different than that for any child undergoing cardiac surgery.

OPERATIONS

Palliative procedures

INDICATIONS

Palliative procedures are rarely required in patients with CC-TGA unless severe subpulmonary obstruction is present in infancy, or, inversely, a large VSD exists with an unobstructed pulmonary outflow tract, resulting in congestive heart failure during early infancy.

SYSTEMIC-TO-PULMONARY SHUNTS

In young infants with severe cyanosis, a palliative systemic-to-pulmonary shunt may be indicated to augment pulmonary blood flow in preparation for subsequent anatomical correction or, in cases of hypoplasia of one ventricle, staged management of single ventricle.

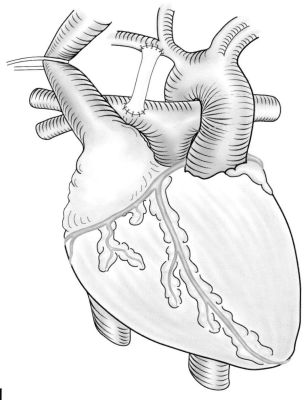

1

1 A median sternotomy is preferred for insertion of a systemic-to-PA shunt. This approach provides access to the arch vessels and branch pulmonary arteries independent of aortic arch position and branch distribution. After the sternotomy is completed, the pericardium is opened in the midline and the dissection extended to expose the innominate and subclavian artery. In situs solitus, the main pulmonary trunk is to the right and posterior to the aorta. The right PA is easily dissected between the ascending aorta and superior vena cava. In infants younger than 3 months of age, we prefer to use a 3.5-mm thin wall Gore-Tex graft sewn end-to-side from the base of the subclavian artery at the origin of the innominate artery with the distal end of the shunt inserting into the right PA near the main pulmonary trunk.

In neonates, the ductus may be left open, allowing it to close spontaneously after prostaglandins are discontinued. In cases in which a large ductus exists, ligation is preferable at the time of shunt insertion to prevent pulmonary overcirculation, low diastolic pressure, and, possibly, necrotizing enterocolitis. A single chest drain is left in the mediastinum, and the pericardium is only partially closed to prevent pericardial fluid accumulation and, potentially, tamponade after surgery.

PULMONARY ARTERY BANDING IN INFANTS WITH PULMONARY OVERCIRCULATION

In neonates or young infants with unrestricted pulmonary flow and signs of congestive heart failure, restriction of pulmonary blood flow can be achieved by inserting a constricting band at the level of the main pulmonary trunk. The goal is to provide a physical restriction to pulmonary blood flow to prevent overcirculation of the pulmonary bed, at the expense of systemic blood flow. Thus, a physiological improvement is achieved without the need for a complex intracardiac repair, which can be deferred for several months.

2 The approach is also a midline sternotomy because this approach provides access to the posteriorly placed pulmonary artery. Dissection around the pulmonary trunk should be done just below the takeoff of both branches and should be limited to prevent band migration. The width of the band should be 4 mm to avoid encroaching onto the cusps of the pulmonary valve, because distortion of the pulmonary valve may preclude anatomical repair later in infancy. Silicone-covered Dacron mesh is ideal material for banding because it has minimal stretch and does not adhere to the PA wall, facilitating band removal at the time of repair. Two methods of banding a pulmonary artery are commonly used. In one method, the band is tightened to a distal PA pressure of approximately 50 per cent of systemic pressure, monitoring arterial oxygen saturation, which should be maintained at more than 80 per cent. The second method uses a regression formula described by Albus and colleagues. In this technique, the band circumference around the PA is determined by a preset value, based on anatomical diagnosis (usually 20–22 mm), then adding 1 mm/kg weight of the infant (younger than 6 months of age) to the circumference.

Monitoring pulse oxymetry or arterial blood gases to maintain a hemoglobin oxygen saturation higher than 80 per cent is also necessary because other factors such cardiac index, hematocrit, and pulmonary vascular resistance affect systemic blood oxygen content. The band should be fixed to the pulmonary adventitia to prevent migration and distortion of one of the branch pulmonary arteries.

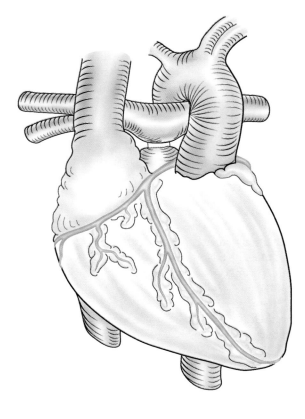

2

Anatomical repair

The goal of an anatomical repair of CC-TGA is to leave the anatomical left ventricle supporting systemic circulation and the anatomical right ventricle connected to the pulmonary circulation. To accomplish this goal, the systemic venous inflow must be rerouted from its entry into the right atrium towards the posterior and leftward positioned tricuspid valve and morphological right ventricle. This step involves baffling of the systemic venous return towards the left atrium using either atrial tissue, as in a Senning procedure, or autologous pericardium, as in the Mustard operation. The technique for achieving ventricular arterial concordance depends on the presence and degree of pulmonary or subpulmonary obstruction.

In the majority of patients, a large VSD is present adjacent to the AV valves, and at least moderate subpulmonary obstruction also exists. Because the subpulmonary obstruction is usually due to a combination of AV valve tissue and conal septum, enlargement of this area usually results in injury to the AV valve or complete heart block from damage to the conduction tissue, which runs in the subpulmonary region. Ventriculoarterial concordance in these patients can be achieved by diverting LV flow through the VSD towards the aorta, creating an interventricular tunnel, similar to a Rastelli procedure for d-transposition. Right ventricle to PA continuity is then achieved with a conduit from the infundibulum of the right ventricle to the transected pulmonary trunk, usually to the left of the aorta. The pulmonary arteries can be mobilized to the left of the aorta in cases of mesocardia to facilitate insertion of the RV to the PA conduit.

In children without subpulmonary obstruction, with or without a ventricular septal defect, ventriculoarterial concordance can be achieved by an arterial switch procedure involving transection and reconnection of the great arteries to their respective ventricles, reimplanting the coronary arteries into the neoaorta, and closure of the ventricular septal defect.

ANATOMICAL REPAIR OF CONGENITALLY CORRECTED TRANSPOSITION OF THE GREAT ARTERIES WITH VENTRICULAR SEPTAL DEFECT AND SUBPULMONARY OBSTRUCTION

VENTRICULOTOMY

3 To gain access to the VSD and subaortic area, a longitudinal ventriculotomy in the infundibulum of the anatomical right ventricle is made, extending to the subaortic area. Care must be taken to stay to the left of the left anterior descending coronary artery and not to extend the incision too close to the aortic valve annulus because the sinuses of Valsalva frequently extend below the edge of the right ventricular muscle. The VSD can then be identified, and AV valve chordal attachments should be noted.

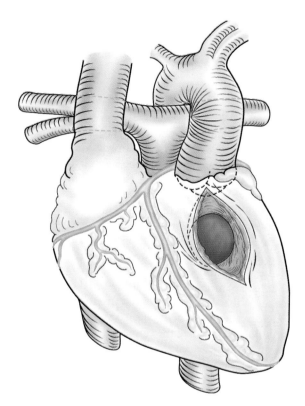

3

4a, b

Straddling chordae across the VSD from either AV valve may preclude a ventriculoaortic tunnel unless the chordae can be reimplanted, maintaining AV valve competence. A tube graft of knitted Dacron is then chosen with a diameter similar to the size of the VSD. The tube graft is then cut in an oblique angle and opened length wise to serve as the roof of the intracardiac tunnel. The Dacron is fixed posteriorly to the junction of the two AV valves directly using a running monofilament suture, and the suture line is continued circumferentially around the VSD, staying at least 5 mm away from the crest of the anterior superior border of the VSD to avoid injury to the conduction system. The distal end of the baffle is sewn around the aortic valve annulus to complete the tunnel.

PULMONARY TRANSECTION AND RIGHT VENTRICLE TO PULMONARY CONNECTION

The main pulmonary trunk is transected at the top of the commissures with the proximal pulmonary root oversewn with interrupted reinforced myofilament sutures. The pulmonary valve leaflets should be incorporated by the sutures to obliterate the supravalvar space because this area may be a source of thrombus formation and potential emboli late after surgery. Alternatively, the semilunar valve leaflet can be excised before closing the proximal pulmonary stump. The main PA and branches are then dissected circumferentially to mobilize them towards the left of the aorta to facilitate connection with the right ventricle-to-PA conduit. The pulmonary arteriotomy can be extended into the left PA branch to facilitate conduit implantation.

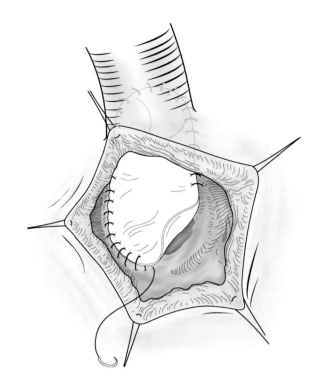

4a

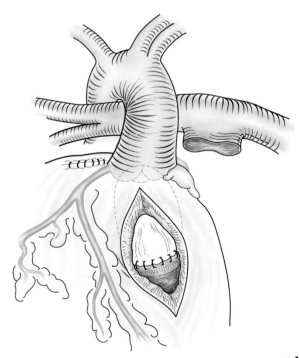

4b

5 To connect the right ventricle to the pulmonary trunk, in most cases a valved conduit is used to minimize pulmonary regurgitation. We prefer to use an aortic or pulmonary homograft with the full length of the artery to reach the native pulmonary arteries, avoiding circumferential synthetic tube grafts as extensions because these can result in early obstruction from neointimal proliferation. The right ventricle-to-PA conduit is usually positioned to the left of the aorta. Opening the left pleural space and mobilizing the pericardium leftward and posteriorly facilitate positioning of the conduit. Care must be taken to avoid injury to the phrenic nerve during this maneuver. Mobilization of the pericardium also facilitates rotation of the ventricular apex towards the left, displacing the conduit leftward and away from the sternum to avoid compression. The proximal end of the conduit is then sewn directly to the edge of the ventriculotomy posteriorly. A gusset of autologous pericardium treated with glutaraldehyde or Gore-Tex can be used to form the roof of the right ventricle to conduit connection.

ATRIAL REROUTING PROCEDURE

To complete the anatomical repair of CC-TGA, in addition to establishing ventricular arterial concordance, venous return must be rerouted to the appropriate ventricle. Conceptually, this goal involves diverting systemic venous return (inferior vena cava and superior vena cava) to the tricuspid valve situated posteriorly, including the coronary sinus in the baffle. By exclusion, the pulmonary veins are able to drain into the anterior ventricle (morphological left ventricle), which is now connected to the aorta. This step is accomplished using either native atrial tissue (Senning operation) or with baffles created with autologous pericardium. In this section, we describe the baffling procedure with pericardium (Mustard operation) because it is applicable to patients with levocardia and dextrocardia in which the right atrium can be small making a Senning procedure difficult.

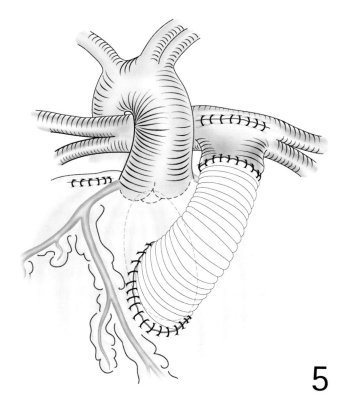

5

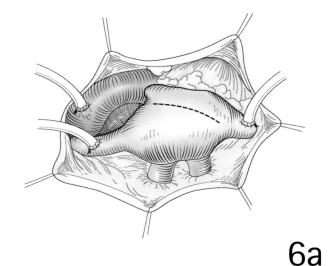

6a

ATRIAL SEPTECTOMY

6a, b To permit unobstructed flow of caval return posteriorly towards the tricuspid valve, the interatrial septum must first be resected. To avoid injury to the conduction tissue, the medial extent of the septal excision ends at the superior limbus or tendon of Todaro. The superior resection margin extends to the superior caval orifice, ending in the mid portion of the orifice. The septectomy extends laterally to the level of the pulmonary vein orifice including the edge of the crista terminalis. The coronary sinus is unroofed towards the mid portion of the mitral valve. This maneuver enlarges the inferior caval baffle and maintains the coronary venous return in the systemic venous circulation.

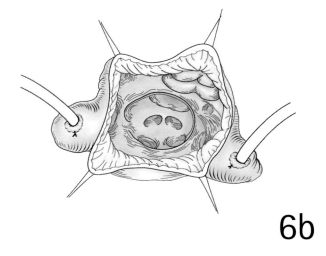

6b

ATRIAL BAFFLE

7 A dumbbell-shaped pericardial patch is then prepared using autologous pericardium. The pericardial patch is harvested from the anterior pericardium and extended from the left to the right phrenic nerve. In most patients, adequate pericardium is present to create both baffles. The length and width of the baffle is determined by the patient's size. However, the goal is to maintain a uniform size from the caval orifice to the tricuspid valve. The posterior suture line of the baffle is started by first attaching the mid portion of the baffle to the atrium between the left pulmonary veins and left atrial appendage. The suture lines are continued rightward around both caval orifices leaving adequate room for left pulmonary vein drainage towards the right-sided atrium. The anterior portion of the baffle is shorter than the posterior; therefore, the patch must be trimmed at this point. This step is facilitated by starting the suture line in the interatrial septum near the tendon of Todaro and extending it towards the caval orifices. Once the baffle is completed, the atriotomy can be closed. At this point, confirming that pulmonary venous flow can enter the mitral valve without obstruction is important. If insufficient right atrial free wall is present, the pulmonary venous pathway can be enlarged with a patch of pericardium or Cortex material, extending from the atrial appendage to the right pulmonary veins.

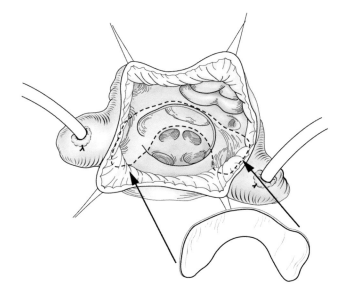

7

ANATOMICAL REPAIR OF CONGENITALLY CORRECTED TRANSPOSITION OF THE GREAT ARTERIES WITH OR WITHOUT VENTRICULAR SEPTAL DEFECT AND *WITHOUT* SUBPULMONARY OBSTRUCTION

ARTERIAL SWITCH PROCEDURE

In children with CC-TGA who do not have significant sub-pulmonary obstruction and have a well formed pulmonary valve, ventriculoarterial concordance can be established by switching the great arteries and reimplanting the coronaries to the neoaorta, analogous to anatomical repair of simple transposition. As in children with simple transposition, consideration of coronary artery distribution and position with respect to the pulmonary root is important in planning this part of the operation. In most cases, the left coronary artery rises anteriorly giving rise to the left anterior descending and circumflex branches, which in patients with CC-TGA courses towards the right. The right coronary artery arises posteriorly, coursing in the AV groove of the anatomical right ventricle, which is to the left of the midline.

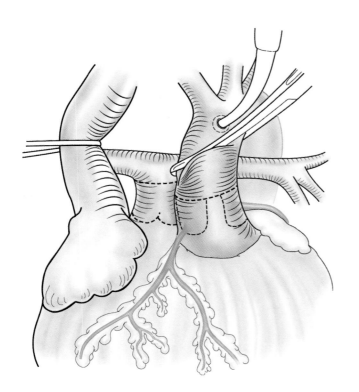

8 The technique of arterial switch in patients with CC-TGA requires mobilization of the ascending aorta, which is L-malposed. Therefore, arterial cannulation should be done at the level of the innominate artery or transverse arch. The pulmonary trunk arises posterior and rightward of the aorta, and the main PA is usually short. The pulmonary trunk is transected at the level of the takeoff of the right PA, with the branch pulmonary arteries being extensively dissected, particularly towards the right to permit mobilization leftward to accomplish the anatomical connections. The coronary arteries are removed as large buttons contain nearly the entire sinus of Valsalva. Dissection can be extended to the level of the bifurcation of the left coronary artery. In cases in which there is a large conal branch originating from a left anterior descending or from the right coronary artery, division of the conal branch facilitates translocation of the coronary buttons to the neopulmonary root.

8

9 As is the case with simple transposition, the coronary buttons usually end up above the level of the neoaortic valve at the sinotubular junction or above. An aortic end-to-end anastomosis is then performed connecting the ascending aorta to the neoaortic root, usually anterior to the right pulmonary artery. The defect left in the neopulmonary root from removal of the coronary buttons is then repaired with autologous glutaraldehyde-treated pericardium. The patch should have sufficient length to extend the neopulmonary root to reach the branch pulmonary arteries, which have been mobilized to the left of the ascending aorta. In older children, owing to the lack of mobility of the branch pulmonary arteries, the neopulmonary trunk may not reach the PAs directly, and an interposition tube graft may be necessary. In these cases, we have used a valveless pulmonary or aortic homograft.

Closure of the VSD, if present, can be done through the neoaortic root before completion of the arterial switch or, alternatively, through the right atrium retracting the mitral valve leaflets. Due to the anterior-superior position of the conduction system, the superior edge of the VSD patch is positioned to the right of the crest of the septum to avoid injury to the conduction tissue (see closure of ventricular septal defect in the section 'Nonanatomical (physiological) repair').

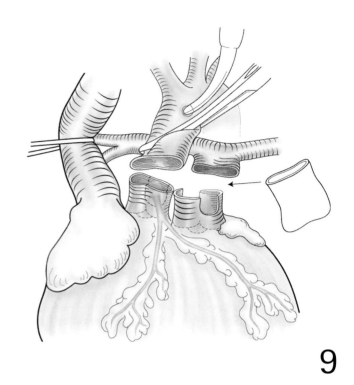

9

Nonanatomical repair

Nonanatomical repair of CC-TGA refers to operative procedures that repair hemodynamical defects and result in a two-ventricle repair; however, the morphological right ventricle remains the systemic ventricle. Examples include S,L,L with isolated VSD, and more commonly, S,L,L, VSD, and subpulmonary obstruction. In these children, a 'physiological' repair can be achieved by simply closing the VSD, or in cases with subpulmonary obstruction, adding a left ventricle-to-PA conduit. Concerns about the development of late complications such as systemic (tricuspid) AV valve regurgitation and right (systemic) ventricular dysfunction have resulted in these procedures being performed less frequently. Nevertheless, circumstances exist in which this approach is indicated, such as children with S,L,L and

a restrictive VSD, and S,L,L with VSD and dextrocardia in which the RV infundibulum is directly behind the sternum and potentially compressing the RV-PA conduit.

CLOSURE OF VENTRICULAR SEPTAL DEFECT

In children with CC-TGA who have a VSD with a mild to moderate degree of subpulmonary obstruction, an option for achieving a two-ventricle repair is simply to close the VSD, leaving the morphological right ventricle supporting the systemic circulation. Our preference has been to perform an anatomical repair; however, if the VSD is small or restrictive, VSD closure may be an option to consider as a physiological, nonanatomical two-ventricle repair.

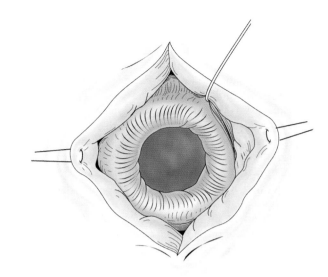

10a, b In children with levo- or mesocardia, the approach to the VSD can be visualized through a right atriotomy, retracting the mitral valve leaflet to expose the VSD which is usually posterior and directly beneath the mitral valve leaflets. In children with dextrocardia and situs solitus, visualizing the VSD from the right atrium can be difficult because the ventricular mass is in front. In these cases, if the ventricles cannot be rotated leftward sufficiently, then a ventriculotomy in the morphological left ventricle may be necessary to expose the VSD. To determine the safest place for the ventriculotomy, inserting a digit into the morphological left ventricle may be helpful to identify the area between the two papillary muscles and make the incision directly between the two, extending from the base of the ventricle towards the apex. This maneuver affords direct exposure to the VSD, which is closed in the same fashion as previously described. Alternative strategies for exposing the VSD include transecting the aorta, which is usually large in older patients, and closing the VSD on the right ventricular side of the septum. Alternatively, in situs inversus, the VSD can be exposed via the left atrium. Incisions in the right ventricular infundibulum should be avoided because this ventricle remains systemic in this type of nonanatomical, two-ventricle repair.

10a

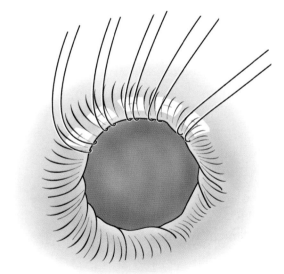

10b

10c Because the conduction tissue is anterior and courses on the superior crest of the septal defect, the VSD patch should be attached to the morphological right ventricular side of the defect crossing over to the morphological left ventricle posteriorly.

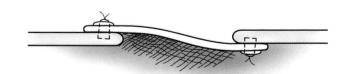

10c

Single-ventricle management of congenitally corrected transposition of the great arteries

Contraindications to a two-ventricle repair in children with CC-TGA include (1) severe hypoplasia of one ventricular chamber, straddling of the AV valves such that closure of the VSD or diversion of the flow through the septal defect to the aorta is not possible without impairing normal valve function, and (2) unusual cases in which the complexity of a two-ventricle repair due to unusual anatomy make single-ventricle management a more attractive alternative. Examples of the latter include children with CC-TGA, VSD, severe subpulmonary obstruction, and isolated dextrocardia in whom the right ventricle-to-PA conduit is directly beneath the sternum and likely to be significantly compressed. Another example is children with moderate hypoplasia of the morphological right ventricle in whom a significant portion of the ventricle will be occupied by the LV to aortic intracardiac baffle, leaving a relatively small ventricular chamber to support pulmonary circulation. In these cases, cavopulmonary connection is a good alternative and is usually accomplished by a staged procedure. Initial bidirectional cavopulmonary connection (unilateral or bilateral depending on the number of superior cavae) can be done within the first 6–8 months of life (see Chapter 44 page 629).

Completion of the cavopulmonary connection is usually done between 2 and 4 years of age and involves creation of a lateral tunnel in the right atrium to extend the inferior cava to the PA confluence or using an extracardiac tube graft to connect the inferior vena cava to the PA (see Chapter 43 page 619). In cases in which moderate hypoplasia of the morphological right ventricle exists, a combination of both approaches may be preferable. This combination would include a bidirectional cavopulmonary connection to connect superior caval blood flow to the pulmonary circuit. Inferior caval blood flow is diverted to the tricuspid valve using an intra-atrial baffle, and right ventricular outflow-to-PA continuity is established with a right ventricle-to-PA conduit similar to the anatomical repair described previously for CC-TGA, VSD, and subpulmonary stenosis.

POSTOPERATIVE CARE

Postoperative management of children having undergone anatomical two-ventricle repair is similar to that of any child having undergone a major cardiac surgical procedure. Intraoperative assessment of residual defects including residual shunts at atrial or ventricular level, obstruction in any of the baffle pathways, and AV valve regurgitation is a critical component of the repair. Residual defects or incomplete repair imposes an additional workload on the ventricle and is one of the common causes of low cardiac output in the immediate postoperative period, resulting in a higher risk for morbidity and mortality. Hemodynamic assessment in the operating room can be accomplished by transesophageal echocardiography in addition to sampling superior caval and PA hemoglobin oxygen saturation to search for significant residual shunts. Conduit obstruction can be difficult to detect, particularly when conduit compression by the sternum occurs when the chest is closed. A high index of suspicion based on conduit position and a sudden increase in atrial pressures when closing the sternum should be an indication of conduit compression. An attempt should then be made to shift the heart or conduit to one side of the sternum. In infants, leaving the sternum open until mediastinal edema resolves may prevent conduit compression.

All children undergoing anatomical or nonanatomical repair should have temporary pacemaker wires because transient or permanent complete AV block is a known risk factor in these patients.

OUTCOME

Mortality

The operative (30 day) mortality for corrective procedures varies between 0 and 10 per cent with the number of patients being less than 30 in most series. These results compare favorably with earlier reports of operative mortality rates of 15–20 per cent for nonanatomical, two-ventricle procedures, however, no reports of direct comparisons are available.

The risk of a single-ventricle procedure such as a total cavopulmonary connection is the same for this group of patients as for single-ventricle lesions. Although in theory having two ventricles contributing to cardiac output should provide a benefit, analysis of early mortality with Fontan procedures does not support this contention. Whether long-term outcome or exercise capacity is better in the S,L,L patients with two normal-size ventricles remains speculative because no specific information is available at this time.

Postoperative complications

Complete heart block from injury to the anteriorly positioned AV node and His bundle remains higher for this defect than for corrective procedures in children with d-loop cardiac anatomy. As the intracardiac anatomy and location of the conduction tissue has become more widely known and the experience of surgeons has increased, the incidence of complete AV block has decreased. Current reports describe rates between 0 and 10 per cent.

Conduit obstruction occurring early is relatively rare with anatomical repairs when the apex of the ventricle is leftward. Dextrocardia with situs solitus is a risk factor for conduit obstruction and is considered by many surgeons to be a relative contraindication to two-ventricle repair unless the conduit can be positioned away from the sternum. Reoperation rates vary with the type of repair performed at the first procedure. However, if a conduit is used, freedom from reoperation is less than 50 per cent by 8 years after surgery.

FURTHER READING

Di Donato, R.M., Wernovsky, G., Jonas, R.A., Mayer, J.E. Jr, Keane, J.F., Castaneda, A.R. 1991. Corrected transposition in situs inversus. Biventricular repair of associated cardiac anomalies. *Circulation* 84, III193–9.

Imamura, M., Drummond-Webb, J.J., Murphy, D.J. Jr, *et al.* 2000. Results of the double switch operation in the current era. *Annals of Thoracic Surgery* 70, 100–5.

Karl, T.R., Weintraub, R.G., Brizard, C.P., Cochrane, A.D., Mee, R.B. 1997. Senning plus arterial switch operation for discordant (congenitally corrected) transposition. *Annals of Thoracic Surgery* 64, 495–502.

Termignon, J.L., Leca, F., Vouhe, P.R., *et al.* 1996. 'Classic' repair of congenitally corrected transposition and ventricular septal defect. *Annals of Thoracic Surgery* 62, 199–206.

Van Praagh, R., Papagiannis, J., Grunenfelder, J., Bartram, U., Martanovic, P. 1998. Pathologic anatomy of corrected transposition of the great arteries: medical and surgical implications. *American Heart Journal* 135, 772–85.

van Son, J.A., Danielson, G.K., Huhta, J.C., *et al.* 1995. Late results of systemic atrioventricular valve replacement in corrected transposition. *Journal of Thoracic and Cardiovascular Surgery* 109, 642–52.

55

Persistent truncus arteriosus

MARTIN J. ELLIOTT MD, FRCS
Senior Lecturer of Surgery, Institute of Child Health, University College; Consultant Cardiothoracic Surgeon, Cardiac Unit, Great Ormond Street Hospital for Children National Health Service Trust, London, UK

ROBERT CESNJEVAR MD
Cardiothoracic Surgeon, Zentrum fuer Herzchirurgie, Universitaetsklinik Erlangen-Nuremberg, Erlangen, Germany

HISTORY

Truncus arteriosus is an uncommon congenital anomaly accounting for 1–4 per cent of patients born with congenital heart disease. First described by Wilson in 1798, anatomical classifications were introduced by Collett and Edwards based on the presence of a main pulmonary trunk or the separation of the pulmonary arteries from the arterial trunk in 1949. A widely used classification has been the scheme developed by Van Praagh in 1965, which describes four subtypes with and without the presence of a ventricular septal defect (VSD). The detailed morphology is reviewed by Professor Robert H. Anderson in chapter 38 'Anatomy of congenital heart disease'.

Classification

1 Van Praagh classification

Type A: VSD present
Type B: VSD not present

1 Partially formed aortopulmonary septum (main pulmonary artery [PA] segment present)
2 Absent aortopulmonary septum (both pulmonary arteries originate directly from the aorta)
3 Absence of one PA branch from the trunk (ductal origin of one PA)
4 Interrupted aortic arch associated with truncus arteriosus.

In the past, patients were palliated by single or bilateral PA banding followed by definitive repair at a later age. This approach resulted in a high early mortality and morbidity. McGoon reported the first single-stage repair in 1968 using a valved homograft. Paul Ebert from San Francisco demonstrated, in a classic series published in 1984, that primary repair in infancy could be performed with a low mortality (11 per cent) and advocated this as the preferred approach. Primary one-stage repair is now the treatment of choice, but even now few centers have achieved the results that Ebert produced so long ago.

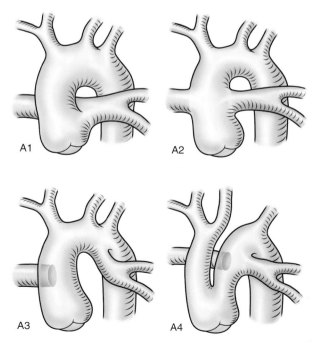

A1 A2 A3 A4

1

PRINCIPLES AND JUSTIFICATION

The majority of infants born with truncus arteriosus present with severe congestive heart failure within the first week of life. Without surgical treatment, a 75–85 per cent mortality occurs during the first year of life. Excessive pulmonary blood flow results in severe pulmonary vascular disease very early in life. Further 'runoff' from the truncal artery into the low resistance pulmonary circuit can result in a low diastolic blood pressure and, thus, decreased coronary perfusion, affecting ventricular performance. Corrective surgery should be undertaken once the diagnosis is established, certainly within the first month of life. Operative risk increases after 100 days of life, and some experts suggest that waiting until after 7 days of age is best. In the presence of severe truncal valvar regurgitation or aortic arch interruption, emergency surgery may be needed.

PREOPERATIVE ASSESSMENT AND PREPARATION

Echocardiography usually establishes the diagnosis without difficulty. Assessment of truncal valve function, coronary arterial origins, aortic arch anatomy, and pulmonary arteries is crucial. On the rare occurrence of late referral, when irreversible pulmonary vascular disease needs to be ruled out or when echocardiography is inconclusive, cardiac catheterization may be warranted. If pulmonary vascular disease is identified, detailed physiological studies on pulmonary vascular resistance and its manipulation may be helpful for postoperative management.

If a child needs preoperative resuscitation and ventilatory support, careful clinical assessment is needed. Avoiding an acute decrease in pulmonary vascular resistance, which could alter ventricular performance, is important. Indeed, to maintain adequate diastolic pressure, management is directed at maintaining a degree of pulmonary vascular resistance by reducing ventilatory rates, using smaller tidal volumes, and increasing pulmonary vasoconstriction with lower inspiratory oxygen (F_{IO_2}). Thus, the situation is very like a preoperative 'Norwood' for duct-dependent hypoplastic left heart syndrome.

ANESTHESIA

Anesthetic management does not differ from operations for most congenital heart defects. Manipulations that increase the already excessive pulmonary blood flow should be avoided. A significant number of patients with persistent truncus arteriosus have DiGeorge syndrome; therefore, irradiated blood products must be used to avoid graft-versus-host reactions after blood transfusions. Blood calcium concentrations need particular attention intra- and postoperatively.

OPERATION

Surgical approach

The heart is exposed via a median sternotomy. The thymus (if present) is excised, taking care to avoid damage to the phrenic nerve. The pericardium is opened longitudinally, and a patch is harvested if needed. The aorta is dissected beyond the innominate artery. The pulmonary arteries are mobilized, and vessel loops are placed around both branch pulmonary arteries but are not tightened at this stage. A ligature is placed around the duct (if present) for later ligation. The external anatomy (in particular the coronary arteries) must be assessed.

Conduct of cardiopulmonary bypass

Circulatory arrest is best avoided. The aorta is cannulated at the level of the transverse arch, and bicaval venous return is established, so that circulatory arrest can be avoided during the intracardiac repair. Venous cannulation is best done via the right atrium in small children. Some surgeons prefer to use venous return via a single angled cannula in smaller children (less than 1.5–2.0 kg), and the patient is cooled slowly down to 18°C over 20 minutes. Vacuum-assisted venous drainage permits the use of smaller venous cannulae for adequate venous return and may permit bicaval cannulation even in very small infants.

2 As soon as bypass is initiated, the pulmonary arteries must be snared closed (we use looped vascular slings [vessel loops]) to prevent run-off into the pulmonary circulation. Such run-off, associated with a drop in diastolic blood pressure, could cause significant cardiac or cerebral hypoperfusion.

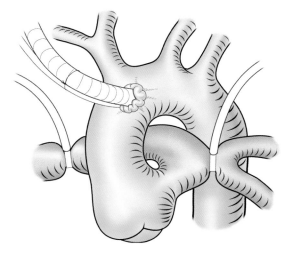

2

Pulmonary artery detachment from truncus arteriosus

The aorta is cross-clamped as high as possible, and cardioplegic solution is infused before transection of the common arterial trunk. Continued occlusion of branch pulmonary arteries ensures that cardioplegia perfuses the coronary arteries. If significant truncal valve incompetence exists, the trunk should be opened and cardioplegic solution infused directly into the coronary arteries with a small cannula. Retrograde cardioplegia delivery via the coronary sinus may also be used. The line of incision should be chosen carefully so as not to damage the coronary ostia, which may originate higher than usual, even from the branch pulmonary arteries. Sudden ST-segment changes on snaring the pulmonary arteries or failure to deliver adequately antegrade cardioplegia should alert the surgeon to this possibility.

3a-d For detachment of the pulmonary arteries from the aorta, a number of important steps should be performed. The first step is to observe the coronaries, their origin, and course, because abnormal origin of the coronary arteries is not infrequent. The second step is the inspection of the pulmonary arteries, their origin, and course. This inspection allows the surgeon to make a decision as to how to make the detachment of the pulmonary arteries from the trunk. Our preferred approach is simple transverse transection of the aorta, starting slightly above the origin of the pulmonary arteries from the common trunk, making an incision approximately halfway around the aorta. This maneuver provides excellent exposure of the PA origins, coronary artery anatomy, and the truncal valve. The incision is continued around the pulmonary arteries, leaving a generous cuff around their origins.

After placing stay sutures of 6/0 Prolene above each commissure, the truncal valve is assessed, and a repair or replacement is undertaken if required. Aortic reconstruction after a transection approach may be complicated because of the mismatch between the proximal aorta and the much smaller distal aorta. A small anterior incision in the distal aorta allows the placement of a small anterior patch if needed, at a convenient position away from the coronaries.

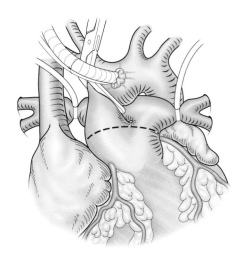

3a

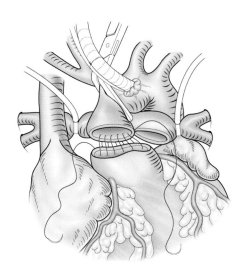

3b

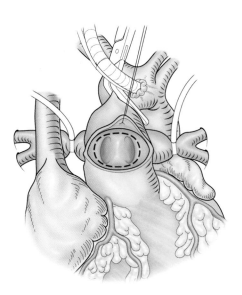

3c

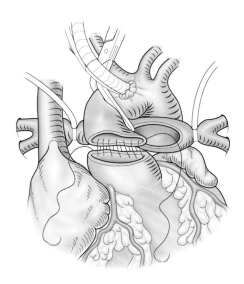

3d

4 However, in most circumstances the reanastomosis can be performed easily by making minor alterations to the continuous suture line, for example using a horizontal mattress suture proximally and a vertical mattress suture distally.

The alternative method of separation is to dissect and detach the PA from the aorta. This approach is most suitable for a true type I truncus arteriosus, in which the pulmonary arteries have a common origin. However, this method runs the risk of damaging important structures such as the left coronary ostium, the aortic sinuses, and the truncal valve itself. Dissection has to be taken slowly and carefully. Detachment by this technique leaves a hole in a difficult posterior and leftward position.

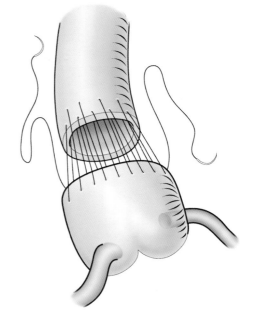

4

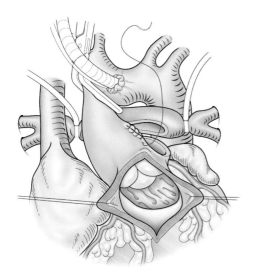

5a

5a, b The pulmonary arteries are excised from the common trunk with a generous cuff, and the defect in the aorta is closed either primarily or with a patch. A patch is usually required to avoid distortion, particularly of the truncal valve and coronary arteries.

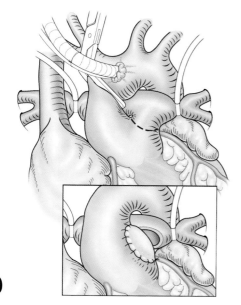

5b

Truncal valve repair/replacement

Mild-to-moderate truncal valve regurgitation can be well tolerated and may improve postoperatively after corrective surgery. Significant truncal valve stenosis (gradient greater than 30 mm Hg) and severe truncal valve regurgitation often necessitate surgery to the valve. As with all other heart valves, repair is better than replacement if it can be done successfully.

Truncal valve stenosis

The stenotic truncal valve is often thickened and dysplastic. Thus, principles learnt from the surgical management of congenital aortic stenosis (e.g. commissurotomy and shaving [thinning] techniques) can be applied.

Truncal valve regurgitation

6a–d Recent publications from the Cleveland Group have provided very helpful new techniques for truncal valve repair. In quadricuspid valves, repair may be possible by reducing the number of leaflets. Quadricusp valves can also be remodeled by excising the smallest cusp. The created defect is closed with pledgetted subcommissural sutures.

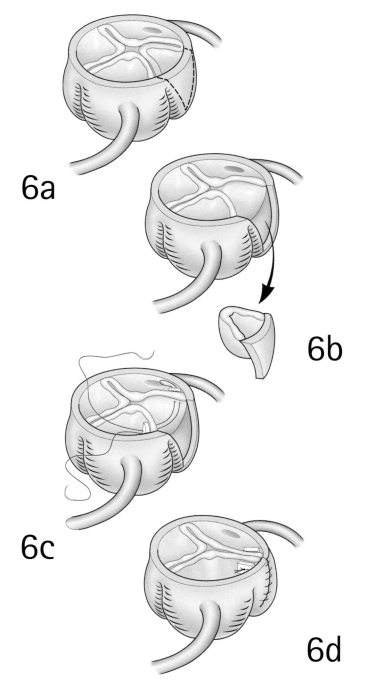

7a–d If repair of the truncal valve fails, valve replacement may need to be undertaken. In this setting, a primary aortic root replacement using a cryopreserved homograft is probably the only viable procedure (Figures a–d). The homograft should be sized to the age of the child; therefore, preoperative echo diagnosis is mandatory, because the homograft has to be ordered in advance. We have used homografts as small as 6 mm in 1.5 kg children and sizes from 10–15 mm in children weighing up to 5 kg. If an aortic homograft is inserted, the mitral leaflet can sometimes be used to close the VSD (Figure c). The coronary arteries are excised from the truncal wall and reimplanted onto the homograft using fine suture material (Figures a–d). The right coronary artery is best sited after filling the aortic root with cardioplegia to identify the sinuses better.

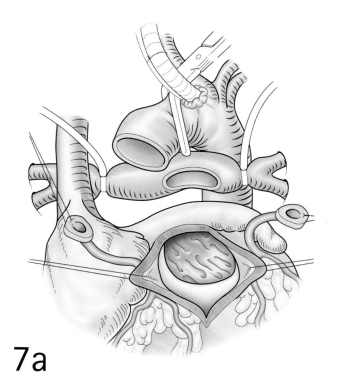

7a

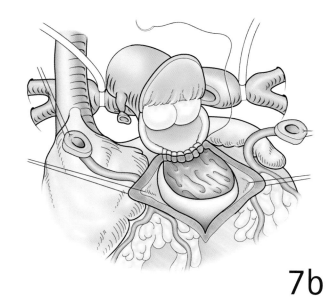

7b

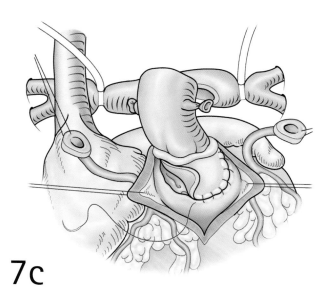

7c

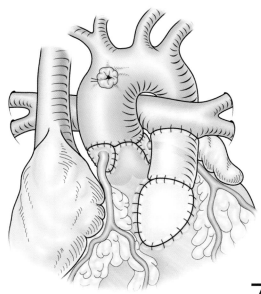

7d

Closure of ventricular septal defect

The VSD is approached through a vertical right ventricular infundibular incision between stay sutures (5/0 Prolene) approximately 0.5 cm apart and 1 cm below the truncal valve (which is closer than one expects). Care must be taken not to damage any crossing major coronary artery branches. The incision in the right ventricle (RV) should be large enough to create a good outlet for the conduit, but not so large as to damage the function of the RV. Gentle retraction of the incision using eyelid, nerve root retractors, or special VSD retractors gives good exposure of the VSD. The truncal valve can be inspected through the ventriculotomy to ensure that no damage has been done. Any obstructing right ventricular muscle bundles are divided, leaving the supporting apparatus for the tricuspid valve intact.

8 The VSD may be muscular (approximately 70 per cent) or perimembranous (approximately 30 per cent). In the more common muscular defects, suturing in this area can be performed without risk to the conduction tissue. A patch of Gore-Tex, Dacron, bovine pericardium, or glutaraldehyde-treated autologous pericardium can be used to close the defect to direct left ventricular blood to the aorta. The size of the patch should be big enough not to obstruct the pathway towards the aorta and to avoid truncal valve distortion. Our preference is to close these defects with interrupted 5/0 Surgilene sutures, reinforced with Teflon pledgets. The muscle in these small neonates is often very friable. At the upper part of the VSD the sutures are passed from the inside to the outside, leaving the pledgets on the outside of the heart. Usually, three or four stitches need to be placed like this.

If the VSD is perimembranous, then the placement of the sutures in the depth of the RV is similar to a transventricular approach for a perimembranous VSD in tetralogy of Fallot. The interrupted Teflon-pledgeted sutures can be placed by passing the needle through the open tricuspid valve, inserting the suture through the atrial aspect of the anteroseptal leaflet close to the annulus of the tricuspid valve. The tricuspid valve annulus itself is avoided, bringing the sutures into the ventricular cavity.

Three sutures are placed in this fashion, leaving the Teflon pledgets on the atrial side. The remainder of the VSD closure can proceed as usual. The conduction tissue sits at the inferior border, where the muscular rim meets the tricuspid valve. At this point a further suture should be placed *away* from the margin of the VSD, behind the chordae, to avoid damage of the bundle.

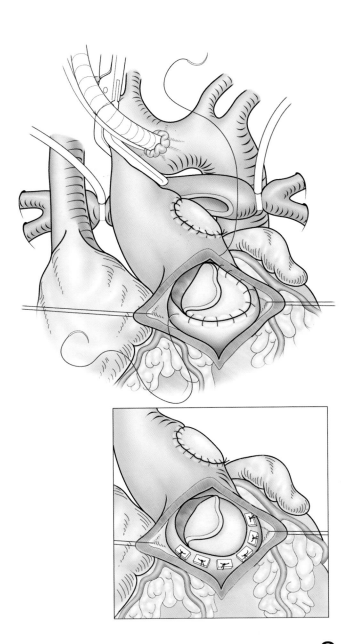

8

Atrial septal defect/Patent foramen ovale

A simple patent foramen ovale (PFO) is left open, and a larger concomitant atrial septal defect can be closed partially so as to leave the equivalent of a small PFO. This opening can be very useful in the postoperative period during pulmonary hypertensive episodes to maintain cardiac output by diverting some desaturated blood to the left atrium. If forward failure of the RV occurs and blood flow to the lungs is reduced, right ventricular and central venous pressures increase. Cardiac output can be maintained up to a certain level by right-to-left shunting through the PFO ('blue output is better than no output').

If the decision is not to leave a PFO, deairing of the left side of the heart could then be undertaken, leaving a vent in the right superior pulmonary vein. The cross-clamp is taken off, and the rest of the procedure is done on the beating heart to reduce aortic cross-clamp time. If the PFO is going to be left open, the right atrium needs to be closed before removal of the cross-clamp.

Insertion of right ventricle-to-pulmonary artery conduit

After completion of the intracardiac repair, the left ventricle is deaired, and RV-to-PA continuity is restored with a cryo-preserved homograft or other suitable conduit (Contegra, Medtronic, Inc; Shellhigh No-React VascuPatch). Placing an intracardiac sucker in the right atrium is useful to obtain a bloodless field for suturing.

Most centers use valved conduits, because several studies suggest that the use of a nonvalved conduit is another risk factor for adverse outcome. Some individual surgeons report good results from direct connection (described later). Pulmonary homografts seem to do better in the mid-term than aortic homografts. The choice of conduit size is very important and should match the size of the child. Excessively large conduits can produce an adverse hemodynamic outcome and are of no advantage in duration of valve survival. Closure of the chest may be made impossible as the conduit may be compressed after delayed chest closure.

9 If a homograft of an appropriate size is not available, then a slightly larger one could be downsized by converting it from a tricuspid valve to a bicuspid valve, removing one of the cusps with the associated circumference of conduit and resuturing the homograft longitudinally. Smaller homograft sizes (6–10 mm, adjusted to the patient's body weight) are not disadvantageous and should be preferred because of better postoperative hemodynamic tolerance and no increased risk of early failure. The valve is often best placed distally, close to the bifurcation to avoid sternal compression, although opening of the left pleura may help in positioning. The distal anastomosis to the pulmonary arteries is constructed during rewarming using fine suture material (7/0 Prolene). If the pulmonary arteries are tiny, a bifurcated pulmonary homograft as a spatulated onlay allows extension into each branch to widen narrow segments. The conduit should lie without excess length to avoid kinking at the distal end. Next, the posterior proximal conduit wall is sutured directly to the ventriculotomy. A strip of Teflon, pericardium, or Dacron can be used to buttress the suture line. The anterior aspect is augmented with a patch of autologous or bovine pericardium. Gore-Tex, Dacron, and other materials can be used to create a large enough hood for the RV-to-conduit connection.

In a number of patients, a direct anastomosis of PA–right ventricular outflow tract (RVOT) incision may be used, as proposed by Barbero-Marcial *et al* (1990). The pulmonary arteries must be thoroughly mobilized to allow the partition wall of the distal transected main PA to be anastomosed to the upper end of the incision in the RVOT. A Lecompte (French) maneuver may be needed to achieve this goal. Once the posterior wall has been anastomosed, the anterior part of the RVOT–PA connection can be roofed with autologous or heterologous pericardium, creating a valveless connection.

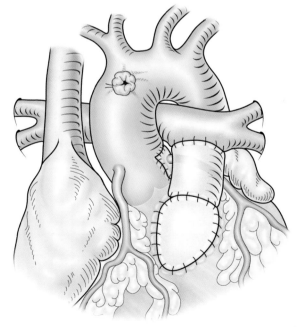

9

Truncus arteriosus with discontinuous pulmonary arteries

10a-d Occasionally, the left PA originates from the ductus arteriosus, and the right PA arises from the truncus arteriosus. Both arteries are detached from their aortic connections. The larger artery is connected to the homograft with an end-to-end anastomosis, and the other is sewn end-to-side to the newly constructed PA.

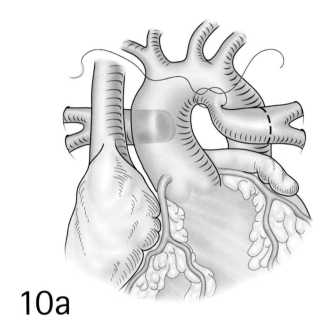

10a

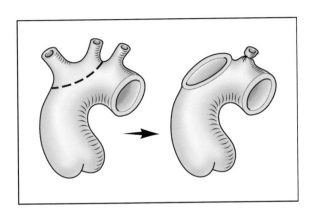

10b

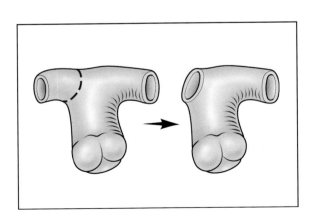

10c

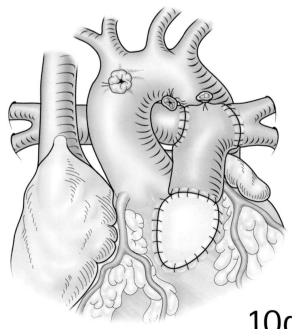

10d

11 Alternatively, a bifurcated pulmonary homograft can be used. Continuity is restored with an end-to-end anastomosis. Suturing the back wall of the two pulmonary arteries together provides the patient with a bifurcation of native tissue.

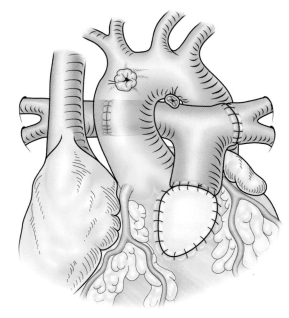

11

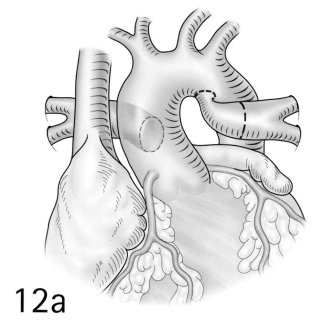

12a

12a–c The anterior aspect is enlarged using the bifurcated homograft as an onlay-patch.

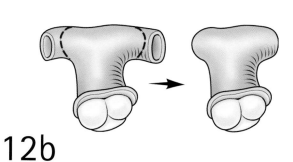

12b

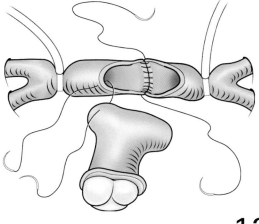

12c

Truncus arteriosus with interrupted aortic arch

13 Approximately 10 per cent of patients present with aortic arch interruption. All three types of interruption have been described, but interruption between the common left carotid and subclavian artery (interruption of aortic arch type B) is found most commonly. After extensive mobilization of the ascending and descending aorta, the pulmonary arteries, the ductus, and the head and neck vessels, the repair is undertaken under deep circulatory arrest. The patient's temperature is lowered to 18°C, the circulation arrested, and the head vessels snared. If one wishes to avoid deep hypothermic circulatory arrest, antegrade perfusion of the right carotid artery can be achieved by repositioning the aortic cannula at reduced flow to approximately 10mL/kg/minute. The truncal root is transected as described above. Ductal tissue is resected from the descending aorta. Continuity between the small ascending aorta and normal sized descending aorta can be achieved in several ways.

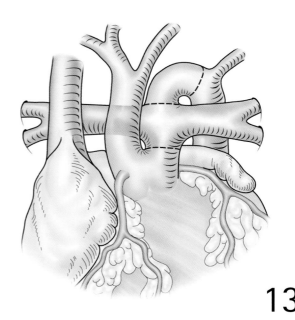

13

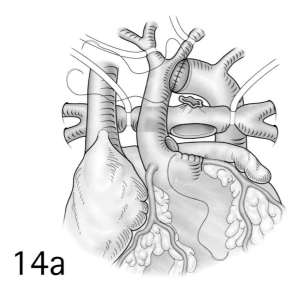

14a

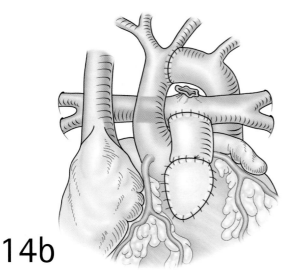

14b

14a, b End-to-end anastomosis is feasible if the gap between the two vessels is not too large. Extensive mobilization of the head and neck vessels and the descending aorta can be improved by disconnecting the left subclavian artery in some rare patients.

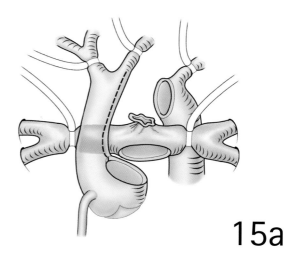

15a

15a, b and 16 The hypoplastic ascending aorta and aortic arch can be enlarged with a homograft patch after end-to-end connection of the posterior vessel wall.

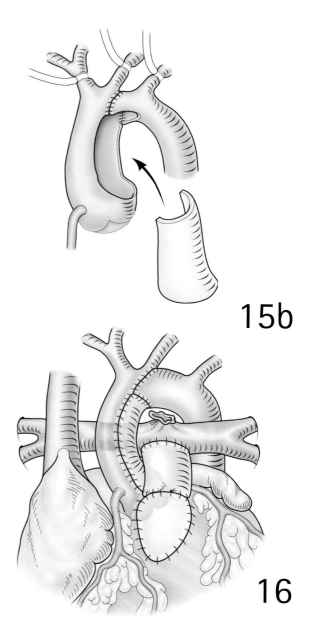

15b

16

POSTOPERATIVE CARE

Intraoperatively-placed monitoring lines (PA, left atrium) are used to assess postoperative hemodynamic variables of the patients. Most infants require some form of inotropic support with low doses of dopamine or dobutamine for approximately 48 hours. High doses of inotropes (particularly adrenaline) and pulmonary vasoconstrictors should be avoided. Patients are kept paralyzed or heavily sedated for 24–72 hours to avoid a pulmonary hypertensive crisis. Typical triggers such as hypercarbia, hypoxia, acidosis, and unnecessary manipulations must be avoided. The core temperature is maintained below 37.5°C by active cooling if necessary to avoid arrhythmias. Junctional ectopic tachycardia is treated with further cooling and sequential or amiodarone pacing if required.

Vasodilators, such as nitroglycerine, nitroprusside, prostaglandin and, most effectively, nitric oxide, can be used when PA pressures are elevated. Since early repair has become established, pulmonary hypertensive crises have become rare in the postoperative period, which has reduced the procedure-related mortality and morbidity significantly.

OUTCOME

The operative risk is somewhere between 10 and 20 per cent, even in experienced centers. Important risk factors are severe truncal valve incompetence, interrupted aortic arch, coronary artery anomalies, and older age at repair (more than 100 days old) in most large series. Early repair dramatically reduces the incidence of pulmonary hypertensive crises in the postoperative period; and thus, the overall results have improved.

Follow-up data spanning more than 20 years after surgical repair of truncus arteriosus are now available. Large studies confirm that hemodynamic results and long-term survival are excellent. The major potential of morbidity and mortality after the initial repair is related to reoperations such as conduit replacements or procedures on the truncal valve.

Replacement of obstructed, calcified RV-to-PA conduits is common several years (mean, 5.5 years) after the initial operation. Surprisingly, the incidence of conduit replacement is not related to the size of the first placed conduit, whereas aortic allografts fail earlier than pulmonary allografts. Obstructive lesions in the pulmonary artery can be ballooned and stented.

Worsening regurgitation or stenosis of the dysplastic truncal valve may make repair or replacement necessary during follow-up of these children. A significant number of children develop aneurysmatic enlargement of the newly constructed aortic root, requiring root replacement with a Bentall-type procedure.

FURTHER READING

Barbero-Marcial, M., Riso, A., Atik, E., Jatene, A. 1990. A technique for correction of truncus arteriosus types I and II without extracardiac conduits. *Journal of Thoracic and Cardiovascular Surgery* **99**, 364–9.

de Leval, M.R. 1994. Persistent truncus arteriosus. In *Surgery for congenital heart defects*. 2nd edition. Philadelphia, PA: Saunders, 539–48.

Hanley, F.L., Heinemann, M.K., Jonas, R.A., *et al.* 1993. Repair of truncus arteriosus in the neonate. *Journal of Thoracic and Cardiovascular Surgery* **105**, 1047–56.

Heinemann, M.K., Hanley, F.L., Fenton, K.N., Jonas R.A., Mayer, J.E., Castaneda, A.R. 1993. Fate of small homograft conduits after early repair of truncus arteriosus. *Annals of Thoracic Surgery* **55**, 1409–12.

Imamura, M., Drummond-Webb, J.J., Sarris, G.E., Mee, R.B.B. 1999. Improving early and intermediate results of truncus arteriosus repair: a new technique of truncal valve repair. *Annals of Thoracic Surgery* **67**, 1142–6.

Kirklin, J.W., Barratt-Boyes, B.G. (eds) 1992. Truncus arteriosus. In *Cardiac surgery*. New York: Churchill Livingstone, 1131–51.

Spray, T. 1998. Truncus arteriosus. In Kaiser, L.R., Kron, I.L., Spray, T.L. (eds) *Mastery of cardiothoracic surgery*. Philadelphia, PA: Lippincott–Raven, 759–70.

56

Surgery for persistent ductus arteriosus and aortopulmonary window

WILLIAM M. DECAMPLI MD, PHD
Associate Professor of Surgery, University of Pennsylvania School of Medicine; Cardiothoracic Surgeon, The Children's Hospital of Philadelphia, Philadelphia, Pennsylvania, USA

HISTORY

In 1907, Dr. John Munro presented a paper before the Philadelphia Academy of Surgery proposing ligation of the patent (persistent) ductus arteriosus (PDA), but the first clinical attempt at ligation was by Strieder in 1938 for bacterial endocarditis. That patient died from acute gastric dilatation on postoperative day 4. The first successful ligation was performed by Gross later that year. Recognizing the risks of a persistent PDA, Gross and others argued for routine ligation after diagnosis. Over the next 20 years, thousands of ductus ligations were reported, with mortality of 0.5–2.0 per cent. Indications were expanded to include ligation in premature infants with the separate reports of Powell and Decancq in 1963. Video-assisted thoracoscopic (VATS) PDA clip ligation was first reported by Laborde and colleagues in 1993. DeCampli, in 1998, described VATS suture ligation of PDA with routine discharge of the patient on the day of operation.

Aortopulmonary (AP) window was described by Elliotson in 1830. Gross, while operating for a presumed PDA, encountered an AP window and successfully ligated it in 1948. Cooley and associates reported division of an AP window using cardiopulmonary bypass (CPB) in 1957.

PRINCIPLES AND JUSTIFICATION

PDA is the second most common congenital cardiac anomaly, with an incidence of approximately 1.5 per 3 000 live births. The ductus normally closes spontaneously within 72 hours after birth in full-term infants. For reasons still not understood, spontaneous closure occasionally fails to occur. Spontaneous closure after the third month is very unlikely. In premature infants, spontaneous closure is less likely, with approximately 80 per cent patent at 1 week of life in infants weighing less than 1 000 g at birth.

The risks from isolated PDA vary with the amount of blood flow through the ductus. Full-term infants with large PDAs (those associated with an audible 'machinery' murmur, greater than 2 mm in diameter and causing cardiac chamber enlargement) may present with signs of congestive heart failure (CHF) or pulmonary hypertension. Infants and children with small PDAs are usually asymptomatic. Potential late complications from PDAs include bacterial endocarditis and aneurysm formation. If the ductus is large, additional late risks include advanced CHF and pulmonary vascular obstructive disease, the latter leading clinically to Eisenmenger's syndrome. Despite the advent of antibiotic prophylaxis of endocarditis, approximately 42 per cent of patients with untreated PDA are dead by 45 years of age.

Premature newborns are at risk for complications of end organ prematurity. These complications may be exacerbated by the abnormal hemodynamics associated with PDA. These newborns are relatively refractory to medical management of this hemodynamic pattern.

For infants who are asymptomatic in the neonatal period, isolated PDA should be electively closed after a few months of age, when spontaneous closure is unlikely. Isolated PDA should be closed in older infants, children, and adults when diagnosed, except in patients with Eisenmenger's syndrome, patients with bacterial endocarditis not yet given a trial of antibiotic therapy, or asymptomatic octogenarians. Premature infants with PDA being managed for end-organ dysfunction secondary to prematurity may first undergo a trial of indomethacin therapy at the discretion of the neonatologist. If this therapy is contraindicated, or if it fails to close the ductus, surgical closure is indicated. Closure of isolated PDA usually resolves CHF in infants and reduces symptoms in older patients. Closure usually, but not always, reverses 'reactive' pulmonary hypertension. PDA closure significantly reduces, but probably does not completely eliminate, the risk of endocarditis or aneurysm formation.

Closure of the isolated noncalcified, noninfected PDA is accomplished by one of several methods. These include open ligation or division, VATS ligation, and transcatheter coil occlusion. Currently, all three of these methods are considered acceptable. The mortality is significantly less than 1 per cent. Complications of the surgical approaches include transfusion (less than 1 per cent), pneumothorax (2–5 per cent), wound infection (2 per cent), chylothorax (2 per cent), recurrent nerve injury (2.6 per cent), and recurrence or persistence of flow (5–20 per cent; ligation only). Complications of the coil approach include hemorrhage, coil embolization to the lungs or legs, leg ischemia from femoral artery thrombosis, femoral artery pseudoaneurysm, and recurrence or persistence of flow. PDA closure in the presence of calcification or active endocarditis may require some form of atrio-aortic or CPB, with its attendant risks.

1a–c

AP window is a relatively rare anomaly, found in 0.2 per cent of patients with congenital heart disease. The disorder consists of a direct connection between the ascending aorta and main pulmonary artery. The lesion is thought to arise embryologically from failure of fusion of the proximal and distal AP septum, malalignment of the truncal cushions (from which the proximal septum arises), or abnormal migration of the sixth aortic arches. The most common defect begins within a few millimeters above the semilunar valves on the left wall of the aorta. The most common types are shown in Figure 1. Although frequently found as an isolated defect, AP window can occur with PDA, type A interrupted aortic arch (IAA), ventricular septal defect, or tetralogy of Fallot. In some patients, anomalous origin of either coronary artery from the pulmonary artery can occur.

The physiology of AP window is similar to that of PDA. Occasionally, the defect is restrictive, and patients may present with an asymptomatic murmur. More often, the defect is moderate or large, giving rise to symptoms of CHF and signs of volume overload. As in the case of PDA, later complications can include heart failure, pulmonary hypertension with pulmonary vascular obstructive disease, and endocarditis.

Repair of AP window is indicated at the time of diagnosis to avoid the complications of the lesion listed previously. Generally speaking, associated cardiovascular anomalies can be repaired at the same operation. Although repair without CPB has been reported in the past, the standard approach to repair of AP window is through a median sternotomy using CPB. The risks associated with repair are similar to those of other congenital cardiac anomalies of intermediate complexity repaired with CPB. In patients with a large AP window and

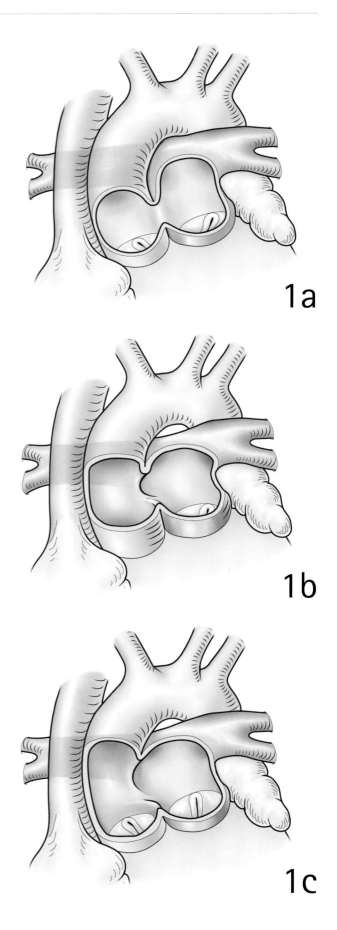

1a

1b

1c

long-standing pulmonary overcirculation, the risk of episodical pulmonary hypertension, possibly requiring advanced therapeutic modalities, is significant.

PREOPERATIVE ASSESSMENT AND PREPARATION

Babies and children suspected of having a patent ductus should undergo echocardiography. This study should be sufficient to establish the diagnosis. Additionally, the echocardiogram should establish the arch anatomy, presence of coarctation, direction of ductal flow, and any associated cardiac anomalies. Premature newborns with PDA should be free of active infection at the time of ligation. Many premature newborns have abnormal coagulation times; an attempt to correct them with fresh frozen plasma subjects them to a volume load and is not necessary before operation.

Older children or adults with large PDA and CHF or with the presence of right-to-left shunting should undergo cardiac catheterization to assess pulmonary resistance. Aortic angiography or magnetic resonance imaging is indicated in cases of ductal or periductal aneurysm or calcified ductus. Patients with acute endocarditis and PDA should undergo a trial of antibiotic therapy. If the infection is controlled, the ductus can be ligated a few months thereafter. If infection cannot be controlled with antibiotics, then prompt ligation is carried out.

Babies should undergo echocardiography to confirm the diagnosis of AP window. The echocardiogram should carefully delineate the location of the window, the anatomy of the branch pulmonary arteries, and the presence of associated anomalies. Occasionally, the anatomy is not clear, in which case cardiac catheterization should be performed. In older children, echocardiography is also usually sufficient to determine the anatomy and physiology. Patients older than young infants with large AP window, CHF, or the presence of associated cardiac anomalies should undergo cardiac catheterization to clarify the hemodynamics.

ANESTHESIA

For low birthweight babies undergoing PDA ligation, 1 U of blood should be available for operation. An arterial monitoring catheter is not necessary, but a pulse oximeter and blood pressure cuff should be placed on the lower extremity. An end tidal CO_2 monitor is useful to determine whether lung retraction is affecting pulmonary blood flow, although this technique is unreliable in small babies. Babies on an oscillator ventilator can undergo operation. In many of these cases, however, the baby can be safely switched to a conventional ventilator for transport to the operating room and for the duration of the operation. Performing the operation in the neonatal intensive care unit is acceptable, provided the staffing and facilities meet standards.

Infants and children undergoing PDA ligation with thoracotomy can undergo standard intravenous anesthetic, but a regional technique, as described by Peterson *et al.*, is also well suited for this operation. Single lung ventilation is preferable but not necessary. This approach can be achieved by selective right mainstem bronchus intubation in small children and by use of a double-lumen tube in children more than approximately 25 kg in weight. When the VATS technique is used, intravenous anesthetic is used and single-lung ventilation is preferred but not required.

In patients undergoing repair of AP window, the anesthetic considerations for CPB apply. For the patient with pulmonary hypertension, inhaled nitric oxide occasionally may be necessary.

OPERATIONS

Patent ductus arteriosus in the very-low-birthweight (less than 1000 g) newborn

POSITIONING OF PATIENT AND INCISION

2 The operation can be performed on the patient's warming bed so radiant heat can be applied. A custom-made electrocautery ground pad can be applied to babies as small as 400 g. The right lateral decubitus position is used. The position of the baby on the bed should be biased toward the side of the surgeon. An approximately 2-cm transverse incision is made just caudad to the palpable tip of the scapula.

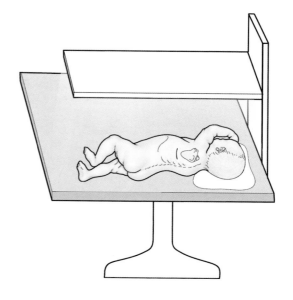

2

EXPOSURE OF THE DUCTUS

The chest wall muscles can be mobilized and preserved, or the latissimus muscle can be partially divided. The pleura is entered. Care should be taken to avoid violation of the visceral pleura, as this violation causes an air leak and the necessity of a chest tube. A rib retractor is placed.

3 The lung lobes are swept anteriorly by the first assistant using two rubber-coated malleable retractors. The position of these retractors is determined by the surgeon, as the assistant cannot see in the wound, and is based on exposure and the hemodynamic and ventilatory status of the patient, which can change rapidly. The ductus arteriosus is readily identified as the structure that the recurrent nerve loops around.

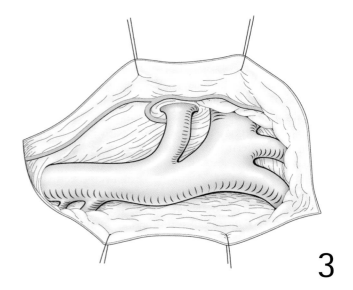

3

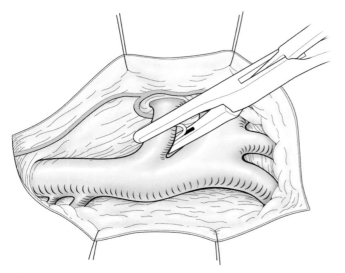

4

CLIP LIGATION

4 Using low-power needlepoint cautery, small incisions are made in the pleural reflection just caudad and cephalad to the ductus toward its aortic end. A Jacobson clamp is then used to gently and bluntly dissect to the deep (medial) margin of the ductus. The ductus itself should not be dissected out, nor should it be grasped or otherwise be put on traction. The course of the recurrent laryngeal nerve is determined. An appropriate size metal clip on a manual applier is carefully positioned around the ductus at its aortic end and then applied without traction on the ductus. Spring-loaded or 'Autoclip' applicators should never be used. A rise in blood pressure in the lower extremity is confirmed.

CLOSURE

Hemostasis is confirmed, then the lung retractors are removed. If the lung was injured during the procedure, an 8-Fr catheter or 10-Fr pleural tube is placed and set to 15-cm water suction. The pleural reflection over the aorta does not need to be reclosed. The ribs are reapproximated with three 2/0 absorbable stitches during manual inflation of the lungs, then the soft tissue layers are closed with running absorbable suture.

TORN DUCTUS

If bleeding from the ductus occurs, a 'peanut' gauze should be used to directly compress the tissue. Blood should be made ready to infuse by the anesthesiologist. The thoracotomy incision is enlarged as needed, and the chest is suctioned of blood. The aorta proximal and distal to the ductus is quickly mobilized, and curved occluding clamps are applied at both locations. Bleeding should now be controllable with direct pressure. A small Potts or 'C-clamp' is applied on the pulmonary artery side, or the peanut gauze is held in place by the assistant. The ductal orifice at the aorta is obliterated with a running 6/0 polypropylene (Prolene) suture, then the aortic clamps are released. The pulmonary artery end of the defect can be repaired with a running 6/0 Prolene stitch either with the clamp in place or by slowly rolling the peanut gauze off the defect.

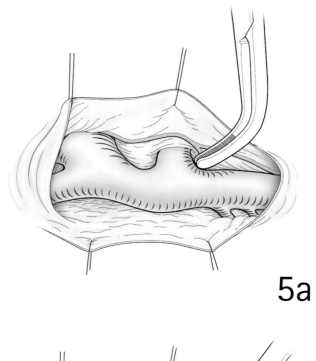

Patent ductus arteriosus ligation in patients weighing more than 1000 g

EXPOSURE AND DUCTAL MOBILIZATION

5a, b 'Double' or 'triple ligation' is performed in all but the smallest infants. The positioning, incision, and exposure of the ductus is performed as described in the sections 'Positioning of patient incision' and 'Exposure of the ductus.' Somewhat more dissection is carried out cephalad and caudad to the ductus, and the pedicle containing the vagus and recurrent nerves is mobilized more medially. Traction sutures may be placed on this pedicle. A right-angle instrument is passed medial to (underneath) the ductus toward its pulmonary artery end. This maneuver may require some patience, as the pleural reflection is relatively firm. Viewing this dissection from the caudad position, one should confirm that the instrument tip is deep to the ductus and superficial to the recurrent nerve.

5a

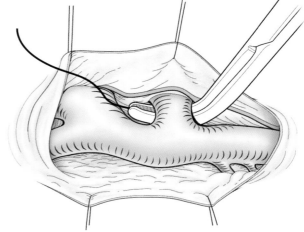

5b

PLACEMENT OF PURSESTRING SUTURE AND LIGATION

6a Next, a 5/0 monofilament Prolene pursestring stitch is taken around the aortic base of the ductus, taking only bites of adventitia. The needles are then cut off, and each free end is brought under the ductus.

6b, c The ductus is then ligated with the pursestring suture. If the ductus is somewhat large, some surgeons prefer to temporarily apply a clamp across the aortic isthmus to lower the pressure in the ductus while tying down the first suture. Gentle lateral traction is then applied to the aorta, and a free tie or second pursestring suture is secured toward the pulmonary artery end.

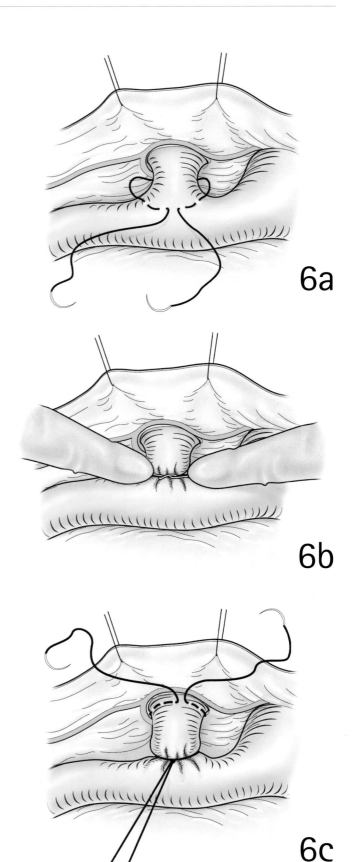

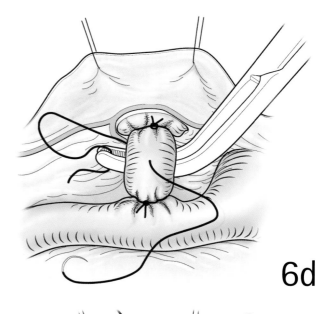

6d

6d–f A clip or transfixion suture should be added as a third ligature if ductal length is sufficient.

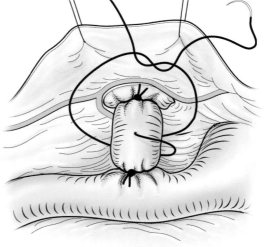

6e

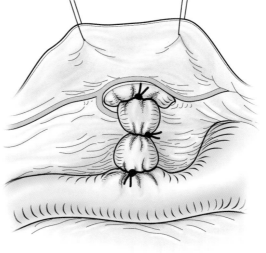

6f

Ligation and division for large ductus

Division of the ductus should be performed whenever the ductus is so short as to make it difficult to place two ligatures separated by at least a few millimeters. In this case, the vagus nerve pedicle flap should be mobilized thoroughly and traction sutures placed on its edges. The ductus, isthmus, and proximal descending aorta are mobilized. In particular, the aorta should be retracted anteriorly and dissection under the ductus performed under direct vision.

APPLICATION OF CLAMPS

7a A multi-toothed, atraumatic partial occlusion clamp is then placed across the aorto-ductal junction, with the handles caudad. A similar straight clamp is then placed across the ductus, keeping the recurrent nerve medial. Traction should not be placed on these clamps. On the contrary, they should be 'pushed into' the pulmonary artery and aorta to avoid slippage.

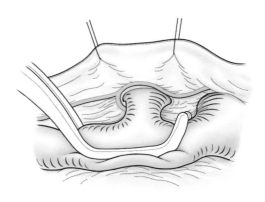

7a

7b Alternatively, occlusion clamps are placed on the aorta proximal and distal to the ductus when the latter is very short.

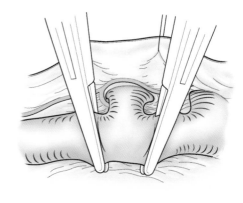

7b

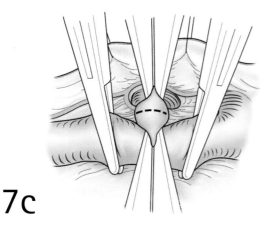

7c

7c, d The ductus is then divided and each end oversewn with 5/0 Prolene suture using a mattress technique followed by an over-and-over stitch.

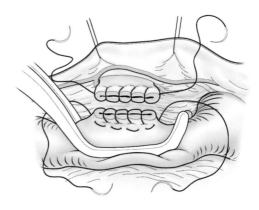

7d

Patent ductus arteriosus ligation using video-assisted thoracoscopic technique

The technique of VATS ligation of PDA can be applied, in principle, to any ductus that does not need to be divided. Evidence of pulmonary adhesions, ductal calcification, or recent endocarditis are contraindications to using the technique. Proper training in the general techniques of video-assisted surgery is, of course, essential.

8 Specialized instruments allow safe, efficient exposure and ligation of the ductus. The instruments shown here were developed by Pilling-Weck (King of Prussia, PA) and include (A) 'fan' lung retractor, (B) ring forceps, (C) tissue grasper, (D) clip applier, (E) 'diamond-dusted' suture grasper, (F) right angle, (G) suture scissors, (H) large right angle, (I) tissue scissors, (J) small grasper, and (K) small clip applier. Additionally, a cautery device and a 2.5–5.0 mm zero degree angle thoracoscope with attached camera are used. The technique described herein is the one used at the Children's Hospital of Philadelphia for patients weighing 2 kg or more.

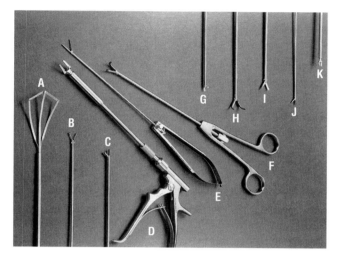

8

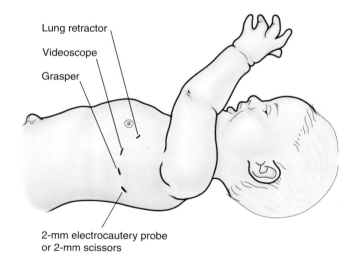

Lung retractor

Videoscope

Grasper

2-mm electrocautery probe or 2-mm scissors

9

POSITION OF PATIENT AND LOCATION OF INCISIONS

9 The patient is placed in the standard position for a left thoracotomy, with the area of the fourth, fifth, and sixth interspaces prepped. Standard thoracotomy instruments should be on the operating table, in case conversion to open thoracotomy is necessary. Two units of blood should be available. Four small (5 mm) incisions are made as shown. The most anterior incision (site 1) is at the posterior axillary line, the third interspace. The second (site 2) is just anterior to the scapular tip, the fourth interspace. The most posterior incision (site 4) lies between the medial edge of the scapula and the vertebral column. The last incision (site 3) lies between the latter two. Each incision is deepened by muscle-splitting blunt dissection, then the pleura is entered. A 5-mm port is placed at site 2, and a thoracoscope is advanced. The lung retractor is placed through site 1. The retractor sweeps the upper lobe in an inferomedial direction. If the lower lobe obscures the juxtaductal area, a second fan retractor can be placed through site 1. A grasper is placed through site 3, and the cautery through site 4. The camera or the retractor, or both, can be held by an adjustable support bar to avoid the necessity of two assistants or can be manipulated by a robot.

DISSECTION OF DUCTUS

10a With the juxtaductal area exposed, the pleural reflection on the aorta is grasped and opened along the aorta with cautery. The anterior flap is developed with blunt and sharp dissection, and the ductus is exposed. An appropriate balance of blunt and sharp dissection further mobilizes the cephalad and caudad borders of the ductus. A standard cotton-tipped applicator placed through sites 3 or 4 is useful for blotting blood and for blunt dissection.

10b A right-angle instrument is used, coming from the cephalad border, to undermine the ductus. This step requires patience, as the medial connective tissue ('behind' the ductus) is firm. The thoracoscope should focus on the caudad border of the ductus to assure the right angle is passing through the proper plane.

LIGATION

10c The right angle is used to pass a No. 1 polyfilament silk tie around the pulmonary end of the ductus. Smaller gauge suture material tends to fray with the instrument tie technique. The ductus is ligated using an intracorporeal instrument tie technique. The preferred instruments for this maneuver are a pair of nonratcheted suture graspers with diamond-dusted jaws, as shown previously. The first two throws form a sliding knot. The third throw forms a square knot with the second, and the fourth throw forms a square knot with the third. Although this tie may not always completely occlude the ductus, it serves to gather up ductal tissue for precise clip ligation without entrapment of the recurrent nerve.

APPLICATION OF CLIP

10d The thoracoscope is now replaced via a port into site 3. A nasal speculum is used to spread parallel to the rib through site 2 so that the clip applier can be advanced into the chest. The aorta is retracted laterally with the grasper through site 4, then the clip is advanced onto the aortic end of the ductus and fired. Care is taken to have a good thoracoscopic view of the ductus during this phase and not to exert traction on the ductus by the applier.

Hemostasis is checked. A transesophageal echocardiogram is obtained to confirm ductal closure. An additional clip can be applied if residual ductal flow is detected. All instruments are removed except the thoracoscope. An 8-Fr pigtail catheter is placed using the Seldinger technique. The lung is then re-inflated, and the thoracoscope is removed. The wounds are closed in two layers using absorbable sutures, and small bandages are applied. The patient is turned to the supine position and if no active air leak or excessive drainage is present, the pleural catheter is removed. The patient is awakened, extubated, and taken to the recovery area. In a few hours, when the patient is able to get out of bed, void, and take liquids, he/she is discharged from the hospital.

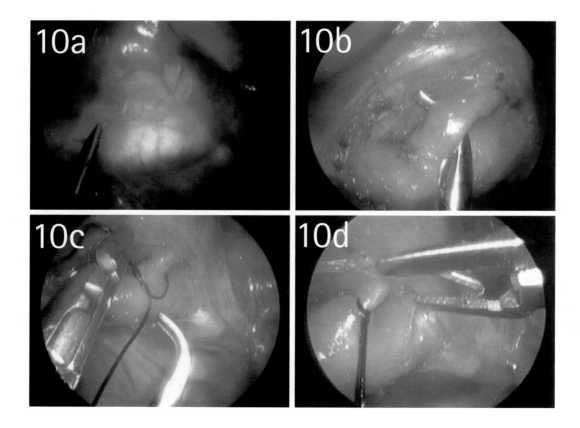

Calcified ductus

In the older adult patient or the patient with a history of endocarditis, the ductus and/or periductal area may be calcified. Simple ligation may be difficult or hazardous. Division may also be unwise if clamps cannot be applied to calcified or friable pulmonary arterial or aortic tissue. In this case, a full or partial upper-median sternotomy is performed, and the patient placed on CPB using a single two-stage venous cannula. Ductal flow, if prolific, should be controlled with tourniquets around the branch pulmonary arteries or, occasionally, by direct pressure on the ductus. The patient is cooled.

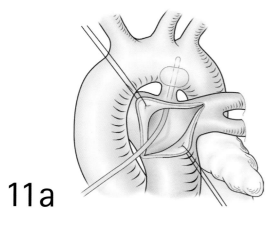

11a

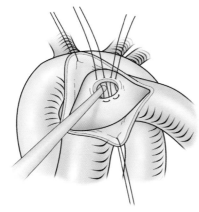

11b

TRANSPULMONARY CLOSURE

11a If the ductal orifice is small, mild hypothermia is induced, and the main pulmonary artery is opened distally, extending slightly onto the left branch. Bleeding is controlled using a short period of low-flow CPB. Alternatively, a balloon catheter can be used to occlude the ductal flow.

11b The ductal orifice is closed within the pulmonary artery primarily, or using a polytetrafluoroethylene patch. If the ductal orifice is large, or if extensive débridement is necessary to treat endocarditis, it may be preferable to use a short period of deep hypothermic circulatory arrest. With this technique, one should control the innominate and left carotid arteries, cross-clamp the aorta, and arrest the heart, as air may enter the orifice during the repair. After patch placement, the flow is increased, the aorta is deaired adjacent to the cannula site, then the carotid tourniquets and aortic cross-clamp are removed. During rewarming, the pulmonary artery is closed with running Prolene sutures.

TRANSAORTIC CLOSURE

12 An alternative technique has been described by Johnson and Kron in which the ductal orifice is closed from within the aorta, applying clamps to the aorta proximally and distally. Ductal flow is controlled by a balloon catheter or by use of full CPB through the thoracotomy. This approach, however, may not be as reliable as the pulmonary artery approach for the severely calcified or friable ductus or juxtaductal aortic tissue.

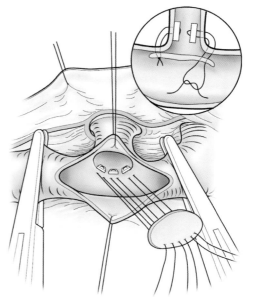

12

Repair of aortopulmonary window

EXPOSURE AND CANNULATION

13a A median sternotomy is performed. For an isolated AP window, single venous cannulation is sufficient. The aortic cannula is placed near the innominate artery orifice. CPB is initiated, then the branch pulmonary arteries are controlled with tourniquets. The patient is cooled to 28°C. The aorta is cross-clamped, and cardioplegia is given.

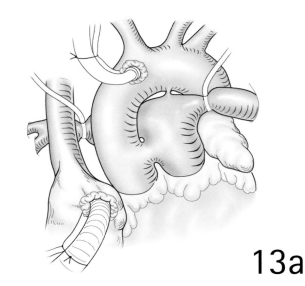

13a

OPENING OF WINDOW AND PATCH CLOSURE

13b, c The anterior border of the AP window is opened along its length, representing one-third to one-half of the circumference. Within the lumen, the coronary ostia should be located. If a coronary artery is located close to or within the pulmonary artery lumen, then the patch that closes the window must baffle the aortic flow to that ostium. Occasionally, a coronary button must be formed and transferred to the appropriate position. A prosthetic patch is used to close the communication. Its anterior edge is sandwiched between the walls of the aorta and pulmonary artery. The aortic root is vented through the cardioplegia catheter, and the cross-clamp is removed. The patient is warmed. CPB is weaned at 37°C.

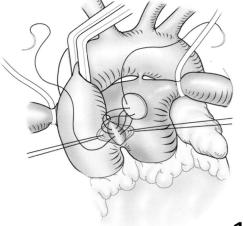

13b

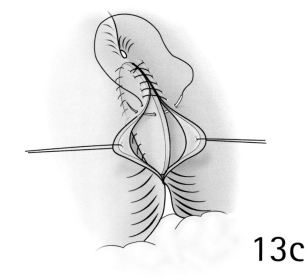

13c

EXPOSURE AND CANNULATION FOR AORTOPULMONARY WINDOW WITH INTERRUPTED AORTIC ARCH

14a In the case of AP window and IAA, single venous cannulation is used. CPB is begun, the branch PAs are occluded, and the patient is cooled to 18°C over 15–20 minutes. Tourniquets are placed around the arch branch vessels, and a cardioplegia catheter is placed. At 18°C, pump flow is stopped, the aorta is cross-clamped, and cardioplegia solution is given. The arch vessel tourniquets are tightened, and the aortic cross-clamp, aortic cannula, and PA tourniquets are removed. Alternatively, low flow to the brain can be maintained through a cannula inserted directly into the innominate artery.

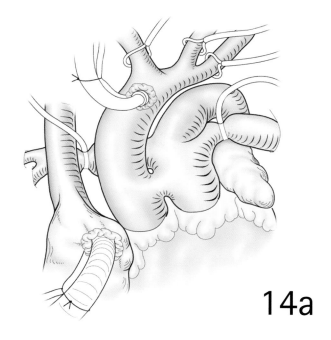

14a

14b The AP window is divided, again with careful attention given to the location of the coronary ostia. The ductus arteriosus is ligated on the pulmonary artery end then divided. The pulmonary artery defect is repaired with a homograft patch. The aortic defect is extended along the arch up onto the left carotid artery (type B IAA) or left subclavian artery (type A IAA). Ductal tissue is trimmed from the distal aorta, then the latter is opened up into the left subclavian artery (type B IAA).

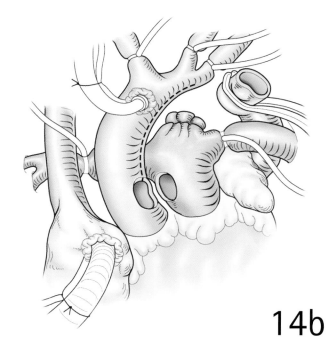

14b

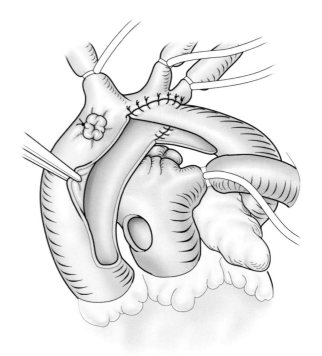

14c

ARCH RECONSTRUCTION

14c, d The two vessels are sutured together, augmenting the arch as needed with a homograft patch. The arch is distended with saline, then the cannula is replaced. The cardioplegia catheter is used as a vent, and CPB is restarted with warming. CPB is weaned at 37°C. The umbilical artery catheter, together with a right radial arterial catheter or direct measurement through the aortic cannula provides a measure of the transaortic gradient.

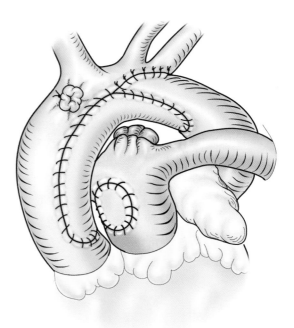

14d

POSTOPERATIVE CARE

Low-birthweight neonates undergoing PDA ligation are returned to their preoperative ventilatory settings. Pain is controlled by small doses of intravenous morphine. A drain tube, if placed, is removed in 12–24 hours. The most common early complication is pneumothorax, manifested by hypoxemia and increased inspiratory pressure requirements. This problem is treated with catheter drainage. Pleural effusion is infrequent and is also treated with catheter drainage. Wound infection is treated with drainage, and antibiotic treatment is begun according to wound culture results. Recurrent ductal flow is rare. If the residual shunt is small, it is left alone, and consideration is given to coil embolization beyond infancy. Residual large shunts are treated with surgical re-ligation. Recurrent nerve palsy can cause aspiration in small infants. If aspiration occurs with oral feeding, nasal tube or gastrostomy feeding is used until the infant is stronger. Rarely, secretions are aspirated, mandating chronic airway control (tracheostomy). Teflon injection of the vocal cord is performed beyond infancy.

The older patient undergoing ligation of an isolated PDA should be mobilized within hours of the procedure. Pain is controlled with small doses of intravenous morphine sulfate, oral acetaminophen, or, when a thoracotomy has been performed, agents administered through an epidural catheter. The chest tube can be removed within 24 hours, and the patient can be discharged in 1 or 2 days. When VATS is used, the patient can usually be discharged on the day of surgery, and oral acetaminophen provides good pain control.

Postoperative care of the infant after AP window repair (and associated anomalies) follows the general guidelines of infant care after CPB. Important residual lesions should be sought and repaired at the time of the original operation. Large AP windows in older infants and children subject the patient to the risk of pulmonary hypertension. This problem can be treated by maintaining adequate sedation, and mechanical ventilation and paralysis if necessary, during the initial 24 hours' recovery from operation. Nitric oxide should be available to treat recurrent or refractory episodes.

OUTCOME

The outcome after simple PDA ligation is good. Early mortality, even in premature infants is nearly zero. Late mortality in premature infants is related to associated pulmonary disease, but is now less than 10 per cent. Most normal weight infants and children undergoing PDA ligation go on to have a normal life expectancy. Older adults with calcified ductus or ductal aneurysm have higher risk of death and complications, often related to associated cardiovascular disease.

Outcome after repair of isolated AP window is good. Several studies containing between 6 and 12 patients had zero early mortality. Mortality is increased when associated lesions require repair, such as IAA. Late morbidity is also related to associated lesions, such as recurrent arch obstruction after repair of AP window with IAA.

FURTHER READING

DeCampli, W.M. 1998. Video-assisted thoracic surgical procedures in children. In Spray, T.L. (ed.), *Pediatric cardiac surgery annual 1998 of the seminars in thoracic and cardiovascular surgery*. Philadelphia: WB Saunders, 61–73.

Gaynor, J.W, *et al*. Aortopulmonary window and aortic origin of a pulmonary artery. In Mavroudis, C. and Backer, C.L. (eds), *Pediatric cardiac surgery*, 3rd edition. St. Louis: Mosby, in press.

Johnson, A.M., Kron, I.L. 1988. Closure of the calcified patent ductus in the elderly: avoidance of ductal clamps and shunts. *Annals of Thoracic Surgery* 45, 572.

McElhinney, D.B., Reddy, V.M., Tworetsky ,W., Silverman, N.H., Hanley, F.L. 1998. Early and late results after repair of aortopulmonary septal defect and associated anomalies in infants <6 months of age. *American Journal of Cardiology* 81, 195–201.

Peterson, K.L., DeCampli, W.M., Pike, N.A., Robbins, R.C., Reitz, B.A. 2000. A report of two hundred twenty cases of regional anesthesia in pediatric cardiac surgery. *Anesthesia and Analgesia* 90, 1014–19.

Tkebuchava, T., Von Segesser, L.K., Vogt, P.R., *et al*. 1997. Congenital aortopulmonary window: diagnosis, surgical technique and long-term results. *European Journal of Cardiothoracic Surgery* 11, 293–7.

57

Coarctation of the aorta: repair of coarctation and arch interruption

ERLE H. AUSTIN III MD
Professor of Surgery, University of Louisville School of Medicine; Chief of Cardiothoracic Surgery, Kosair Children's Hospital, Louisville, Kentucky, USA

HISTORY

Crafoord was the first to successfully repair coarctation of the aorta in 1944. The techniques of resection and end-to-end anastomosis had been thoroughly studied in laboratory animals by Gross, who soon followed with his own clinical success in 1945. The procedure had been limited to older children until 1955, when Mustard succeeded in repairing the lesion in a newborn infant. Resection and end-to-end anastomosis in small infants, however, often resulted in inadequate vessel growth at the circumferential suture line, leading to a high incidence of recurrent coarctation. In response to this problem, Waldhausen introduced the subclavian flap technique in 1966. Other surgeons, emphasizing the need to resect all ductal tissue, continued to obtain satisfactory results with the end-to-end technique. Neither technique specifically addressed the problem of arch hypoplasia, which was being seen at an increased frequency as more neonates with critical coarctation came to surgery. The maintenance of ductal patency with prostaglandin E_1, introduced by Elliott in 1975, permitted stabilization of many newborns who otherwise would not have survived to surgical intervention. Zannini and colleagues in 1985 introduced the concept of an extended end-to-end anastomosis to deal with the hypoplastic aortic arch.

The first successful repair of an interrupted aortic arch was performed by Samson in 1955 in a 3-year-old child with type A interruption. The child's ventricular septal defects were closed 4 years later when cardiopulmonary bypass became available. Simultaneous repair of the interrupted arch and ventricular septal defect was performed by Barratt-Boyes in 1970 using a period of deep hypothermic circulatory arrest and a Dacron conduit to bridge the interruption. Complete single-stage repair with direct primary anastomosis of the interrupted segments and closure of the ventricular septal defect was first performed successfully by Trusler in 1975.

PRINCIPLES AND JUSTIFICATION

Congenital obstruction of the aortic arch encompasses a broad spectrum from discrete coarctation distal to the left subclavian artery through tubular hypoplasia of the aortic arch to complete arch interruption. The presence of coarctation or arch interruption is sufficient indication for operative repair. The clinical presentation and natural history of coarctation segregates into two groups – infants presenting in the first weeks of life and children diagnosed after 3 months of age.

Neonates and very young infants typically present with severe congestive heart failure that can rapidly progress to acidosis and death. More than one-third of these infants have an associated cardiac anomaly such as ventricular septal defect, transposition of the great arteries, or some form of univentricular heart. The outcome without repair in neonates with coarctation or interrupted arch is almost uniformly fatal.

In contrast, older infants and children rarely have associated defects, are often asymptomatic, and may go undiagnosed until a routine physical examination uncovers upper extremity hypertension and diminished lower extremity pulses. Repair of coarctation is indicated in these older children and young adults to avoid the long-term complications of upper body hypertension, which include aortic dissection, hypertensive heart failure, atherosclerosis, myocardial infarction, and cerebral vascular disease.

Careful preoperative assessment of aortic anatomy by echocardiography and/or angiography is required to determine the exact site of obstruction and the degree and sites of associated arch hypoplasia. Associated cardiac defects must also be identified with these studies. In older children and young adults, satisfactory imaging of the aorta may be obtained using computed tomography or magnetic resonance imaging. The image obtained must provide a reliable measurement of the ascending aorta, the proximal arch (between the innominate artery and the left carotid artery), the distal arch (between the left carotid and the left subclavian artery), and the isthmus (between the left subclavian artery and the ductus or ligament).

The overriding principle of surgical repair is to maximally reduce afterload on the systemic ventricle by eliminating any obstruction to flow between the ascending and descending aorta. Ideally, therefore, at the completion of the repair, no pressure gradient should exist between the left ventricle and the descending aorta. The operative technique chosen should result in a pathway that is at no point less than 50 per cent of the diameter of the ascending aorta just before the innominate artery. As a rule of thumb in neonatal repairs, the final minimum pathway diameter in millimeters should be no less than the infant's weight in kilograms plus 1 (i.e. a diameter of at least 4.6 mm in a 3.6-kg infant).

PREOPERATIVE ASSESSMENT

Newborns with coarctation or interrupted aortic arch require nonelective operation after a period of stabilization with prostaglandin E_1. Other resuscitative techniques including mechanical ventilation, pharmacological paralysis, sodium bicarbonate, inotropic agents, and diuretics are also used to stabilize the child. If ductal patency cannot be achieved and acidosis worsens despite these measures, operative repair is performed emergently.

Asymptomatic infants undergo elective repair after 6 months of age after ductal remodeling has stabilized. Older infants and children with discrete coarctation are repaired electively at the time of diagnosis. Waiting until 3–5 years of age is unnecessary.

ANESTHESIA

All procedures are performed with general orotracheal anesthesia. Intraoperative monitoring should include a right radial arterial line. Placement of the arterial line in the left radial or in either femoral artery results in loss of the waveform during the period of aortic cross-clamping. If an umbilical artery line is present in a neonate, it is left in place to permit direct measurement of the post-repair flow gradient. A right radial artery catheter is still required for monitoring during the repair.

A left thoracotomy without cardiopulmonary bypass is the approach of choice for the majority of coarctation repairs. Rectal and/or nasopharyngeal temperature is monitored, and the patient is allowed to cool to as low as 34°C for spinal cord protection during the period of aortic clamping.

A median sternotomy with cardiopulmonary bypass and a brief period of deep hypothermic circulatory arrest is used for most cases of interrupted aortic arch, coarctations requiring concomitant intracardiac repairs, and coarctations with hypoplasia of the proximal arch that cannot be safely approached from a left thoracotomy. With this approach, the patient is cooled actively on cardiopulmonary bypass to 18°C for the period of hypothermic circulatory arrest required to repair the arch.

OPERATIONS FOR DISCRETE COARCTATION

Resection with end-to-end anastomosis

This technique is most commonly applied to infants and young children with discrete coarctation and a normal aortic arch.

1a, b After performing a left posterolateral muscle-sparing thoracotomy via the fourth intercostal space, the lung is retracted anteriorly and inferiorly. The parietal pleura overlying the aorta is incised from the descending aorta up along the subclavian artery dividing the superior intercostal vein between ligatures. The pleura is tacked up to further retract the lung and to create an operative 'well.' The vagus and recurrent laryngeal nerves are identified and carefully preserved. The aorta is dissected and mobilized from the left carotid artery to the second set of intercostal arteries. Although not always necessary, one or two levels of intercostals may be ligated (clipped) and divided to facilitate mobilization, clamping, and anastomosis. Because the ligamentum occasionally is patent, it is ligated. A vascular clamp is placed proximally across the aorta and base of the subclavian artery, and distally across the descending aorta. The coarctation segment is excised leaving wide orifices proximally and distally. A double-armed polypropylene suture is used to perform the posterior portion of the anastomosis sewing from the inside beginning with the ends apart. The clamps are used to approximate the vessels, and the anterior portion of the anastomosis is completed with the other arm of the suture. The caliber of the suture is adjusted to the size of the patient. A 7/0 suture is used in neonates and a 4/0 suture in young adults with intermediate choices for patients in between these ages. The anterior segment of the anastomosis may be performed with interrupted sutures to prevent pursestringing and to minimize narrowing. Interrupting a portion of the suture line may also permit diameter growth, although fine caliber polypropylene (6/0 and 7/0) tends to fracture over time after adequate healing has occurred and, as evidenced by the arterial switch experience, is unlikely to limit growth.

1c At completion of the anastomosis, the distal clamp is released first, and the suture line is carefully inspected. Any significant bleeding is controlled with additional simple sutures. The proximal clamp is slowly released. An excellent pulse should be visible and palpable in the distal aorta. When concern exists, distal aortic pressure can be directly measured using a needle through a fine pursestring. When adequate hemostasis is achieved, the pleura is closed over the repair with a continuous suture of fine polypropylene or Dexon. After placing a single chest tube, the lung is reexpanded, and the thoracotomy incision is closed in the standard manner.

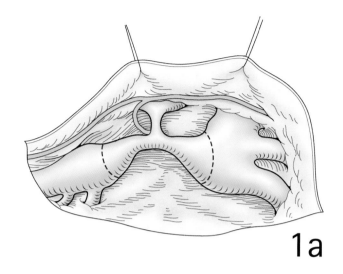

1a

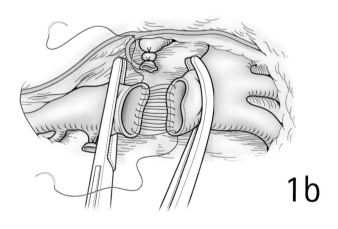

1b

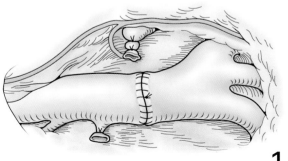

1c

Resection with insertion of tubular Dacron graft

2 In young adults and older patients, the area of coarctation may be long and/or the mobility of the aorta too restricted to allow a tension-free primary anastomosis. In these cases, a tubular graft of Dacron is inserted to bridge the gap. The size graft chosen should match the diameter of the descending aorta. Polypropylene (4/0 or 5/0) is used for the two suture lines.

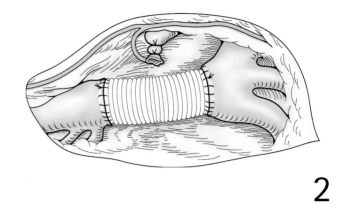

2

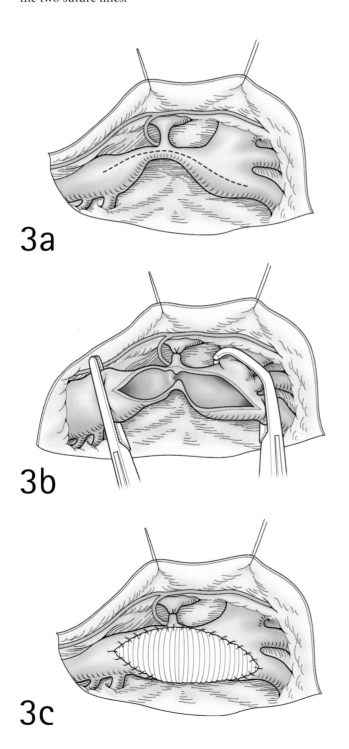

3a

3b

3c

Patch aortoplasty

Another technique used is the placement of a diamond-shaped patch across the segment of narrowing. Because aortoplasty can be performed quickly, it may be the procedure of choice when coarctation repair must be performed emergently in a desperately ill infant whose ductus cannot be reopened with prostaglandin E_1. This technique is also used in older children and young adults.

3a–c After dissecting the area of the coarctation as well as the distal arch, subclavian artery, and proximal descending aorta, the ligamentum is tied, and clamps are placed. The aorta is incised longitudinally across the area of coarctation. A coarctation membrane is typically encountered at the narrowest point. This fibrous thickening should be left intact, because resecting it tends to significantly weaken the aortic wall at this point. A large diamond-shaped patch is then fashioned from autologous or heterologous pericardium (neonates) or from a Dacron tube graft (older children or adults). The patch is sewn in place with a continuous polypropylene suture. The posterolateral aspect of the anastomosis is sewn first within the vessel. The anastomosis is completed, bringing the two suture ends together on the anteromedial aspect of the patch.

Patch aortoplasty offers a reproducible and easily performed correction of coarctation with excellent short-term results. Unfortunately, the technique has been associated with a high incidence of late aneurysm formation. For that reason, this author prefers to use resection and tubular graft insertion for older patients requiring coarctation repair.

Subclavian flap aortoplasty

This technique was introduced to eliminate the circumferential scar thought to be responsible for recurrence noted after resection and end-to-end anastomosis in small infants. Flap aortoplasty is primarily used in infants younger than 3 months of age who do not have arch hypoplasia. This procedure requires less overall dissection than the end-to-end technique and avoids tension on the suture line. On the other hand, the primary blood supply to the left arm is interrupted, potentially affecting its growth, and abnormal ductal tissue is retained, presenting the potential for recurrent coarctation or late aneurysm formation.

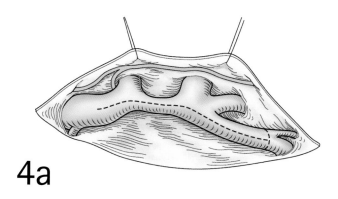

4a

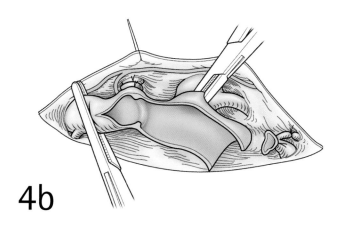

4b

4a–c With this technique, in addition to the usual exposure, the subclavian artery is dissected to the point of its first branch, usually the vertebral artery, which is ligated. The subclavian artery is ligated at this point. After ligating the ductus arteriosus, a proximal clamp is applied across the arch between the left carotid and left subclavian artery. A distal clamp is placed at least 1 cm distal to the coarctation. A longitudinal incision is made beginning in the descending aorta and is carried across the coarctation and the isthmus and along the lateral border of the subclavian artery, which is divided just proximal to the ligature. If a discrete intimal shelf exists, it may be carefully excised, but care must be taken to preserve the aortic media. The subclavian flap is then folded down into the aortic incision with a loose stay suture and sewn into place with a running suture of 7/0 polypropylene.

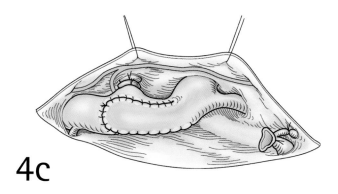

4c

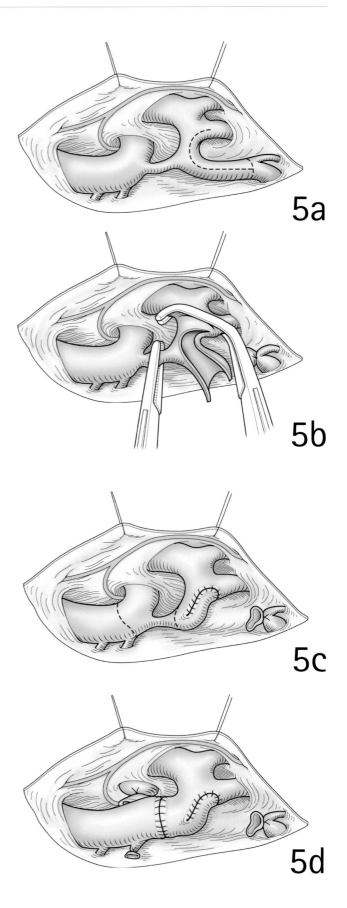

OPERATIONS FOR COARCTATION WITH ARCH HYPOPLASIA

Reverse subclavian flap aortoplasty

When the site of arch hypoplasia is confined to the segment between the left carotid artery and the left subclavian artery, this technique may be used in combination with the standard resection and anastomosis procedure.

5a–d For all procedures dealing with arch hypoplasia, the dissection proximally and distally must provide extensive mobilization of the head vessels and the descending aorta. The arch is clearly exposed to the base of the innominate artery, and the distal aorta is dissected down to the fourth set of intercostals. The left subclavian artery is ligated just before it branches, as previously described. A curved clamp is placed between the innominate artery and the left carotid in such a way as to occlude the left carotid distally. A second clamp is placed across the aortic isthmus, allowing distal perfusion through the ductus arteriosus if it is open. The subclavian artery is divided proximal to the ligature and is incised along its medial border onto the superior aspect of the distal arch to the base of the left carotid artery. The flap of subclavian artery is turned in a reverse direction into the proximal aortic incision and sewn into place with 7/0 polypropylene. The distal clamp is removed from the isthmus, and the proximal clamp is repositioned just distal to the left carotid. The ductus is now ligated, a second clamp is placed across the descending aorta, and a standard coarctation resection and end-to-end anastomosis is performed.

Resection with extended end-to-end anastomosis

When arch hypoplasia extends proximal to the left carotid artery, a reverse subclavian technique does not eliminate the arch obstruction, and a more extensive approach is required. The extended end-to-end approach is now preferred by many surgeons because it results in complete removal of all ductal tissue and preserves normal blood flow to the left arm. This technique does, however, present a greater degree of technical difficulty and requires more extensive dissection to achieve a tension-free anastomosis.

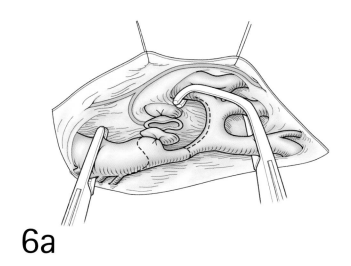

6a

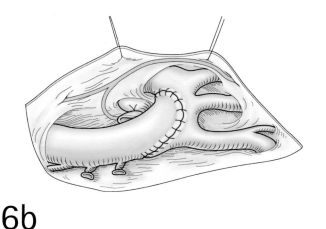

6b

6a, b After thorough dissection and mobilization of the head vessels, isthmus, ductus arteriosus, and descending aorta, the ductus arteriosus is ligated and divided. This step often improves exposure of the most proximal arch, including the distal ascending aorta and innominate artery. A large curved clamp is then positioned in such a way as to include the left subclavian artery, the left carotid artery, and part of the innominate artery. The tip of the clamp is positioned well down the left wall of the ascending aorta, but it must not obstruct flow to the innominate artery. If a significant change in the radial artery tracing occurs with application of the clamp, it must be repositioned. Other methods to assure unobstructed cerebral blood flow include palpation by the anesthesiologist of the right carotid or right temporal artery and/or assessment of a pulse oximeter placed on the right ear. Although not commonly available, continuous transcranial Doppler monitoring of the right middle cerebral artery provides the most reliable feedback regarding cerebral blood flow during this critical period. A second clamp is placed across the mobilized descending aorta, often including several intercostal vessels. The coarctation is completely excised, and an incision is made along the undersurface of the aortic arch to within a few millimeters of the tip of the clamp. Failure to bring this incision proximal to the origin of the left carotid artery is likely to result in a residual flow gradient. The orifice of the descending aorta is enlarged with a posterior longitudinal incision to match the extent of the opened aortic arch and to receive the tongue of the arch containing the left subclavian artery. An anastomosis is performed with 7/0 polypropylene, beginning medially and posteriorly with the vessels separated, then approximating the two clamps to reduce tension as the anastomosis is completed. A continuous suture technique is usually satisfactory, although interrupted simple sutures can be used for the anterior aspect of the anastomosis.

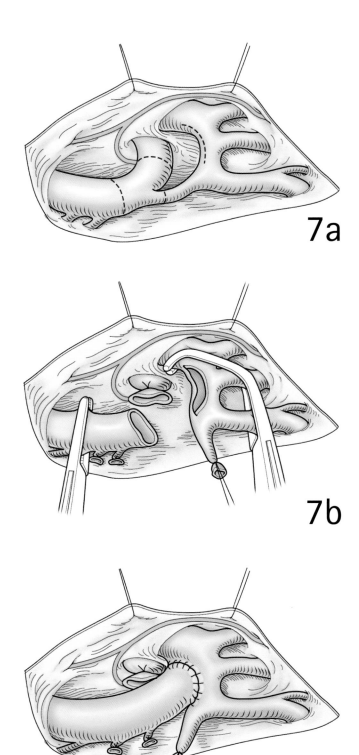

End-to-side anastomosis to the aortic arch

An end-to-side anastomosis of the divided descending aorta to the underside of the proximal aortic arch has recently evolved as a modification of the extended end-to-end technique. This procedure is designed to assure apposition of normal aortic tissue at the site of anastomosis as well as to bypass all hypoplastic structures proximal to the discrete coarctation.

7a–c Initial exposure, dissection, and extensive mobilization are carried out as in the extended end-to-end technique; however, after ligation and division of the ductus arteriosus, the aortic isthmus is ligated. After a distal descending aorta clamp is placed, the aorta is divided distal to the coarctation, leaving no ductal tissue at the edge of the divided descending aorta. Lateral traction on the isthmus provides excellent exposure for placement of the arch clamp, which is placed as proximally as possible, preserving innominate artery flow. A longitudinal incision is made on the underside of the aortic arch beginning only millimeters from the tip of the clamp and is brought distally to a length slightly larger than the cross-sectional diameter of the descending aorta. An end-to-side anastomosis is performed with 7/0 polypropylene, bringing the descending aorta up to the underside of the arch.

OPERATIONS FOR INTERRUPTED AORTIC ARCH

Repair of simple interrupted arch with ventricular septal defect

Although an interrupted aortic arch can be repaired in stages, currently the preferred approach is a single-stage complete repair with primary anastomosis of the descending aorta to the side of the ascending aorta and ventricular septal defect closure. The procedure is performed through a median sternotomy and requires cardiopulmonary bypass and a brief period of deep hypothermic circulatory arrest. If the head vessels that come off of the ascending aorta are large enough, a small (6- or 8-F) cannula is placed in one of the carotid arteries to provide antegrade cerebral blood flow while the aortic anastomosis is performed. This technique eliminates the requirement for circulatory arrest but may give rise to overperfusion of the brain and may result in stenosis at the cannulation site. Because the aortic anastomosis is easy to perform in an expeditious fashion, the use of circulatory arrest in this circumstance introduces minimal risk and greatly facilitates this portion of the procedure.

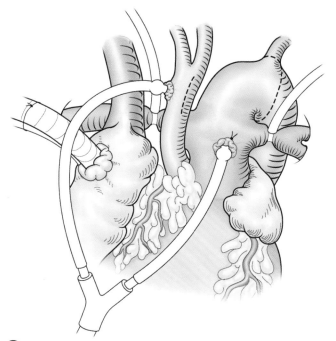

8a

8a After routine median sternotomy, the thymus, if present, is excised and the pericardium opened. The brachiocephalic vessels, branch pulmonary arteries, ductus arteriosus, and the proximal portion of the descending aorta are thoroughly dissected. The recurrent laryngeal nerve should be clearly identified and protected. To achieve relatively uniform and complete cooling, two 8-F arterial cannulas are used, one in the ascending aorta and one in the main pulmonary artery or ductus. The ascending aortic cannula is positioned in the right lateral aspect directly opposite the anticipated site of the aortic anastomosis. Tourniquets are placed around the right and left pulmonary arteries or around the duct to be tightened at commencement of cardiopulmonary bypass to direct flow from the second cannula through the ductus to the descending aorta. Venous cannulation can be single or double, depending on the surgeon's preference. If closure of the ventricular septal defect requires exposure through the right atrium, double venous cannulation will permit this visualization while on cardiopulmonary bypass.

8b Once cardiopulmonary bypass has been instituted, further mobilization of the aortic branches is performed while the patient is cooled to 18°C. Although the left subclavian artery can be preserved in type B interruption, ligation and division of this vessel improves mobility of the descending aorta and minimizes tension on the final anastomosis. If an aberrant right subclavian artery exists, this vessel should also be ligated and divided. When rectal and tympanic temperatures reach 18°C, bypass is discontinued. Tourniquets around the innominate and carotid arteries are tightened, whereas those around the pulmonary artery branches are removed. Cardioplegic solution is infused into the aortic root, and the arterial cannulas are removed. The ductus is ligated and divided where it joins the descending aorta. All ductal tissue is excised. Placing a small C-clamp on the descending aorta at this point helps pull the divided end up to the level of the ascending aorta. After a longitudinal incision is made on the left posterior aspect of the ascending aorta, an end-to-side anastomosis is performed with 7/0 polypropylene suture. If very little circulatory arrest time has elapsed at this point, the ventricular septal defect is closed before reinstituting bypass. Alternatively, cerebral and systemic blood flow can be resumed at this point by reinserting one of the arterial cannulas into the aortic site and recommencing bypass. An additional dose of cardioplegic solution is infused into the aortic root for the ventricular septal defect closure. Systemic rewarming can begin at this point.

8c, d In most cases, the ventricular septal defect is best approached through a transverse incision in the proximal main pulmonary artery, just distal to the pulmonary valve. Using interrupted pledget-reinforced mattress sutures of 5/0 Tevdek, a Dacron or pericardial patch is positioned such that its superior margin is placed on the left ventricular side of the conal septum to promote deflection of the conal septum away from the left ventricular outflow tract. Once the ventricular septal defect is closed, the interatrial septum should be inspected, and any large communication closed down to the size of a 4-mm patent foramen ovale. After appropriate deairing, the clamp on the aortic root is removed, and the pulmonary and atrial incisions closed in a routine fashion. A left atrial line is typically placed for postoperative monitoring. When the patient is adequately rewarmed (36°C), separation from cardiopulmonary bypass is usually accomplished with minimal inotropic support.

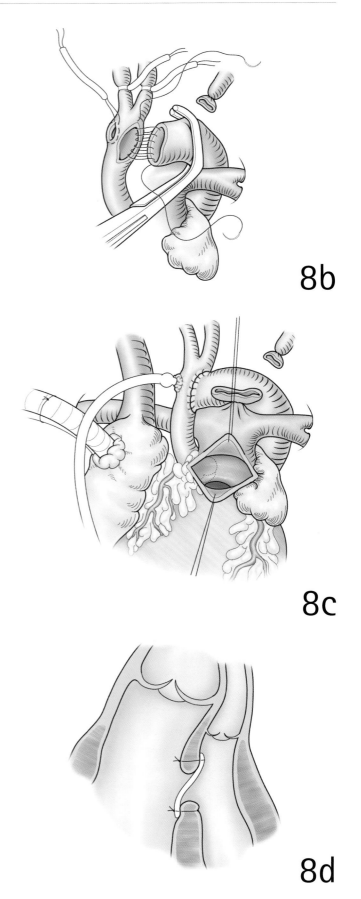

8b

8c

8d

Repair of interrupted aortic arch with truncus arteriosus

9a–d Other than ventricular septal defect, truncus arteriosus is the most common co-existent cardiac anomaly associated with interrupted aortic arch. When these two lesions coexist, operative repair can successfully address both lesions. Arterial cannulation is simplified with the use of a single cannula placed in the distal ascending aorta or main pulmonary artery component of the trunk. The branch pulmonary arteries are occluded with tourniquets at the initiation of cardiopulmonary bypass. Once a temperature of 18°C is reached, the head vessels are occluded, and circulatory arrest is achieved. The ductus is ligated and divided, and the pulmonary artery component of the truncus is separated from the truncal root. The ascending aorta is incised to include the first 5 mm of the left carotid artery. All ductal tissue is removed from the descending aorta, but the left subclavian artery is left in place. An incision in the base of the left subclavian artery of approximately 5 mm is made. With adequate mobilization of the left carotid and left subclavian arteries and the proximal descending aorta, the incisions in the left subclavian and left carotid arteries are brought together with 7/0 polypropylene. A gusset of allograft pulmonary artery or aorta, similar to that used in first stage reconstruction for hypoplastic left heart syndrome, is then implanted to create the lesser curvature of this aortic reconstruction from truncal valve to descending aorta. At this point, the arterial cannula is replaced, cardiopulmonary bypass is resumed, and the patient is rewarmed. Closure of the ventricular septal defect is then performed through a longitudinal incision in the right ventricle, just below the truncal valve. Continuity between the right ventricle and the pulmonary artery bifurcation is achieved with a valved pulmonary or aortic allograft.

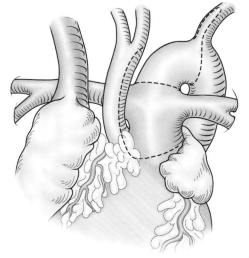

9a

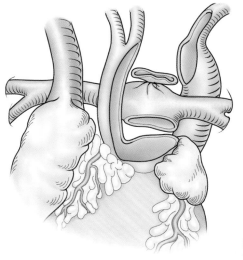

9b

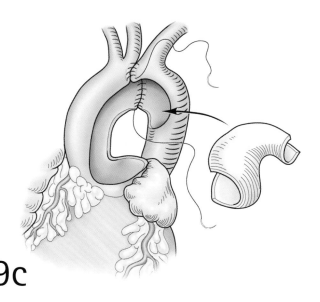

9c

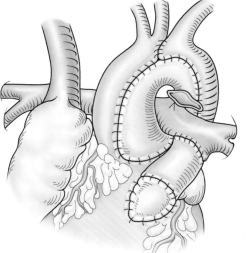

9d

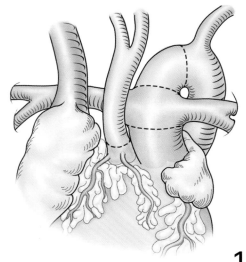

10a

Repair of interrupted aortic arch with transposition of the great arteries

10a–c When interrupted aortic arch is associated with transposition of the great arteries or Taussig-Bing anomaly (double-outlet right ventricle with subpulmonic ventricular septal defect), arch reconstruction is combined with an arterial switch procedure. To address the marked disparity in the size of the great vessels in these patients, the arch repair is performed by dividing the ascending aorta just above the sinuses of Valsalva and swinging it to the left and posteriorly to be anastomosed end-to-end to the descending aorta. A longitudinal incision is made in the underside of this neoaortic arch. The large proximal neoaorta with its implanted coronary buttons is then anastomosed to this incision in an end-to-side fashion. After resumption of bypass, the ventricular septal defect is closed through a right ventriculotomy, the atrial septal defect is closed through a small right atriotomy, and the proximal neopulmonary artery is anastomosed to the pulmonary bifurcation or right pulmonary artery with (anterior-posterior great arteries) or without (side-by-side great arteries) a Lecompte maneuver.

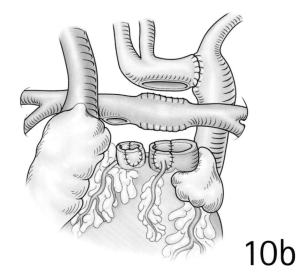

10b

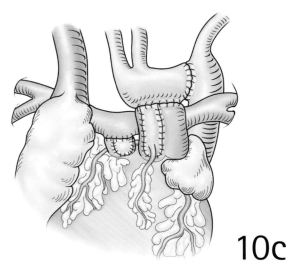

10c

POSTOPERATIVE CARE

Care of patients after repair of coarctation differs little from that for any patient after a thoracotomy. The chest tube is generally removed on the first postoperative day. Systemic arterial hypertension is common and is generally treated with intravenous nitroprusside for the first 24 hours if the systolic blood pressure exceeds 120 mm Hg in neonates or 150 mm Hg in older patients. The patient is then rapidly weaned off of the nitroprusside as an oral beta-blocker (e.g. propranolol) or angiotensin-converting enzyme inhibitor (e.g. captopril) is begun. Some patients are discharged on these agents, which are to be discontinued some time over the first 3 postoperative months. Neonates with residual cardiomegaly, especially those with cardiovascular lesions, such as a ventricular septal defect, may also require digoxin and a diuretic at discharge.

Neonates and young infants are allowed to feed within the first 24 hours after coarctation repair. Older patients may have abdominal discomfort within the first few postoperative days secondary to some degree of splanchnic vasospasm. In these patients, oral intake should be instituted slowly. Occasionally, abdominal distension may require nasogastric decompression and intravenous fluids. A chest radiograph is obtained before discharge to rule out the occasional chylothorax which, if present, is treated conservatively with chest tube drainage and a diet restricted in fat.

As with coarctation, the postoperative management of neonates after repair of interrupted aortic arch and ventricular septal defect is relatively routine. To minimize hemodynamic lability, the infant is paralyzed and anesthetized with a continuous infusion of fentanyl (10–15 µg/kg per hour) for the first 24 hours. Beginning on the first postoperative day, these agents are weaned and progress toward extubation occurs over the next 48–72 hours. Infants with DiGeorge syndrome (common in infants with type B interruption) are likely to exhibit significant hypocalcemia in the postoperative period. Ionized calcium levels, therefore, must be frequently monitored and treated accordingly with infusions of calcium chloride or gluconate. After successful extubation, oral nutrition is begun, and caloric intake is increased as tolerated until the infant is feeding well and gaining weight appropriately. Most infants require digoxin and a diuretic at discharge and for the first few months postoperatively.

OUTCOME

Hospital mortality after coarctation repair in newborns with simple coarctation with or without a ventricular septal defect is less than 5 per cent. The mortality is significantly increased, however, if other major cardiac defects, especially other obstructive lesions of the left heart–aorta complex, are also present. Hospital mortality for repair of simple coarctation in older infants, children, and young adults is less than 1 per cent. Recurrent coarctation requiring reoperation or balloon angioplasty occurs in 3–9 per cent of neonates and in less than 1 per cent of older children or adults. In a recent multicenter study of neonatal coarctation repair, no significant difference in recoarctation rate was noted between the techniques of resection and end-to-end anastomosis and the subclavian flap operation. In this study, the recoarctation rate after patch aortoplasty, however, was significantly higher at 21 per cent.

Most reports describing outcomes after repair of interrupted arch and ventricular septal defect are from single institutions with relatively small patient numbers and significant variation in hospital mortality. The Congenital Heart Surgeons Society did conduct a multi-institutional study enrolling 183 neonates with this lesion between 1987 and 1992. In this study, the hospital mortality for repair was 27 per cent. More recent experience reported from single institutions indicates that hospital mortality for repair of this lesion currently ranges between 5 and 15 per cent. Residual or recurrent obstruction of the repaired aortic arch requiring reintervention occurs in 15–20 per cent of patients with a peak time of occurrence 4 months after the initial repair. In most cases, percutaneous balloon dilation provides satisfactory relief.

FURTHER READING

Jonas, R.A., Quaegebeur, J.M., Kirklin, J.W., Blackstone, E.H., Daicoff, G. 1994. Outcomes in patients with interrupted aortic arch and ventricular septal defect. A multiinstitutional study. Congenital Heart Surgeons Society. *Journal of Thoracic and Cardiovascular Surgery* 107(4), 1099–113.

Liddicoat, J.R., Reddy, V.M., Hanley, F.L. 1994. New approach to great-vessel reconstruction in transposition complexes with interrupted aortic arch. *Annals of Thoracic Surgery* 58(4), 1146–50.

Luciani, G.B., Ackerman, R.J., Chang, A.C., Wells, W.J., Starnes, V.A. 1996. One-stage repair of interrupted aortic arch, ventricular septal defect, and subaortic obstruction in the neonate: a novel approach. *Journal of Thoracic and Cardiovascular Surgery* 111(2), 348–58.

Quaegebeur, J.M., Jonas, R.A., Weinberg, A.D., Blackstone, E.H., Kirklin, J.W. 1994. Outcomes in seriously ill neonates with coarctation of the aorta. A multiinstitutional study. *Journal of Thoracic Cardiovascular Surgery* 108(5), 841–4.

Rajasinghe, H.A., Reddy, V.M., van Son, J.A., *et al.* 1996. Coarctation repair using end-to-side anastomosis of descending aorta to proximal aortic arch. *Annals of Thoracic Surgery* 61(3), 840–4.

Serraf, A., Lacour-Gayet, F., Robotin, M., *et al.* 1996. Repair of interrupted aortic arch: a ten-year experience. *Journal of Thoracic and Cardiovascular Surgery* 112(5), 1150–60.

58

Congenital anomalies of the aortic arch

DUKE CAMERON MD

Chief of Pediatric Cardiac Surgery, Professor of Surgery, The Johns Hopkins Medical Institutions, Baltimore, Maryland, USA

HISTORY

Abnormalities of the aortic arch are rare congenital anomalies commonly known as *vascular rings*, a term coined by Gross in 1945. The first report of a vascular ring was by Hommel in 1737, who described a double aortic arch. The first successful treatment of a vascular ring was by Gross in 1945, who also performed the first innominate artery 'pexy' to the sternum for innominate artery compression syndrome in 1948. Recent advances for the most part have been in non-invasive diagnostic imaging.

1a, b An understanding of embryological origins is probably more important in the treatment of aortic arch anomalies than in any other group of congenital cardiovascular diseases. The Edwards classification system, based on the progression of a double arch to a single one, is the most widely used. Early in development, six pairs of aortic arches connect the ventral and dorsal aortae, although at no time do all six coexist. These arches variously recede, fuse, and remodel to form the typical left-sided aortic arch and its major branches. Inappropriate persistence or resorption of these arches may result in a vascular ring. Most of the first, second, and fifth arches regress, whereas the third pair evolve into the carotid arteries. The sixth arches become the pulmonary arteries, and the seventh intersegmental arteries become the subclavian arteries. The ventral portion of the left fourth arch becomes the ductus arteriosus, usually on the left side because of involution of the right fourth arch. The 'sidedness' of the aortic arch is determined by which fourth arch persists, usually the left. A double arch is the result of bilateral persistence of the fourth arches.

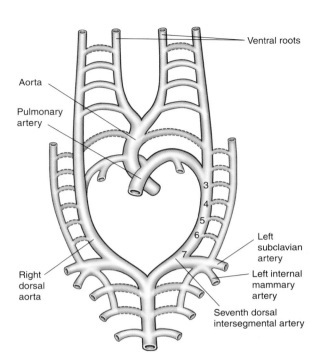

1a

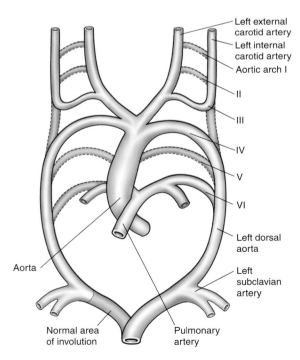

1b

PRINCIPLES AND JUSTIFICATION

Vascular rings typically present because of compression of the trachea or esophagus. The former is manifest as stridor, tachypnea, or frequent respiratory infections, whereas the latter leads to dysphagia or aspiration. The presence of symptoms is sufficient indication for surgery; the asymptomatic patient is rarely identified and probably best left untreated. Most patients present within the first 2 years of life.

PREOPERATIVE ASSESSMENT AND PREPARATION

The goals of evaluation and treatment are the following:

1. Confirm the diagnosis of vascular ring
2. Characterize the anatomy of the ring to plan the operative approach
3. Divide the ring and mobilize the compressed structures

Clinical history and examination

The initial clinical presentation is usually intolerance of feeds or respiratory distress, sometimes triggered by trivial pulmonary infection. Physical findings are frequently absent, but examination may reveal noisy breathing, wheezing, tachypnea, cough, or retractions.

Imaging

CHEST RADIOGRAPH

The plain chest film should show the side of the aortic arch; ambiguity suggests a double arch. Infiltrates and hyperinflation raise the possibility of tracheobronchial compromise. The lateral chest film should be reviewed for narrowing of the tracheal air column.

BARIUM ESOPHAGRAM

Historically, the barium esophagram has been the most powerful tool used to confirm the diagnosis and even to delineate the anatomy of the ring, and in many centers it remains so.

CHEST TOMOGRAPHY/MAGNETIC RESONANCE IMAGING

Chest tomography and magnetic resonance imaging produce striking images, but they may miss short atretic arch segments. Small infants may require sedation and intubation for these studies, which carry significant risk in a patient with airway compromise.

ECHOCARDIOGRAPHY

Approximately 20 per cent of vascular ring patients have congenital heart disease, an incidence that justifies routine echocardiographic screening. Imaging of the ring itself is often possible, and precision is improving with experience.

ENDOSCOPY

Although not usually necessary, bronchoscopy may confirm the site of airway compression and evaluate the severity of malacia. Mainly, it is useful in the setting of innominate artery compression of the trachea. Esophagoscopy is rarely necessary, but may be useful to evaluate other potential diagnoses.

ANGIOGRAPHY

Catheterization is rarely necessary for diagnosis; but, as with echocardiography, it may be part of the evaluation of concomitant congenital heart disease.

ANESTHESIA

General anesthesia and endotracheal intubation are routinely used. In older children and adults, a double-lumen endotracheal tube or 'bronchial blocker' with one-lung ventilation can improve operative exposure. Bilateral radial artery pressure monitoring and intraoperative palpation of the carotid arteries may help to determine which limb of the double arch should be divided in cases in which neither limb is strongly dominant. Spinal catheters for perioperative narcotic infusion minimize post-thoracotomy pain and ease ventilation.

OPERATION

General principles

2a, b Left thoracotomy is the preferred incision for almost all vascular rings. The exceptions are right thoracotomy for innominate artery compression, anomalous origin of the right subclavian artery from a left-sided descending thoracic aorta, and double aortic arch with a right-sided descending thoracic aorta or right-sided ligamentum arteriosum.

Median sternotomy is chosen for repair of concomitant congenital heart disease and pulmonary artery sling (not covered in this chapter). Posterolateral thoracotomy should be serratus-sparing and usually should be performed through the fourth intercostal space. The mediastinal pleura is incised posterior to the vagus nerve, and the major aortic branches are dissected out. No vascular structures should be divided until all are identified with certainty and the hemodynamic consequences of division known from pressure monitoring catheters or carotid palpation. The ligamentum is divided even if not part of the ring. Fibrous bands are lysed, and the trachea and esophagus are freed from surrounding tissues. Kommerell's diverticulum should be dissected out and, if necessary, resected or 'pexed' to the prevertebral fascia. Lymphatic leaks should be controlled by suture or biological sealant.

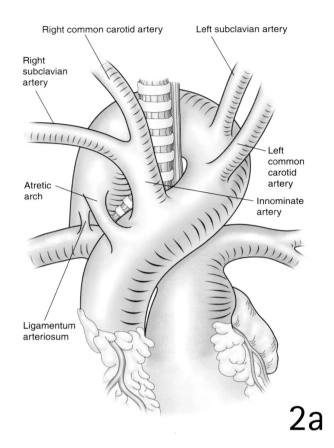

2a

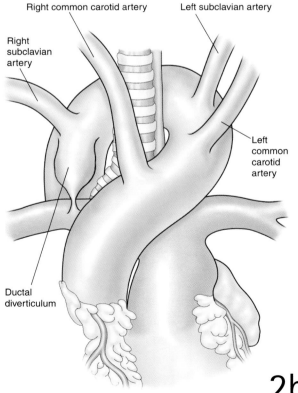

2b

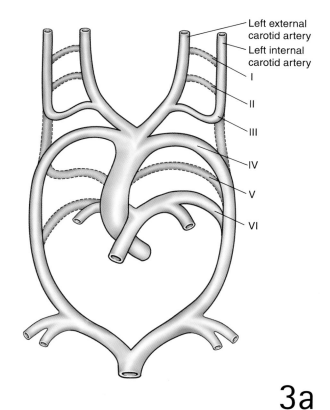

Left external carotid artery

Left internal carotid artery

I

II

III

IV

V

VI

3a

Double aortic arch

3a, b Persistent left and right fourth arches result in an encircling ring formed by an anterior and leftward arch and a posterior and rightward arch that join to form the descending aorta posteriorly. In 75 per cent of cases, the right and posterior arch is the dominant one. The left subclavian and carotid arteries usually arise from the smaller left arch. Atretic or hypoplastic segments occur in the lesser arch approximately a third of the time and can be anywhere along the arch's curve, but are usually distal at the junction with descending aorta. In 15 per cent of cases, the left arch is dominant, and in the remaining 10 per cent, the arches are of equal size.

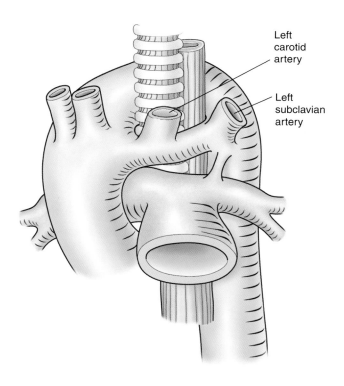

Left carotid artery

Left subclavian artery

3b

4a, b

After mobilization of the arches, the ligamentum, esophagus, and trachea, the lesser arch should be text occluded, typically at the apparently atretic portion. Preservation of brachiocephalic flow is confirmed. Clamps are applied to the narrowest part of the lesser arch, the segment divided, and each end oversewn with continuous polypropylene suture in two layers. The arches are then reflected away from the trachea and esophagus, which are mobilized completely. The ligamentum is divided between ligatures.

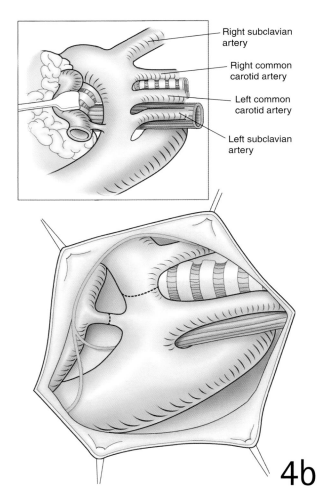

Right subclavian artery

Right common carotid artery

Left common carotid artery

Left subclavian artery

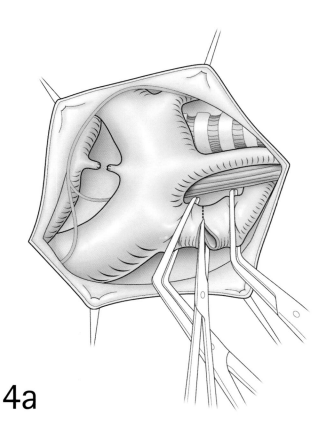

4a

4b

Right aortic arch/left ligamentum

5a–d In this situation, the aorta passes to the right of the trachea and esophagus, coursing posteriorly and leftward behind them, and then usually descends on the left. The ring is formed by a left-sided ligamentum between the left subclavian artery or descending thoracic aorta, depending on the pattern of branching of the ascending aorta. Treatment is simple division of the liga-mentum and mobilization of the aorta and branches. If there is mirror image branching (which is the common pattern), the ligamentum inserts under the innominate artery, and no ring is formed. Similarly, in the rare instances in which the aorta descends on the right and the ligamentum connects the arch undersurface to the right pulmonary artery, no ring exists.

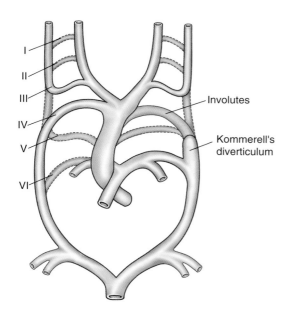

5a

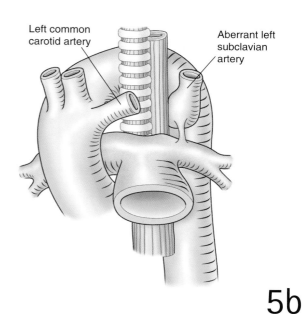

5b

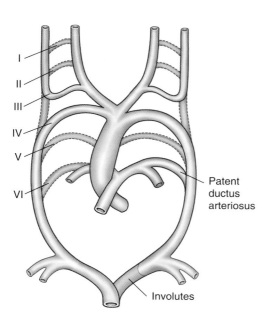

5c

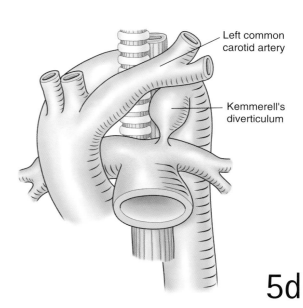

5d

Aberrant right subclavian artery

6a, b The aberrant right subclavian artery arising from a leftward descending thoracic aorta is the most common aortic arch anomaly. As with innominate artery compression, this entity is not a true vascular ring, but may cause compression nonetheless. Most patients with this entity are asymptomatic. Through a right thoracotomy, the subclavian artery may be ligated, divided, and mobilized in infants and small children. In older patients, or when a large vertebral artery arises from the anomalous subclavian artery, reimplantation of the vertebral artery to the ascending aorta is recommended. A prosthetic interposition graft is sometimes necessary.

Aberrant left subclavian artery

When the left subclavian artery arises anomalously from a right-sided arch, it may compress the esophagus as it passes posteriorly and to the left, being drawn anteriorly by the left-sided ligamentum. Division of the ligamentum is usually sufficient; but, as it is the mirror image situation to the above (anomalous right subclavian artery from the contralateral descending thoracic aorta), division and reimplantation may be required.

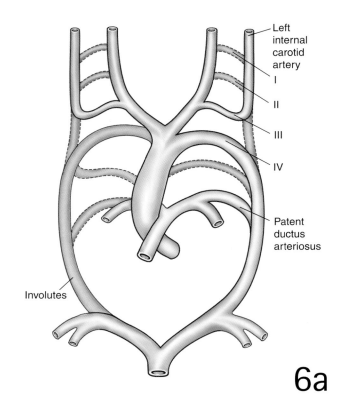

Left internal carotid artery

I

II

III

IV

Patent ductus arteriosus

Involutes

6a

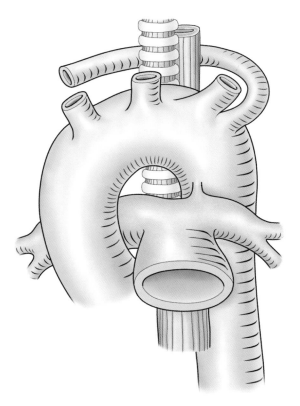

6b

Innominate artery compression

7a–c In innominate artery compression (which, strictly speaking, is not a vascular ring), the innominate artery arises from the aortic arch far to the left. The body of the innominate artery is thus stretched across the anterior tracheal wall and compresses the airway as it passes rightward. Via right thoracotomy, the right lobe of the thymus is excised, and the adventitia of the anterior wall of the innominate artery is fixed to the periosteum of the sternum, elevating the artery off the trachea, which is dissected from the posterior wall of the artery. Reimplantation may be necessary if the thoracic inlet is compressed so that insufficient room exists to 'pexy' the artery to the sternum.

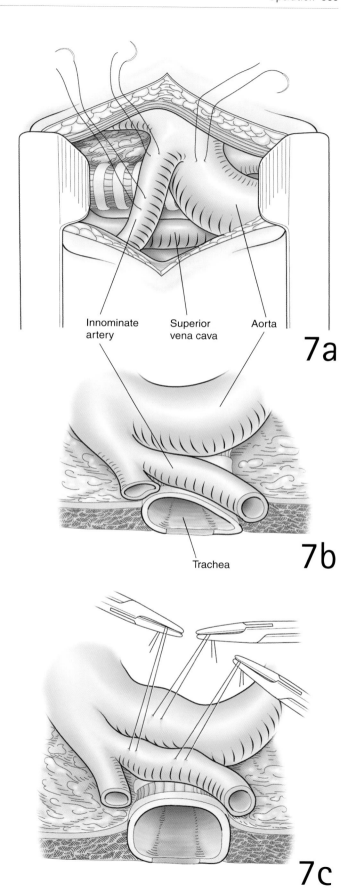

7a

Innominate artery   Superior vena cava   Aorta

7b

Trachea

7c

POSTOPERATIVE CARE

Early extubation is possible in most cases, but should be followed by careful attention to pulmonary toilet, airway humidification, treatment of bronchospasm, and pain control. Potential concerns about recurrent laryngeal or phrenic nerve injury should be communicated to the intensive care unit team. Management of chest drains and the thoracotomy wound are the same as for other thoracotomy patients.

OUTCOME

Operative mortality is low (less than 5 per cent) but not zero. Deaths are usually related to coexistent cardiac disease or severe tracheomalacia. Complications include hemorrhage, infection, esophageal and tracheal leaks, and chylothorax. Relief of symptoms occurs in 70–80 per cent of patients, slightly greater in those with esophageal compression and slightly less in those with tracheal compression. Benefit of surgical division of the ring may not be immediate, as some patients require several months to achieve their ultimate result. Persistent or recurrent symptoms beyond several months should prompt re-evaluation for incomplete mobilization of compressed structures from surrounding fibrous bands, Kommerell's diverticulum, esophageal stricture, or irreversible airway damage.

FURTHER READING

Arciniegas, E., Hakimi, M., Hertzler, J.H., *et al.* 1979. Surgical management of congenital vascular rings. *Journal of Thoracic and Cardiovascular Surgery* **77**, 721–7.

Backer, C.L., Ilbawi, M.N., Idriss, F.S., *et al.* 1989. Vascular anomalies causing tracheoesophageal compression. *Journal of Thoracic and Cardiovascular Surgery* **97**, 725–31.

Chun, K., Colombani, P.M., Dudgeon, D.L., *et al.* 1992. Diagnosis and management of congenital vascular rings – a 22-year experience. *Annals of Thoracic Surgery* **53**, 597–603.

Edwards, J.E. 1948. Anomalies of the derivatives of the aortic arch system. *Medical Clinics of North America* **32**, 925.

Gross, R.E. 1945. Surgical relief for tracheal obstruction from a vascular ring. *New England Journal of Medicine* **233**, 586.

Woods, R.K., Sharp, R.J., Holcomb, G.W., *et al.* 2001. Vascular anomalies and tracheoesophageal compression: a single institution's 25-year experience. *Annals of Thoracic Surgery* **72**, 434–9.

59

Hypoplastic left heart syndrome

THOMAS L. SPRAY MD
Alice Langdon Warner Professor of Surgery, Department of Cardiothoracic Surgery, University of Pennsylvania School of Medicine; Division
Chief of Cardiothoracic Surgery, The Children's Hospital of Philadelphia, Philadelphia, Pennsylvania, USA

HISTORY

The term *hypoplastic left heart syndrome* (HLHS) has been used to describe a group of cardiac malformations that consists of hypoplasia or absence of the left ventricle and hypoplasia of the ascending aorta. In the most extreme form, HLHS refers to aortic valvar atresia, with a very diminutive ascending aorta and diminutive left ventricle. Like other single ventricle malformations of the heart, HLHS has a circulation dependent on patency of the ductus arteriosus and obligatory mixing of pulmonary and systemic venous blood. The single ventricle (in this case, an anatomic right ventricle) supplies the pulmonary circulation by the branch pulmonary arteries and the systemic circulation via the patent ductus arteriosus. Flow in the ascending aorta is usually primarily retrograde, and in aortic atresia, the ascending aorta acts as a common coronary artery supplying coronary perfusion.

HLHS is the most common severe congenital heart defect, representing 7–9 per cent of all congenital heart anomalies diagnosed within the first year of life; if left untreated, HLHS is virtually always fatal, accounting for 25 per cent of all cardiac deaths in the first week of life. Early attempts to provide palliative therapy for infants with HLHS were described by

Cayler and Freedom. Continuity was created between the right ventricle and descending aorta by placement of a graft, and pulmonary arterial banding was used to limit pulmonary blood flow. Initial attempts, however, were unsuccessful, due primarily to distortion of the pulmonary vascular bed. Evolution of these initial therapies, however, continued, and much of the development of successful first stage reconstruction is credited to Dr. William I. Norwood, who gradually refined and developed the surgical principles that have led to successful outcomes. Neonatal heart transplantation, pioneered by Leonard Bailey and his colleagues, has been used as an alternate form of therapy; however, the limitation of donor heart availability and the increased success with staged reconstruction operations have made primary transplantation less desirable. The first successful palliation operations with staged reconstruction operations as described by Norwood have changed little over the past 20 years; however, recently several technical modifications have been proposed to limit the use of prosthetic material in the reconstruction and to decrease the use or duration of deep hypothermic circulatory arrest.

PRINCIPLES AND JUSTIFICATION

The principle of the staged reconstruction operations for HLHS is similar to that for other single ventricle malformations of the heart. The goals of the first stage reconstructive procedure (known commonly as the Norwood procedure) are (1) the creation of an unobstructed connection between the systemic ventricle (the right ventricle) and the aorta in a fashion that permits growth; (2) regulation of pulmonary blood flow to permit growth of the pulmonary vascular bed and to limit the development of pulmonary vascular obstructive disease while minimizing the volume load on the single ventricle; and (3) creation of an unobstructed interatrial communication to avoid restriction of the pulmonary venous return to the heart. These principles must be performed technically in such a fashion as to prevent distal arch obstruction and limit or interfere with coronary perfusion. Because successful first-stage reconstruction creates a situation where pulmonary blood flow is dependent on an aortopulmonary shunt, the single right ventricle is subjected to increased volume load as the entire systemic and pulmonary cardiac output passes through the right atrium, right ventricle, and pulmonary artery to the aorta. Tricuspid valve regurgitation can be a consequence of either ischemic damage due to the diminutive aorta supplying coronary blood flow or to true coronary anomalies, or it can be a secondary effect of the increased volume load. Significant tricuspid regurgitation may require intervention at the first or second stage operation and, if associated with severe ventricular dysfunction, may be an indication for conversion to transplantation as a second stage operation.

Satisfactory completion of the first stage operation creates a somewhat unstable physiological situation, with shunt-dependent pulmonary blood flow and significant volume load on an anatomical right ventricle. For this reason, a second stage reconstruction operation (performed at 3–6 months of age) consisting of either a bidirectional Glenn shunt or hemi-Fontan procedure (see Chapter 44 'Bidirectional Glenn and hemi-Fontan procedures') is undertaken to decrease the volume load of the single ventricle and improve effective pulmonary blood flow. The third stage in the reconstruction, as in other single ventricle malformations, is a modification of the Fontan-Kreutzer procedure. The systemic and pulmonary circulations are separated, often with the use of a single fenestration to permit right-to-left shunting at the atrial level to maintain ventricular preload in the postoperative period and during times of stress or elevated pulmonary vascular resistance.

PREOPERATIVE ASSESSMENT AND PREPARATION

As in other single ventricle malformations with duct-dependent physiology, signs of HLHS may be minimal. Tachypnea and mild cyanosis are the primary early signs. HLHS often is not diagnosed until ductal constriction has begun, when systemic perfusion is severely compromised and metabolic acidosis, organ dysfunction, and shock evolve. If the ductal patency is maintained and the atrial septal defect is unrestrictive, significant pulmonary overcirculation can occur, resulting in a severe volume-loaded ventricle and congestive heart failure, which also leads to systemic organ dysfunction and metabolic acidosis with compromised peripheral perfusion. In rare cases, a severely restrictive atrial communication is present (2–5 per cent of cases), and in these patients, severe hypoxemia with a congestive pattern on chest x-rays is present; these patients may require emergent intervention to create a more unrestrictive atrial communication in the catheterization laboratory or in the operating room.

The diagnosis of HLHS is confirmed by two-dimensional echocardiography with color flow Doppler mapping, and cardiac catheterization is rarely necessary unless intervention is required to create less restriction at the atrial septal level or to document unusual pulmonary venous return. In patients without severe restriction of venous return at the atrial level, dilation of the atrial septal defect should not be undertaken, as the procedure increases the pulmonary blood flow and can potentially cause hemodynamic deterioration in another stable balance of pulmonary and systemic blood flow. Echocardiographic examination can evaluate the degree of hypoplasia of the aortic arch, the retrograde flow in the ascending aorta, the presence or absence of coarctation in most cases, and the presence or absence of significant tricuspid valve regurgitation and restriction at the atrial septal defect.

Initial medical support after birth in infants with HLHS involves maintaining patency of the ductus arteriosus and balancing the pulmonary and systemic blood flows to prevent significant abnormalities of systemic perfusion or of pulmonary overcirculation. Prostaglandin E_1 is infused at a low dose (0.025–0.05 µg/kg per minute) to maintain patency of the ductus arteriosus. In patients who have no apnea as a consequence of prostaglandin infusion, maintenance of normal ventilation is preferable by permitting the patient to breathe spontaneously on room air. If mechanical ventilation is necessary, ventilation with 21–30 per cent oxygen to prevent pulmonary consolidation is preferable, and high oxygen gas mixtures are avoided to prevent pulmonary vasodilation. Blending carbon dioxide or nitrogen into the gas mixture on the ventilator may occasionally be useful to increase pulmonary vasoconstriction and improve systemic cardiac output. If ventricular dysfunction is present, low doses of inotropic agents may be used; however, the lowest possible levels of inotropic support should be sought to limit the effects of unbalancing the systemic and pulmonary vascular resistance. Ventricular function generally recovers after initial acidosis and hemodynamic compromise has been corrected, and addition of diuretics and digoxin is often useful before and after surgery to help deal with the volume effects on the single ventricle as pulmonary resistance decreases. Judicious use of these agents may permit a significant period of stabilization and improvement in patients with HLHS to allow recovery of renal and hepatic function and assessment of neurological status. In addition, noncardiac malformations can be assessed. Despite significant volume loads, the resuscitated single ventricle can provide quite stable physiology for several days to weeks before surgical intervention. Surgery is generally performed nonemergently after the hepatic and renal function have normalized.

ANESTHESIA

Anesthesia for infants with HLHS can require delicate manipulations to systemic and pulmonary resistances during the anesthetic induction and maintenance. Anesthesia is achieved with administration of narcotic agents (fentanyl, 10 µg/kg) and muscle relaxant (pancuronium or variant, 0.2 mg/kg). Nasotracheal intubation is performed for a more stable airway postoperatively. If the patient has unrestricted pulmonary blood flow, care is taken to avoid high oxygen gas mixtures to maintain the stable balance of pulmonary and systemic resistance. As anesthesia-induced vasodilation occurs, addition of nitrogen or carbon dioxide to the gas mixture may be necessary to maintain systemic perfusion in this critical stage. Monitoring with an umbilical arterial and venous line is used, and blood gases are monitored frequently to correct imbalances in perfusion and acidosis.

OPERATION

1a–c
Exposure is performed through a midline sternotomy incision, and the majority of thymic tissue is excised to gain access to the superior mediastinum and the arch vessels from the aorta. The pericardium is opened in the midline. Because of the significant volume loading of the ventricle and hypothermia (body temperature is generally 34°C due to low room temperature in the operating room), the myocardium can be extremely irritable and even minor retraction or irritation of the ventricle can result in instability and ventricular fibrillation. Therefore, care is taken to avoid manipulation of the ventricle as much as possible during the dissection, which is done with low-power electrocautery (Figure 1a). The very diminutive ascending aorta is separated from the pulmonary artery to which it is adherent down proximal to the takeoff of the right pulmonary artery, and then the entire arch of the aorta is mobilized, including the head vessels, which are encircled with sutures and snares for control. The ductus arteriosus is mobilized, as is the descending thoracic aorta beyond the ductus, with care being taken to avoid direct retraction on the ductal tissue, which is friable and can easily cause hemorrhage. The pulmonary bifurcation is also mobilized freely, and the right and left pulmonary arteries are encircled with sutures and tourniquets for control when bypass is initiated. After mobilization of these structures, pursestring sutures are placed in the proximal main pulmonary artery below the pulmonary bifurcation and in the right atrial appendage for cannulation for cardiopulmonary bypass (Figure 1b). After heparinization, the pulmonary artery and right atrium are cannulated, and the patient is begun on cardiopulmonary bypass and cooled to a nasopharyngeal temperature of 18°C. After initiation of bypass, the tourniquets on the right and left pulmonary arteries are tightened to prevent pulmonary blood flow during the cooling phase of the operation. Cooling is done for an optimal time to determine the length of the modified Blalock-Taussig shunt used to control pulmonary blood flow. A polytetrafluoroethylene tube graft of an appropriate size (3.4–4.0 mm in diameter) is cut at this time, because the anatomical relationships of the innominate artery and the right pulmonary artery can be readily identified. A diagonal cut is made for the proximal graft, a partial occluding vascular clamp is placed on the innominate artery proximally, and the proximal anastomosis of the graft is created to a longitudinal arteriotomy using a running 7/0 monofilament suture. At this time, the vascular clamp can be released and the flow though the shunt assessed to ensure that unrestricted inflow into the shunt is occurring (Figure 1c).

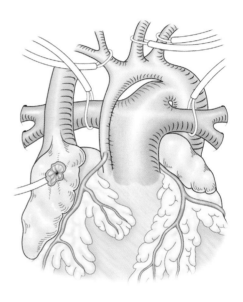

1a

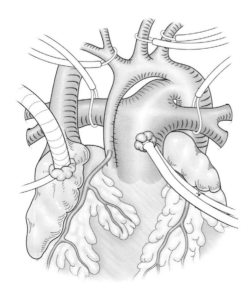

1b

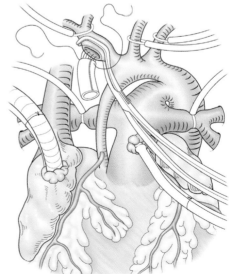

1c

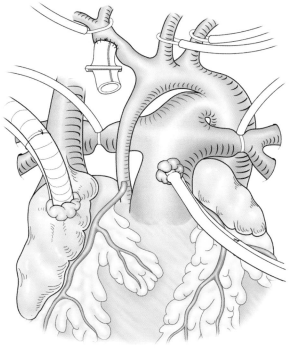

2a

2a, b The shunt is then controlled with a hemoclip during the remainder of the procedure or, in alternative techniques, the shunt can be cannulated and bypass continued to maintain perfusion of the arch during the remainder of the operation. Cardioplegia is connected to a side arm in the arterial cannula and, after cooling to 18°C has been achieved over a 15–20 minute period, the circulation is arrested, and the tourniquets on the arch vessels are tightened.

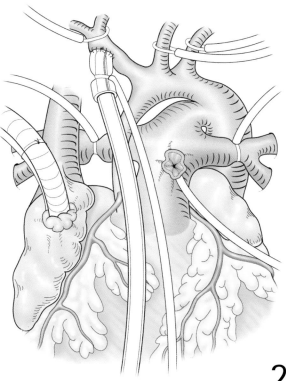

2b

3a–c A clamp is placed on the descending thoracic aorta below the ductal insertion site. Cardioplegia can then be injected retrograde through the aortic cannula and ductus into the ascending aorta to provide diastolic arrest of the heart. The aortic cannula is then removed, as is the venous cannula after venous blood has been returned to the reservoir. The tourniquets on the pulmonary arteries are then removed, and the ductus arteriosus is ligated and divided distally on the aortic end (Figure 3b). Working through the atrial pursestring suture, the atrial septum can be widely excised; however, if exposure is limited, a right atriotomy incision is made and the septum primum, which is commonly displaced to the left, can be excised to create a widely unobstructed atrial opening (Figure 3c). The atrium is then closed with monofilament suture.

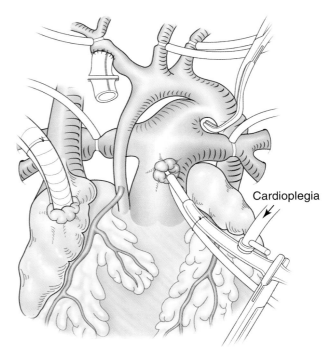

Cardioplegia

3a

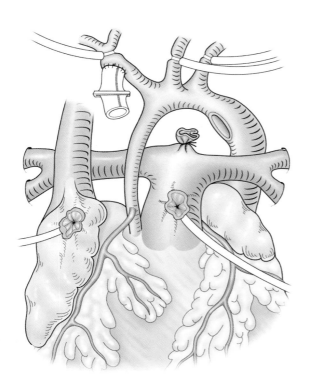

3b

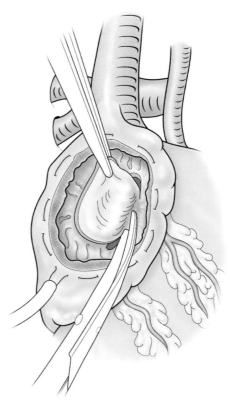

3c

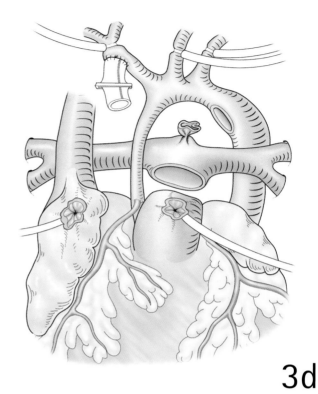

3d

3d–e Next, the pulmonary artery is divided transversely at the origin of the right pulmonary artery (Figure 3d). This incision leaves slightly more pulmonary artery on the left side, unless the cut is made in an oblique fashion up to the origin of the left pulmonary artery. Making the pulmonary artery transection at the origin of the right pulmonary artery ensures that the connection between the proximal pulmonary artery and aorta is high enough to avoid sewing near the coronary artery origin from the diminutive ascending aorta. The bifurcation of the pulmonary arteries is then closed primarily if the pulmonary arteries are large or, more commonly, the bifurcation is closed with an oval-shaped patch of pulmonary homograft material using a running monofilament technique (Figure 3e).

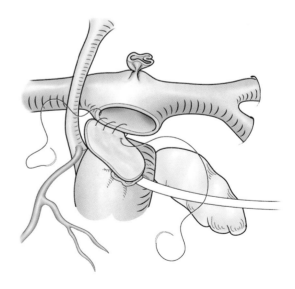

3e

4 The pulmonary bifurcation has been reconstructed in an optimal time to create the distal anastomosis of the shunt to the origin of the right pulmonary artery at the takeoff from the main pulmonary bifurcation. This technique permits the shunt to connect more medially behind the reconstructed aorta and avoids having to create this anastomosis with the aorta reperfused and the large neoaorta making exposure difficult. Meticulous shunt creation is an important part of the Norwood operation to avoid cyanosis or early shunt thrombosis. Next, an incision is made in the medial aspect of the diminutive ascending aorta and carried across the undersurface of the arch or the aorta beyond the last of the ductal insertion sites.

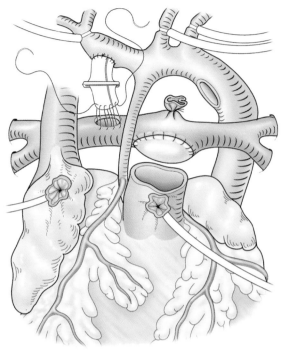

4

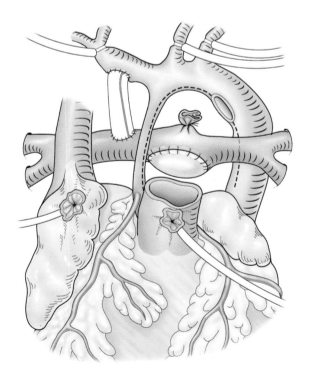

5a

5a–d Ductal tissue is débrided, and the ridge of coarctation opposite the ductus is excised if present (Figure 5b). Proximally, the incision is carried down to the level of the transection of the pulmonary bifurcation. In some cases a small incision into the proximal pulmonary artery to allow adequate connection between the pulmonary artery and ascending aorta may be necessary to prevent compression of the aorta (Figure 5c). The proximal pulmonary artery is then sutured delicately to the diminutive ascending aorta with interrupted 7/0 monofilament sutures to prevent a pursestring effect and to create meticulous hemostasis at this critical junction (Figure 5d). At this time, it must be assured that no restriction to inflow into the coronary arteries is present. Mobilization of the tissue between the aorta and pulmonary artery is present so that epicardial adhesions do not potentially kink the origin of the coronary arteries when the neoaorta expands.

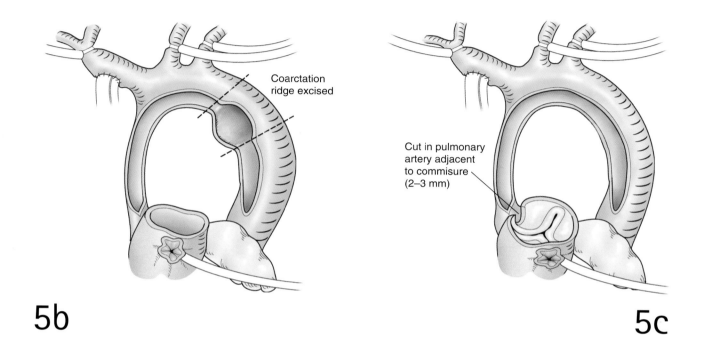

Coarctation
ridge excised

5b

Cut in pulmonary
artery adjacent
to commisure
(2–3 mm)

5c

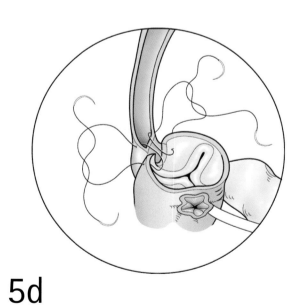

5d

6a–c The final stage of reconstruction is creation of an unobstructed aortic arch by augmenting the arch with a patch of pulmonary homograft material and running monofilament suture. The geometry of this patch is complex (Figure 6a) and care must be taken to avoid a patch so redundant that as systolic pressure increases, twisting of the reconstruction to the right occurs, causing either impingement on the origin of the innominate artery and limitation of inflow into the shunt and other head vessels (Figure 6b) or twisting in the descending aorta causing a distal arch obstruction (Figure 6c).

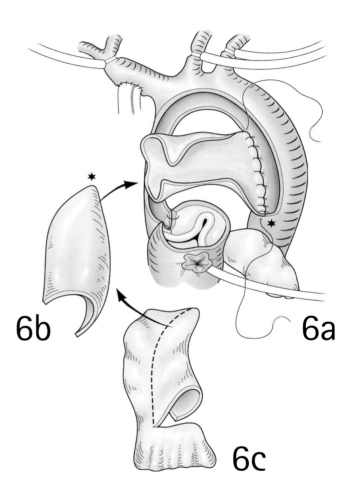

6d In general, making the patch too narrow rather than too wide is preferable. The posterior part of the pathway is generally smaller in length than the anterior portion, and the patch is generally scooped out on the inferior incision to prevent excessive length, which can cause kinking of the pulmonary artery at the connection to the patch and restriction to ejection from the heart with creation of neoaortic insufficiency through the pulmonary valve. Variations in the patch tailoring are necessary for variations of HLHS in which the ascending aorta is larger than in aortic atresia or where the arch of the aorta is well developed to avoid too redundant a patch with the previously mentioned complications (Figure 6d).

After completion of the reconstruction, air is evacuated from the heart by injection of saline into the right atrial cannulation site and evacuation out of the aortic cannulation site. Then, the venous and arterial cannulae are reinserted. The infant is then placed back on cardiopulmonary bypass and rewarmed to 37°C, and the tourniquets on the arch vessels are released. At this time, myocardial perfusion can be assessed to ensure that no restriction to coronary inflow exists, and good myocardial function should promptly return. Significant dilation of the heart at this stage generally requires assessment, because, if present, distortion of the pulmonary valve and neoaortic insufficiency needs to be addressed. After rewarming has been completed, atrial lines are brought through the chest wall and positioned in the pursestring suture in the right atrial appendage for pressure measurement and volume infusion, and the patient is started on low dose inotropic support consisting of dopamine at 3 µg/kg per minute. Milrinone is commonly used, and the patient is loaded with this drug in the bypass circuit to create vasodilation and improve right ventricular performance. Other centers have used powerful alpha-blocking agents, such as phenoxybenzamine, to accomplish the same purpose. For maintenance of systemic perfusion, decreasing elevated systemic resistance which would otherwise increase shunt flow and lead to myocardial dysfunction is critical. Ventilation is initiated at high tidal volumes to ensure the elimination of atelectasis and to minimize pulmonary resistance. The hemoclip is then removed from the shunt, and the patient is rapidly weaned off cardiopulmonary bypass. Modified ultrafiltration is routinely used in our center to decrease myocardial edema, improve systolic ventricular performance, and minimize the volume load on the circulation in the early postoperative period. After cannulae are removed from the heart and hemostasis is secured, the chest is drained; and generally, the sternum is closed before transport to the intensive care unit. If concerns exist about myocardial function or if hemorrhage is a concern, the chest is left open, and a polytetrafluoroethylene patch is used to approximate the skin edges.

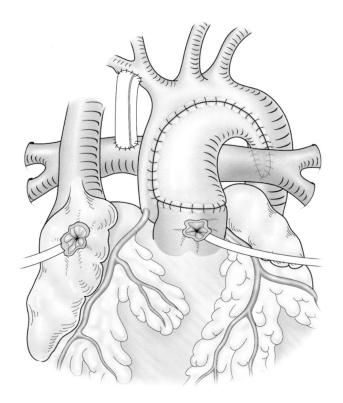

6d

7a, b Occasionally, variations in operative technique are used depending on the particular cardiac anatomy. If the aorta and pulmonary artery are transposed or, in cases in which the aorta is large in relation to the pulmonary artery, reconstruction of the aortic arch may be simplified by division of the aorta and pulmonary artery proximally with side-to-side connection over a short distance, followed by augmentation of the aortic arch with a triangular-shaped patch of cryopreserved pulmonary homograft material. The aorta is reconstructed to the double-barrel exit from the heart using continuous monofilament suture. This approach avoids potential distortion and twisting of the reconstructed arch and can avoid too large a patch with a possible compression of the posteriorly-located bifurcation.

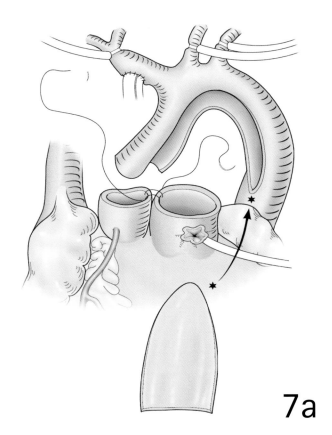

7a

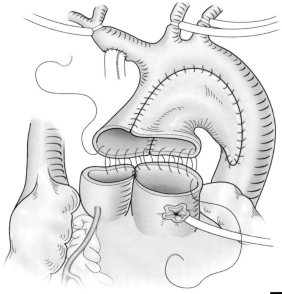

7b

8a, b An additional modification avoids the use of most prosthetic material in the arch reconstruction. In this approach, rather than reconstruction of the aortic arch with cryopreserved homograft material, a direct connection is performed between the proximal pulmonary artery and the undersurface of the aortic arch. In this procedure, the arch vessels must be extensively mobilized to allow them to come down to the pulmonary artery, and the division of the pulmonary artery is created high enough towards the origin of the right pulmonary artery so that the diminutive ascending aorta does not have to be pulled up so far that kinking of the tiny ascending aorta, which acts as a common coronary vessel, occurs. Problems with coronary inflow have led may centers to divide the diminutive ascending aorta and reimplant it directly onto the anterolateral aspect of the pulmonary artery with interrupted or running monofilament sutures to avoid this complication.

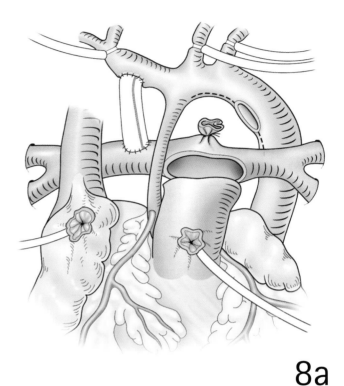

8a

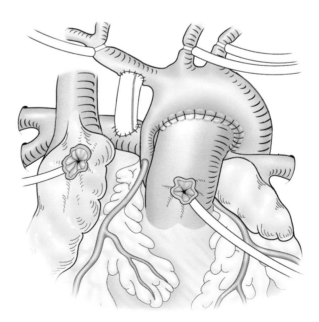

8b

9a, b If significant coarctation is present, division of the distal aorta beyond the subclavian artery and excision of all ductal tissue with direct connection posteriorly before arch reconstruction is also advisable to avoid leaving ductal tissue, which can reconstruct and cause recurrent arch obstruction.

A recent modification of the stage one operation for hypoplastic left heart syndrome developed by Sano uses a right ventricle-(RV) to-pulmonary artery (PA) shunt instead of an aortopulmonary shunt to provide pulmonary blood flow. This modification has the advantage of providing systolic antegrade flow into the pulmonary arteries and avoiding diastolic runoff into the pulmonary vascular bed that may decrease the diastolic pressure and potentially decrease the coronary perfusion pressure. The Sano modification has gained rapid acceptance in many centers due to an improvement in early postoperative stability in patients in whom the RV-to-PA connection has been established. The early postoperative elevation of systemic vascular resistance which causes low cardiac output after the standard stage one Norwood operation has less physiologic impact with an RV-to-PA shunt, where the elevated systemic resistance results actually in improvement in forward flow into the pulmonary vascular bed as the right ventricular pressure increases. The theoretical disadvantages of the use of an RV-to-PA shunt are the need for an incision in the right ventricular infundibulum (which may have impact on long-term right ventricular function) and the potential for narrowing of the shunt at the origin from the right ventricle due to the thick ventricular muscle.

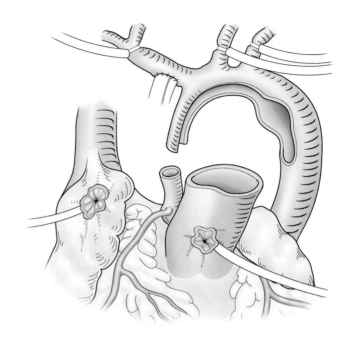

9a

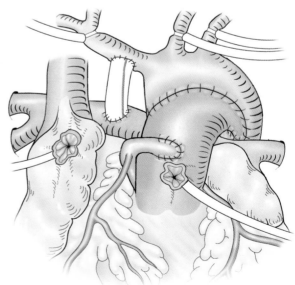

9b

10a, b The arch reconstruction is performed with the Sano modification in the standard fashion; however, instead of creating a PTFE tube graft from the innominate artery to the right pulmonary artery, a 5-mm tube of PTFE material is anastomosed to the pulmonary bifurcation directly using running suture. The pulmonary bifurcation is closed partially, and then the distal anastomosis of the shunt created, which brings the entrance of the shunt superiorly into the pulmonary bifurcation to avoid interference with the reconstructed neoaorta and to allow for good growth of the pulmonary bifurcation. The shunt is then beveled to an appropriate length, and an incision is made in the infundibulum of the right ventricular outflow tract (Figure 10b). After excision of a small amount of muscle from the edges of the incision, the proximal anastomosis is created using running suture.

When using the Sano modification, no obstruction to the inflow of the right ventricle-to-pulmonary artery shunt should be present and the length of the shunt should be tailored appropriately so that it does not push posteriorly and cause kinking and potential occlusion of the pulmonary bifurcation. Postoperative diastolic pressures are higher than in the standard Norwood operation using this technique; however, systolic pressures are often slightly lower. In addition, oxygen saturations may be higher with the RV-to-PA connection; however, the higher oxygen saturations are well-tolerated and 'steal' of coronary flow does not occur in diastole as has been seen in the standard Norwood aortopulmonary shunt connection.

A further modification of the technique involves the limited use or the lack of use of circulatory arrest. This approach can be done by initial cannulation of the pulmonary artery through the ductus arteriosus with snaring of the ductus to maintain systemic perfusion or creation of the proximal modified Blalock-Taussig shunt before initiation of bypass with cannulation of the shunt for arterial inflow. In general, creation of the proximal shunt anastomosis is difficult without distortion of a very diminutive ascending aorta and temporary myocardial dysfunction; therefore, bypass support is generally preferable. The proximal anastomosis of the modified Blalock-Taussig shunt is created to the origin of the innominate artery. Then, with a brief period of circulatory arrest, cannulation is moved to the distal end of the shunt to provide retrograde flow into the innominate artery to perfuse the brain and, through collaterals, the distal vascular bed. Snares are tightened on the carotid and subclavian vessels, and the descending aorta is clamped while flow is maintained at approximately 30 per cent of normal. Monitoring of radial perfusion pressures is advisable when this technique is used. Venous return is evacuated either through a patent venous cannula or sump suction placed in the right atrium. With this technique, perfusion can be maintained through the arch with some distal perfusion maintained during the reconstruction of the aortic arch. After reconstruction of the aortic arch is complete, arch cannulation can be performed, and the distal anastomosis of the shunt is created to the pulmonary arteries during rewarming.

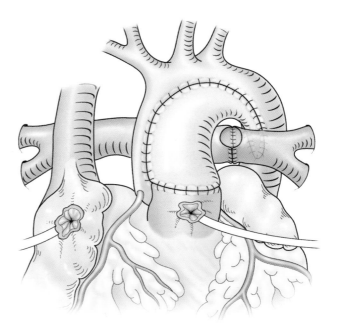

10a

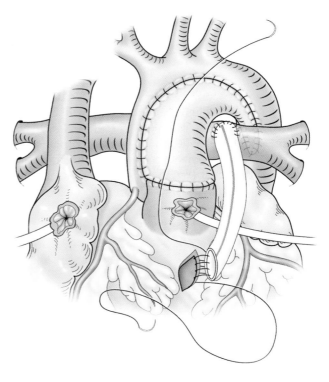

10b

POSTOPERATIVE CARE

The major advancement in the management of patients with HLHS has been the refinement of postoperative care, which has decreased the occurrence of early myocardial dysfunction and cardiovascular collapse.

Maintenance of systemic vascular perfusion by vasodilation of the systemic vascular bed is the primary goal in the early postoperative period. Early approaches to balancing systemic and pulmonary circulations after the first stage reconstruction operation focused on preventing pulmonary overcirculation by limiting pulmonary blood flow with manipulation of vascular resistance. Oxygen was rapidly decreased; and occasionally, carbon dioxide was blended into the gas mixture to raise pulmonary vascular resistance. However, elegant studies performed by Tweddell and associates have suggested that the pulmonary blood flow is restricted by the shunt sufficiently so that significant manipulation of pulmonary vascular resistance is rarely necessary. Oxygen is weaned as appropriate to nontoxic levels of less than 40 per cent as the patient recovers from the operative procedure and, with a satisfactory size shunt, weaning to 30–40 per cent oxygen can generally be done fairly rapidly. However, strict attention to base deficit is important, and significant development or progression of base deficits suggests significant systemic perfusion abnormalities that require intervention with increasing inotropic support or more significant vasodilation, or both. The use of vasodilatory inotropes such as milrinone has significantly improved the maintenance of systemic output while improving right heart function, and our current preference is to use 3 µg/kg per minute of dopamine for baseline inotropic and renal support and to add 0.5–1.0 µg/kg per minute of milrinone support to improve vasodilation and systemic output postoperatively. Ventilation is maintained with slight hypocarbia in the 35–38 mm Hg range to prevent alveolar hypoxemia and hypercarbia, and high tidal volumes are generally used to prevent atelectasis. The infant is kept sedated and paralyzed overnight, although patients who are in good condition preoperatively and have a stable balance of systemic and pulmonary flow can be allowed to awaken and extubate within 24–48 hours after surgery. Nutritional support is begun as early as possible after surgery, initially with intravenous and, subsequently, enteral feeds as tolerated.

OUTCOME

The surgical results of the first-stage reconstruction operation for HLHS have progressively improved. In a recent report of the entire experience with HLHS from 1984 to 2000 from The Philadelphia Children's Hospital, approximately 1000 consecutive infants underwent staged reconstruction operations. Results improved in each 2- to 3-year time interval over that period, such that current operative survival for first-stage reconstruction is approximately 80 per cent with additional interstage mortality of 3–5 per cent. Patients at extremely low birth weight (less than 2 kg) have been noted to have a slightly higher operative mortality; however, other anatomic features (e.g. aortic atresia versus aortic stenosis subgroups) have not been associated with increased operative risk. Survival after the first-stage operation is related to risk factors that include prematurity, low birth weight, organ system dysfunction, and associated genetic syndromes. Patients with no significant risk factors who present in good condition for surgical intervention have survival approaching 90 per cent or more for first-stage reconstruction, and early mortality is now related primarily to noncardiac abnormalities such as necrotizing enterocolitis, neurological dysfunction, or infection. Analysis of long-term results has shown that, after second-stage reconstruction at 3–6 months of age, the intermediate-term survival is excellent with little late decremental survival over the follow-up period extending out to approximately 15 years. The hemi-Fontan, bidirectional Glenn, and Fontan procedures' mortality has also dramatically improved for HLHS patients, such that mortality of less than 1 per cent is currently noted in both the second- and third-stage operations at our center. Therefore, with optimal intraoperative and postoperative management in infancy, the patient with HLHS has a significant opportunity for survival and reasonable quality of life.

Recent studies on neurological outcome after staged operation suggest that patients with HLHS are at risk for neurodevelopmental delay for multiple reasons such as cyanosis, congestive heart failure, and pre-existing central nervous system abnormalities, in addition to the effects of cardiopulmonary bypass and hypothermic circulatory arrest. Children with HLHS scored statistically lower than non-HLHS children with single ventricles on scales of infant development and intelligence quotient testing; however, the majority remain in the normal range. Verbal tests tend to have higher scores than motor skill tests, as has been noted in other patients with congenital heart disease who undergo surgical intervention. The primary determinant of poor neurodevelopmental outcome is the presence of genetic syndromes or the presence of a seizure disorder in the perioperative or preoperative period. As techniques for management in the pre- and postoperative period improve and with modification of surgical technique which may limit circulatory arrest periods and improve systemic output postoperatively, continued improvement and neurological outcomes can be expected.

FURTHER READING

Bove, E.L., Lloyd, T.R. 1996. Staged reconstruction for hypoplastic left heart syndrome. Contemporary results. *Annals of Thoracic Surgery* **224**, 387–94.

Hoffman, G.M., Ghanayem, N.S., Kampine, J.M., *et al.* 2000. Venous saturation and the anaerobic threshold in neonates after the Norwood procedure for hypoplastic left heart syndrome. *Annals of Thoracic Surgery* **70**, 1515–21.

Mahle, W.T., Spray, T.L., Wernovsky, G., *et al.* 2000. Survival after reconstructive surgery for hypoplastic left heart syndrome: a 15-year experience from a single institution. *Circulation* **102[Suppl III]**, III-136–III-141.

Tweddell, J.S., Hoffman, G.M., Fedderly, R.T., *et al.* 2000. Patients at risk for low systemic oxygen delivery after the Norwood procedure. *Annals of Thoracic Surgery* **69**, 1893–9.

Weinstein, S., Gaynor, J.W., Bridges, N.D., *et al.* 1999. Early survival of infants weighing 2.5 kilograms or less undergoing first-stage reconstruction for hypoplastic left heart syndrome. *Circulation* **100[Suppl II]**, II-167–II-170.

Weinstein, S., Gaynor, J.W., Wernovsky, G., *et al.* 1998. Survival of low birth weight infants undergoing Stage I Norwood reconstruction for hypoplastic left heart syndrome or single ventricle physiology. *Circulation* **98[17 Suppl I]**, 62.

60

Coronary anomalies

J. WILLIAM GAYNOR MD

Assistant Professor of Surgery, University of Pennsylvania School of Medicine; Assistant Surgeon, Department of Cardiothoracic Surgery, The Children's Hospital of Philadelphia, Philadelphia, Pennsylvania, USA

Most common variations in the number, origin, and distribution of the coronary arteries are of intellectual interest only. Although clinically significant congenital coronary artery anomalies are rare, they may result in myocardial ischemia, left ventricular dysfunction, and sudden death. Important anomalies include anomalous origin of a coronary artery from the pulmonary artery, anomalous course of a coronary artery between the pulmonary artery and aorta, and coronary artery fistulae.

ANOMALOUS ORIGIN OF A CORONARY ARTERY FROM THE PULMONARY ARTERY

The most important coronary anomaly is anomalous origin of the left main coronary artery (LMCA) from the pulmonary artery. Anomalous origin of the LMCA from the pulmonary artery occurs more frequently than anomalous origin of the right coronary artery (RCA). Anomalous origin of both the LMCA and RCA from the pulmonary artery is very rare and almost uniformly fatal. Rarely, either the left anterior descending coronary artery (LAD) or the circumflex coronary artery may arise separately from the pulmonary artery. Associated anomalies are uncommon. Without surgical correction, anomalous origin of the LMCA is usually lethal during infancy with a mortality of 90 per cent by 1 year of age.

Children with anomalous origin of the LMCA from the pulmonary artery usually develop symptoms after closure of the ductus arteriosus and the postnatal fall in pulmonary vascular resistance. Before ductal closure, pulmonary artery pressure is elevated, and perfusion of the anomalous coronary artery is maintained. The clinical course after ductal closure is determined largely by the presence or absence of collaterals from the RCA to the left coronary system. If the collaterals are inadequate, myocardial ischemia and ventricular dysfunction result from inadequate perfusion. If the collaterals are adequate, perfusion of the left coronary system is maintained; however, as the pulmonary vascular resistance falls, a significant left-to-right shunt develops from the RCA to the pulmonary artery with progressive dilatation of the RCA and left coronary systems. Children with significant collaterals may survive past infancy, but they usually develop progressive left ventricular dysfunction. Severe mitral regurgitation is often present secondary to papillary muscle dysfunction and ventricular dilation.

1a–c

The origin of the anomalous LMCA may be located almost anywhere on the main pulmonary artery or branch pulmonary arteries. Most commonly, the anomalous LMCA originates from the rightward posterior sinus (facing) of the pulmonary artery; however, the anomalous coronary may originate from the left or posterior (nonfacing), or rarely, from the anterior (facing) sinus of the main pulmonary artery. An anomalous RCA most commonly originates from the anterior portion of the pulmonary artery.

The first successful surgical therapy for anomalous origin of the LMCA from the pulmonary artery was simple ligation of the anomalous artery. Ligation prevents the left-to-right shunt and allows perfusion of the left ventricle through collaterals from the RCA. However, because of concern over early mortality and an increased risk of late sudden death, a variety of techniques were developed to create a dual coronary artery system, including bypass grafting with the left subclavian artery, the internal mammary artery, and saphenous vein. Takeuchi and associates described creation of an aorto-pulmonary window and intrapulmonary artery baffle using a flap of pulmonary artery to direct blood from the aorta to the anomalous coronary. In recent years, direct reimplantation of the anomalous coronary into the aorta has become the procedure of choice at most centers.

Because of the high mortality associated with medical therapy in these children, surgical intervention is indicated at the time of initial diagnosis. The goal of surgery is restoration of a two coronary system. Severe left ventricular dysfunction and mitral insufficiency are not contraindications to revascularization in infants because significant recovery usually occurs. Mitral valve repair is rarely indicated at the time of the initial procedure. Even if severe mitral regurgitation is present preoperatively, the severity of mitral regurgitation almost always improves following reimplantation. In rare occurrences, transplantation may be necessary if ventricular function does not improve after reimplantation.

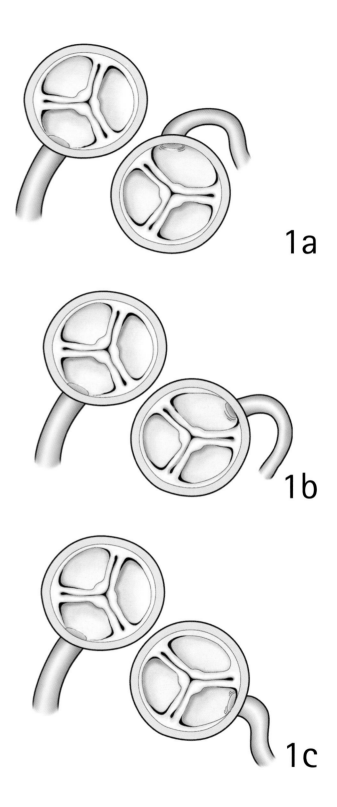

OPERATION FOR ANOMALOUS ORIGIN OF CORONARY ARTERY FROM THE PA

Aortic reimplantation

After induction of anesthesia and placement of monitoring lines, the chest is prepped and draped. A median sternotomy is performed, and the thymus is resected. The pericardium is opened and suspended with stay sutures. The ventricle is usually dilated with significant dysfunction secondary to myocardial ischemia and mitral regurgitation. Contact with the myocardium should be minimized until the patient is placed on cardiopulmonary bypass (CPB) to avoid ventricular fibrillation.

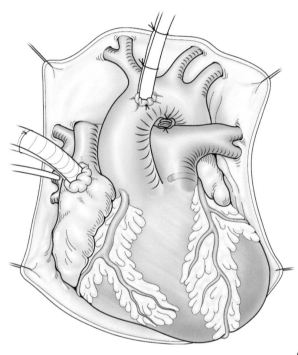

2 The aortic pursestring suture is placed distally, near the innominate artery, and a pursestring suture is placed in the right atrial appendage. Heparin is administered, the aorta is cannulated, a single right atrial cannula is inserted, and CPB is initiated. The operation may be performed using either continuous low-flow CPB with moderate hypothermia (25°–30°C) or deep hypothermic circulatory arrest (18°C) in very small infants. A left ventricular vent should be placed via the right superior pulmonary vein to decompress the dilated left ventricle.

2

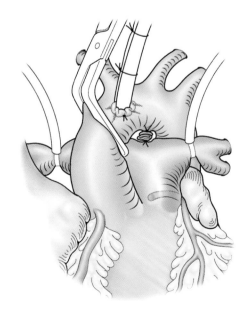

The pulmonary artery is mobilized, and the epicardial course of the left coronary artery carefully inspected. If the anomalous coronary originates far to the left or anteriorly on the pulmonary artery, direct reimplantation may not be possible. The aorta is fully mobilized, as are the right and left pulmonary arteries. The ligamentum arteriosum is ligated and divided to improve mobility of the pulmonary artery. Tourniquets are placed around the right and left branch pulmonary arteries.

3 A cannula is placed in the ascending aorta for administration of cardioplegia solution. The aorta is cross-clamped, and cold cardioplegia solution is administered via the aortic root. Occlusion of the branch pulmonary arteries with tourniquets prevents run-off of cardioplegic solution into the lungs. Alternatively, the ostium of the coronary artery may be compressed and occluded.

3

4 The pulmonary artery is opened transversely immediately above the sinotubular junction. The orifice of the anomalous coronary is identified, and the pulmonary artery is divided. The coronary ostium is excised from the pulmonary artery, as in the arterial switch operation, with a generous button of arterial wall. If the coronary ostium is located near a commissure, takedown of the commissure may be necessary to excise the coronary button. The excised pulmonary artery wall allows extension of the proximal end of the coronary, so that the anastomosis can be constructed without tension. The proximal portion of the coronary artery is mobilized using cautery, with care being taken to avoid small branches.

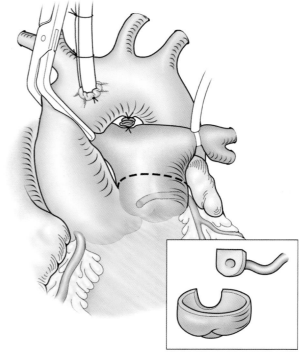

4

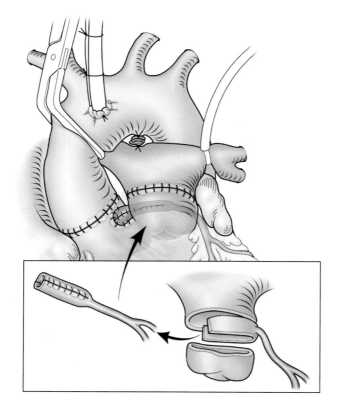

5 If the anomalous coronary arises anteriorly from the pulmonary artery, a portion of the pulmonary artery wall may be excised and used to create a tubular extension of the coronary artery.

5

6a The aorta is opened transversely just above the sinotubular junction. The incision is carried posteriorly above the left posterior sinus. The sinus is incised vertically to accept the coronary button. The coronary button is carefully aligned with the incision in the aorta to avoid twisting or kinking. Alternatively, a medially based trap door incision may be performed as in the arterial switch operation to reduce tension on the anastomosis.

6b The anastomosis begins at the most inferior aspect of the coronary button, which is attached to the most inferior portion of the incision in the sinus with a continuous suture of 7/0 Prolene. The suture line is carried to the top of the incision anteriorly and posteriorly. The aorta is closed with a continuous suture 7/0 Prolene, which is tied to the coronary button suture as the anastomosis is completed. After completion of aortic closure, cardioplegic solution is administered via the aorta root. The anastomosis is inspected to insure adequate filling of the coronary artery.

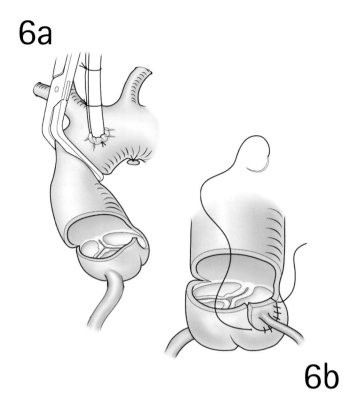

6a

6b

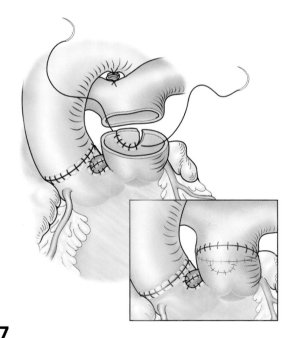

7

7 The defect in the pulmonary artery is usually repaired with a patch of autologous pericardium. The reconstructed proximal pulmonary artery is then anastomosed to the distal pulmonary artery confluence with a continuous suture of 7/0 Prolene. Occasionally, the pulmonary artery may be repaired with a direct anastomosis of the proximal pulmonary artery to the distal pulmonary artery confluence. If a commissure was taken down during excision of the coronary button, the pulmonary artery should be reconstructed with pericardium and the commissure resuspended. The aortic cross-clamp is removed, and the patient is rewarmed. If preferred, the cross-clamp may be removed before pulmonary artery reconstruction to decrease the ischemic time.

The left ventricle is inspected to assess perfusion and function. The suture lines are inspected for hemostasis. Right and left atrial lines are inserted for pressure monitoring and drug administration. Atrial and ventricular pacing wires are also placed. After full rewarming, the patient is separated from CPB, and modified ultrafiltration is performed. The electrocardiogram should be monitored during reperfusion and after separation from bypass for evidence of ischemia. Temporary inotropic support is often necessary in infants or children with severe preoperative left ventricular dysfunction. Support with a left ventricular assist device or extracorporeal membrane oxygenation may occasionally be necessary in the postoperative period.

Modified Takeuchi repair

An alternative method for repair of the anomalous origin of the LMCA from the pulmonary artery is the intrapulmonary artery tunnel or Takeuchi repair. In the original repair, an aorta-pulmonary window was created, and a portion of the anterior pulmonary wall was used to create a baffle directing blood from the aorta to the ostium of the anomalous coronary. In the modified repair, the baffle is constructed with a polytetrafluoroethylene (Gore-Tex) patch. This technique may be particularly useful if the origin of the coronary artery is located leftward on the pulmonary artery. Creation of a baffle may not be possible if the ostium is located near a commissure or arises from a branch pulmonary artery. Complications of the Takeuchi repair include baffle obstruction, baffle leaks, and supravalvar right ventricular outflow tract obstruction.

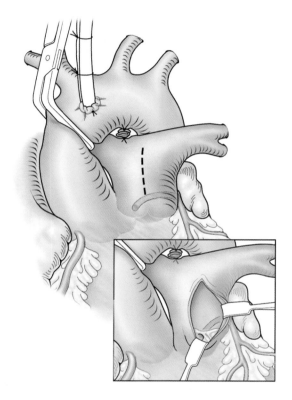

8 The modified Takeuchi repair may be performed with either continuous low-flow CPB (25°–30°C) or deep hypothermic circulatory arrest (18°C). Cannulation is performed as for direct reimplantation, with a left ventricular vent to decompress the ventricle. Cardioplegia is administered via the aortic root with occlusion of the branch pulmonary arteries. After cardioplegic arrest of the heart, an anterior longitudinal pulmonary arteriotomy is performed. The ostium of the aberrant coronary artery is identified.

9 Using a punch, a 5-mm diameter opening is made in the aorta above the sinotubular junction, on the leftward aspect of the aorta. If any question exists concerning placement of the aortic opening, an anterior aortotomy should be performed, and the punch hole should be performed under direct vision to avoid damage to the aortic valve. Placement of the aorto-pulmonary window above the sinotubular junction allows the baffle to angle downward into the sinus if the coronary ostium is located deep within the sinus.

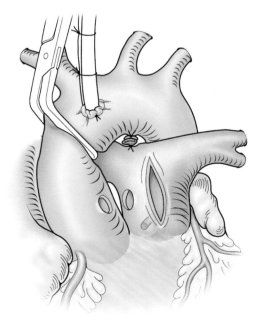

9

10 A similar punch-hole is made in the pulmonary artery directly opposite the punch-hole in the aorta, and an aorta-pulmonary window is created with a continuous suture of 7/0 Prolene.

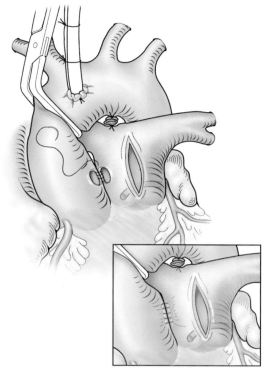

10

11 A 4-mm polytetrafluoroethylene graft is split longitudinally and tailored to an appropriate length. This graft is used to create an intrapulmonary tunnel, baffling blood from the aorto-pulmonary window to the coronary ostium. The suture line begins at the coronary ostium and is continued inferiorly along the pulmonary artery wall to the aorta-pulmonary window. The suture line is completed by starting again at the coronary artery ostium and completing the superior portion of the baffle.

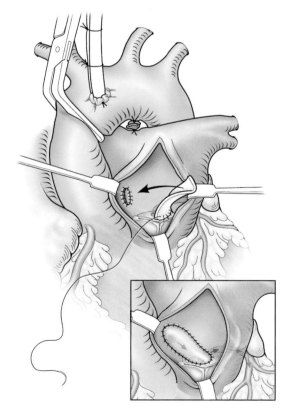

11

12 After creation of the baffle, the pulmonary artery should be repaired with a patched autologous pericardium to avoid supravalvar right ventricular outflow tract obstruction. The cross-clamp is removed, and the patient is rewarmed. Monitoring lines are inserted, and the patient is separated from CPB as after direct reimplantation.

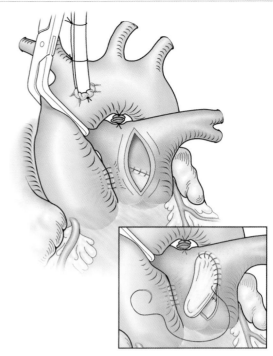

12

Additional procedures for anomalous origin of a coronary artery from the pulmonary artery

Coronary bypass grafting with the left subclavian artery, saphenous vein, or left internal mammary artery has been used for treatment of anomalous origin of the LMCA from the pulmonary artery. The most common indication for use of a left internal mammary artery graft is creation of a dual coronary system after a previous ligation or because of stenosis or occlusion after a previous attempt at repair. Because of the risk of occlusion and poor long-term results, saphenous vein should be used only if no other conduit is available.

If anomalous origin of the LAD is present, excision of the ostium of the coronary artery with a portion of the pulmonary artery may be possible to create a tube graft to elongate the coronary artery for implantation. However, as the origin of the LAD is frequently anterior on the pulmonary artery, this maneuver may be difficult. The reimplanted artery may drape over the pulmonary artery and is at increased risk of occlusion. An alternative procedure is ligation with left internal mammary artery grafting. Isolated origin of the left circumflex coronary artery from the pulmonary artery is rare, and the optimal therapy (ligation or reimplantation) is not known. In patients with anomalous origin of the RCA from the pulmonary artery, the coronary artery usually arises anteriorly from the pulmonary artery. Direct reimplantation is the treatment of choice.

ANOMALOUS COURSE OF A CORONARY ARTERY BETWEEN THE AORTA AND PULMONARY ARTERY

Anomalous course of a coronary artery between the aorta and pulmonary artery occurs when the RCA or LMCA arises from a separate ostium in the opposite sinus and courses between the great vessels. An anomalous course also occurs when a single coronary arises from the right aortic sinus and the LMCA or LAD passes between the great vessels or when a single coronary arises from the left aortic sinus and the RCA courses between the great vessels. Because the coronary artery is positioned between the great vessels, myocardial compression and ischemia may occur, especially during exercise. When two ostia are present in the same sinus, the ostium of the anomalous coronary artery is frequently abnormal and slit-like. Anomalous course of a coronary artery between the aorta and pulmonary artery is associated with a high incidence of sudden death, particularly with exercise. These patients are often asymptomatic until an episode of syncope or sudden cardiac death. The incidence and natural history of anomalous course of a coronary artery between the great vessels are unknown. Surgical intervention is indicated in any patient with angina, syncope, or sudden death who is found to have an anomalous course of the coronary between the great vessels. The indications for surgery in asymptomatic patients have not been defined.

When two ostia are present, repair of this defect consists of enlargement and remodeling of the anomalous ostium to prevent compression between the great vessels and to relieve the ostial obstruction. Bypass grafting may not be successful as normal flow usually is present in the coronary artery; and, thus, an increased risk of poor flow and occlusion in the graft exist secondary to competitive flow. However, when a single coronary artery exists and the LMCA or RCA courses between the great vessels, relief of obstruction by reimplantation or remodeling of the ostium may not be possible, and bypass grafting may be the only therapeutic option.

OPERATION FOR ANOMALOUS COURSE OF A CORONARY ARTERY

Remodeling of abnormal ostium

A median sternotomy is performed, the pericardium is opened, and the anatomy is inspected. The aorta is cannulated near the innominate artery, and a two-stage venous cannula is inserted via the right atrial appendage. CPB with moderate hypothermia is instituted, and a left ventricular vent is placed in the right superior pulmonary vein. A cannula for administration of cardioplegia solution is placed in the ascending aorta. The aorta is cross-clamped, and cold cardioplegia solution is administered.

13a, b After an adequate arrest is obtained, a transverse aortotomy is performed, and the coronary ostia are identified. The origin of the anomalous coronary is usually small and slit-like. Because the anomalous coronary usually arises from the opposite sinus, detachment of the aortic valve commissure may be necessary to remodel and enlarge the ostium.

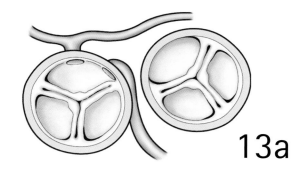

13a

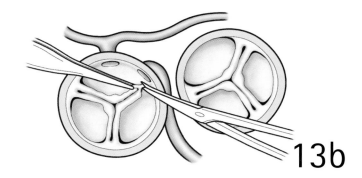

13b

13c After detachment of the commissure, the slit-like ostium is opened along the longitudinal axis of the coronary artery, and a portion of the common wall between the aorta and coronary is excised.

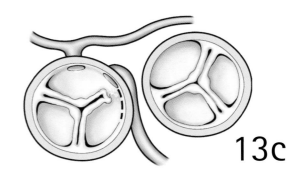

13c

13d

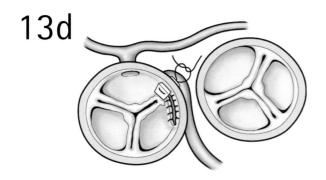

13d The intimal surfaces are approximated with sutures of 7/0 or 8/0 Prolene. The aortic valve commissure is resuspended with a pledgeted suture.

The aortotomy is repaired. The cross-clamp is removed after deairing, and the patient is rewarmed. The electrocardiogram is monitored for signs of ischemia. Monitoring lines are inserted. The patient is separated from CPB in the usual fashion.

CORONARY ARTERY FISTULAE

A coronary artery fistula is a communication between a coronary artery and a cardiac chamber, the coronary sinus, the vena cavae, a pulmonary artery, or a pulmonary vein. Coronary artery fistulae may arise from the right or left coronary artery. The most common sites of termination are the right ventricle and the right atrium. Most fistulae arise from a coronary artery with an otherwise normal distribution; they may arise in the midportion of the vessel with a normal vessel continuing past the origin or they may arise at the most distal portion of the vessel as an end artery.

Most patients with coronary fistulas are asymptomatic, and the fistula is discovered during an evaluation for a murmur. Rarely, the fistula may "steal" flow from the coronary circulation; however, angina is uncommon. The natural history of coronary fistulae has not been fully delineated; however, fistulae are most likely present early in life and gradually increase in size. All patients with symptomatic fistulae should undergo closure. Patients with very small fistulae may not require surgical closure; however, they should be followed because progressive enlargement may occur.

OPERATION FOR CORONARY ARTERY FISTULAE

Technique of operation ostium

The coronary artery anatomy must be clearly defined before surgical closure and before the operation is individualized. Many fistulae can be closed without the use of CPB and frequently can be ligated or oversewn at their origin or termination. Transcatheter coil embolization has been used for closure in some coronary artery fistulae.

14a After a median sternotomy, the thymus is resected, and the pericardium is opened. The coronary artery is carefully inspected, and the distribution of the coronary arteries at the site of the enlarged vessel is noted. If the fistula is located at the distal end of a coronary artery and no viable myocardium exists distal to the fistula, the fistula may be closed by ligation without the use of CPB. The ligature is placed around the coronary artery immediately proximal to the fistula, and the fistula is occluded temporarily. The heart is observed for signs of ischemia. If no signs of ischemia are present and myocardial perfusion remains adequate, the ligature is tied.

If the fistula arises from the midportion of a coronary artery and the course cannot be fully defined, CPB should be used. The cannula is placed in the ascending aorta, both venae cavae are cannulated, and CPB is initiated. If opening a coronary artery or cardiac chamber is necessary, cardioplegic arrest should be used. The fistula should be compressed during administration of cardioplegia to prevent run-off into the heart. If inadequate arrest is not obtained because of run-off into the fistula, retrograde administration of the cardioplegia solution may be helpful.

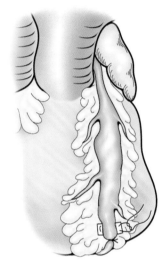

14a

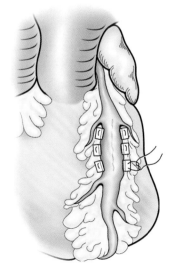

14b

14b A variety of techniques may be used to close the fistula. If the fistula arises from the midportion of the dilated aneurysm of coronary artery, the fistula's communication may be obliterated by placing multiple pledgeted sutures beneath the coronary artery with care being taken to avoid compromising the distal perfusion.

15 Alternatively, the enlarged coronary artery may be opened, the fistula identified, and oversewn from within the coronary artery. The coronary artery is closed primarily. If distal perfusion of the coronary bed is compromised and the fistula is closed, coronary artery bypass grafting may be necessary.

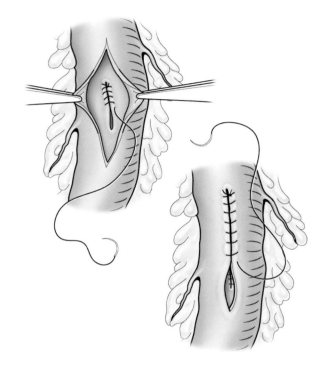

15

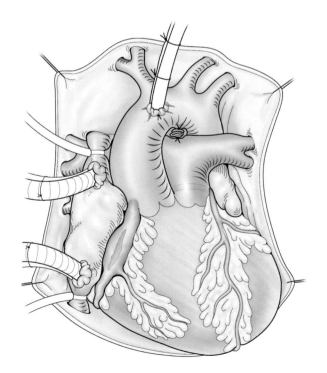

16

16 If the fistula terminates in the right atrium, right ventricle, or other cardiac chamber, the fistula may be closed directly from within the chamber.

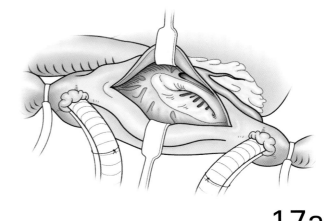

17a

17a, b A right atriotomy is performed, and the termination site of the fistula is identified. Administration of cardioplegia solution may be helpful for localization. The termination site of the fistula may be closed primarily or with a pericardial patch.

After complete closure of the fistula, the cross-clamp is removed. The patient is rewarmed. The electrocardiogram is monitored for signs of ischemia. Intraoperative echocardiography may be helpful to assess myocardial function and to document closure of the fistula.

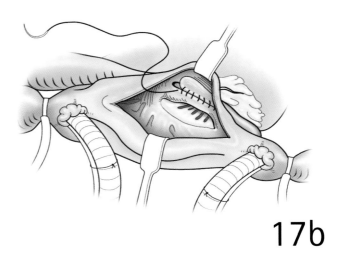

17b

OUTCOME

Outcomes following surgical repair of anomalous coronary artery arising from the pulmonary arteries have improved significantly, even in patients with significant left ventricular dysfunction and mitral regurgitation. Overall survival should be greater than 90%. Mitral valve repair is rarely necessary, even in patients with significant preoperative mitral regurgitation. There is little data available on the long-term outcome in these patients, particularly in terms of left ventricular function and late mortality. The existing data, however, suggests that establishment of a two coronary system is associated with improved survival and improved left ventricular function compared to simple ligation of the anomalous artery.

Operative mortality for repair of a coronary with an anomalous course between the aorta and the pulmonary artery should be minimal. However there is very little data on the long-term prognosis for these patients. It is unclear if these reconstructive techniques reduce the incidence of syncope and sudden cardiac death. Mortality following surgery after closure of coronary artery fistulae should be minimal with a low incidence of recurrence and excellent long-term outcome.

FURTHER READING

Backer, C.L., Stout, M.J., Zales, V.R., et al. 1992. Anomalous origin of the left coronary artery. A twenty-year review of surgical management. Journal of Thoracic and Cardiovascular Surgery 103, 1049.

Davis, J.T., Allen, H.D., Wheeler, J.J., et al. 1994. Coronary artery fistula in the pediatric age group: a 19-year institutional experience. Annals of Thoracic Surgery 58, 760.

Gaynor, J.W. 1998. Coronary artery anomalies in children. In Kaiser, L.R., Kron, I.L., Spray, T.L. (ed.), Mastery of Cardiothoracic Surgery. Boston: Little, Brown and Company.

Rinaldi, R.G., Carballido, J., Giles, R., et al. 1994. Right coronary artery with anomalous origin and slit ostium. Annals of Thoracic Surgery 58, 828.

Turley, K., Szarnick, R.J., Flachsbart, K.D., et al. 1995. Aortic implantation is possible in all cases of anomalous origin of the left coronary artery from the pulmonary artery. Annals of Thoracic Surgery 60, 84.

Vouhé, P.R., Tamisier, D., Sidi, D., et al. 1992. Anomalous left coronary artery from the pulmonary artery: results of isolated aortic reimplantation. Annals of Thoracic Surgery 54, 621.

Index